The Clinical Education and Supervisory Process

in Speech-Language Pathology and Audiology

The Clinical Education and Supervisory Process

in Speech-Language Pathology and Audiology

Editors

Elizabeth S. McCrea, PhD, CCC-SLP, F-ASHA

Clinical Professor Emerita
Indiana University
Bloomington, Indiana

Judith A. Brasseur, PhD, CCC-SLP, F-ASHA

Professor Emerita
California State University, Chico
Chico, California

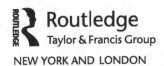

Routledge
Taylor & Francis Group

NEW YORK AND LONDON

Cover Artist: Lori Shields

First published in 2020 by SLACK Incorporated

Published in 2024 by Routledge
605 Third Avenue, New York, NY 10158

and by Routledge
4 Park Square, Milton Park, Abingdon, Oxon, OX14 4RN

Routledge is an imprint of the Taylor & Francis Group, an informa business

Library of Congress Control Number:2019945418

ISBN: 9781630915292 (hbk)
ISBN: 9781003523031 (ebk)

DOI: 10.4324/9781003523031

DEDICATION

To our colleagues and students who have inspired and sustained us in the pursuit of excellence in clinical education and the supervisory process.

And to our spouses, David and Ben, who have always encouraged and supported every personal and professional journey we have taken.

But, most of all to Jean L. Anderson who began it all.

CONTENTS

ACKNOWLEDGMENTS

The first mention of supervision and supervisor responsibilities appeared in the literature of the professions in 1937 in the *Journal of Speech and Hearing Disorders*; 30 years later, the first American Speech-Language-Hearing Association (ASHA) Convention presentation was made by Adah Miner in 1967. The decades since have documented a consistent and burgeoning interest in the fundamental importance of the clinical education and supervisory processes to the education and training of students and, ultimately, to the integrity of the services they provide.

During the time period between the early 1980s and early 2000s, the knowledge base in supervision in speech-language pathology and audiology enjoyed a flurry of development. A primary and motivating influence on this development was the Council of Supervisors in Speech-Language Pathology and Audiology (CSSPA), which was the predecessor to Special Interest Group 11, Administration and Supervision. CSSPA, following the leadership of Jean L. Anderson, sponsored five national conferences on supervision and the supervisory process; a highlight of each of these conferences was the presentation and discussion of research by members of the council and publication of conference papers in a proceedings of each conference. Paralleling these conferences, doctoral students who studied the supervisory process with Jean L. Anderson at Indiana University were completing dissertations that also contributed to the body of basic research. This body of research resulted in dissertations, several journal articles, innumerable presentations at national and regional conferences, and three books on supervision, including the first edition of this book in 2003. These initiatives began the refinement of the understanding of the critical factors in clinical education and supervision methodology in speech-language pathology and audiology and their relationship to supervisory effectiveness.

We owe thanks for all of the work represented in this edition of *The Clinical Education and Supervisory Process in Speech-Language Pathology and Audiology* to the many colleagues and friends with whom we worked to build the knowledge base to support ethical and effective professional practice in supervision. There are simply too many to name individually, but the doctoral students with whom we studied at Indiana University, fellow members of CSSPA and Special Interest Group 11, and, most especially, the indomitable Jean L. Anderson deserve as much credit for this work as do either of the editors. None of this would have been possible without their time, intellect, and contributions.

Special thanks are necessary to all of the contributing authors who have helped to contemporize this edition by addressing the challenges posed by five unique supervision constituent groups (speech-language pathology graduate students, audiology externs, clinical fellows, support personnel, and professionals transitioning in the workplace) as well as the challenges inherent in interprofessional education and practice in communication sciences and disorders. In addition, chapters on ethical practice in supervision and research strategies for studying the clinical education and supervisory round out the content for what we hope will be a primary resource for anyone serving as a supervisor and their supervisees.

—*Elizabeth S. McCrea, PhD, CCC-SLP, F-ASHA*
—*Judith A. Brasseur, PhD, CCC-SLP, F-ASHA*

ABOUT THE EDITORS

Elizabeth S. McCrea, PhD, CCC-SLP, F-ASHA is a clinical professor emerita of the Department of Speech and Hearing Sciences at Indiana University. She retired from the university in 2011. As a member of the department's faculty, she was both a didactic and clinical educator. She taught courses in the clinical process, professional issues, clinical education, and the organization and administration of public school communication disorders programs. She was also a clinical instructor in the department's R. L. Milisen Speech and Language Clinic at Indiana University, with an emphasis on children's speech sound and language disorders and language-learning disorders. Dr. McCrea was director of the R. L. Milisen Speech and Hearing Center for almost a decade and coordinator of the department's externship program in speech-language pathology until her retirement. Before joining the faculty, Dr. McCrea was a pediatric speech-language pathologist in both school-based and hospital settings.

Dr. McCrea received both the bachelor's and PhD degrees in speech and hearing sciences from Indiana University and the master's degree from the University of Virginia. During her PhD study at Indiana, she worked with, and was mentored by, Jean L. Anderson. She was recognized as a distinguished alumna by the Indiana University Department of Speech and Hearing Sciences and received the honors of the Indiana Speech and Hearing Association. She is an ASHA Fellow and served the Association as both Vice President for Academic Affairs (2009-2011) and as President in 2014.

In addition to her teaching and administration, Dr. McCrea's research focused on identifying the parameters of best practice in clinical education and supervision; this work contributed to the foundation for the development of ASHA's technical and knowledge and skill documents for clinical education and supervision, as well as to the profession's standards for appropriate supervision. She was the principal investigator of a $326,000 4-year personnel preparation grant from the U.S. Department of Education centered on developing leadership personnel in clinical education in the professions. She is the coauthor of *The Supervisory Process in Speech-Language Pathology and Audiology* and contributed to a chapter on clinical education and supervision in *Professional Issues in Speech-Language Pathology and Audiology* (3rd edition), edited by Lubinski and Golper. She has presented over 50 peer-reviewed or invited papers at national and state meetings on the clinical education process and effective behavior of both supervisors and supervisees within the process.

Judith A. Brasseur, PhD, CCC-SLP, F-ASHA is a professor emerita of the Communication Arts and Sciences Department at California State University (CSU), Chico. She retired from the university in 2010 after 30 years in the Communication Sciences and Disorders (CMSD) program, where she taught undergraduate and graduate courses and supervised on and off campus, with an emphasis on children's speech sound, fluency, and language disorders. She held administrative roles in the CMSD program both as program coordinator for 9 years and clinic director for 7 years. In addition, for 19 years she directed the doctoral incentive programs for underrepresented students on the Chico campus that operated through CSU, Chico's Graduate School, part of the California State University system-wide effort to increase the number of underrepresented students who progress through the educational pipeline and obtain doctoral degrees and careers in academe. In addition, from 1988 through 1997, she was co-principal investigator for the prestigious Patricia Roberts Harris Fellowship Program Awards with $520,000 funded by the U.S. Department of Education for Chico master's students in biological sciences, computer science, geography, and speech-language pathology.

Dr. Brasseur earned the bachelor's and master's degrees from Indiana State University and the PhD degree from Indiana University in 1980, where she and Elizabeth McCrea studied with and were mentored by Jean L. Anderson. From the time she completed her terminal degree, Dr. Brasseur has been active in state and national professional organizations, including ASHA. She served a term on ASHA's Council on Academic Accreditation (2007-2010), is currently a member of ASHA's Special Interest Group 11, Administration and Supervision Coordinating Committee, and editor of *Perspectives*. In addition, she is chair of the Petitioning Group for Specialty Certification in Supervision. Dr. Brasseur is a fellow of both ASHA and the California Speech-Language-Hearing Association (CSHA).

Dr. Brasseur's research involved investigations in treatment for functional child articulation and phonological disorders and best practices in clinical supervision. She was principal investigator of a $112,082 2-year personnel preparation grant from the U.S. Department of Education to provide a three-part, 9 credit-hour training program for off-campus supervisors, funded for a third year by the university. She is coauthor of *The Supervisory Process in Speech-Language Pathology and Audiology*, has also presented over 50 peer-reviewed or invited presentations at state and national meetings, and has more than 30 publications to her credit.

Contributing Authors

Mindi Anderson, PhD, APRN, CPNP-PC, CNE, CHSE-A, ANEF, FAAN (Chapter 10)
Associate Professor
Graduate Simulation Coordinator
Director of the Healthcare Simulation Program (MSN Post-Graduate Certificate)
Simulation MSN Program and Health Care Simulation Graduate Certificate
University of Central Florida College of Nursing
Orlando, Florida

Mary L. Casper, MA, CCC-SLP, F-ASHA, FNAP (Chapter 15)
Corporate Rehabilitation Consultant
Manor Care
Rockville, Maryland

Mark DeRuiter, MBA, PhD, CCC-A/SLP, F-ASHA (Chapter 16)
Associate Department Head for Clinical Education
Department of Speech-Language-Hearing Sciences
The University of Arizona
Tucson, Arizona

Donna Fisher Smiley, PhD, CCC-A, F-ASHA (Chapter 12)
Audiology Supervisor/Audiologist
Arkansas Children's Hospital
Little Rock, Arkansas

Sarah Ginsberg, EdD, CCC-SLP, F-ASHA (Chapter 16)
Professor
Speech-Language Pathology Program
Department of Special Education
Eastern Michigan University
Ypsilanti, Michigan

Melanie W. Hudson, MA, CCC-SLP, F-ASHA (Chapter 13)
National Director
EBS Healthcare
West Chester, Pennsylvania

Cheryl Messick, PhD, CCC-SLP, F-ASHA (Chapter 11)
Vice Chair for Academic Affairs
Department of Communication Sciences and Disorders
University of Pittsburgh
Pittsburgh, Pennsylvania

Wren Newman, SLPD, CCC-SLP, F-ASHA (Chapter 9)
Chair, Department of Speech-Language Pathology
Dr. Pallavi Patel College of Health Care Sciences
Nova Southeastern University
Fort Lauderdale, Florida

Cynthia McCormick Richburg, PhD, CCC-A (Chapter 12)
Professor and AuD Program Coordinator
Communication Sciences and Disorders
Wichita State University
Wichita, Kansas

Heather L. Thompson, PhD, CCC-SLP (Chapter 14)
Assistant Professor/SLPA Program Coordinator
Department of Communication Sciences and Disorders
California State University
Sacramento, California

A. Lynn Williams, PhD, CCC-SLP, F-ASHA, F-NAP (Chapter 10)
Associate Dean and Professor
College of Clinical and Rehabilitative Health Sciences
East Tennessee State University
Johnson City, Tennessee

PREFACE BY JEAN L. ANDERSON

Although supervision has long been a component of the profession of speech-language pathology and audiology, the study of the supervisory process has been largely ignored until recently. In the past few years, however, a surge of interest has resulted in published articles, convention presentations, continuing education offerings, books, and activities of the American Speech-Language-Hearing Association (ASHA). This book will make a statement about where the profession stands in its implementation of the supervisory process as a major influence in the preparation of future speech-language pathologists and audiologists and the delivery of service to clients. It will propose a continuum of supervision, offered as a framework upon which supervisors and their supervisees may place themselves as they work together, and through which they can examine, "dissect," and discuss the process. It is hoped that the presentation of the continuum and the accompanying material will encourage members of the profession to view the supervisory process as an important and appropriate area for self-study. Additionally, it is hoped it will help make clearer the many questions that exist about the effectiveness of supervisory methodologies and stimulate active research to seek answers to those questions.

This book has been written mainly for the many people in speech-language pathology and audiology who have been or may be plunged into the role of supervisor without opportunity to think about it or study it. Speech-language pathologists and audiologists often become what I call "overnight supervisors"—one day a clinician, the next a supervisor. Many are thrust into the role without preparation, sometimes without much choice, and nearly always without much role definition from the organizations for which they work or within themselves. Often they have little opportunity to talk with anyone about supervision and are forced to draw upon their own past experiences as supervisees, positive or negative, as a source for the development of their own techniques and methodologies. I hope that this book will help them and all the other supervisors to make supervision manageable. I hope that it will encourage them to think about the process and increase their knowledge of themselves and their supervisory procedures. I hope supervisors will perceive supervision as a process that can and must be studied, just as we expect our clinicians to study the clinical process. I hope, too, that student supervisees in educational programs will study the book and that it will serve two purposes for them: to help them understand their role as supervisees, and to prepare them for the time in the not-too-distant future when they will probably be supervisors themselves.

This book has been "happening" to me since long before I began seriously to put the words on paper. A series of events led to my interest in the supervisory process, but a few of them stand out as probably the most significant. The first was my own introduction in to supervision, when I, too, became an overnight supervisor of a student in school practicum assignment that was not defined and for which there were no guidelines.

The second experience, and possibly the most significant, was the opportunity to serve as a state supervisor of speech-hearing-language programs in a department of education. In this position I was able to spend several days a week for several years observing and talking with speech-language pathologists in the schools, program supervisors, and administrators as well as university personnel. Often I talked with clinicians who were serving as supervisors of "student teachers" with little or no guidance from universities about their responsibilities, and I learned about their questions. My experiences in this position led me first to concern about their number of "leaderless" programs, that is, those in which there was no leadership from a person within our discipline. My attention first focused on this administrative aspect—what the ASHA Committee on Supervision was later to call *program management*. However, that attention soon turned to the *process*, later termed *clinical teaching* by the ASHA Committee. My interest in the process came as a result of the dawning realization that, when visiting and observing first- or second-year, or even more experienced, clinicians I could often guess correctly where they had done their "student teaching," as the school practicum experience was then called, because of the obvious modeling that took place. Through this realization, I became aware of the impact that the teaching aspect of supervision has on the development of professionals and the significance of that impact on their future clients. In other words, I began to ask myself these questions: If each generation of clinicians does exactly what its supervisors do, where are we going in terms of the kind of service we will deliver to our clients in the future? Is there something in this teaching aspect of supervision that makes the difference between clinicians who become clones of their supervisors and clinicians who are able to go beyond their supervisors and become independent, autonomous clinicians that we profess to produce in our educational programs? Is there something in the supervisory experience that makes the difference and, if so, what is it?

The third important influence on my developing concern about how we, as a profession, were dealing with the supervisory process came when I had the privilege of becoming the chair of the first ASHA Committee on Supervision of Speech Pathology and Audiology. It was through the data-gathering done by the Committee that I fully realized the magnitude of the profession's lack of recognition of the importance of this process that affects all of us at some time. Further, the enormity of our neglect of the dedicated and frustrated members of the profession who were serving in the important role of supervisor became clear and was well documented by the first position statement of the Committee (ASHA, 1978).

The fourth event was the opportunity to develop a doctoral-level program at Indiana University in which students could study the supervisory process, learn to prepare other supervisors, and conduct research on supervision. The interaction with the students in that program and the research we completed have been an important dimension of my own development.

Thus, a long journey that began with the sudden assignment of a student on the school practicum those many years ago has culminated in the struggle to produce this book. In the words of Alice in Wonderland, I have become "curiouser and curiouser" about the dynamics of the process, and about what I call the professional/political issues that have prevented, or at least not encouraged, the study of this important facet of our profession.

I make no claim for having found the answers to all the questions. Certainly I do not wish to proclaim that this book provides the answers for everyone. I only hope that it provides some encouragement for others to ask more questions about supervision—individually as supervisors or collectively as a profession. The book has become a statement of what I believe to be important in the supervisory process. Some of it is supportable by data, some by consensus, some by common sense. Not everyone will agree with what I say. None of it should go unchallenged, for we have only begun to scratch at the complexities of the process.

It was my somewhat nebulous objective at one time to produce a book that would bring together a spectacular review of what has been written in all the helping professions about supervision. This effort would have resulted in a lengthy tome that would not necessarily have been definitive, alas, I have learned that many of those disciplines to which I had thought to turn— assuming that they had discovered the answer to the mystery of supervision— are not much better off than we are. Therefore, I have included only that material from other professions that is pertinent to specific points. I have drawn particularly, as will be seen, on the work in education by Blumberg, Cogan, and Goldhammer. But a funny thing has happened on the way to getting this book on paper! We have begun to develop a body of literature of our own over the past few years. It is literature that ranges over a broad continuum of importance and quality, but nevertheless it is ours, and it is developing rapidly to answer our own questions.

A few clarifications are necessary for the reader. One is related to the title, which includes "audiology." Why, you may ask, is a speech-language pathologist writing about supervision in audiology? The answer is that I believe the supervisory process is the same for the two areas of practice within the discipline. Differences, if they exist, will be more related to the position of supervisor and supervisee on the continuum, or to such factors as the differences between the needs of supervisees in the diagnostic process and in the therapeutic process. Not all audiologists will agree with me, but nevertheless I hope there will be much in this book that they will find useful.

Another clarification is necessary in relation to some of the examples provided in the book. My own professional background is in the schools, the school practicum, and the university program, so many of the examples come from those settings. I wish to emphasize here, however, as I do throughout the book, my unwavering belief that the *process* of supervision has more commonalities than differences across sites and situations. Therefore, readers are invited to apply the examples to their own experience.

The reader who is looking for statistical validation for the effects of any method of supervision will be disappointed with this book. So will the reader who is looking for unequivocal support for **the** way to supervise. Neither will be found here, nor in any other source. Despite my confidence in the value of the approach to the supervisory process presented in this book, I am the first to acknowledge that is has not been validated. It is an approach that makes sense to me and is actually used by many supervisors now, whether or not they conceptualize it in the same way I do. The methodology proposed herein should be "weighed and measured" carefully, however, to determine its validity.

We are, I think, in a wonderful period of evolution in the study of the supervisory process. It is my wish that this book will contribute to that evolution.

—*Jean L. Anderson,*
From the original edition, 1988

Reference

American Speech and Hearing Association. (1978). Current status of supervision of speech-language pathology and audiology [Special report of the Committee on Supervision in Speech-Language-Pathology and Audiology.]. *Asha, 20*, 478-486.

FOREWORD BY JEAN L. ANDERSON

In the 15 years since the publication of the first edition of this book, many highly motivated and dedicated professionals in speech-language pathology and audiology have directed their attention to the significance of high quality supervision in educational programs and in the work setting. In conjunction with the efforts of individuals, the American Speech-Language-Hearing Association has continued the work begun in the late 1960s. The organization and operation of several conferences on various components of supervision led to the establishment in 1974 of a Committee on Supervision in Speech-Language Pathology and Audiology. Since that time, the output of conferences, sets of guidelines and research reports on this complex process have increased in quantity and quality.

We have made much progress since 1988 in recognizing the importance of studying the supervisory process, of upgrading its quality, and in accountability. There is much more to be done.

In the preface to the first edition, I detailed my long and challenging journey to the book. I am grateful to Elizabeth S. McCrea and Judith A. Brasseur for continuing that journey. They were two of the many thoughtful, inquisitive, questioning doctoral students who were willing to experiment along with me, who could tolerate uncertainty and recognize the need that I saw. I am proud of all of my former students who participated with me in my search. I am especially grateful to these two for making this tremendous effort to perpetuate my thoughts and words and bring their own into the equation.

I also stated that we were "in a wonderful period of evolution in the study of the supervisory process." I trust that this book will be another step in that evolution.

—Jean L. Anderson
From the 2003 edition

Editors' Note: Jean died on June 8, 2016 at 96 years old.

INTRODUCTION

Formal ASHA activity related to the clinical education and supervisory process began in 1974 with the appointment of the first ASHA Committee on Supervision. The Educational Standards Board and the Professional Standards Board developed requirements for supervision in 1980 and 1983, respectively; these standards have since been updated by both the Council on Academic Accreditation and the Council for Clinical Certification. In 1985, the ASHA Executive Council approved the position statement: Clinical Supervision in Speech-Language Pathology and Audiology; this position statement recognized supervision as a distinct area of professional practice and was the first formal statement of the tasks and competencies for supervisors within the supervisory process in the professions. Subsequently, in 2008, another ASHA Committee on Supervision reinforced the notion of supervision as a distinct area of professional practice, restated the fundamental tasks and competencies of clinical educators and supervisors, and underscored the importance of preparation of supervisors. The updated position statement, new technical report and new knowledge and skills documents were approved by ASHA's Executive Board. More recently, the 2013 ASHA Ad Hoc Committee on Supervision again emphasized the need for training of supervisors and identified requisite knowledge and skills for supervisors of five unique supervision constituencies: students in university training programs or in off-campus/externship placements; audiology students in their final externship; clinical fellows; professionals transitioning to a new area of practice or entering the workforce; and support personnel. In May 2016, 80 years after the first reference of supervision in the literature of the profession(s), the Ad Hoc Committee on Supervision Training issued its final report, which identified a systematic plan for the preparation and training of supervisors to be implemented over the next 6 years, "culminating in an increased number of audiologists and speech-language pathologists trained in supervision" (ASHA, 2016). In addition, the report also outlined training goals for each of the five supervision constituencies identified in the 2013 Ad Hoc Supervision Committee Report. The 2013 and 2016 reports and concomitant recommendations were both approved by the ASHA Board of Directors.

The supervisory process in speech-language pathology and audiology continues to challenge those who practice it, especially those who are thrust into the role of supervisor and clinical educator without much, if any, opportunity to think about or study it. In the intervening 30 years since Anderson's first edition of this work and the 15 since McCrea and Brasseur's second, research findings and conceptual application of Anderson's Continuum Model of Supervision continue to find their way into the literature of the professions, supplemented more recently by applications of the clinical education and supervisory process from allied health disciplines. The purpose of this edition of the book is to preserve and summarize, as completely as possible, the foundation and substance of the Continuum Model for a new generation of supervisors and supervisees and to integrate the information of the last decade and a half into their consideration of it. Chapters 1 through 7 introduce the model and address each aspect of it from both a theoretical as well as a practical application perspective. Chapter 8 addresses the importance of accountability within the clinical education and supervisory process and the importance of preparation of supervisors for their role as supervisors. Chapter 9 speaks to the ethical parameters of supervision and clinical education. Chapter 10 focuses on the challenges of interprofessional education and practice with regard to clinical education and supervision. Chapters 11 through 15 focus on the special issues attendant on the full consideration of the process in the five special supervision constituencies identified in the report of the 2013 ASHA Ad Hoc Committee on Supervision. Lastly, and importantly, Chapter 16 reinforces the importance of continued research into the clinical education and supervision process and suggests both qualitative and quantitative methodologies to implement it.

The clinical education and supervisory processes continue to evolve in the professions. Beginning in 2020, the Council for Clinical Certification will require that coursework in supervision/clinical education be documented in the application for the Certificate of Clinical Competence. In addition, any member of the profession who supervises students in training will similarly need to document continuing education in supervision/clinical education in order to provide that supervision. It is our hope that *The Clinical Education and Supervisory Process in Speech-Language Pathology and Audiology* will continue this evolution as it informs and supports the supervisory practice of both supervisors and supervisees as they work together to enhance their knowledge and skill in this important activity which is fundamental to the integrity of the professions' training practices.

—*Elizabeth S. McCrea, PhD, CCC-SLP, F-ASHA*
—*Judith A. Brasseur, PhD, CCC-SLP, F-ASHA*

REFERENCE

American Speech-Language-Hearing Association. (2016, May). *A plan for developing resources and training opportunities in clinical supervision* [Final report of the ASHA Ad Hoc Committee on Supervision Training]. Retrieved from https://www.asha.org/uploadedFiles/A-Plan-for-Developing-Resources-and-Training-Opportunities-in-Clinical-Supervision.pdf

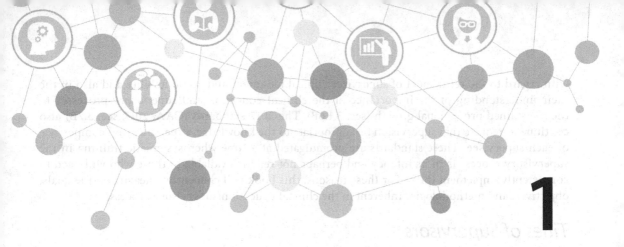

Introduction to the Process
Putting Things in Context

Elizabeth S. McCrea, PhD, CCC-SLP, F-ASHA and
Judith A. Brasseur, PhD, CCC-SLP, F-ASHA

DESCRIBING SUPERVISION AND SUPERVISORS

In 1978, American Speech-Language-Hearing Association (ASHA) issued a special report that divided the tasks of supervisors into two categories: *clinical teaching* and *program management.* The report defined each category as separate aspects of the role while stating that each supervisor's professional activity may include behaviors from each category. It defined clinical teaching as "the interaction between supervisor/supervisee in any setting which furthers the development of clinical skills of students or practicing clinicians as related to changes in client behavior" and program management as "those activities that relate to the administration or coordination of programs, for example, scheduling, budgeting, program planning, employing, or dismissing personnel" (ASHA, 1978, p. 479).

The discussions in this book will center mainly on clinical teaching, although many of the principles presented are applicable to program management as well. Clinical teaching, as it has been defined, should be at the center of supervisory process in any setting. It may receive greater emphasis in the educational program, but it also includes the procedure through which the growth and development of clinicians is supported after they enter the workforce. Clinical teaching is certainly a crucial component of any program, even though program management may become the predominant responsibility of the supervisor of a service delivery program.

The revised standards for the accreditation of academic programs in speech-language pathology and audiology imply a significantly greater emphasis on the importance of the clinical teaching and supervisory process in the development of supervisee self-reflective abilities (Council on Academic Accreditation in Audiology and Speech-Language Pathology [CAA], 2017, sec. 3.1.1B)

McCrea, E. S., & Brasseur, J. A. *The Clinical Education and*
Supervisory Process in Speech-Language Pathology and Audiology (pp 1-7).
© 2020 Taylor & Francis Group.

with regard to the refinement of supervisee clinical judgment and accountability and also in the their understanding of the importance of the clinical education and supervisory processes to their sustained professional growth (sec. 3.1.6B). The 2017 standards (CAA, 2017, sec. 3.7B) also continue to require that supervision be appropriate to the knowledge, experience and competence of each supervisee. These standards are promulgated at a time when systematic training in the supervisory process is in its infancy and perhaps not readily available to those who will need to competently implement them. For these reasons, this book will concentrate heavily on the goals, objectives, and methodologies inherent in the clinical education/supervisory process.

Titles of Supervisors

A variety of labels have evolved to identify persons who have historically been identified as supervisors. These alternative labels include clinical educator, clinical instructor, preceptor, and mentor, and reflect the complexities of professional education and practice in clinical disciplines. These complexities are precipitated in large part by increasingly diverse students in training, rapidly changing workplace demands, increased complexity of clinical populations, an expanding continuum of service personnel, and increased public and employer expectations of graduates.

McAllister (2000) suggested that the terms *clinical educator* and *clinical education* more appropriately characterize the skills and applications necessary to support the development of the knowledge and skills contained in the revised training program accreditation standards. The use of these terms implies the sharing of knowledge from clinical educator to and with the student in training. In addition, Fish and Twinn (1997) suggested that the clinical educator has the responsibility to function across a wide variety of educational interactions with students, each of which requires the use of different combinations of supervisory knowledge and skills by the clinical educator.

Both the 2013 ASHA Ad Hoc Committee on Supervision (AHCS) and the 2016 ASHA Ad Hoc Committee on Supervision Training (AHCST) recognized the variety of labels used to identify professionals who complete many of the tasks historically associated with supervision no matter where or with whom it occurs; however, for the purposes of this book the generic title supervisor/supervision/supervisory process will be used. This label is consistent with the conclusion of the 2016 AHSCT report, which recognizes that more specific terminology may be used in specific professional settings. The use of the generic label is also in deference to its use within the official documents of the profession. The reader is cautioned, however, to understand that the writers' use of *supervisor*, *supervision*, and *supervisory process* is in deference to history only and that the focus of this book is more fully captured in the concept of clinical education and the work of clinical educators.

SETTINGS FOR SUPERVISION

Speech-language pathologists and audiologists are prepared by colleges and universities where their experiences include clinical work with communicatively disordered individuals. This clinical phase of their preparation is supervised by certified professionals in programs operated on campus or in cooperative off-campus placements. The professionals prepared in this way ultimately provide services to communicatively disordered persons in a variety of settings: public schools; clinics; acute care hospitals; subacute, rehabilitation, and extended care centers; long-term care and skilled nursing facilities; private practice; homes; and other agencies and institutions. At any point in their career, in any of these varied settings, a speech-language pathologist or audiologist may also become a supervisor.

Educational Programs

In college and university programs, supervisors teach, facilitate, support, and monitor students' application of academic knowledge to the solution of problems of disordered communication and service delivery in the interest of optimal service to current and future clients. Most of this applied teaching takes place in clinical programs operated by colleges or universities in conjunction with their academic programs. Supervisors in such programs operate within a number of difference frameworks, depending on the particular organizational and structure of the program in which they work. Some are full-time supervisors employed for this purpose alone, while for others, supervision is only a part of their responsibilities, which may also include clinical work, academic teaching, administration, or research.

Off-Campus Practicum

The off-campus practicum, where students are assigned to service delivery settings to obtain clinical experience, is part of a total educational program. Some colleges and universities use off-campus sites more extensively than others in order to meet the CAA standards, which require experience across the spectrum of communication disorders and the lifespan. Two types of supervisors are typically involved in these off-campus experiences. One is the *site supervisor* whose primary responsibility is the provision of clinical services to the clients being served by the employer. This individual assumes the additional role of supervisor for a particular students from a college or university for a specified period of time. The second type of supervisor involved in the off-campus practicum is employed by the college or university to serve as a liaison between the campus program and off-campus site personnel. The *university supervisor* performs a variety of tasks, ranging from site selection and assignment of students to on-site observations, and has a different degree of responsibility for the supervision and education of the student, depending on the structure of the total educational program and the nature of and proximity to the off-campus site.

Service Delivery Settings

In settings where the main objective of the organization is the delivery of services to clients/patients, supervision is the process through which these services are developed, monitored, improved, and evaluated. The functions of supervisors in these settings vary greatly, and may include, among other duties, maintaining the quality of services to clients and patients through program organization and management, monitoring and evaluating services, ensuring compliance with regulatory regulations, and being responsible for the ongoing professional development of speech-language pathologists employed by the facility. Such supervisors may or may not be involved with students assigned to their programs by their college or university for off-campus practicum experiences, with persons completing their clinical fellowship (CF) or final audiology externship, or with speech-language pathology assistants.

The Clinical Fellowship

Many speech-language pathologists mentor their colleagues during the CF. The CF is 9 months of full-time professional or equivalent part-time practice after the master's degree is obtained and is a time in which the speech-language pathologist is mentored by an individual who holds the Certificate of Clinical Competence (CCC) from ASHA. The CF is assumed to be a capstone experience during which the clinical fellow is mentored by the supervisor and is one of the requirements for granting the CCC. Program supervisors or other speech-language pathologists who hold the CCC may be asked to mentor persons who are completing a CF in their own facility or in another program. In these cases, contact between the supervisor and the CF candidate is usually more intermittent than in situations in which the clinical fellow is on site.

Final Audiology Externship

The entry-level degree for the profession of audiology is a clinical doctorate known as the Doctor of Audiology (AuD). The advent of this requirement meant that audiology students no longer completed a CF after graduation. Currently, AuD students complete a culminating externship experience as part of degree requirements, typically in the final year of their program. The person in charge of transitioning students from the educational phase to the professional phase is the preceptor, who is a licensed audiologist. CAA standards require experience in a variety of clinical settings, populations and age groups (CAA, 2017, sec. 3.6A). Further, standards mandate that the type and structure of clinical education be commensurate with the development of an individual's knowledge and skills (sec. 3.7A). Students who want to pursue the ASHA Certificate of Clinical Competence in Audiology (CCC-A) must obtain 1,820 hours of clinical experience with preceptors who hold CCC-A.

Other Types of Supervisory Settings

Some supervisors function at the state or regional level, mainly in education agencies and health departments. Their roles may be administrative, regulatory, or consultative and may affect the individual speech-language pathologist and audiologist more indirectly than directly.

Another supervisory setting exists where speech-language pathology assistants are employed to support and/or extend the delivery of services by the speech-language pathologist. When assigned an assistant, a speech-language pathologist assumes the role of supervisor in relation to the work done by the assistant. ASHA (2013) has adopted guidelines for the training, credentialing, use and supervision of assistants to guide the supervisors in these situations.

As interprofessional practice becomes a more routine approach to the delivery of care to clients and patients, speech-language pathologists and audiologists may find themselves in a supervisory position with professionals from other disciplines. For example, speech-language pathologists may become supervisors in rehabilitation centers where they are responsible for physical and occupational therapists and their work, or they may find themselves in interdisciplinary settings where their function is to work with supervisors from other disciplines to provide collaborative care to clients and patients or to meet organizational objectives.

COMPLEXITIES OF THE SUPERVISORY PROCESS

Everyone in speech-language pathology and audiology participates in the supervisory process at some time, certainly as a supervisee and frequently as a supervisor. The "web of supervision" is a complex one in which professionals may be involved in many different types of supervisory interactions throughout their careers or at any one time. The nature of these interactions varies greatly across time and between situations and each of these interactions can vary within itself due to the diversity of the situation and those participating in it. Even after obtaining the CCC, speech-language pathologists and audiologists will interact with a variety of persons who will have supervisory or administrative responsibility for them. They may, in turn, supervise individuals during a CF, students in off-campus practicum, or assistants, and may, at some point, become a supervisor themselves in the context of their work setting.

A final aspect of this supervision web is that nearly every person who is a supervisor is also a supervisee to someone else, necessitating another change of roles. The web of supervision is one that has different subtleties and dynamics associated with the variables inherent in each of its strands. Consequently, it is important for those involved in it to have reasoned approach to the spinning it.

Demographic Data

It has always been difficult to obtain demographic date about supervisors in speech-language pathology and audiology. Although ASHA annually asks members to indicate their primary and secondary activity on the membership survey, the total number of professionals who are participating in some form of supervision has never been clearly documented. ASHA membership and affiliate counts for year-end 2017 documented a total certified membership of 182,719 (ASHA, 2018b). Of the 151,631 who reported their primary employment function, 1.5% indicated that their primary activity was as a "supervisor of clinical activity." However, this is only part of the picture. Currently, there are 348 accredited and candidate programs in speech-language pathology (273) and audiology (75) in the United States (Council of Academic Programs in Communication Sciences and Disorders and the ASHA, 2017). Assuming an average enrollment of 34 master's students in speech-language pathology each year in 273 institutions, each of whom must accrue 350 supervised clinical contact hours, 25% to 50% which must be observed, training programs need to generate a minimum of 812,175 supervised hours each year, out of a total 3,248,700 clinical hours. Further in 2017, 7,848 new certification applications were received at the end of the CF in speech-language pathology (ASHA, 2018a). Each of these experiences required 18 supervisory contacts for a total of 141,264 supervisory activities. Clearly, these numbers speak to the intensity of the contribution supervisors make to the education and training of new members of the profession and imply involvement of more than 1.5% of the membership, probably in part-time supervisory situations (e.g., off-campus practicum, CF).

Although the size of the membership has quadrupled since the first edition of this book (1988), when it was 49,878, these data about the numbers of professionals engaged in supervision are unfortunately slightly less positive than those reported by Anderson (1988) 30 years ago. She indicated that in 1986, 3.1% of professionals indicated that their primary professional activity was supervision. The current data suggest there is an increase in the numbers of professionals who are supervising in a part-time capacity.

Purposes of Supervision in the Professions

Villareal (1964), in reporting on a conference called by ASHA to discuss guidelines for supervision of clinical practicum, cited the report of one subcommittee of the conference when he wrote, "The role of an effective supervisor should transcend the mere monitoring of the student's clinical activities. It should include informal teaching of clinical content, the demonstration of clinical techniques, and mature counseling of the student in relation to his clinical training" (p. 14). Van Riper (1965) said that students are turned into clinicians through supervision. Anderson (1970), in a meeting of school program supervisors, stated, "The major roles of the supervisor are to manage, evaluate and innovate programs for the communicatively handicapped children and youth within the community. At all times the welfare of children with speech, hearing or language disorders is the reason for the supervisor's activities" (p. 152). Turton (1973) said, "Supervision can be viewed as a process wherein one person is responsible for changing the knowledge and skill of another" (p. 94). Ward and Webster (1965), in discussing the training of clinicians, said, "Clinical supervision is conceived as an interactive process between student and supervisor in which both are working together to find the most productive ways of effecting the diagnostic or therapeutic relationship" (p. 104).

Writing about supervision in audiology, Rassi (1978) defined clinical supervision as clinical teaching and said, "It's aim is to teach a student in a one-on-one situation how to apply his academic knowledge in a practical clinical setting as he functions in that setting. The ultimate goal is to transform the student into an independent clinician" (p. 9).

A Definition of Supervision for the Professions

It is clear that there are a variety of personal concepts built into all of the statements about the purposes of supervision and the role of the supervisor with some common threads running through them all. To add to this array, the following definition of the supervisory process is offered as the basis for the remainder of this book.

> Supervision is a process that consists of a variety of patterns of behavior, the appropriateness of which depends upon the needs, competencies, expectations, and philosophies of the supervisor and the supervisee and the specifics of the situation (task, client, setting and other variables). The goals of the supervisory process are the professional growth and development of the supervisee and the supervisor, which it is assumed will result ultimately in optimal service to clients. (Anderson, 1988, p. 12)

Despite the fact that this description of the supervisory process was first introduced 30 years ago, it is consistent with the notion of clinical education and of the goals of clinical educators that McAllister identified in 2000. Even more importantly perhaps, the goals of the process explicated in the first edition of this work are now embodied in the standards for accreditation of academic programs, which require that the "type and structure of clinical education are commensurate with the development of the knowledge and skill of each student" (CAA, 2017). The 2008 ASHA Technical Report on clinical supervision in speech-language pathology expanded Anderson's definition (1988) in stating that:

> Professional growth and development of the supervisee and supervisor are enhanced when supervision or clinical teaching involves self-analysis and self-evaluation. Effective clinical teaching also promotes the use of critical thinking and problem-solving skills on the part of the individual being supervised. (ASHA, 2008, p. 4)

In addition, supervision must support the student's abilities in self-reflection and the development of reasoned clinical decision making across the knowledge base of the professions. Furthermore, the dynamics of this definition of the supervisory process provide a platform for lifelong learning and refinement of one's own knowledge and skill as a supervisor.

Summary

Supervision in speech-language pathology and audiology is a pervading and complex activity within the professions. Although it is accepted that many individuals are involved in supervision, complete demographic data are limited. The stated purposes of the supervisory process vary among individuals; however, this book is based on the premise that the objective of supervision is to develop independent professionals who, by means of their own professional knowledge and self-awareness as a service provider and supervisor or supervisee, can think critically, solve problems, and provide optimal services to communicatively disordered persons.

REFERENCES

American Speech and Hearing Association. (1978). Current status of supervision of speech-language pathology and audiology [Special report of the Committee on Supervision in Speech-Language-Pathology and Audiology.]. *Asha, 20,* 478-486.

American Speech-Language-Hearing Association. (2008). *Knowledge and skills needed by speech-language pathologists providing clinical supervision* [Technical report]. Retrieved from https://www.asha.org/policy/TR2008-00296

American Speech-Language-Hearing Association. (2013a). *Knowledge, skills and training considerations for individuals serving as supervisors.* [Final report of the Ad Hoc Committee on Supervision]. Retrieved from https://www.asha.org/uploadedFiles/Supervisors-Knowledge-Skills-Report.pdf.

American Speech-Language-Hearing Association. (2018a). *2018 CFCC update.* Presented at CAPCSD, Austin, TX. Retrieved from https://www.asha.org/uploadedFiles/CFCC-2018-Update.pdf

American Speech-Language-Hearing Association. (2018b). *ASHA summary membership and affiliation counts, year-end 2017.* Retrieved from https://www.asha.org/uploadedFiles/2017-Member-Counts.pdf

Anderson, J. (Ed.). (1970). *Proceedings of conference on supervision of speech and hearing programs in the schools.* Bloomington, IN: Indiana University.

Anderson, J. (1988). *The supervisory process in speech-language pathology and audiology.* Boston, MA: College-Hill.

Council of Academic Programs in Communication Sciences and Disorders and the American Speech-Language-Hearing Association. (2017). *Communication sciences and disorders (CSD) education survey national aggregate data report 2016-2017 academic year.* Retrieved from https://www.asha.org/uploadedFiles/2016-2017-CSD-Education-Survey-National-Aggregate-Data-Report.pdf

Council on Academic Accreditation in Audiology and Speech-Language Pathology. (2017). *Standards for accreditation of graduate education programs in audiology and speech-language pathology.* Retrieved May 21, 2018 from http://caa.asha.org/wp-content/uploads/Accreditation-Standards-for-Graduate-Programs.pdf

Fish, D., & Twinn, S. (1997). *Quality clinical supervision in the health care professions: Principled approaches to practice.* Oxford, England: Butterworth Heinemann.

McAllister, L. (2000). *Where are we going in clinical education? A review of current status and some theoretical and philosophical guideposts for new directions.* Proceedings of the Council of Academic Programs in Communication Sciences and Disorders 2000 Conference. Minneapolis, MN: The Council of Academic Programs in Communication Sciences and Disorders.

Rassi, J. (1978). *Supervision in audiology.* Baltimore, MD: University Park Press.

Turton, L. (Ed.). (1973). *Proceedings of a Workshop on Supervision in Speech Pathology.* Ann Arbor, MI: University of Michigan, Institute for the Study of Mental Retardation and Related Disabilities.

Van Riper, C. (1965). Supervision of clinical practice. *Asha, 3,* 75-77.

Villareal, J. (Ed.). (1964). *Seminar on guidelines for supervision of clinical practicum.* Washington, DC: American Speech and Hearing Association.

Ward, L., & Webster, E. (1965). The training of clinical personnel: II. A concept of clinical preparation. *Asha, 7,* 103-106.

i This chapter is a revision of that appearing in the 2003 edition of this book.

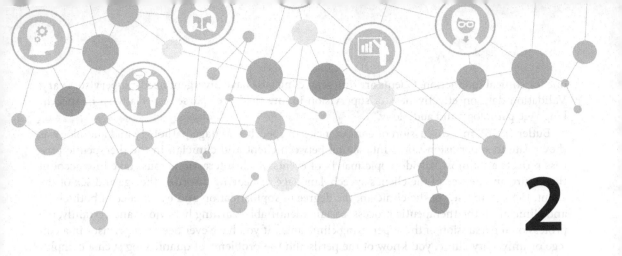

2

The Continuum Model of Supervision

Elizabeth S. McCrea, PhD, CCC-SLP, F-ASHA and
Judith A. Brasseur, PhD, CCC-SLP, F-ASHA

IS THERE A METHODOLOGY?

Perhaps the most reliable fact about supervision in speech-language pathology and audiology is that, until recently, the vast majority of supervisors operate without much preparation for the process (Anderson, 1973, 1974, 1980; American Speech-Language-Hearing Association [ASHA], 1978; Schubert & Aitchison, 1975; Stace & Drexler, 1969). Very few training programs offer coursework in the supervisory process as part of their curricular offerings for the master's or doctoral degree. Similarly, despite the continuing education activities of first, the Council of Supervisors in Speech-Language Pathology and Audiology and now, Special Interest Group 11, Administration and Supervision as well as individual convention and conference contributions from members and information on the ASHA Practice Portal, there have been no systematic professional development activities sponsored by ASHA.

What was true over 40 years ago still is, in great measure, true today; however, the environment may be about to change. The Council of Academic Programs in Communication Sciences and Disorders (CAPCSD; 2013) recommended that systematic training initiatives for those engaged in the supervision of clinical practicum within graduate programs be developed. A 2016 CAPCSD initiative (www.capcsd.org) sparked the development of web-based professional development modules to promote best practices in clinical supervision which are available to member programs of the Council in support of their on- and off-campus supervisors. In addition, the 2016 Ad Hoc Committee on Supervision Training (ASHA, 2016) recommended that ASHA develop systematic training for supervisors across five specific supervision constituencies by 2020. In spite of these important developments, the search for a specific supervisory methodology is still as elusive as is

McCrea, E. S., & Brasseur, J. A. *The Clinical Education and Supervisory Process in Speech-Language Pathology and Audiology* (pp 9-43). © 2020 Taylor & Francis Group.

one for clinical interaction. Clients are different; clinicians have divergent needs; supervisors vary. Validation data on effectiveness of supervision in any field are sparse, especially so in speech-language pathology and audiology.

Butler (1976), in a discussion of competencies in speech-language pathology and audiology as they relate to supervision said: "Interaction between client and clinician in the therapeutic process reflects an almost kaleidoscopic matrix of events. Such interactions must take into account the nature and degree of the client's speech, language or hearing disorder, the age and sex of the client, the age and sex of the clinician, the degree of sophistication and experience of both client and clinician in the therapeutic process, certain identifiable learning behaviors, and certainly, the professional persuasion of the supervising clinician.… If you have ever been a supervisor in a college or university clinic, you know of the perils and the problems of quantifying such a complex matrix" (p. 2).

The supervisor of a service delivery program in no less vulnerable to these complexities. Fisher (1982) addressed the issues in supervising professional personnel in the schools and stated that "the responsibility requires a multitude of skills in human interaction, motivation, and leadership in developing professionals. The role of the supervisor is vastly different from the role of a speech-language pathologist in this respect. In essence, when a person becomes a supervisor, this person changes professions" (p. 54). This same challenge is attendant upon the supervisory process in healthcare as well and is increasingly important in interprofessional education and practice settings. Although most supervisors in the professions probably see themselves as speech-language pathologists first, Fisher's statement underscores the range of skills that are important to the process of supervision and that are important to supervisors' abilities to mediate knowledge and skill as clinicians with their supervisees.

Gouran (1980) recognized the fact that supervision remains something of an art and said, "Recommendations related to the practice of supervision should be viewed in probabilistic terms" (p. 87). He further noted that there would be a number of expectations for any set of recommendations and it would not be prudent to develop or implement standard operating procedures for all situations. Weller (1971) asserted that a single methodological approach is impossible; rather supervisory functions related to problems should be identified and methodologies appropriate to each should be proposed.

DEVELOPMENT OF SUPERVISORY BEHAVIORS

In the presence of so many situational variables and relatively little (but increasing) "how to supervise" information, what forms the basis for the actions of professionals when they become supervisors? How do supervisory behaviors or styles develop? Obviously, past experiences in human interaction influence behaviors toward people in all situations. A major focus in the way supervisors interact with those in less dominant positions in the supervisor-supervisee relationship may be the way in which they have been dealt with by others who have held dominant positions over them, such as parents, teachers, siblings, or others. Similarly, much of the perception of the role of the supervisor and the behaviors of persons who find themselves in that role probably have come from interactions with their own supervisors, if not modeled from behaviors of those supervisors.

In addition to personal experiences, supervisory behavior may be influenced by a variety of other means. Popular media, both print and visual, have often depicted stylized characterizations of those with supervisory responsibility. More often than not, they are examples of highly directive and controlling behavior. Some supervisors may have read books and articles from other fields about leadership and management and tried to apply that content within the dynamics of their own situation. Policies and organizational structure of the workplace may also influence the way in which supervisors develop their own style. Productivity pressures, organizational philosophy, delegation of responsibility, and other organizational variables may directly influence the way in which supervisors perceive and carry out their roles. Last, although perhaps even more fundamentally, each supervisor's personal characteristics and interpersonal relationships will determine to a great extent the kind of supervisory behavior and interaction style each person adopts. Generally speaking then, individual approaches of supervisors have developed in response to a variety of experiences rather than as a result of a study of the supervisory process, reflections of one's own behavior as a supervisor, or the application of theoretical models and research findings. Still today, the development of supervisory behaviors and individual style likely occurs, more often than not, by happenstance than by strategic design.

LITERATURE FROM OTHER DISCIPLINES

The study of supervision is made more complex because of its existence in so many areas of endeavor; however, there is significant overlap among the helping professions, which makes it important to consider the contributions of each. A complete review of this literature would result in a voluminous text and, so, isn't possible here. However, for additional substantive areas of thought , please consider:

- Scientific management (Taylor, 1911)
- Hawthorne studies (Mayo, 1933)
- Human relations management (Hampton, Summer, & Webber, 1982; Hersey & Blanchard, 1982; Hersey, Blanchard & Johnson, 2012; Kelly, 1980; Pascale & Athos, 1981; Peters & Waterman, 1982; Reitz, 1981; Tannenbaum, 1966)
- Motivation and personality (Maslow, 1954)
- Participative management (McGregor, 1960; Argyris, 1962)

Situational Leadership

Gouran (1980) implied that there is not one best way to supervise. This concept of adaptive leadership or *situational leadership*—that is, not one best style but the most effective style for the situation (Gouran, 1980; Hersey & Blanchard, 1982; Hersey, Blanchard & Johnson, 2012; Reitz, 1981) is probably the most significant theoretical model from other disciplines when the variables inherent in the definition of supervision in speech-language pathology and audiology are considered. The *leadership contingency model* developed by Fiedler (1967) stated that, although there are more or less effective styles of leadership, they are not effective in every situation. The three major situational variables identified by Fiedler in determining the appropriateness of a style of leadership were 1) leader-member relations, 2) degree of structure in the task, and 3) the power and authority their position provides.

Gouran (1980) also suggested that too many people who have supervisory responsibilities function "within narrowly or stereotypically conceived notions of what constitutes 'good supervision'" (p. 93). He maintained that practices based on this erroneous conception as "injurious to the task of clinical supervision." He presented the work of Farris (1974) who identified four supervisory styles: collaboration, domination, delegation, and abdication. The appropriateness of each style is determined by relative capabilities of the supervisor and supervisee to deal independently with a specific kind of demand. Gouran further stated several principles that are applications of Farris' ideas about the relationship between supervisory style and circumstantial influences:

- No one style of supervision is best.
- A supervisor must be prepared to deal differently with different supervisees.
- Within any given supervisor-supervisee relationship, circumstances may require periodic changes in style.

- Adoption of an inappropriate style in relation to a particular situational demand will reduce chances for achieving the supervisor's and supervisee's mutually shared goals.
- The measure of success in effective supervision is not the extent of the supervisor's influence on the supervisee, but the extent in which their interaction contributes to the achievement of specified objectives.

Hersey and Blanchard (1982) proposed a *situational leadership theory* utilizing the terms *task behavior* and *relationship behavior* to describe leadership style. Any leadership style is made up of some combination of task or relationship behaviors. Task behavior is defined as the extent to which the leader provides direction, organizes roles and activities, and specifies how they are to be achieved; relationship behavior is the extent to which the leader establishes and maintains personal relationships with the followers that are supportive and facilitative. It is the interaction of style and environment that makes leadership effective or ineffective; therefore, no one style is appropriate in all situations. Hersey and Blanchard further proposed that the level of maturity (Argyris, 1962) of the follower is a variable that must be considered in relation to the task. Maturity is defined by Hersey and Blanchard as the ability to set high but attainable goals, the ability and willingness to take responsibility, and having the education and experience to complete a task or job effectively. Because maturity will vary among people or within a group, the leaders must know the level of maturity in determining the appropriate style. Hersey and Blanchard's model includes four behavioral styles and presents an important parallel to the continuum of supervision proposed in this book:

1. *Telling* (high task-low relationship): The leader defines roles and tasks
2. *Selling* (high task-high relationship): Direction is still provided but it is accompanied by more two-way communication and socioemotional support to encourage communication
3. *Participative* (high relationship-low task): Facilitative, shared decision making
4. *Delegating* (low relationship-low task): The follower "runs own show"

Thus, Hersey and Blanchard (1982) proposed that when the follower is immature in relation to a task, the appropriate style will be high task-low relationship, that is, the leader will be more involved in organizing and directing in relation to the task. "As the individual or group begins to move into an above average level of maturity, it becomes appropriate for leaders to decrease not only task behavior but also relationship behavior" (p. 163). In other words, as the follower works more independently, socioemotional support is not as necessary and there is less direction and more delegation by the leader. Style, then, changes as followers become more able to set goals and accomplish tasks independently.

Much of the early work in supervision in audiology and speech-language pathology focused on the orientation and behavior of supervisors that they brought to the process of clinical supervision. During the last 3 decades, however, interest also grew in the development and progression of supervisee competence as a result of instruction and experience. Several theorists proposed models that described this progression and cognitive and behavioral development of students or supervisees as a result of instruction and practice. The supervisor's responsibility in these models is to strategically structure and mediate the supervisee's experiences to support their demonstration of skill and the achievement of increased competence.

Five-Stage Model of Adult Skill Acquisition

Dreyfus and Dreyfus (2004) proposed a five-stage model that suggests students learn and develop competence across tasks through didactic instruction and practice. The model was originally developed in the mathematical and engineering sciences but has found application in both medical and nursing education. These stages, with adaptation in speech-language pathology and audiology, include:

- *Novice*: The learner demonstrates little knowledge or experience to support practice, is often inflexible, and is generally not self-aware nor reflective. The instructor needs to provide rules and procedures and needs to decompose a task or plan so the learner can practice in a "context free" environment.
- *Advanced beginner*: The learner begins to be self-analytic and reflective of his or her own behavior and its effect on behavior of others, and begins to demonstrate some capacity at modifying behavior based on its consequences. The learner is gaining experience but needs to preplan and overplan to be able to modify behavior and simplify tasks in real time.
- *Competent*: The learner understands demands, dynamics, and management needs within a task or situation, is aware of his or her own behavior in context and can modify it to achieve enhanced outcomes. The learner is emotionally involved. Increased experience, knowledge, and skills can make the learner feel overwhelmed at times, but he or she has to learn to "cope with crowdedness."
- *Proficient*: The learner is able to understand the totality of the situation or problem and is able to independently design and implement a solution The learner can identify unexpected challenges and uses analytical problem solving to identify and implement strategies to address them. He or she uses self-analysis and reflection and takes responsibility for behavior.
- *Expert*: The learner intuitively and accurately sees the "big picture" and accurately uses knowledge and experience to address tasks. He or she is willing to go beyond existing paradigms to address problems, and fully engages self-analysis and reflection to sustain professional growth.

The model emphasizes the notion that skill development within tasks and situations is a function of context and the development of perspective and intuition within those tasks.

Conscious Competence and the SQF Model of Supervision

More contemporarily, The *S* (supervision) *Q* (questioning) *F* (feedback) model of supervision (Barnum, Guyer, Levy, & Graham, 2009), which has its foundations in the *conscious competency* model of Howell and Fleischman (1982), suggested that there are four stages of adult learning, each of which is characterized by different aspects of consciousness (awareness) and competency:

- *Unconscious incompetence*: The learner is unaware of what they do not know.
- *Conscious incompetence*: The learner is becoming aware of what they do and do not know.
- *Conscious competence*: The learner understands his or her own knowledge and skill level and increasingly understands what must be done or be evident in their behavior to achieve greater competence.
- *Unconscious competence*: The learner's demonstration of knowledge and appropriate skill is fluid and relatively effortless.

Barnum and Guyer (2015) describe strategic and intentional strategies to move learners from unconscious incompetence to conscious competence across situations and tasks that are important to professional skill sets. The amount and type of supervision is contingent on the learner's knowledge and skills, urgency with which a specific task must be completed and consequences for the learner and her or his client. Questioning strategies predicted on Bloom's taxonomy are used by the supervisor as important to foster critical thinking and decision making on the part of the learner while "feedback is used to confirm, guide and correct clinical reasoning and professionalism" (Mormer & Messick, 2016, p. 11). The utilization of each of these strategies is situationally based and predicated upon the learner's demonstrated knowledge and skill.

LEADERSHIP AND SUPERVISION IN EDUCATION

At a time that this research on leadership and supervision was developing in other disciplines, a parallel stream of supervision theory and research was emerging in education. Often borrowing from the management literature, but more frequently related to the teaching aspect of supervision, this parallel development probably had an even stronger impact on supervision in speech-language pathology and audiology than that of the business literature.

Research on the behaviors of teachers in the classroom during the 1970s influenced attitudes toward the study of supervision. Flanders (1967, 1969) was among the first to maintain that direct behavioral styles are less productive in the problem-solving activities in the classroom than indirect styles. Generally, Flanders concluded from his studies that children learn better from teachers who did not dominate but were flexible in their behavior and those who could be indirect or direct as indicated by a particular situation.

Studies of Indirect and Direct Behavior

The indirect-direct concept was applied to the study of the supervisory process by Blumberg and Weber (1968), Blumberg and Amidon (1965), Blumberg, Amidon, and Weber (1967), and Blumberg and Cusick (1970). Influenced by Flanders (1967) and Bales (1950, 1951), Blumberg and his associates maintained that the exclusive use of direct behaviors in supervision increased defensiveness on the part of supervisees. Blumberg (1974, 1980) also recognized that most texts on supervision did not address what happens between supervisor and supervisees in the supervisory interaction. He and his associates conducted extensive inquiries about the human relationship aspect of supervision, particularly direct and indirect dimensions of the supervisor's behavior. Blumberg's investigations were based on Gibb's (1969) work on defensive communication, in which he identified six bipolar communication behaviors that were either *support inducing* or *defense inducing*. Behavior that was support inducing, Gibb said, was oriented toward problem solving, spontaneity, equality, provisionalism, empathy, and description. Behavior that was defense inducing was oriented toward control, strategy, superiority, certainty, neutrality, and evaluation.

Blumberg (1974, 1980) equated Gibb's (1969) defense-inducing behaviors with direct supervisory behaviors, such as giving opinions, telling, criticizing, suggesting change, and evaluating. Support inducing behaviors were equated with indirect supervisory behavior and included accepting and clarifying teachers' questions, praising teacher behavior, asking teachers for their own opinions and suggestions, and discussing teachers' feeling about the relationship between the supervisor and supervisee. In other words, Blumberg contended that these Direct-Indirect Styles communicate a totally different attitude about the teacher-supervisee interaction. Direct behaviors communicate that the supervisor wishes to control the teacher, exclude the teacher from problem solving, sees evaluation by the supervisor as the main function of observation, and does not value the worth of the teacher in the teaching role. Indirect behaviors communicate a concern for the teacher as a person, a desire for collaborative problem solving and a recognition of the teacher's personal and professional growth.

Using these categories of indirect and direct behaviors, Blumberg and Amidon (1965) investigated whether teachers could discriminate between specific types of behavior of their supervisors. Results of this study made it clear that a one-dimensional approach to supervisory behavior was too simplistic. From this study, the authors developed the following set of four supervisory styles that Blumberg and his colleagues use in subsequent studies.

- *Style A*: High direct-high indirect. Supervisors were perceived by teachers as emphasizing both direct and indirect behavior, telling and criticizing but also asking and listening.
- *Style B*: High direct-low indirect. Supervisors were perceived by teachers as doing a great deal of telling and criticizing but very little asking or listening.

- *Style C*: Low direct-high indirect. Supervisors were perceived by teachers as rarely telling or criticizing but emphasizing the asking of questions, listening, and reflecting back the teacher's ideas and feelings.
- *Style D*: Low direct-low indirect. Supervisors were perceived as passive and not doing much within the interaction.

Blumberg and his associates also found that perception of these supervisory styles made a difference in the way teachers viewed their interaction with their supervisors (Blumberg & Weber, 1968). The results presented support for a mix of the two styles of behavior but with a strong tendency to prefer high amounts of indirect behavior and are an important base for the study of supervisory methodologies. Teachers in these studies perceived more positive interpersonal relationships with their supervisors under the two styles containing the most indirect behavior (styles A and C). Teachers gave positive evaluations of their interpersonal relationships with their supervisors when they perceived the interaction consisted of telling, suggesting and criticizing as well as reflecting and asking for information and opinions (style A) or when there was little telling and much reflecting and asking (style C). Negative attitudes resulted from perceptions of supervisory behavior as predominately telling with little reflecting or asking (style B) or when the supervisor was perceived as passive (style D).

Teachers in these studies also indicated that they were able to obtain more insight about themselves, both as teacher and as a person, if supervisors used a high degree of indirect behavior with some direct (again a combination of style A and C). Thus, Blumberg stated, "This finding suggests that hearing about oneself is probably most productive, not only when the supervisor (or other helping agent) questions, listens, and reflects back what he hears, but also when he does a bit of telling and gives feedback" (Blumberg, 1974, 1980, p. 67). Behavioral styles D and B were not seen by teachers as contributing to learning about themselves.

When supervisors were perceived to use style B, the teachers understandably perceived their supervisors to be more oriented toward control than problem solving; teachers under this treatment felt the need to be more strategy oriented and less spontaneous and they felt that supervisors were more oriented toward superiority than equality and toward certainty than provisionalism. Also, teachers felt their interaction was more dominated by evaluation of their behaviors than toward description of behavior. All of these behaviors are equated with defense-inducing behavior.

At the same time, teachers whose supervisors were seen to operate under style C perceived the highest degree of empathy and productivity and the least degree of defense-inducing behaviors. Thus, said Blumberg (1980), "Our spoken expectations that style C would result in communicative freedom and high productivity while style B would reflect defensiveness and low productivity were met" (p. 69).

Other similar findings by Blumberg and Cusick (1970) present support for the use of direct and indirect behaviors, together with the first definitive discussion of behaviors and data to dispute the value of the Direct Style. Their findings support the need to look carefully at the effects of the Direct and Indirect Styles and the probably need to analyze one's own behavior supervisory behavior on the basis of these styles.

Interpersonal Approach

Meanwhile at Teacher's College, Columbia University, Dussault (1970) proposed a middle-range theory of supervision in the education of student teachers that was based on Carl Rogers' theory of therapy and personality change. Dussault discussed the relationships that exist between therapy and the teaching function of supervision and developed a theory that parallels Rogers' writings and in brief, states that if facilitative interpersonal conditions exist during the supervisory conference that certain changes will be observed supervisee behavior.

Dussault (1970) clearly differentiated between the *evaluative* function of supervision and the *teaching* function. Evaluation, he said, is the process of assessment or judgment about the person's readiness to assume professional responsibilities. The teaching function, on the other hand, is the process of helping the student acquire the competencies necessary to fulfill those professional responsibilities. Thus, he made a distinction between evaluation as feedback and guidance and evaluation as judgmental assessment.

Clinical Supervision

At about the same time, Cogan (1973) and Goldhammer (1969) began advocating a style of supervision called *clinical supervision*. Their approach to supervision, although not supported by evidence at the time, was decidedly more specific and more related to the analysis of actual supervisor behavior than any previous thinkers and writers. The methodology employs shared interaction between supervisor and supervisee, based on objective data, that is, data collected and analyzed by both supervisor and supervisee. *Clinical*, a term rarely found in the education literature up to this time, was used by both writers to describe supervision as not referring to the pathological but to describe "supervision up close" (Goldhammer, 1969, p. 54)—the one-to-one relationship between supervisor and teacher. There is a strong emphasis on the desirability of teachers and supervisors to be "supportive and empathetic; to perfect technical behaviors and concepts from which they are generated; to increase efficiencies of learning and becoming; to treat one other decently and responsibly and with affection; to engage with one another, honestly" (pp. 55-56).

Cogan (1973) described the genesis of the clinical supervision methodology with students in the Master of Arts in Teaching Program at Harvard in the late 1950s and indicated it grew out of the dissatisfaction of many students with the nature of the supervision they experienced during their own training. Cogan also defended the use of the word "clinical" and said "it was selected precisely to draw attention to the emphasis placed on the classroom observation, analysis of the in-class events, and the focus on the teachers' and students' in-class behavior (pp. 8-9). Cogan formulated the eight phases in this cycle of supervision:

1. Phase 1: Establishing the student-teacher relationship
2. Phase 2: Planning with the teacher
3. Phase 3: Planning the strategy of the observation
4. Phase 4: Observing the interaction
5. Phase 5: Analyzing the teaching-learning processes
6. Phase 6: Planning the strategy of the conference
7. Phase 7: The conference
8. Phase 8: Renewed planning

Goldhammer (1969) proposed five similar stages for the clinical supervisory process:

1. Preobservation conference
2. Observation
3. Analysis and strategy
4. Supervision conference
5. Preconference analysis (postmortem)

Both Cogan's (1973) and Goldhammer's (1969) methodologies definitely mandated recognition of the contributions of supervisor and supervisee in the supervisory process. In a revision of Goldhammer's earlier work, Goldhammer, Anderson, and Krajewski (1980) called supervision "that place of instructional supervision which draws its data from first-hand observation of actual teaching events and involves face-to-face (and other associated) interaction between the supervisor and teacher in the analysis of teaching behaviors and activities for instructional improvement" (pp. 19-20).

Cognitive Coaching

Costa and Garmston (1985a) posited an approach to supervision that they called *cognitive coaching*. It is an approach that supports informed teacher decision making that finds it roots in the ideas of Cogan (1973) and Goldhammer (1969) about clinical supervision (a relationship to foster the teacher's freedom to act self-sufficiently) rather than an approach to supervision that actually is teacher evaluation in disguise. Their rationale was their belief that the teaching act can best be described as a constant stream of decisions and any teacher behavior used is the result of a decision, either conscious or unconscious. Teachers make many decisions each day about students, curriculum, and teaching strategy. "A supervisory process, therefore, should help teachers make better decisions about instruction. Cognitive Coaching is intended to enhance those intellectual skills which contribute to educationally sound decision making" (p. i).

In Costa and Garmston's (1965b) thinking, the supervisor is seen as a mediator of teachers' intelligent behavior. To stimulate the teachers' intellectual skills, the supervisor must call attention to discrepancies between intended and actual learning outcomes and pose problems designed to invite more than response based on memory (Fishler, 1971). For example, cognitive coaches ask questions to facilitate teacher thinking, inference building, self-evaluation and self-prescription: How do you think the student did in meeting the objective? What data seem to support your decision? What do you think the problem is? "The supervisor's questions and statements can be designed to elicit specific cognitive functions that produce data, identify relationships and generalizations to help resolve the problem" (Costa & Garmston, 1965b, pp. 72-73). They suggested a supervisory process which consists of four phases:

- *Auditing*: Planning and clarification of goals, objectives, strategies
- *Monitoring*: Gathering data about student and teacher performance
- *Validating*: Analysis and reflection on student and teacher performance in which cause-and-effect relationships between teacher performance and student achievement are considered
- *Consulting*: Evaluating appropriateness of goals and teaching strategies, prescribing alternative strategies, and developing insight into the supervisory process.

The writings of Blumberg (1974), Cogan (1973), Goldhammer (1969), Goldhammer et al. (1980), and Costa and Garmston (1985a, 1985b) exerted significant influence on the writers of this book as well as on Jean Anderson, the author of the original edition. Although the proposal for supervision that will be presented here is different from that proposed by them, it draws heavily from their writings for concept development and support. Readers are invited to read their original works carefully.

SUPERVISORY APPROACHES IN THE PROFESSIONS

The literature in the professions of speech-language pathology and audiology has descriptive research and theoretical approaches to define the practice of supervision in both disciplines. While this body of work may be considered historical at this point, it is important to maintain it as a record of the early history of the interest in and study of the supervisory process.

Descriptive Findings

There is a fairly large body of information about supervisory conferences in speech-language pathology from many sources. These studies identified a definite pattern found in the dynamics of the conferences in these studies (Blumberg, 1980; Culatta, Colucci, & Wiggins, 1975; Culatta & Seltzer, 1976, 1977; Dowling & Shank, 1981; Hatten, 1965; Irwin, 1975, 1976, 1981; McCrea, 1980; Pickering, 1982, 1984; Roberts & Smith, 1982; Russell, 1976; Schubert & Nelson, 1976; Seeley, 1973;

Shapiro, 1985; Smith, 1977; Smith & Anderson, 1982; Tufts, 1983; Weller, 1971). The details of the studies will be provided later as appropriate but if the data from these conferences are combined and the reader conjectures about a typical supervisory conference in speech-language pathology (there are no specific data about audiology conferences), the description of a typical conference would be something like this:

- The conference is brief, probably less than 30 min.
- The supervisor assumes a dominate role, doing most of the talking, initiating and structuring of discussion, thereby setting the tone for the entire conference.
- Topics change frequently.
- Much of the content of the conference consists of the supervisee "rehashing" what happened in the therapy session, most often without data to support the discussion, and the supervisor making most of the suggestions about strategies to be used in the future.
- Supervisors do not spend much time asking the supervisee for suggestions about future action.
- Very little explanation, elaboration, justification, clarification, or summaries of statements (all behaviors that enhance communication) are made by either the supervisor or supervisee.
- Supervisors use praise or other supportive behaviors to create a positive socioemotional climate, which probably is perceived by the supervisee as reinforcement of certain behaviors.
- Discussion probably deals with maintenance or procedural topics such as discussion of anxieties, defensiveness, or other affective issues being avoided.
- Emphasis in discussion is on the teaching-therapy process or the client, not on the supervisor or supervisee. The supervisory process is seldom discussed.
- Very few evaluative statements are made about the supervisee, perhaps because the supervisors assume that supervisees can utilize the discussion of the client to learn about their own behavior.
- Supervisor style will be much the same from one conference to another, regardless of the supervisee's experience, expertise, or expectations.
- Supervisees are usually passive participants in the conferences and seldom ask questions, initiate a topic or ask for justification. Instead, they react and respond to the supervisors. Their responses tend to be short, most likely agreeing with the supervisor.
- Supervisees' needs for indirect behavior from the supervisor and their own participation are probably not met.
- As with supervisors, supervisees utilize simple utterances without justification and they do not provide reinforcement for supervisor .

Because there was such overwhelming evidence that this was what happens in conferences, this type of interaction will be referred to as *traditional* supervision.

Theoretical Positions

Although less extensive, the fields of speech-language pathology and audiology have produced a number of suggested approaches to the supervisory process Most reveal influences of work in other disciplines.

Probably the first in-depth look at the complexities of preparing clinical personnel came over 5 decades ago in two thoughtful articles by Ward and Webster (1965a, 1965b). Perhaps not so well known except to those specifically interested in the study of supervision and the preparation of speech-language pathologists and audiologists, these articles should be required reading for everyone in the professions because they raised issues that have not yet been thoroughly resolved. Ward and Webster (1965a) probed "the nature of the human encounter" and stressed the importance of providing proper conditions for growth and change for students as is done for clients, and for developing "concepts of training in which students may gain repeated experience in exploring and exercising their own humanness" (p. 39). Ward and Webster (1965b) defined clinical supervision as "an interactive process between student and supervisor in which both are working together to find the most productive ways of effecting the diagnostic or therapeutic relationship" (p. 104). Supervisors, they believed, must be willing to examine their own attitudes and relationships—the first mention in the literature that both supervisor and clinician behaviors need the same kind of focus given to client behavior.

A Rogerian orientation to the relationship between supervisor and supervisee was proposed by Carracciolo, Rigrodsky, and Morrison (1978). Based on Carl Rogers' (1961, 1962) work on client-centered therapy and Dussault's (1970) middle-range theory of supervision, the authors suggested that the same facilitative interpersonal conditions that most speech-language pathologists or audiologists would agree are important to facilitate change in client behavior are also relevant to the supervisory process. These facilitating behaviors, if offered to the supervisee by the supervisor, will "provide a psychosocial environment which enables the student to develop into a competent, secure and independent professional clinician" (Carracciolo, Rigrodsky, & Morrison, p. 286). Further discussion of this approach by Carracciolo and colleagues suggested that the supervisor, while needing to utilize the nondirective, facilitative orientation to establish a relationship conducive to growth, must also play another role. This role is a more directive one, "when the supervisor must be more directive with respect to giving information to the student, making judgments of the student's behaviors and establishing requirements and standards" (p. 288).

At the same time that interest in the supervisory process in speech-language pathology was growing, a parallel interest was developing in audiology. An approach to supervision by Rassi (1978) utilized a framework of competency-based instruction that includes skills in testing, writing, and interpersonal and decision-making areas. Her definition of supervision is "clinical teaching in which the student is taught in a 'one-on-one' situation how to apply his academic knowledge in a practical clinical setting as he functions in that setting. The ultimate goal is to transform the student into an independent clinician" (p. 9). Later, Rassi (1985, 1987) provided arguments for differences between supervision in audiology and speech-language pathology. She felt the preponderant diagnostic nature of work inherent in the practice of audiology dictates a different approach to supervision and requires competency-based instruction.

Schubert (1978) suggested an approach to supervision based on the use of an interaction analysis system, the Analysis of Behavior of Clinicians, which will be discussed in Chapter 5. The Integrative Task Maturity Model of Supervision (ITMMS), presented by Mawdsley (1985) at an ASHA convention was an ingenious combination of Hersey and Blanchard's (1982) Situational Leadership Model, the Wisconsin Procedure for Appraisal of Clinical Competence (Shriberg et al., 1975) and Cogan's (1973) clinical supervision model. It includes a system for analyzing appropriate supervisory styles and specific techniques to be utilized at different levels of maturity. Crago and Pickering (1987) published a book that discussed several facets of the supervisory process with a major emphasis on its interpersonal aspects.

Farmer and Farmer (1989) promoted a Trigonal Model of Communication Disorders Supervision, which identified three components of the supervisory process. In addition to positing the model itself, they proposed specific activities to implement it which were consistent with its theoretical constructs.

Gillam and Pena (1995) and Gillam (1999) suggested an approach to clinical education that is rooted in Vygotsky's (1978) social constructivist theory of learning in which supervisors demonstrate and mediate the ideals and practices that are valued by the professions. In the initial stages of their training, student clinicians are assigned to supervisors who function as master clinicians and who model and interpret clinical behavior for students during an initial period of highly structured, specific observation. Gradually, supervisors should encourage participation at a comfortable, yet challenging, level and should provide a bridge for generalizing skills and approaches from familiar to novel. This approach is perhaps best described as an apprenticeship model of supervision and has real utility in a downward extension of the model of supervision proposed in this book—undergraduate practicum and supervision of assistants who will provide direct service to patient and clients.

Dowling (1992, 2001) authored two books that also enhanced the literature base in the supervisory process in speech-language pathology. They both were predicated on a broad, interdisciplinary compilation of theory and research in leadership and supervision with an expanded focus on the application of information to clinical supervision in speech-language pathology and audiology (ASHA, 1985a) and the continuum of supervision developed by Anderson (1988).

Walden and Gordon-Pershey (2013) suggested a model of supervision based on Jarvis' (2006) principles of adult learning theory and integrated them with Bloom's Taxonomy (Anderson & Kratwohl, 2001). This approach incorporates Jarvis' learning responses of non-learning, non-reflective learning, reflective learning, and overlays them on the cognitive processes described by Bloom. As learners gain in reflectivity, they move from presumption and rote practice to memorization and practice, to reflective learning. The learner increasingly evidences responsibility for her or his own learning and professional growth; engages in critical evaluation of professional information and practices; uses her or his own original thinking in an effort to learn what to do, when to do it, how to do it and why to do it, all of which are fundamental to clinical problem-solving.

THE CONTINUUM OF SUPERVISION IN SPEECH-LANGUAGE PATHOLOGY AND AUDIOLOGY

The definition and description of the supervisory process in Chapter 1 emphasizes the growth of both supervisor and supervisee. Expansion of this idea leads to the notion of supervisors as facilitating supervisees' ability to reach a level of independence in which their relationship is one of peer consultation and collaboration. This conceptualization of the supervisory relationship is in contrast to the early descriptive data that identified the traditional approach to supervision detailed earlier in this chapter. It is, however, a process that is consistent with those described by Blumberg (1980), Cogan (1973), Goldhammer (1969), Goldhammer and colleagues (1980), Costa and Garmston (1985a, 1985b), and the clinical education process identified by McAllister (2000). Indeed, it is also a process that is consistent with the framework and cognitive and behavioral outcomes of both Dreyfus & Dreyfus' (1986, 2004) Five Stage Model of Skill Acquisition as well as Howell and Fleischman's (1982) Model of Conscious Competency. The remainder of this chapter will discuss a continuum of supervision in which the goal is the type of supervisory practice that is appropriate to the student's level of knowledge, experience, and competence and that will help develop a speech-language pathologist or audiologist who is self-reflective and able to practice independently (ASHA, 2016). Further, this continuum is applicable to the professional whose continued growth is necessary to meet the demands of the professions' scope of practices and the ethical commitment to quality (and continuous quality improvement) in order to fulfill requirements of Principles I and II of the ASHA (2016) Code of Ethics.

It will become immediately clear that the continuum model recognizes that there is not just one way to supervise and function as a clinical educator. In fact, the model is predicated on the belief that supervision and clinical education employ different strategies and styles of interactions that are appropriate at different times and points in the process. Strategy and style are determined by the variables inherent in the process—the needs, expectations, competencies and philosophies of both supervisor and supervises as well as the variables associated with the setting (task, client, organizational structure, etc.). The model offers a structure for supervisors and supervisees to examine their own philosophies about supervision, identify their own behaviors, and determine what changes they want and need to make. As a result, it suggests an approach of continuous improvement that can span a career from preprofessional training as a supervisee through the clinical fellowship to the development of independent and successful clinical and supervisory practice.

Stages of the Continuum

The continuum of supervision is based on the assumption that professionals will be involved in some supervisory or consultative experience for the duration of their professional lives and that the expectations and needs of supervisees change throughout this period of time. The continuum is composed of three stages:

- Evaluation Feedback
- Transitional
- Self-Supervision

The continuum mandates a change over time in the amount and type of involvement of both supervisor and supervisee within the process. As the degree of dominance of the supervisor decrease, participation by the supervisee increases across the continuum. As they move into the Self-Supervision Stage, the balance changes to reflect an interaction between peers. Each stage and is appropriate style will be discussed briefly here, with more detailed discussion to follow in succeeding chapters.

Perhaps the most significant feature of the continuum that must be fully appreciated is that none of the stages are time-bound. Individual supervisees may be found at any point of the continuum throughout their training or careers, depending on the personal and professional situational variables. Some may never reach the Self-Supervision Stage and other may begin well beyond evaluation feedback.

It is assumed that the continuum applies to both speech-language pathology and audiology. In fact, Rassi (1978), in discussing supervision in audiology, presented a similar continuum that identified eight possible levels of supervision beginning with detailed explanation accompanied by demonstration to the final level where the student is working independently with monitoring and suggestion provided by the supervisor only when necessary. Rassi stated, "Each succeeding level requires less active participation by the supervisor, while at the same time, the student's direct involvement and attendant responsibilities increase" (p. 15). It is also likely that within each level, there will be a shift in the supervisor-supervisee balance of interaction as well.

Evaluation-Feedback Stage

This is the stage that aligns most directly with Dreyfus and Dreyfus' (2004) novice stage or the unconscious incompetency and unconscious competent stage of Howell and Fleishman (1982). This is where the beginning supervisee may be found or the supervisee who is working with a new type of client or one who has just entered a new setting. The supervisee who is unknowledgeable or has difficulty applying academic information to the clinical process, often called the "marginal or at-risk student" may perseverate at this stage. Unprepared for clinical interaction for whatever reason, without the ability to be self-reflective about what they do not know, unable to problem solve, overwhelmed by the dynamics of a given situation, or being accustomed to being told what to do, supervisees at this stage assume a very passive role. (Supervisees may be placed at this stage by supervisors who have inaccurate perceptions of a student or who perceive their role to be strictly that of instructor or evaluator.)

Whatever the reasons for the dynamics of the Evaluation-Feedback Stage, the goal for both supervisor and supervisee is to work together to move quickly from this point. Hersey and Blanchard (1982) identified eight variables that influence the amount and degree of supervisor involvement:

- Supervisee's clinical competencies (e.g., technical knowledge, practical skill, and ability to apply them)
- Supervisee's psychological maturity and commitment (e.g., degree of self-confidence, ability to be self-reflective, motivation, and self-respect)
- Supervisee's perception of supervisor's expertise

- Supervisee's expectations of what the supervisor should or should not be able to do and provide
- Styles and expectations of the supervisor' superior or boss
- The colleagues with whom a supervisor interacts on a regular basis
- Organizational and institutional expectations, goals, policy, and philosophy
- Amount of time

Transitional Stage

The Transitional Stage follows the Evaluation-Feedback Stage and aligns with the advanced beginner, competent, and proficient stages of Dreyfus and Dreyfus (2004) and the unconscious competent and conscious incompetence stages of Howell and Fleischman (1982). It is perceived as the place where the supervisee has reached a level of competency (knowledge and skill) and the supervisor has achieved an attitude that results in participation by both in collaborative problem solving and peer interaction. Supervision in this stage is a shared process. The supervisee is not able to operate entirely independently but is moving along the continuum in that direction.

At this stage, supervisees are able to participate in varying degrees in decision making. They are becoming self-reflective and analytical of their own clinical behavior and action. They are learning to plan future strategies and actions on the basis of their analyses, to make modifications during their clinical interactions, to actively problem solve, and to collaborate within the supervisory conference. Most importantly, the supervisor is able to allow the supervisee to assume these responsibilities. As the supervisory dyad moves along the continuum, the interaction increasingly approaches the peer interaction described by Cogan (1973) with the ultimate goal of independence and self-supervision. Supervisees move back and forth within the Transitional Stage, depending on many variables, but most especially those of experience, task, and setting. Some supervisees may have knowledge and skills that enable them to begin their supervisory experiences at any point within the Transitional Stage. For example, some may have had many hours of experience with language impaired children and be able to work independently with them but may find it necessary to move back into the Evaluation-Feedback Stage and receive more direct and structured input from their supervisor when they encounter their first client with traumatic brain injury. Such situations may occur in either the educational setting or the service delivery setting, but the key is that when they do, the supervisees are able to "recover" their position in the Transitional Stage sooner rather than later because of their previous experiences and their understanding of themselves as clinicians, their enhanced abilities at self-reflection and their growing understanding of themselves as clinicians.

Self-Supervision Stage

Self-Supervision is defined as a stage in which supervisors have the ability to accurately analyze their clinical behavior and its outcomes and to alter it based on that analysis. It is the stage that is consistent with Dreyfus & Dreyfus' (2004) expert stage and the Howell and Fleischman's (1982) consciously competent stage. It denotes a level of independence in problem solving in which supervisees are no longer dependent on supervisors for the observation, analysis, and feedback about their clinical work; they are fully self-reflective of and about their own status. It is the stage in which supervisees become responsible for their own professional growth and can think outside the box in regard to meeting the needs of a particular client or patient; they are willing to go beyond traditional management paradigms to address client needs and to use date to document outcomes. It is also the stage in which supervisees become responsible for their own continued professional growth but yet still desire peer interaction and collaboration and consultation. As rapidly as research and regulation are changing the dynamics of clinical service delivery, consultation and collaboration are becoming increasingly important professional skills.

Implications of the Continuum

The continuum has important implications in terms of expectations of professionals during their educational program and after they leave it. Some supervisees may not reach the independence of the Self-Supervision Stage across the spectrum of age and disorders for which they must be trained or they may not reach independence in relation to certain aspects of it despite the efforts of the training program. This then becomes a question of accountability for the program. If the supervisee enters an externship, the clinical fellowship, or the work force at a point on the continuum below the Self-Supervision Stage, the supervisor in this situation must then implement the supervisory style relevant to that point. Supervisors must demonstrate the flexibility that will enable them to adjust their behaviors as they move back and forth along the continuum with their supervisees. The task of identifying the place at which the supervisor and supervisee should be operating and the behaviors that make up the appropriate style will be the focus of the much of the remainder of this book.

Appropriate Styles for Each Stage

The appropriate style for each of the continuum is determined by the level of skills demonstrated by the supervisee and the nature of the task as related to the client. The supervisor's flexibility in adapting to these variables also affects the appropriateness of the interaction.

Direct-Active Style

The Direct-Active Style of supervisor behavior is most appropriate for the Evaluation-Feedback Stage of the continuum. It embodies what might be thought as stereotypical supervisor behavior: critiquing, directing, telling, evaluating. In this style, the supervisor is in a superior and controlling position while the supervisee is in a passive, at best respondent, role. Direct-Active supervisor style is analogous to the S1 style of supervision described by Mormer and Messick (2016) and consists of coaching and directing supervisor behavior.

The style at its extreme demonstrates maximum control and responsibility in the supervisor's role; dependence and minimal participation in the supervisee's role. It is the high direct-low indirect style of Blumberg (1980) and the style of choice of many supervisors. According to the literature, it is comparable to the high task-low relationship stage of Hersey and Blanchard (1982). It may be appropriate, depending on the needs of the supervisee in relation to the client or specific setting. The frequency with which it is used may depend on the perceptions that both supervisor and supervisee have of their role in the supervisory process. Some supervisors may hold a firm conviction that direct behavior produces greater change in supervisees and, therefore, prefer the style.

Available time is perceived by some as the variable that influences the use of this style by the supervisor more than any other (Irwin, 1976). Those who use this reason say that joint problem solving, which is the characteristic of the Collaborative or Consultative Style, takes time that supervisors do not have, especially today in settings where billable hour productivity is an important dynamic. Supervisors may feel that it is necessary to be more directive with supervisees in the interest of the client and the bottom line when time is limited. This assumption has not been empirically tested, however, and the ramifications of time spent engaging in supervision are not known.

Although it is clear that there are situations in which the supervisee is in the Evaluation-Feedback Stage and the direct style is appropriate, especially with the unskilled or inexperienced student, the decision to use the Direct-Active Style must be carefully made. A number of questions need to be asked and answered to help determine if this style is indeed appropriate:

- By whose judgment is the supervisee determined to be inexperienced or unskilled?
- On what basis has the judgment been made that the supervisee is in the Evaluation-Feedback Stage?

- Has the judgment been made on the basis of objective data?
- Is the judgment merely the result of the subjective appraisal of the supervisor, potentially biased by her or his own experiences and preferences?
- Is this the supervisor's style with all supervisees?

This style used exclusively has certain hazards. Theoretical writing and research on leadership and human interaction clearly negate the use of any single style for all situations because of differences in supervisee, supervisor, and situation (Gouran, 1980). Once potential outcome of the overuse of this style is the phenomenon of modeling. Although a certain amount of directing, suggesting, modeling by supervisors may be necessary, appropriate, even desirable at times, it also may be a deterrent to the growth and development of the supervisee. The constant shaping of the supervisee's behavior to accommodate that of the supervisor based on what her or his own performance would be in similar situation, has the potential to stifle supervisee growth and perhaps, even create a mirror image of the supervisor. The purpose of supervision is not to clone supervisees into mirror images of supervisors and certainly is not consonant with the current ASHA CFCC 2014 or CAA 2017 standards 3.7A/B and their emphasis on the development of self-reflective behavior. In fact, it works against the development of critical thinking and problem-solving professionals who are able to develop efficacious systems for delivery of service.

Confusion About Direct-Indirect

Those who have studied the supervisory process have been introduced to the direct-indirect concept and certain misconceptions have grown up around it. Its characteristics have been distorted from the original description by Blumberg (1974) and its use has been subject to a variety of interpretations. Additionally, a value judgment has been placed on the two styles in some instances—direct supervisory behavior is wrong, indirect is right—which is not at all consistent with the results of early research.

Perhaps it would be more productive to describe these behaviors as active and passive rather than direct and indirect to more accurately and precisely capture the behavior of both supervisors and supervisees. Accordingly, a supervisor's behavior may be direct-active, characterized by descriptors of direct behavior; indirect-active characterized by the purposeful behaviors that encourage problem solving, such as asking for opinions and suggestions, accepting or expanding supervisee ideas or asking for rationale and justification of supervisee statements; indirect-passive, characterized by listening and waiting for supervisees to process ideas and problem solve; or passive, characterized by not listening, providing little or no input and not responding to supervisee requests. Similarly, an active supervisee would participate by collecting and analyzing data, initiating discussion, problem solving, questioning, giving opinions, and requesting rationale and justification for supervisor statements. A passive supervisee would be listening, accepting, asking for direction and guidance, seeking strategies and waiting for direction from the supervisor.

The early researchers, particularly in education, made no allowances for a direct supervisor style but they were writing about the supervision of the professionally employed teacher. Supervisors must allow for the fact that some supervisees will need varying amounts of direct-active assistance in learning how to begin their journey to becoming independent professionals. There are times when supervisors will legitimately need to provide specific direction and demonstration. In reality, what becomes important in terms of the continuum is the balance of direct and indirect supervisor behavior and the appropriateness of that balance to a situation and all of its dynamics.

Collaborative Style

The Collaborative Style is the style appropriate for moving away from Evaluation-Feedback Stage through the Transitional Stage to Self-Supervision. This style is a dynamic, problem-solving process in which supervisor and supervisee work together in support of the professional growth of each other to achieve optimum quality of service for clients and patients. The supervisors' role

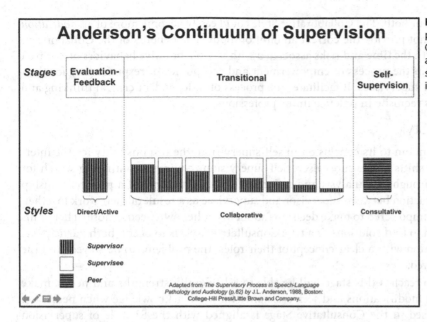

Anderson's Continuum of Supervision

Stages	Evaluation-Feedback	Transitional	Self-Supervision

Styles	Direct/Active	Collaborative	Consultative

▦ Supervisor

☐ Supervisee

▤ Peer

Adapted from *The Supervisory Process in Speech-Language Pathology and Audiology (p. 62)* by J.L. Anderson, 1988, Boston: College-Hill Press/Little Brown and Company.

Figure 2-1. A visual composite of the stages of the Continuum of Supervision and their appropriate supervisor and supervisee interactional styles.

is less direct but not inactive and is reflective of the S2 level of supervision identified by Mormer and Messick (2016). Both participants assume responsibility and provide input in varying degrees at different times about the clinical and supervisory processes. Goals are jointly established. The supervisor poses questions, provides feedback but also encourages input from the supervisee, accepts the supervisee's contributions and ideas, problem solves with the supervisee, and recognizes and respects the worth of the supervisee as a developing professional and as a person. The supervisee, in turn, accepts responsibility for participation in the clinical and supervisory process, provides input, accepts suggestions, questions the supervisor, requests rationale and justification for supervisor statements, engages in self-analysis and problem solving, and works toward independence. The supervisor, though responsible for structuring and facilitating the interaction, is not the only responsible individual within the interaction and does not make all the decisions or provide all of the information. Rather, supervision is seen as a joint process in which the supervisor and supervisee share responsibilities and interact as collaborators to meet common goals. As progress continues along the continuum, the degree of participation of each individual is altered as shown in Figure 2-1. This becomes what Kurpius, Baker, and Thomas (1977) termed *increased ownership* by the supervisee in the joint experiences of supervision. The aim of the Collaborative Style is to move away from direct supervisor and passive supervisee as rapidly as possible to involve the supervisee in decision making. Supervisors should continue to have input however. They must share their expertise and experience, but not to the exclusion of meaningful participation by the supervisee.

Carracciolo and colleagues (1978) described this mix of situations and behaviors when they said that the supervisor plays two roles; a nondirective one that enables the student to express ideas without fearing judgment or penalty; and a directive one that gives information when appropriate, establishes standards and guidelines, and makes judgements when appropriate.

> The speech-language pathology supervisor must, therefore, be sensitive to the continuously changing needs of the supervisee within any given moment of the supervisory conference period and must be able to match the supervisory behavior to the supervisee's needs and expectations. (Blumberg, 1978, pp. 25, 288)

As in the Evaluation-Feedback Stage, there may be hazards. If the proper place on the continuum is not identified accurately, supervisors may expect supervisees to operate beyond their level, resulting in frustration or both. The Collaborative Style could easily become more of an *abdication style* if supervisors do not provide the correct amount of input. The benefits of the Collaborative Style, however, are worth the time and risks associated with it. Collaborative behaviors on the part of supervisors can begin the process of empowerment and acceptance of responsibility for their behavior on the part of supervisees. It facilitates the process of independent critical thinking and problem solving that is requisite in practice in the professions.

Consultative Style

Following the continuum to its conclusion in self-supervision, the responsibility for the inter-action or process now shifts to the supervisee. Self-supervision requires a continuing search for professional growth through self-analysis and reflection. It suggests more of a peer relationship and a cooperative interaction between supervisor and supervisee as a result of their work together. The supervisee is now empowered to make decisions about his or her own needs, those of her or his client, and can proceed to find solutions. If a true Consultative Style is to occur, both participants must enter the interaction with a clear concept of their roles, the problems to be solved, and the procedures to be followed.

The supervisee who reaches this stage will be able to self-identify strengths and needs, make appropriate behavioral modifications and seek assistance for further knowledge when necessary. Supervisor behavior used in the Consultative Stage is aligned with the S3 style of supervision described by Mormer and Messick (2016). It consists of delegating to the supervisee as well as listening, supporting, problem solving, and when appropriate, making suggestions. As with other stages, self-supervision is not time bound, and therefore, the Consultative Style may be utilized at appropriate times in the educational program, the off-campus placement, the clinical fellowship experience, or the employment setting.

Scripts of the three styles of supervision in hypothetical conferences can be found in Appendix 2-1.

Place on the Continuum

A composite of the stages of the continuum and their appropriate styles is seen in Figure 2-1. Determining the level at which the supervisor and supervisee are functioning and therefore, the appropriate style to use, is a decision that requires insight and analysis on the part of both partici-pants. It is somewhat analogous to the assessment process used to determine the need of the clients and patients and will be discussed in Chapter 4. Although individuals may enter the continuum at any point or move back and forth along it, depending upon situational variables, it is the continu-ous movement toward the ultimate objective of independence that is critical.

Most supervisors would probably say that this continuum does represent the manner in which they engage their supervisees, that they do treat supervisees differently, that they do change their style depending upon the knowledge and skill of the supervisee, and that their style is a collabora-tive one. Research has not supported this contention. The historical body of literature indicates that supervisors most frequently use a Direct-Active Style and do not change their behavior over time, even when they perceive that they do (Culatta & Seltzer, 1976; Culatta, Colucci, & Wiggins, 1975; Dowling & Shank, 1981; Hatten, 1965; Irwin, 1975, 1976, 1981; McCrea, 1980; Pickering, 1979, 1981a, 1981b, 1982, 1984; Roberts & Smith, 1982; Russell, 1976; Schubert & Nelson, 1976; Shapiro, 1975; Smith, 1977; Smith & Anderson, 1982; Tufts, 1983; Underwood, 1973). Despite the fact that these data are historical, very little systematic training of supervisors has occurred until very recently and so it is more likely than not the supervisors do misperceive themselves and do demonstrate a predominate single supervisory style over time and across supervisees. This mis-conception should provide momentum for not only training in the supervisory process but for supervisors' abilities to be both analytical and reflective about their behavior within the process.

Components of the Supervisory Process

In 1985, the Position Statement on Clinical Supervision (ASHA, 1985b) recognized supervision as a distinct area of expertise and professional practice and stipulated that special skills are needed to function as a competent supervisor and clinical educator. This position statement, updated in 2008, and a technical report and knowledge and skills documents were added (ASHA, 2008a, 2008b, 2008c). The knowledge and skills document identities eleven core areas of knowledge and associated skills, which together form the basis of contemporary practice in the supervisory process. With the knowledge base identified, those seeking to supervise now need a process. Practically speaking, we know what we need to do, but how to implement these skills involves understanding the components of the supervisory process and how to implement them to effect the professional growth and development of not only supervisees, but supervisors as well.

The continuum introduced previously in the chapter consists of three stages: Evaluation-Feedback, Transitional, and Self-Supervision. While all of the stages and their facilitating supervisor styles are important, it is the Transitional Stage with its collaborative supervisory style that is the pivot point for the development of supervisor and supervisee self-awareness and professional development. This style has several components to its implementation—understanding the supervisory process, planning, observing, analyzing, and integrating. The point on the continuum at which the supervisory dyad is working will determine the amount of time spent on each component, the nature and degree of input from supervisor and supervisee, and the operational specifics of each supervisory interaction.

Understanding the Supervisory Process

An important premise of this book is that supervisors need to be prepared for their role. Another is the need for collaboration between supervisor and supervisee in the process. It follows then that supervisees need preparation for their role. For some, preparation is nonexistent. For others, it may consist of a brief discussion or a unit of study in a pre-practicum course. Whatever previous information has been shared, it is important to discuss the supervisory process itself at the beginning of every new supervisory experience and throughout the supervisory relationship.

Each person brings to the total supervisory experience her or his own previous experience, needs, expectations, concerns, and goals. Because supervisors and supervisees often have different perceptions of the same interaction (Blumberg, 1980; Culatta et al., 1975; Smith & Anderson, 1982), it is important for the two to discuss the supervisory interaction throughout their work together. If there is a lack of congruency about goals and procedures at any point, attempts can be made to clarify them. For example, one way to begin to implement the Collaborative Style is the use of strategic questioning strategies by the supervisor. If, however, the supervisee perceives that the supervisor's role is to tell them what they did right or wrong, evaluate them, provide strategies on what to do next, not ask them what they think, there is likely to be an incongruence, which may disrupt the supervisory relationship and the learning that should take place (Larson, 1981). A discussion about the process into which the supervisor and supervises are about to embark, preparation of the supervisee for her or his own role in the current experience and sharing expectations and objectives will help alleviate any confusion that might arise due to the misunderstanding of perceptions about the work to be done. This discussion should continue throughout the supervisory relationship and process as needs and goals are altered, levels of awareness and expertise change, and new insights or problems arise.

Planning

Supervisees spend a great deal of time planning for the client and patient. Supervisors spend time educating their students in this aspect of the planning process. The focus on the patient and client is not new and certainly fundamental to the success of the clinical interaction but other planning is needed as well in order to implement the continuum. *Joint planning* is required: planning for the clinical process (planning for the client, planning for the clinician) and planning for the supervisory process (planning for the supervisee, planning for the supervisor). Planning for the client and patient is not new. Planning for the clinician may not be new for many; however, planning for the supervisory process itself may be a novel task for most supervisors and supervisees and is addressed in this stage.

Observing

Historically, clinicians are evaluated by their supervisors based on notes written during the supervisor's observation of them at work with a client and patient. These comments and evaluations are communicated to the clinician in a variety of ways (verbally, immediately after a session, written notes or checklists given to a clinician for discussion in a conference later). Observation should not be the time when evaluation takes place.

Observation and evaluation are two separate entities for effective supervision. Observation is the place where real objectivity begins in the supervisory process. During observation, data are collected and recorded by both the supervisor and supervisee for subsequent analysis and interpretation, which then lead to evaluation. A good operational definition of observation is conveyed by editing Cogan's (1973) definition: those operations by which individuals make careful, systematic scrutiny of the events and interactions occurring during clinical or supervisory sessions; the term also applies to the record made of these events and interactions (p. 134).

Analyzing

The analysis stage of the supervisory process is the bridge between observation and evaluation. The objective data collected during the observation mean little by themselves. It is in the analysis component that the supervisor and supervisee begin to make sense of the data (Cogan, 1973; Goldhammer, 1969). The data are examined, categorized, and interpreted in relation to the change or lack of change in the client or clinician and supervisee. Analysis comes naturally from the planning and observation stages because if planning is well done, both supervisor and supervisee will have determined exactly what data will be collected and what will be done with them.

A fundamentally important aspect of the analysis stage is the joint responsibility for analysis or interpretation of the data. This is when supervisees begin to self-analyze and reflect, to problem solve in regard to their own behavior, and to look for the relationship between their behaviors and those of the patient or client.

Integrating

At various points throughout each supervisory experience, content of the continuum components must be integrated through some form of communication between the supervisor and supervisee. Typically, this occurs in a conference which can be done face-to-face on an individual basis or in a group. Conferences, especially early in a supervisory experience, occur on a regular basis and combine the products of the understanding, planning, observing, and analyzing components to facilitate critical thinking, problem solving, reflective thinking, and professional growth. It is a time for both supervisor and supervisee to concentrate not only on the outcomes achieved for the client or patient but on the outcomes of their work together as a supervisory dyad.

PRACTICAL RESEARCH IN SUPERVISION

The 1985 Position Statement on Clinical Supervision in Speech-Language Pathology and Audiology (ASHA, 1985b) identified for the first time, the tasks and competencies fundamental to competent practice in supervision (and clinical education). The 13th task identified in the statement was the ability to demonstrate research skills in the clinical or supervisory process and included five competencies:

1. Ability to read, interpret, and apply clinical and supervisory research
2. Ability to formulate clinical or supervisory research questions
3. Ability to investigate clinical or supervisory research questions
4. Ability to support or refute clinical or supervisory research findings
5. Ability to report results of clinical or supervisory research and disseminate as appropriate (e.g., in-service, conferences, publication)

As Ulrich (1990) stated, "The degree to which we are able to carry out this task is very likely to determine our future as an area of specialized expertise and practice" (p. 15). In the course of reading this text, it will become apparent that there is a significant body of research in supervision; however, there remains a great need for continued research in the supervisory process if the knowledge base is to continue to grow. Significant questions continue to emerge from actual practice and it is essential that our practices be based on theories and findings that come from rigorous research. Indeed, in order to meet the transformative challenge of ASHA's Strategic Pathway to Excellence (ASHA, n.d.; Strategic Objective 1—Expand data available for quality improvement and demonstration of value and Strategic Objective 3—Enhance generation, publication, knowledge translation, and implementation of clinical research), it is imperative that supervisory process research continue to be an important part of the contribution to the professions by those engaged in the supervisory process. Admittedly, these strategic objectives were predicated upon the generation of data to support clinical practice and to demonstrate that our worth as professionals to clients and payers but the same is true of those who are supervisors and the fundamentally important work that they do. It is necessary that they begin to generate the data that will permit the integration of knowledge to sustain our practice and demonstrate our value within the educational processes of the professions.

Practical research is essential for supervisors who want to know what they can do to improve the interaction between themselves and their individual supervisees (Strike & Gillam, 1988). Practical supervision research seeks to answer questions about supervisory procedures. Importantly, the Technical Report on Supervision in Speech-Language Pathology (ASHA, 2008) suggests multiple areas of study that would enhance the knowledge base in the supervisory process. For example, the exploration and study of variables inherent in supervisory process interaction such as relationships between certain supervision procedures and various clinician variables (e.g., experience, motivation, gender, age) or techniques for solving difficulties inherent in the supervisory process are fundamental to understanding not only what we do as supervisors but how and when we do it. Most importantly, research efforts must continue in order to further define the parameters of supervisory best practice through the integration of innovation and research into evidence-based practice guidelines.

Generating practical research requires that those involved in the supervisory process also be actively involved in research processes. This may be difficult for a couple of reasons but lack of time to be involved in ongoing research is often cited as a primary challenge. Supervisors may also be inclined to believe that research can only be done by faculty in academic settings who have formal preparation in research methods as well as time to devote to the endeavor. Although those with doctoral degrees in academic settings have the skills needed to design and conduct research, many are not familiar with the supervisory process and the challenges it poses. Likewise, supervisors who have an understanding of the important issues in supervision and daily opportunities to collect relevant data are often not seasoned researchers. Programs that have a focus on master's level preparation grounded in a clinical orientation or those with a focus on doctoral degrees and a research-only focus can perpetuate this dichotomy. The current Standards for Accreditation of Academic Programs in Audiology and Speech-Language Pathology (ASHA, 2017) have the potential to help resolve this dichotomy through their emphasis on the importance of imbuing students with the scientific and research foundations of the discipline. Students who begin their practice with a greater understanding of research methodology not only are better able to apply research findings to support their clinical practice but are also likely to be more confident participants in the research process itself to help answer the questions that will advance not only clinical practice, but practice in the supervisory process as well.

Richardson and Gillam (1994) provided an innovative example of merging clinical research with clinical teaching. They discussed the "sometimes discordant nature of our dual roles as supervisors and researchers that served as frequent sources of tension throughout the study" (p. 204). Combining practicum and research adds a layer of issues to both the clinical and supervisory process. But the kinds of efficacy research that Richardson and Gillam completed with three graduate students and their clients is precisely the type of collaboration that answers important questions and has the potential to instill interest and confidence in research that students need to develop if we are to invigorate research efforts in supervision.

Pickering (2001) offered a thought-provoking perspective on the nature of joint research and collaborative scholarly work. Citing the foundational work of Boyer (1990) in the Scholarship of Teaching and Learning at the Carnegie Foundation for the Advancement of Teaching, she stressed that professionals need to go beyond what is traditionally perceived of as research and broaden their perspective of scholarship. Boyer's four-part model of scholarship includes the scholarship of discovery, integration, application, and teaching. The scholarship of discovery involves the quest for new knowledge. The scholarship of integration provides the way to give meaning to isolated facts and to make connections within and across disciplines. The scholarship of application puts the knowledge gained from discovery and integration into practice. Finally, the scholarship of teaching involves not merely transmitting knowledge but "transforming and extending it as well" (Boyer, 1990, p. 24). Pickering illustrated how clinical educators have used all four kinds of knowledge of scholarship to expand our knowledge base about supervision and added that viewing scholarship in this larger perspective demonstrates how all professionals can be involved in research and scholarly endeavor.

Important Factors to Consider in Designing Future Studies

Naremore (1984) emphasized that because supervision is a process, exploring it demands a multiple focus. Researchers cannot focus on one variable. She stated, "We are dancing around the process with 'it' questions." We need to be cognizant of the multilayered, complex process that is supervision when selecting dependent variables and also realize we cannot study everything at once.

Numerous descriptive studies have provided important information about the supervisory process and developed a foundation for experimental investigation. We need to identify what are the things we do as supervisors that make a difference in the professional growth and development of supervisees. What is effective practice? What are best practices? Is one methodology better than another? What changes do supervisees make as a result of their supervisory experience? What supervisor variables enhance efficiency?

In designing experimental studies to help in the discovery of new knowledge and in making connections between theory and practice, one kind of design is particularly appealing because the methods closely parallel what good clinicians do in their daily practice. Most simply, single-subject designs require establishing a baseline, applying treatment, and systematically collecting objective data relative to treatment. Given the flexibility and relative ease in using single-subject experimental designs (Connell & Thompson, 1986; Hersen & Barlow, 1976; Kearns, 1986; McReynolds & Kearns, 1983; McReynolds & Thompson, 1986; Orlikoff, Schiavetti & Metz, 2015), they would be "user-friendly" for all members of a research team. Furthermore, these designs are appropriate for answering many of the practical research questions suggested in this text. These functional analysis designs clearly allow cause-effect relationships to be demonstrated while avoiding many of the problems often inherent in group experimental design. Importantly, these designs, when combined with and extended by more descriptive and naturalistic research methodologies (see Chapter 16) have the potential to lead to the integration of the four kinds of knowledge identified by Boyer in his early work at the Carnegie Foundation (Boyer, 1990). Each of these four types of knowledge are foundational to not only understanding the dynamics of the supervisory process but also to the continued development of a robust evidence base in support of them, and therefore, their relevance to the process of the supervision in the professions.

REFERENCES

American Speech-Language-Hearing Association. (n.d.). *Strategic pathway to excellence.* Retrieved from https://www.asha.org/uploadedfiles/asha-strategic-pathway-to-excellence.pdf

American Speech-Language-Hearing Association. (1978). Current status of supervision of speech-language pathology and audiology [Special report of the Committee on Supervision in Speech-Language-Pathology and Audiology]. *Asha, 20,* 478-486.

American Speech-Language-Hearing Association. (1985a). ASHA demographic update. *Asha, 27,* 55.

American Speech-Language-Hearing Association. (1985b). *Clinical supervision in speech-language pathology and audiology* [Position statement]. Retrieved from https://www.asha.org/policy/PS1985-00220/

American-Speech-Language-Hearing Association (2008a). *Knowledge and skills needed by speech-language pathologists providing clinical supervision* [Position statement]. Retrieved from https://www.asha.org/policy/PS2008-00295

American Speech-Language-Hearing Association (2008b). *Knowledge and skills needed by speech-language pathologists providing clinical supervision* [Technical report]. Retrieved from https://www.asha.org/policy/TR2008-00296

American Speech-Language-Hearing Association. (2008c). *Knowledge and skills needed by speech-language pathologists providing clinical supervision* [Knowledge and skills]. Retrieved from https://www.asha.org/policy/KS2008-00294/

American Speech-Language-Hearing Association. (2016, May). *A plan for developing resources and training opportunities in clinical supervision* [Final report of the ASHA Ad Hoc Committee on Supervision Training]. Retrieved from https://www.asha.org/uploadedFiles/A-Plan-for-Developing-Resources-and-Training-Opportunities-in-Clinical-Supervision.pdf

Anderson, J. (1973). Supervision: The neglected component of the profession. In L. Turton (Ed.), Proceedings of a Workshop on Supervision in Speech Pathology. Ann Arbor, MI: University of Michigan.

Anderson, J. (1974). Supervision of school speech, hearing and language programs—An emerging role. *Asha, 16,* 7-10.

Anderson, J. (Ed.). (1980). *Proceedings—Conference on Training in the Supervisory Process in Speech-Language Pathology and Audiology.* Indiana University, Bloomington, IN.

Anderson, J. (1988). The supervisory process in speech-language pathology and audiology. Boston, MA: College-Hill.

Anderson, L. W. & Kratwohl, D. R. (Eds.). (2001). *A taxonomy for learning, teaching, and assessing: A revision of Bloom's taxonomy of educational objectives.* New York, NY: Longman.

Argyris, C. (1962). *Interpersonal competence and organizational effectiveness.* Homewood, IL: Richard D. Irwin.

Bales, R. (1950). *Interaction process analysis: A method for the study of small groups.* Reading, MA: Addison-Wesley.

Bales, R. (1951). *Interaction process analysis.* Reading, MA: Addison-Wesley.

Barnum M., Guyer. S., Levy, L., & Graham, C. (2009). Supervision, questioning, feedback model of clinical teaching: A practical approach. In T. Weidner (Ed.), *The athletic trainers' guide to clinical teaching.* Thorofare, NJ: SLACK.

Barnum, M. & Guyer, S. (2015, April). *The SQF model of clinical supervision.* Workshop presented at the Council on Academic Programs in Communication Sciences & Disorders (CAPCSD), Newport Beach, CA.

Blumberg, A. (1974). *Supervisors and teachers: A private cold war.* Berkeley, CA: McCutchan.

Blumberg, A. (1980). *Supervisors and teachers: A private cold war* (2nd ed.). Berkeley, CA: McCutchan.

Blumberg, A., & Amidon, E. (1965). Teacher perceptions of supervisor-teacher interaction. *Administrator's Notebook, 14,* 1-4.

Blumberg, A., Amidon, E., & Weber, W. (1967). *Supervisor-teacher interaction as seen by supervisors.* Unpublished manuscript, Temple University, Philadelphia, PA.

Blumberg, A., & Cusick, P. (1970). Supervisor-teacher interaction: An analysis of verbal behavior. *Education, 91,* 126-134.

Blumberg, A., & Weber, W. (1968). Teacher morale as a function of perceived supervisor behavior style. *Journal of Educational Research, 62*, 109-113

Boyer, E. (1990). *Scholarship reconsidered*. Princeton, NJ: Carnegie Foundation for the Advancement of Teaching.

Brasseur, J. A. (1980). *The observed differences between direct, indirect, and direct/indirect videotaped supervisory conferences by speech-language pathology supervisors, graduate students, and undergraduate students* (Doctoral dissertation). Retrieved from ProQuest Dissertations & Theses Global. (Accession No. 8029212) http://proxyiub.uits.iu.edu/login?url=https://search.proquest.com/docview/303031314?accountid=11620

Brasseur, J. (1981). The observed differences between direct, indirect, and direct/indirect videotaped supervisory conferences by speech-language pathology supervisors, graduate students, and undergraduate students (Doctoral dissertation, Indiana University, 1980). *Dissertation Abstracts International, 41*, 2131B. (University Microfilms No. 80-29, 212)

Butler, K. (1976). *The supervision of clinicians: The three C's...competition, complaints and competencies*. Paper presented at the annual convention of the American Speech and Hearing Association, Houston, TX.

Caracciolo, G., Rigrodsky, S., & Morrison, E. (1978). A Rogerian orientation to the speech-language pathology supervisory relationship. *Asha, 20*, 286-290.

Cogan, M. (1973). *Clinical supervision*. Boston, MA: Houghton Mifflin Co.

Connell, P., & Thompson, C. (1986). Flexibility of single-subject experimental design. Part III: Using flexibility to design or modify experiments. *Journal of Speech and Hearing Disorders, 51*, 214-215.

Costa, A., & Garmston, R. (1985a). Supervision for intelligent teaching. *Educational Leadership*, 70-80.

Costa, A., & Garmston, R. (1985b). *The art of cognitive coaching: Supervision for intelligent teaching*. Sacramento, CA: The Institute for Intelligent Behavior.

Council of Academic Programs in Communication Sciences and Disorders. (2013). *White Paper: Preparation of speech-language pathology clinical educators*. Retrieved from http://scotthall.dotster.com/capcsd/wp-content/uploads/2014/10/Preparation-of-Clinical-Educators-White-Paper.pdf

Council on Accreditation of Graduate Programs in Audiology and Speech-Language Pathology. (2017). *Standards for accreditation of graduate programs in audiology and speech-language pathology*. Retrieved May 21, 2018 from https://caa.asha/org/wp-content/uploads/Accred-Standards-for-Grad-Programs.pdf/

Crago, M., & Pickering, M. (Eds.). (1987). *Supervision in human communication disorders: Perspectives on a process*. San Diego, CA: Little Brown.

Culatta, R., Colucci, S., & Wiggins, E. (1975). Clinical supervisors and trainees: Two views of a process. *Asha, 17*, 152-157.

Culatta, R., & Seltzer, H. (1976). Content and sequence analysis of the supervisory session. *Asha, 18*, 8-12.

Culatta, R., & Seltzer, H. (1977). Content and sequence analysis of the supervisory session: A report of clinical use. *Asha, 19*, 523-526.

Dowling, S. (1992). *Implementing the supervisory process: Theory and practice*. Englewood Cliffs, NJ: Prentice Hall, Inc.

Dowling, S. (2001). *Supervision: Strategies for successful outcomes and productivity*. Boston, MA: Allyn & Bacon.

Dowling, S., & Shank, K. (1981). A comparison of the effects of two supervisory styles, conventional and teaching clinic, in the training of speech and language pathologists. *Journal of Communication Disorders, 14*, 51-58.

Dreyfus, H. & Dreyfus, S. (2004). The five stage model of adult skill acquisition. *Bulletin of Science, Technology and Society, 24*(3), 177-181.

Dreyfus, S. & Dreyfus, H. (1986). *Mind over machine*. New York, NY: Free Press.

Dussault, G. (1970). *Theory of supervision in teacher education*. New York, NY: Teachers College, Columbia University.

Farmer, S., & Farmer, J. (1989). *Supervision in communication disorders*. Columbus, OH: Merrill.

Farris, G. F. (1974). Leadership and supervision in formal organizations. In J. G. Hunt & L. L. Larson (Eds.), *Contingency approaches to leadership*. Carbondale, IL: Southern Illinois University Press.

Fiedler, F. E. (1967). *A theory of leadership effectiveness*. New York, NY: McGraw Hill.

Fisher, L. (1982). Supervision. In R. Van Hattum (Ed.), *Speech-language programming in the schools*. Springfield, IL: Charles C. Thomas.

Fishler, A. S. (1971). Confrontations: Changing teacher behavior through clinical supervision. In L. Rubin (Ed.), *Improving in-service education*. Boston, MA: Allyn and Bacon.

Flanders, N. (1967). Teacher influence in the classroom. In E. Amidon & J. Hough (Eds.), *Interaction analysis: Theory, research, and application*. Reading, MA: Addison-Wesley.

Flanders, N. (1969). *Classroom interaction patterns, pupil attitudes, and achievement in the second, fourth and sixth grades* (Cooperative Research Project No. 5-1055 [OE 4-10-243]). Ann Arbor, MI: The University of Michigan.

Gibb, J. (1969). Defensive communication. *Journal of Communication, 11*, 141-148.

Gillam, R. (1999). ISSUE III: Models of clinical instruction. Adopting an integrated apprenticeship model in a university clinic. In P. Murphy (Ed.), *Council of Academic Programs in Communication Sciences and Disorders—Proceedings of the Annual Conference on Graduate Education* (pp. 97-99). Minneapolis, MN: Council of Academic Programs in Communication Sciences and Disorders.

Gillam, R., & Pena, E. (1995). Clinical education: A social constructivist perspective. In R. Gillam (Ed.), *The supervisor's forum, 2* (pp. 24-29). Council of Supervisors in Speech-Language Pathology and Audiology.

Goldhammer, R. (1969). *Clinical supervision*. New York, NY: Holt, Rinehart and Winston.

Goldhammer, R., Anderson, R., & Krajewski, R. (1980). *Clinical supervision* (2nd ed.). New York, NY: Holt, Rinehart and Winston.

Gouran, D. (1980). Leadership skills for supervisors. In J. Anderson (Ed.), *Conference on training in the supervisory process in speech-language pathology and audiology*. Bloomington, IN.

Hampton, D. R., Summer, C. E., & Webber, R. A. (1982). *Organizational behavior and the practice of management*. Glenview, IL: Scott, Foresman and Co.

Hatten, J. T. (1965). *A descriptive and analytical investigation of speech therapy supervisors-therapist conferences* (Doctoral dissertation). Retrieved from ProQuest Dissertations and Theses Global. (Accession No. 6513735) http://proxyiub.uits.iu.edu/login?url=https://search.proquest.com/docview/302175416?accountid=11620

Hersey, P., & Blanchard, K. (1982). *Management of organizational behavior* (4th ed.). Englewood Cliffs, NJ: Prentice-Hall.

Hersey, P., Blanchard, K. & Johnson, D. (2012). Management of organizational behavior (10th ed.). London, England: Pearson.

Herson, M., & Barlow, D. (1976). *Single case experimental design: Strategies for studying behavioral change*. New York, NY: Pergamon.

Howell, W.C., & Fleischman, E.A. (Eds). (1982). *Human performance and productivity, vol. 2: Information processing and decision making*. Mahwah, NJ: Erlbaum.

Irwin, R. (1975). Microcounseling interview skills of supervisors of speech clinicians. *Human Communication, 4*(Spring), 5-9.

Irwin, R. (1976). Verbal behavior of supervisors and speech clinicians during microcounseling. *Central States Speech Journal, 26,* 45-51.

Irwin, R. (1981). Video self-confrontation on speech pathology. *Journal of Communication Disorders, 14,* 235-243.

Jarvis, P. (2006). *The theory and practice of teaching* (2nd ed.). London, England: Routledge.

Kearns, K. (1986). Flexibility of single-subject experimental design. Part II: Design selection and arrangement of experimental phases. *Journal of Speech and Hearing Disorders, 51,* 204-214.

Kelly, J. (1980). *Organizational behavior*. Homewood, IL: Richard D. Irwin.

Kurpius, D., Baker, R., & Thomas, I. (Eds.). (1977). *Supervision of applied training*. Westport, CT: Greenwood Press.

Larson, L. C. (1981). *Perceived supervisory needs and expectations of experienced vs. inexperienced student clinicians* (Doctoral dissertation). Retrieved from ProQuest Dissertations and Theses Global. (Accession No. 8211183) http://proxyiub.uits.iu.edu/login?url=https://search.proquest.com/docview/303157417?accountid=11620

Maslow, A. H. (1954). *Motivation and personality*. New York: Harper and Bros.

Mawdsley, B. (1985). *The integrative task-maturity model of supervision*. Presentation at the annual meeting of the American Speech-Language-Hearing Association, Washington, DC.

Mayo, E. (1933). *The human problems of an industrial civilization*. New York, NY: The MacMillan Co.

McAllister, L. (2000). *Where are we going in clinical education? A review of current status and some theoretical and philosophical guideposts for new directions*. Proceedings of the Council of Academic Programs in Communication Sciences and Disorders 2000 Conference. Minneapolis, MN: The Council of Academic Programs in Communication Sciences and Disorders.

McCrea, E. S. (1980). *Supervisee ability to self-explore and four facilitative dimensions of supervisor behavior in individual conferences in speech-language pathology* (Doctoral dissertation). Retrieved from ProQuest Dissertations and Theses Global. (Accession No. 8029239) http://proxyiub.uits.iu.edu/login?url=https://search.proquest.com/docview/303031284?accountid=11620

McGregor, D. M. (1960). *The human side of enterprise*. New York, NY: McGraw-Hill.

McReynolds, L., & Kearns, K. (1983). *Single-subject experimental designs in communicative disorders*. Baltimore, MD: University Park Press.

McReynolds, L., & Thompson, C. (1986). Flexibility of single-subject experimental designs. Part I: Review of the basics of single-subject designs. *Journal of Speech and Hearing Disorders, 51,* 194-203.

Mormer, E. & Messick, C. (2016). *Bringing the evidence to clinical education practices*. Pre-conference workshop presented at the American Speech-Language-Hearing Association Convention in Philadelphia, PA, November 16, 2016.

Naremore, R. (1984). *Research methodologies for the supervisory process*. Presentation with J. Anderson, G. DeVane, M. Laccinole, W. Kennan, E. McCrea, D. Ingrisano, & K. Smith at the annual convention of the American Speech-Language Hearing Association, San Francisco.

Orlikoff, R., Schiavetti, N., & Metz, D. (2015). *Evaluating research in communication disorders*. (7th ed.). San Antonio, TX: Pearson.

Pascale, R. T., & Athos, A. G. (1981). *The art of Japanese management*. New York, NY: Warner Books.

Peters, T. J., & Waterman, R. H. (1982). *In search of excellence: Lessons from America's best-run companies.* New York, NY: Harper and Row.

Pickering, M. (1981a). Supervising student teachers: How to provide non-threatening feedback. *Journal of Childhood Coimmunication Disorders, 5*(2), 150-153.

Pickering, M. (1981b). *Supervisory interaction: The subjective side.* Paper presented at the Council of University Supervisors of Speech Pathology and Audiology annual meeting at the ASHA Convention, Los Angeles, CA.

Pickering, M. (1982). *Interpersonal communication in student-conducted therapy sessions.* Paper presented at the annual convention of the American Speech-Language-Hearing Association, Los Angeles, CA.

Pickering, M. (1984). Interpersonal communication in speech-language pathology supervisory conferences: A qualitative study. *Journal of Speech and Hearing Disorders, 49*, 189-195.

Pickering, M. (2001). Scholarship and the clinical educator. *SIG 11 Perspectives on Administration and Supervision, 11*, 11-15. doi:10-1044/aas11.1.11

Rassi, J. (1978). *Supervision in audiology.* Baltimore, MA: University Park Press.

Rassi, J. (1985). Supervision in audiology. In K. Smith (Moderator), *Preparation and training models for the supervisory process* [Short course]. Presented at the annual convention of the American Speech-Language-Hearing Association, Washington, DC.

Rassi, J. (1987). The uniqueness of audiology supervision. In M. Crago & M. Pickering (Eds.), *Supervision in human communication disorders: Perspectives on a process* (pp. 31-54). San Diego, CA: College-Hill.

Reitz, J. (1981). *Behavior in organizations.* Homewood, IL: Richard D. Irwin.

Richardson, A., & Gillam, R. (1994). Efficacy research in university settings: Supervisory issues. In M. Bruce (Ed.), Proceedings of the 1994 International & Interdisciplinary Conference on Clinical Supervision: Toward the 21st century (pp. 202-206). Council of Supervisors in Speech-Language Pathology and Audiology, Cape Cod, MA.

Roberts, J., & Smith, K. (1982). Supervisor-supervisee role differences and consistency of behavior in supervisory conferences. *Journal of Speech and Hearing Research, 25*, 428-434.

Rogers, C. (1961). *On becoming a person: A therapist's view of psychotherapy.* Boston, MA: Houghton Mifflin.

Rogers, C. (1962). The interpersonal relationship: The core of guidance. *Harvard Educational Review, 32*, 116-129.

Russell, L. (1976). *Aspects of supervision.* Unpublished manuscript, Temple University, Philadelphia, PA.

Schubert, G. (1978). *Introduction to clinical supervision.* St. Louis, MO: W. H. Green.

Schubert, G., & Aitchison, C. (1975). A profile of clinical supervisors in college and university speech and hearing training programs. *Asha, 17*, 440-447.

Schubert, G., & Nelson, J. (1976). *Verbal behaviors occurring in speech pathology supervisory conferences.* Paper presented at the annual convention of the American Speech-Language-Hearing Association, Houston, TX.

Seeley, J. U. (1973). *Interaction analysis between the supervisor and the speech and hearing clinician* (Doctoral dissertation). Retrieved from ProQuest Dissertations and Theses Global. (Accession No. 7329608). http://proxyiub.uits.iu.edu/login?url=https://search.proquest.com/docview/302664667?accountid=11620

Shapiro, D. (1985). *Clinical supervision: A process in progress.* National Student Speech-Language-Hearing Association Journal.

Shriberg, L., Filley, F., Hayes, D., Kwiatkowski, J., Shatz, J., Simmons, K., & Smith, M. (1975). The Wisconsin procedure for appraisal of clinical competence (W-PACC): Model and data. *Asha, 17*, 158-165.

Smith, K. J. (1977). *Identification of perceived effectiveness components in the individual supervisory conference in speech pathology and an evaluation of the relationship between ratings and content in the conference* (Doctoral dissertation). Retrieved from ProQuest Dissertations and Theses Global. (Accession No. 7813175) http://proxyiub.uits.iu.edu/login?url=https://search.proquest.com/docview/302869635?accountid=11620

Smith, K., & Anderson, J. (1982b). Relationship of perceived effectiveness to content in supervisory conferences in speech-language pathology. *Journal of Speech and Hearing Research, 25*, 243-251.

Stace, A., & Drexler, A. (1969). Special training for supervisors of student clinicians: What private speech and hearing centers do and think about training their supervisors. *Asha, 11*, 318-320.

Strike, C., & Gillam, R. (1988). Toward practical research in supervision. In J. Anderson, *The supervisory process in speech-language pathology and audiology* (pp. 273-298). Boston, MA: College-Hill.

Tannenbaum, A. (1966). *Social psychology of the work organization.* Belmont, CA: Wadsworth.

Taylor, F. (1911). *The principles of scientific management.* New York, NY: Harper and Bros.

Tufts, L. (1983). *A content analysis of supervisory conferences in communicative disorders and the relationship of the content analysis system to the clinical experience of supervisees* (Doctoral dissertation). Retrieved from ProQuest Dissertations and Theses Global. (Accession No. 8401588) http://proxyiub.uits.iu.edu/login?url=https://search.proquest.com/docview/303266850?accountid=11620

Ulrich, S. (1990). *The supervisory process: Tasks basic to effective clinical supervision. In Clinical supervision across settings: Communication and collaboration* (pp. 9-22). Rockville, MD: American Speech-Language-Hearing Association.

Underwood, J. (1973). *Interaction analysis between the supervisor and the speech and hearing clinician*. (Doctoral dissertation, University of Denver). Dissertation Abstracts International, 34, 2995B. (University Microfilms No.73-29,608)

Vygotsky, L.S. (1978). *Mind in society: The development of higher psychological processes*. Cambridge, MA: Harvard University Press.

Walden, P., & Gordon-Pershey, M. (2013). Supervisor and supervisee perceptions of an adult learning model of graduate student supervision. *Perspectives in Administration and Supervision, 23*(1), 12-21. doi:10.1044/aaa23.1.12

Ward, L., & Webster, E. (1965a). The training of clinical personnel: I. Issues in conceptualization. *Asha, 7*, 38-41.

Ward, L., & Webster, E. (1965b). The training of clinical personnel: II. A concept of clinical preparation. *Asha, 7*, 103-106.

Weller, R. (1971). *Verbal communication in instructional supervision*. New York, NY: Teachers College Press, Columbia University.

 This chapter is a revision of that appearing in the 2003 edition of this book.

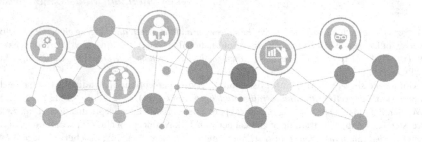

APPENDIX 2-1
SAMPLE SCRIPTS OF INDIRECT, DIRECT-INDIRECT, AND DIRECT SUPERVISORY CONFERENCES

In all three scripts, the clinical problem, therapy strategies and the outcomes of the conference are the same. The scripts differ only in the proportion of direct and indirect behaviors (validated by a panel of five experts, using Blumberg's 1970 Interaction Analysis System to code behaviors every 3 seconds).

KEY:
SR = supervisor
SE = supervisee

Indirect or Consultative Supervisory Style

SR: Hi Ann.... How are you today?

SE: Fine. Were you able to watch my session with Johnny yesterday?

SR: Um hmm.

SE: What did you think about it?

SR: Well, why don't you tell me what you thought about it.

SE: Well, he still isn't getting those /s/s in words…um even though he can do them when they're in a vowel consonant unit…. I'm getting frustrated…. I'm not quite sure what to do because he can produce a vowel plus /s/ without a model from me, and he does it right 90% of the time. But as soon as I give him a word he goes back to his error and he omits the sound.

I thought I had a pretty good program planned…. I mean he is 7 years old and he omits /s/, /z/, sh, ch, zh, and j. So after I decided to work on /s/ and you told me about checking for generalization…and helped me figure out where to start training with him…I thought I'd be on my way.

With the way he is now, I doubt if he'll ever be able to master 10 final /s/ words…much less generalize to untrained /s/ words and other sibilants he omits!

SR: I can tell you're frustrated…and it is frustrating when you think you've got a super plan, and then, for some reason, things don't quite work out the way that you planned. Let's see if we can figure out some things that might help Johnny produce /s/ correctly in final position words.

SE: Okay.

SR: What kinds of strategies do you think might facilitate correct production of /s/ in final position words

SE: I don't know…I've tried everything that I can think of. Do you have any ideas?

SR: Well let's take a look at what you've tried.

SE: Okay, I've shown him pictures that have a final /s/...like "bus," "goose," "base," "race"...well, here are my pictures. [SE shows cards to SR.] Um bus, base, piece, mice, moose, case, geese, goosed, rice, race, and house.

SR: Um hmm. Okay, can you tell me how you've used these pictures?

SE: Well, I've shown him these and asked him to say the words. Um but when I do that, he omits the final sound.

SR: Okay...so you know one thing about Johnny.... You know that showing him a picture card and asking him to say the name doesn't work at this point.

SE: Yea.

[SR writes on paper.]

Stim	Response	RF	Desired result?
1. Present pics	client omits /s/	?	No

SR: Have you tried any other strategies?

SE: Yea. I said the name of the picture and asked him to repeat it five times.... Doing that didn't work either...he still omitted /s/.

SR: Okay.

[SR writes.]

2. Clin models 1 X	client says 5 Xs	interm	No	omits all /s/

Alright...so you know something else about Johnny. You know that providing one model, having him make five attempts, and then giving him feedback doesn't result in correct productions right now. Think about what you know about how people learn. How can you apply what you know about that to your therapy with Johnny?

SE: Hmm. [Silence—SE thinking.] Well, I know about operant conditioning and I know about Bandura's social learning theory.

SR: Okay, let's take one at a time. Um...tell me what you know about operant conditioning.

SE: Well, I know that it involves stimulus—response—reinforcement.

SR: Um hmm...what else?

SE: I know that reinforcement increases a behavior and punishment decreases it.

SR: Um hmm. Can you tell me more about that?

SE: I guess I'm not sure what you're getting at.

SR: What do you know about schedules of reinforcement? How important are the schedules of reinforcement in establishing a new behavior?

SE: Oh! I know.... Um. Uh oh...maybe that's why Johnny didn't get any correct responses in words last time. At first, I should give him feedback after every response. And if his correct production of /s/ increases, then I can say that my verbal feedback is reinforcing.

Oh boy, what a dummy I am. Why didn't I think of that before?

SR: Ann, you're not a dummy...you're just new at this game. Sometimes it's hard to take things that you've learned in class and apply them to what you're doing in therapy. Let's take your rediscovery and write it down as a possible solution for next time.

SE: Okay.

[SR writes.]

SR: Alright, so one possible strategy is that you will give him feedback after each response and see if that increases his correct production of /s/. What kind of feedback do you think you'll have to give him?

SE: Well, I could say "yes and no" or "right and wrong." I don't want him to get discouraged though.... I mean if I always say "no" or "wrong," he might feel bad.

SR: Um hmm. I think that's a valid concern. How do you think you want to handle that?

SE: Hmm [Thinks.] Maybe I could say things like, "No Johnny, you forgot to say /s/ at the end of that word. Watch me, say mice." You know, emphasize the sound.

SR: Yea...emphasize the target, and what you've described also includes giving informative feedback...telling him why a production is incorrect. You've also described modeling.... Um you're going to provide a model before asking him to give it another try.

SE: Yea! [Smiles.] You know, I might even try giving him a model every time.... I mean before I ask him to say a word, I'll name the picture first, and then have him say it. That might work better right now. I mean better than me saying the word once and having him say it five times.

SR: Okay. Let me write all of this down, so we don't forget.

[SR writes and talks while writing.] Let's see...a) Clinician will give informative feedback for client's incorrect productions, b) clinician will provide a model before asking the client to make a subsequent attempt and, c) clinician will provide a model for each presentation of a stim card.

Well, Ann, it looks like you're on your way! Let's take your ideas and develop some specific objectives for your next therapy session. Given these methods, what will your objectives be for your next session on Tuesday?

SE: Hmm. [Looks at paper.] I'm thinking. [Pause.] Well, my overall objective is to have him say 9 out of 10 words correctly on his first attempt in four consecutive sets. That's on my lesson plan you know.

SR: Um hmm. [Nods head.]

SE: So, on Tuesday, if I could get him to say the words correct 70% of the time...producing them right, after I give him a verbal model...I'd say that would be pretty good. Do you think so?

SR: Yes I think um...correct production after a model at 70% proficiency level sounds reasonable to me. Um suppose that after you've completed 10 sets...which would be 1000 trials or productions...that he hasn't met your criteria. What would you think?

SE: Oh no.... I hope that doesn't happen!

SR: Suppose it does.... What would you think?

SE: I think I'd be ready to commit suicide. [Laughs.] I think I should have some aces up my sleeve. I mean I ought to have some other alternative strategies.

SR: Um hmm. [Smiles.]

SE: I'm not sure I know what else I could do. Do you have any suggestions?

SR: Well, you mentioned earlier...when we were talking about how people learn...that you know about operant conditioning and social learning theory. Um.... You've come up with some strategies...based on operant conditioning. Let's see if we can develop some strategies based on what you know about social learning theory.... What do you know about social learning theory?

SE: Well, I know that cognitions, modeling, reinforcement, and feedback are the primary thing that facilitate learning...and I know that modeling is the most powerful.

SR: Um hmm.

SE: I've already incorporated modeling, feedback, and reinforcement into the strategies that I'm planning to use...so I guess I need to think about cognitions.

Direct-Indirect or Collaborative Style

SR: Hi Ann...how are you today?

SE: Fine. Were you able to watch my session with Johnny yesterday?

SR: Um hmm.

SE: What did you think about it?

SR: Well, why don't you tell me what you thought about it.

SE: Well, he still isn't getting those /s/s in words…even though he can do them when they're in a vowel consonant unit.… I'm getting frustrated.… I'm not quite sure what to do because he can produce a vowel plus /s/, without a model from me, and he does it right 90% of the time. But as soon as I give him a word, he goes back to his error and he omits the sound. He is 7 years old and he omits /s/, /z/,ch, sh, zh, and j. So, after we decided to work on /s/ and you told me about checking for generalization…and helped me figure out where to start training with him.… I thought I'd be on my way. With the way he is now, I doubt if he'll ever be able to learn /s/, 10 final /s/ words…much less generalize to untrained /s/ words and other sibilants!

SR: I can tell you're frustrated…and it is frustrating when you think you've got a super plan and then for some reason, um, things don't quite work out the way you planned.… Let's see if we can figure out some things that might help Johnny produce /s/ correctly in final position words.

SE: Okay.

SR: Okay. What kinds of strategies do you think might facilitate correct production of /s/ in final position words?

SE: I don't know.… I've tried everything that I can think of. Do you have any ideas?

SR: First, tell me what you've tried Ann.

SE: Okay, um I've shown him pictures that have a final /s/…like bus, goose, base, race…well, wait, here are my pictures [SE shows pictures to SR.] There's "bus," "base," "piece," "mice," "moose," "case," "geese," "goose," "rice," "race," and "house." I've shown him these pictures and asked him to say the words.… But when I do that, he just omits the final sound.

SR: Ann, in changing from production in syllables to production in words, you left out a few very important details. There are some questions you should ask.

What were your procedures for production in syllables? And what were the procedures that you used when you made the transition to production in words? How are the two sets of procedures different?

SE: Um well, obviously I used syllables first…then I used words. But I don't think that's what you're getting at.

SR: No, it isn't. Let's back up a little bit. Tell me exactly what you did when you started production in words.

SE: When he wasn't able to say /s/ when I showed him the pictures, I changed my strategy. I said the name of the picture and asked him to say it five times…then I told him how many he had right and how many he had wrong. But that didn't help either…he still omitted /s/.

SR: Alright. So you know that providing one model, having Johnny make five attempts and then giving him feedback, doesn't result in correct production right now. Think about what you know about how people learn. How can you apply what you know about that to your therapy with Johnny?

SE: Hmm.… [Silence—SE thinking.]

Well, I know about operant conditioning and I know about Bandura's social learning theory.

SR: Let's talk about one at time. Let's talk about operant conditioning first. What can you tell me about it.?

SE: Well, I know that a behavior is influenced by its consequences.… And when you're trying to get someone to learn a new behavior, you devise small steps that lead to the goal behavior.

SR: Um hmm. What else?

SE: Um you decide what stimuli you will provide…and what the desired response is…and what the consequences of a response will be.… Also, any consequences that increase a behavior is a reinforcement…and any consequence that decreases a behavior is a punishment.

SR: Right. Also consistency is a very important factor.…. Consequences must be provided consistently if you expect to change a behavior. Let's take this framework and analyze the strategies that you've used in your therapy with Johnny.

SE: Okay.

[SR writes]:

STIM	Response	RF	Desired outcome ?
1. Present pics	client omits /s/	?	No
2. Clin models	client says 5 Xs	intermittent	No
1 X	omits all /s/s		

SR: Okay look at this a minute. [SR show notes to SE.] When you were training /s/ syllables, what kind of stimuli and consequences did you provide?

SE: I modeled each time…then I had him make an attempt…and then I gave him feedback. And once he reached criteria for that step, I stopped modeling…but continued to provide verbal feedback after each attempt.

SR: Um hmm. And your feedback acted as a reinforcer because Johnny's correct productions increased. How did you change your strategies when you started training words? [SR points to paper.]

SE: Oh…I know…I changed two things. I changed my method of presenting stimuli…. I stopped providing a model for each attempt…. Also, I didn't provide consistent feedback after his attempts.

SR: So what do you think you'll want to do in your next session?

SE: Well for one thing, every time I show him a picture, I'll say the word first—before I ask him to say it. Um second, I'll give him verbal feedback after every response. And if his correct production of /s/ increases, then I can say that my verbal feedback is reinforcing. I'm going to jot this down. [SE writes.] I should have figured this out…. What a dummy I am!

SR: Ann, you're not a dummy…you're just new at this game. Um, sometimes it's hard to take things that you've learned in class and apply them to what you're doing in therapy. Anyway, now you have two strategies for your next session. [Brief pause.] I think that, in addition to providing consistent feedback, that it would also be helpful if you'd give him informative feedback when he has incorrect responses. I mean, not only let him know when he's wrong…but also let him know why he's wrong.

SE: Hmm.

SR: Can you give me an example of informative feedback, so I know that this is clear to you?

SE: If I model the word "mice" and he responds "mi___", I could say, "No Johnny, you forgot to say /s/ at the end of that word. Watch me, say mice." You know, emphasize the /s/.

SR: Good. You've also described modeling…that is, providing an additional model before asking your client to make a subsequent attempt. Why don't you add those things to your list of strategies?

SE: Okay. [SE writes strategies.] It looks like my sessions next week should be pretty good.

SR: Okay. Let's take these ideas and develop some specific objectives for your therapy sessions. What will your objectives be for your session on Tuesday?

SE: Okay, in my lesson plan, my overall objective is to have him say 9 out of 10 words correctly on his first attempt in four consecutive sets…. That criteria might be a little too high to expect on Tuesday.

SR: I think you're probably right. Um, what do you think would be appropriate criteria?

SE: If I could get him to say the words correctly 70% of the time…producing them right, after I give him a verbal model—I'd say that would be pretty good. Don't you think?

SR: A 70% proficiency level sounds reasonable to me.

SE: Okay. [Silence—thinking.] Um, suppose he doesn't reach the criteria. Say that after 10 sets, or 100 trials, he still can't get 70% correct…. What do you think I should do then?

SR: What do you think you should do?

SE: Hmm…. I suppose I should have some alternative strategies planned.

SR: I think that's a good idea. Do you have any alternatives in mind?

SE: Not anything specific…. I just know that I ought to be able to modify my plan so that I can increase the probability of getting correct responses.

SR: Um, good point. Why don't we back up a bit…. You mentioned earlier, when we were talking about how people learn, that you know about operant conditioning and Bandura's social learning theory. We've developed some strategies—based on operant conditioning. Let's see if we can develop some based on social learning theory…. First, what can you tell me about social learning theory?

SE: Well, I know that cognitions, modeling, feedback, and reinforcement, are the primary things that facilitate learning…. And I know that modeling is the most powerful of all of these.

SR: Um hmm…. And modeling, feedback, and reinforcement have already been incorporated into the strategies that you'll be using next week. So it looks like we need to focus on cognitions.

Direct or Active Supervisory Style

SR: Hi, Ann. How are you today?

SE: Fine. Were you able to watch my session with Johnny yesterday?

SR: Um hmm.

SE: What did you think about it?

SR: Well, I noticed that he still isn't able to produce /s/ in final position words. Let's see…if I'm right, he is able to produce syllables—different vowels plus /s/—without a model from you with 90% accuracy. Is that right?

SE: Um hmm. But I'm getting frustrated…I'm not quite sure what to do because as soon as I give him a word, he goes back to his error…he omits the sound. And I thought I had a pretty good program planned. I mean he is 7 years old and he omits /s/, /z/, sh, ch, zh, and j. And so after you suggested working on /s/ and checking for generalization to untrained /s/ word and the other sibilants—and helped me figure out where to start training him, I thought I'd be on my way. But right now, I doubt if he'll ever learn to say the 10 final position /s/ words that I'm trying to train…much less generalize to untrained items.

SR: Well maybe I can give you some help. I'm sure that I can think of some strategies that would work with Johnny…. After all, that's part of my job…to help you so you can be more effective with Johnny.

SE: Oh good. It's kinda hard for me…because all this is so new to me. And of course, you've had a lot more experience, so you know what works and what doesn't work.

SR: Okay, first tell me what you've tried, Ann.

SE: Okay, well I've shown him some pictures that have a final /s/ like "bus," "goose," "base," "race"… and here are my pictures. [SE show cards to SR.] See, bus, base, piece, mice, moose, case, geese, goose, rice, race, and house.

SR: Um hmm.

SE: Um I've shown him these pictures and asked him to say the words…. But when I do that, he omits the final sound.

SR: Um hmm. But Ann, you've um you've missed an important point. You went from training in syllables…where at first you modeled the syllable, had him make an attempt, then gave him feedback. Once he reached criteria for this step, you stopped modeling, but continued to provide feedback—which acted as a reinforcer…and you did that until he reached criteria. Um, then in making the transition from production in syllables to production in words, you left out a few very important details. Um you gave him one model—asked him to make five attempts—then after all of his attempts, you gave him feedback. [SR looks at clipboard.] In my notes from observing your therapy session yesterday, I wrote down that I needed to talk to you about learning theories, because obviously you've forgotten some things…or you're having trouble applying what you've had in classes to what you're doing in therapy. So that's one of the things I want to discuss with you today. Is that alright with you?

SE: Yes, that's fine.

SR: Okay, first let me review operant conditioning with you. Remember that behaviorists maintain that a behavior is influenced by its consequences. In trying to establish a new behavior, you devise small steps that lead to that goal behavior. You decide what stimuli you will provide… what the desired response is…and what the consequences of a response will be. Any consequence which increases a behavior is a reinforcement…and any consequence which decreases a behavior is a punishment. So you're working with this um stimulus—response—reinforcement paradigm [SR writes and shows to SE].

Consequences must be provided consistently, if you expect to change a behavior. Um, I think consistency may have been part of the reason why Johnny didn't do well in your last session. I think the stimuli that you provided may be the other part of the reason he couldn't successfully produce those final position /s/ words. I would suggest that in your sessions next week, you do two things.

First, give him feedback after every response…that is, provide um consistent consequences. When he's right, let him know. When he's wrong, let him know that too. It might also be helpful to let him know why he's wrong when he has incorrect responses. That is, you give him informative feedback…like, "Johnny, you forgot to say /s/ at the end of the word. Watch me, say mice." Emphasize the final sound.

Second…change the way you are providing the stimulus…give him a verbal model every time. Show him the picture, then you say the word, then ask him to say it.

Do you understand what I mean? Is that clear to you?

SE: Um hmm. I remember talking about that stuff in classes. Now, I think I have a better idea about how to use it in therapy. Um….I mean, your suggestions really were helpful.

SR: Good, good. Also, you want to be sure that you tabulate each one of his responses during your sessions…. That way we can tell if the feedback is acting as a positive reinforcement. Why don't you take a minute and write all of this stuff down, so you don't forget? Um, do you have any questions so far?

SE: No, not right now.

[SE writes:

1. Give feedback to client after each response.

Give informative feedback for incorrect responses.

2. Provide a model with each presentation of stim card.

Also, provide model before requesting subsequent attempt.

3. Tally responses.]

[SE looks at notes] It looks like my sessions next week should be pretty good. Um…in my lesson plan, my overall objective is to have him say nine out of 10 words correctly on his first attempt um this is in four consecutive sets.

So, on Tuesday, I'm not sure if he'll be able to reach that criteria…it might be a little bit too high.

SR: I think you're probably right. I think 90% um is probably a little too high…. I think that you should leave the 90% on four consecutive sets as your overall goal…but on Tuesday, set your objective at 70%. See if he can reach a 70% level of proficiency when you provide a model each time, and when you are providing consistent feedback. That seems like a pretty reasonable expectation for the session.

SE: Yea, it does. Um [Silence; SE thinking] Suppose he doesn't reach criteria…say after 10 sets, or 100 trials, he still can't get that 70% correct…. What do you think I should do?

SR: What do you think you should do?

SE: I probably should have some alternative strategies planned.

SR: I think that's a good idea. Do you have some strategies in mind?

SE: Um, not anything specific…I just know that I ought to be able to modify my plan so that I can increase the probability of getting correct responses.

SR: Good point. That leads to another thing that I wanted to review with you today…. I wanted to talk about operant conditioning and social learning theory. I'd like to show you how you can apply some of the principles of social learning theory to what you're doing in therapy…just like I did with operant conditioning. Then we can talk about some strategies that are based on social learning theory…. Okay, according to social learning theory, what are the factors that facilitate learning?

SE: Um, feedback…cognitions, modeling, and reinforcement.

SR: Um hmm…. Of these factors, which ones have already been incorporated into the strategies that we've discussed today?

SE: Um…modeling, feedback, and reinforcement.

SR: Right…that's good. So, lets focus on cognitions now.

Reprinted with permission from Brasseur, J. A. (1980). *The observed differences between direct, indirect, and direct/indirect videotaped supervisory conferences by speech-language pathology supervisors, graduate students,\and undergraduate students* (Doctoral dissertation). Retrieved from ProQuest Dissertations & Theses Global. (Accession No. 8029212) http://proxyiub.uits.iu.edu/login?url=https://search.proquest.com/docview/303031314?accountid=11620

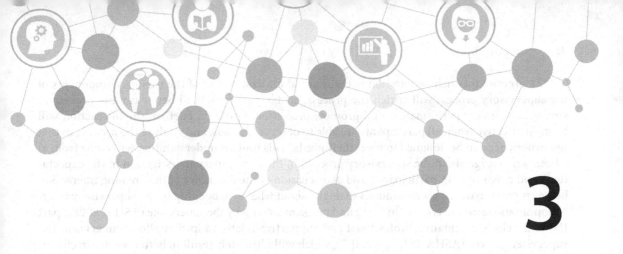

3

Understanding the Supervisory Process

Judith A. Brasseur, PhD, CCC-SLP, F-ASHA and
Elizabeth S. McCrea, PhD, CCC-SLP, F-ASHA

There are many ways to teach people to swim. One is to toss them into the water and hope that they will suddenly acquire the necessary techniques to reach the edge of the pool. At one time, some clinicians were introduced to the clinical process in much the same way—sink or swim! This practice has been modified as a result of requirements set by the American Speech-Hearing-Language Association's (ASHA) Council for Clinical Certification in Audiology and Speech-Language Pathology (CFCC), which call for student observations generally to occur prior to practicum and for supervision commensurate with student's knowledge, skills, and experience. Academic programs typically include certain clinical courses and experiences that orient the neophyte clinician to the intricacies of the clinical process. Introduction to the supervisory process, however, has been "sink or swim" because few programs included direction on the supervisory process. However, new 2017 Council on Academic Accreditation in Audiology and Speech-Language Pathology (CAA) Standards for Professional Practice Competencies in both audiology and speech-language pathology (Std. 3.1.1A and B) necessitate knowledge and skills about the process of clinical education and supervision.

PURPOSE OF THE COMPONENT

This chapter will present ways to a) prepare supervisees for meaningful participation in the supervisory process, and b) communicate about the process throughout the entire period of interaction between supervisor and supervisee.

McCrea, E. S., & Brasseur, J. A. *The Clinical Education and Supervisory Process in Speech-Language Pathology and Audiology* (pp 45-106).
© 2020 Taylor & Francis Group.

The premise for such preparation is that mutual understanding of the various components of the supervisory process will enrich the process, enable participants to better use the process to strengthen clinical performance, and promote professional growth. Further, the interaction will be most effective when all participants are able to observe, discuss, and analyze the process so that the experience can be designed to meet their needs. This mutual understanding will come from a) a basic knowledge about the supervisory process, b) the preliminary investigation of the expectations and needs of both participants, and c) discussion of the dynamics of the ongoing interaction between participants. This continuous dialogue about what is happening in the supervisory interaction should facilitate critical thinking and problem solving by the supervisee (ASHA, 2008c, part III) and help to maintain a professional and supportive relationship that allows supervisor and supervisee growth (ASHA, 2008c, sec. II-7), which will ultimately result in better service to clients.

This first component of the continuum consist of several facets—an awareness of the possible roles of participants, the importance of supervisors and supervisees knowing and understanding each other's needs and expectations as they begin the process, the anxieties that supervisees and perhaps supervisors bring to the process, and the importance of self-knowledge. What will be presented is a method and some strategies for preparing both supervisors and supervisees for an interaction that will best address the needs of all participants in the clinical and supervisory processes—client, clinician, supervisee, supervisor.

The Name of the Game

This Understanding component relates to learning about the basic principles of supervision, but should not be assumed to be relevant only to the beginning of the interaction. The understanding of such a complex set of behaviors is developmental. It is more than an induction phase or an orientation or introduction to the process. It is ongoing and applies across the continuum.

Interpreting is not a satisfactory descriptor of this phase because it is not inclusive enough and it also seems to imply that the supervisor is the sole provider of information, a concept that is inconsistent with the theme of this book. *Rapport* is a term that is used frequently in describing the relationship between clinician and client. It is a desirable objective in the supervisory process; however, what is being discussed here requires a deeper understanding of each other than the usual concept of rapport. Understanding involves in-depth knowledge of and familiarity with the many facets of all the components of the supervisory process, including the thoughts and feelings of the partners in the relationship.

TREATMENT OF THE SUPERVISORY PROCESS IN CONFERENCES

Data from studies of supervisory conferences in speech-language pathology make it clear that conferences traditionally have not included much discussion of the supervisory process or of the needs and behaviors of the supervisees or supervisors who are participating in these conferences (Culatta, Colucci, & Wiggins, 1975: Culatta & Seltzer, 1977; Pickering, 1984; Roberts & Smith, 1982; Shapiro, 1985; Smith & Anderson, 1982b; Tufts, 1983). One can make certain assumptions about that fact. Such discussion may not be perceived as an important component and thus is intentionally excluded from discussion. This assumption seems to be shifting as ASHA and Council of Academic Programs in Communication Sciences and Disorders (CAPCSD) emphasize not only recommended amounts of supervision but also the importance of quality supervision practices (ASHA, 2013, 2016; CAPCSD, 2013). The classic view of the supervisory process as evaluative and supervisor dominated has apparently changed. The need for joint discussion of the process is accepted. New 2017 CAA and 2014 CFCC standards, revised in 2016, policy documents (ASHA, 2008a, 2008b, 2008c), reports (ASHA, 2013, 2016), and papers (CAPCSD, 2013) make it clear that supervisory styles, goals, roles, and responsibilities vary across constituent groups.

Lack of discussion about supervision in conferences may have been that supervisors, who generally control the direction of the conference, did not have an understanding of the components of supervision, and felt inadequate to deal with the topic. Additionally, supervisees historically have not been prepared for supervision in such a way that they are able to either initiate or participate in meaningful discussion. Whatever the reasons, the data consistently indicate that the focus of the conference is on the clinical process, mainly the client but not the clinician.

The appropriateness of this exclusive focus on the clinical process is highly questionable, given that the primary objective of supervision is to facilitate critical thinking and problem-solving skills of the supervisee. Expanding the focus, to encourage interpretation of the supervisory process as a means of contributing to the growth and development of the supervisee and supervisor, should enrich the clinical process as well.

Speech-language pathologists and audiologists have always been concerned about the ability of the client to generalize behaviors acquired in the clinical setting. Of equal concern should be the generalization of behaviors acquired by clinicians in supervisory interactions. However, it appears that supervisees are expected to extrapolate from discussion of the client's behavior to their own to determine the changes they should make in their own clinical performance. Moving supervisees to a stage of conscious competence rather than hoping that generalization will occur necessitates systematic preparation. Further, 2017 CAA Professional Practice Competencies (sec. 3.1.1A and B) were developed because of new professional mandates for interprofessional education and supervision and further substantiate the need for systematic preparation.

Supervisors must attend to the behavior of clinicians as supervisees to engage them in and help them obtain maximum benefits from the supervisory process. This enables them to learn problem-solving techniques that can be generalized to other situations. Supervisors and supervisees must move beyond an exclusive focus on the client and clinical process.

UNDERSTANDING THE ROLES IN THE SUPERVISORY PROCESS

Mutual understanding of participants' roles is an important part of preparation for the supervisory experience (ASHA 2008c, sec. I-1). A role is usually considered to be a set of expectations about the behavior of persons who occupy certain positions in social units or as actions that are perceived as appropriate to certain positions. It is a set of prescriptions for behavior that are shaped by the rules and sanctions of others and by each person's conception of what his or her behavior should be in a certain situation (Biddle & Thomas, 1966).

Preconceived stereotypes about supervisors and supervision, together with the many roles that supervisors and supervisees have available to them and the fact that they may be performing several roles at one time, make it essential to examine the operative roles. If communication is to be open, objectives are to be met, and professional growth is to take place as a result of the supervisory process, that is, if supervision is to be productive, participants should be aware of the role perceptions they have for themselves and each other and the expectations they bring into the supervisory interaction.

Perceived Roles for Supervisors

Supervisors are viewed as assuming a variety of roles, among them that of teacher, overseer, controller, evaluator, and counselor (Hatten, 1965) and decision maker (Schubert, 1978). Cogan (1973) listed six types of relationships between supervisor and supervisee, all of which would demand very different roles for each of the participants: superior-subordinate, teacher-student, counselor-client, helper-helpee, supervisor as evaluator and the "colleagueship" relationship. Weller (1971), in discussing the three functions of counselor, teacher, and trainer, made an important point when he said, "Supervisors can rarely expect to be equally competent in all three functions, yet neither can they afford to be ignorant of any one" (p. 8). Anderson (1988) noted that supervisor roles may include provider of information, questioner, problem solver, evaluator, demonstrator, and facilitator. Other roles commonly cited include coach, role model, mentor, and advocate. Roles should be assumed consciously and should be congruent with the goals of the supervisory process.

Techniques we have used to identify perceived roles for our supervisees and ourselves are to a) write personal definitions of supervision and b) list characteristics of a "good" supervisor and a "good" supervisee. Sharing and discussing these enables us to understand each other's perspective about what we think supervision ought to be. If there is a mismatch between perceived roles and the goals for the supervisory process, this will become apparent in the discussion and modifications can be made. Pannbacker, Middleton, and Lass (1993) surveyed 100 students to identify their perceptions of a "good supervisor." Results revealed that a good supervisor is available, consistent, fair, flexible, and provides feedback while a bad supervisor is late for appointments, has unrealistic expectations, doesn't respect students, and is not clinically competent. Casey's (1985) instrument (Appendix 3-1), based on the 13 tasks and 81 associated competencies for effective clinical supervision in the 1985 ASHA Position Statement allows for systematic assessment of supervisees' understanding of the supervisory process, needs, and expectations. Having students review tools that have been designed to for supervisor self-assessment or evaluation at the onset of the supervisory experience is another method to determine what is important to the supervisee. For example, at the beginning of a term, supervisees could complete Step 1 in Casey's self-assessment from their perspective by ranking the importance of each competency.

Importance of Shared Expectations

Expectations are the perceptions of appropriate behavior for one's own role or the role of others and, as such, are a potent influence on the individual's behavior as well as on how he or she believes others should behave. To speak of shared expectations implies that each individual perceives his or her own and others' roles similarly (Biddle & Thomas, 1966). This is considered an important prerequisite to communication and to meeting objectives, especially in the supervisory relationship. "Leaders must either change their style to coincide with followers' expectations or change followers expectations" (Hersey & Blanchard, 1982, p. 132). If supervisors and supervisees operate from different sets of assumptions about what should take place between them, then communication barriers are raised even before the interaction begins (Blumberg, Amidon & Weber, 1967). Discrepancies between expectations and perceptions of what actually happened lead to confusion and conflict.

After an extensive review of the literature on education students' expectations, Tihen (1983) noted: "If there is a discrepancy between the supervisee's expectations and the supervisor's actual behavior, both the performance of the supervisee, and the satisfaction which he or she derives from the supervisory process may be negatively affected" (p. 7). In a more recent comprehensive review of expectations across professions, Christodoulou (2016) noted that being aware of supervisee expectations and having a willingness to adapt to varying and/or changing expectations is essential for establishing an effective working relationship. Victor (2013) emphasized, "expectations stated at the onset of the supervisory process will result in diminished conflict" (p. 80). To avoid uncertainty, confusion, lack of direction, frustration, and stress, and to establish a positive supervisory relationship, it is imperative to clarify roles, expectations, and needs of both supervisees and supervisors. **In fact, sharing of goals and objectives, defining needs and expectations, and clarification of the differences and similarities in perceptions of roles may well be one of the most important components of the entire supervisory interaction, probably forming the pattern for the entire relationship**. It is also reasonable to assume that needs, expectations, and perceptions are not static, and are altered by maturity, experience, and the influence of the many variables within each situation. Therefore, there is a need for continuing exploration of perceived role, as well as expectations and needs, in every supervisory relationship as it progresses through a semester, a year, or an ongoing situation such as an employment setting. The ability to establish joint communication regarding expectations and responsibilities in the clinical and supervisory processes is an important competency for establishing and maintaining an effective relationship.

EXPECTATIONS FOR SUPERVISION

Speech-Language Pathology and Audiology Research

The literature contains many studies that identify the expectations and needs of supervisees and the extent to which they are met. Much of this literature is overlapping and some is contradictory and equivocal. A few important themes emerge and provide insights about the wide variety of expectations that may be present in any situation.

Supervisor Skills

Russell (1976) asked student supervisees to indicate their perception of the importance of 65 different behaviors and also to indicate what behaviors were actually exhibited by their supervisors. Her subjects listed being treated fairly and impartially; being encouraged to question, disagree, and express their ideas; being guided to make clinical decisions; being provided with constructive feedback; having supervisors perceive and be responsive to clinician's feedback and evaluation; and having supervisors demonstrate flexibility and adaptability as the most valued supervisor behaviors. Interestingly enough, when Russell's supervisees were asked what supervisors do most frequently, "treating the clinician in a fair and impartial manner" was the only actual behavior that emerged from the most valued list. Discrepancies between expectations and reality were greatest in terms of supervisor's attention to clinician needs, feelings, and problems and to evaluation.

Some researchers have looked at needs or expectations of speech-language pathology students at different experience levels. Myers (1980) found beginning students ranked supervisor enthusiasm and interest, demonstration, and being provided the theoretical bases and rationales underlying therapy techniques as more important than most advanced clinicians. As students gained experience, technical needs decreased in importance but affective needs remained constant throughout the educational program and across experience levels. Russell and Engle (1977) and Dowling and Wittkopp (1982) found differences between experienced and less experienced students, indicative of the changing needs of students. In their investigation across six universities, Dowling and Wittkopp found that assistance in writing lesson plans and the need for more frequent observations were given greater value by less-experienced clinicians, whereas the more-experienced clinicians wished to assume increased responsibility for the client.

Larson (1981) examined both need and expectations and found similar expectations in her inexperienced (no clinical hours) and experienced (over 150 hours) supervisees; inexperienced, however, had slightly higher expectations and stronger needs. Both groups expected to ask questions, participate in conferences, express opinions, have their ideas used, and have supervisors be supportive. Both needed to have their point of view considered and to have assistance with client goals and therapy strategies.

Tihen (1983) studied three levels of clinicians. He examined the importance attached to five categories of expectations and whether the clinicians perceived their supervisors attaching similar or dissimilar importance to the same categories. Tihen found, as did other investigators, that inexperienced clinicians expected more direction from supervisors than the more experienced groups. As clinicians gained experience, they placed greater value on the expectations related to their own responsibility in the supervisory process. Tihen concluded that clinicians enter the supervisory process without priorities for their expectations of supervisors and that their priorities develop as a function of supervised practice. Further, he proposed that knowledge of supervisees' expectations profiles would assist a supervisor in planning an experience that is more compatible with needs.

Larson's and Tihen's scales (Appendixes 3-2 through 3-4) are useful tools for analyzing supervisee needs and expectations. Supervisees' responses can be compared with those of the supervisor and provide a focus for subsequent discussion and clarification.

Mandel (2015) surveyed differences in expectations between supervisors, first semester (novice) clinicians and students entering their second clinical experience, using Tihen's (1983) scale as her dependent measure. Results revealed discrepancies in expectations across the three groups. Novice clinicians had strong expectations for direct instruction, having supervisors demonstrate diagnostic techniques and working cooperatively to develop therapy plans and select diagnostic tools. Second semester clinicians had increased expectations for cooperative learning and supervisor feedback. They also trended toward some independence and an understanding of the importance of self-evaluation. Both supervisee groups expected their supervisors to provide direct support throughout the experience. Across groups, supervisors felt more strongly about encouraging students to discuss feelings regarding practicum and having a sense of humor. They also had higher expectations for independence and self-evaluation than both student groups.

Edrich's (2014) examined knowledge, attitudes and expectations of 38 off-campus supervisors following a 3-hour online workshop on the supervisory process. She used Tihen's (1983) Expectation scale, Powell's (1987) Attitudes Toward Clinical Supervision scale and a questionnaire she developed to test knowledge as her dependent measures. Results of her dissertation study revealed significant changes in knowledge but no effect on participants' expectations or attitudes as a function of the training. The content of the workshop focused on knowledge about the supervisory process and findings supported the effectiveness the training. Edrich reported that supervisors had high expectations prior to training, resulting in a ceiling effect. She also stated, "long-term and substantial changes in attitudes are not likely to happen as a result of a 1- or 2-day training workshop that focuses on increasing knowledge and understanding" (p. 51).

These collective findings suggest that supervisees do change in terms of their perception of need and the expectations for supervision as they move along the continuum. Preferences for a direct or indirect style of supervision, which reflects the amount of supervisor involvement has been studied extensively in education (Blumberg, 1974, 1980; Blumberg & Amidon, 1965; Copeland, 1980, 1982; Copeland & Atkinson, 1978) and somewhat in speech-language pathology (Nilsen, 1983; Smith, 1977; Wollman & Conover, 1979). Most novices seem to prefer a directive style, one in which their supervisors initiate, criticize, give suggestions and opinions, and help them reach immediate solutions to problems. With experience, however, supervisees appear to prefer a more indirect style, characterized by supervisor questioning, reflecting the supervisees' ideas and feelings, and listening. This is perhaps not surprising, but the question that supervisors must ask themselves is whether or not their supervisory approaches are compatible with these changes. The literature suggests that supervisory styles do not adjust to changing expectations of supervisees (Blumberg, 1974, 1980; Copeland, 1980, 1982; Culatta & Seltzer, 1977; Nilsen, 1983; Roberts & Smith, 1982; Smith, 1977). Supervisors continue to use a Direct-Active Style, regardless of supervisee needs or preferences. And, although Edrich (2014) did not assess supervisor style, her results suggest that changes requiring changes in attitudes and expectations, which obviously would be needed to modify one's style, may require direct training.

Supervisors in Gordon-Pershey and Waldon's (2013) investigation expressed a need to use a combined Direct-Indirect Style. These five supervisors indicated a need for both nondirective and directive practices—at times providing instruction while at other times facilitating reflective practice by encouraging inquisitiveness, thoughtfulness, and insightfulness (p. 19). The researchers provide an augmented model of adult experiential learning with a decision tree that supervisors could use to move students to increased levels of independence and reflective practice. The findings of Fencel and Mead's (2017) qualitative study of factors that constitute positive and negative supervisory relationships also suggest that a combined Direct-Indirect Style is preferable. Analysis of interviews of nine graduate interns who had completed at least two rotations revealed, "the factors most likely to result in a positive clinical experience included constructive feedback, respect, positive regard, clear expectations and structured clinical guidance" (p. 17). These students wanted supervisors to be clear and straightforward in discussing expectations and responsibilities; lack of clarity is a source of anxiety.

Mastriano, Gordon, and Gottwald (1999) studied expectations from the beginning and end of a semester for 10 supervisors and 35 supervisees at two universities using an adaptation of Larson's (1981) scale. Factor analysis revealed four significant factors with regard to the roles assumed by a supervisor: instructor, mentor, personal facilitator, and the person who helps transfer responsibility for treatment to the supervisee. Interestingly, at the end of the semester the 52 dyads evidenced lower levels of agreement on items that described how actively involved the supervisor should be in the supervisory process but higher levels for how active the supervisee should be. The results substantiate "the need for supervisors and supervisees to engage in some formal assessment of each participant's expectations at the outset of any supervisory relationship" and to periodically review them throughout the supervisory experience. Christodoulou (2016) also affirmed the need to share expectations at the beginning of an experience. Lulai and DeRuiter (2012) provide a structure and tools for supervisors in medical settings to prepare before a student arrives at the practicum site to clarify expectations and facilitate planning.

Broyles, McNeice, Ishee, Ross, and Lance (1999) compared perceptions of effective supervision strategies for 49 supervisors and 197 graduate students from 11 universities. Neither years of supervisory experience nor accrued clock hours of experience influenced the perceptions of the groups. Of the 43 items examined, supervisors and student clinicians reported the following strategies as most effective: demonstrates and models clinical techniques during a therapy session; models professional behavior; and creates an atmosphere of mutual respect and sharing of attitudes, feelings, beliefs, and philosophies. Supervisors' and supervisees' perceptions of effective supervision strategies significantly differed on observation and self-evaluation strategies. At least 12 supervisors reported they did not use the following strategies: requires written agreement to ensure follow through; gives a summary rating sheet within 1 week of a session; gives gestural guidance/cues during a session; holds regularly scheduled group supervision conferences; requires joint analysis of audio or video recorded sessions; holds supervision conferences upon clinician request; and observes through a closed-circuit television monitor. The scale developed for this study (Appendix 3-5) could be a helpful tool for checking perceptions at the onset and throughout a supervisory experience.

Learning Style Preferences

Recognizing and accommodating differences in both learning styles and communication styles (ASHA, 2008c, sec. II.3 and II.5) are essential to effective communication and a positive supervisory relationship. Understanding how one learns best allows for a more efficient and effective teaching-learning process. Educational research demonstrates that what is best depends on the context, the task and the individual learner. Kolb's (1984) Experiential Learning Theory (ELT) posits a four-stage cycle for adult learning. Each stage has a variety of types of activities that facilitate learning at that particular stage. The cycle begins with a concrete experience—a task to be completed by an individual or team. The second stage involves reflective observation—stepping back from the task and reviewing what has been completed. The third stage is abstract conceptualization—drawing on learner knowledge to interpret events and understand relationships. The fourth stage is active experimentation—learners plan how to implement what they learned into actual practice.

Based on Kolb's (1984) ELT, Honey and Mumford (1992) developed four learning styles or preferences: activist, reflector, theorist, and pragmatist.

Activists learn by doing and like to involve themselves in novel experiences. They enjoy the here and now and will "try anything once." They are open minded and enjoy brainstorming. **Reflectors** like to stand back and observe and ponder experiences from many different perspectives. They collect data and think about it thoroughly before coming to conclusions. They are cautious and like to consider all angles and implications before taking action. They prefer to take a back seat in meetings and discussions. **Theorists** adapt and integrate observations into complex, logical theories. They think problems through step-by-step. They assimilate disparate facts into a cohesive whole. They tend to be perfectionists and value rationality and logic. **Pragmatists** are keen on trying out new ideas, theories and techniques. They search for new ideas and like to experiment with applications. They like to get on with things and act quickly. They are practical.

Identifying one's predominant and preferred style seems to be important in order to partner with an instructor to formulate optimal learning experiences. This self-knowledge will enable the learner to provide a concrete answer to an instructor's query, "What can I do to help you?" It is also advisable to understand and develop the ability to learn using other styles—that is, to be able to use a variety of learning styles. Honey and Mumford (1992) highlighted the association between Kolb's (1982) learning cycle and their four styles. Thus, effective learning will involve movement:

1. *Experiencing*—doing something [activitist]
2. *Reflective observation*—reviewing and thinking about what happened [reflector]
3. *Abstract conceptualization*—analyzing, interpreting, concluding [theorist]
4. *Active experimentation*—planning how to implement what was learned [pragmatist]

Honey and Mumford (1986) developed an 80-item Learning Styles Questionnaire and variations are freely available via a Google search using the key words "Honey and Mumford learning styles questionnaire."

Implications of Adult Learning Styles

Knowles (1984) differentiated between pedagogy, the teaching of children, and andragogy "any intentional and professionally guided activity that aims at a change in adult persons" (p. 50). The two are seen as somewhat similar to the continuum presented in the previous chapter, moving from dependency of the learner in pedagogy to self-directiveness in andragogy. Knowles suggested that an andragogical model of learning be based on several assumptions:

1. Adults need to know why they need to learn something before they begin the process.
2. Adults have a concept of being responsible for their own decisions which may lead to resistance to certain types of educational experiences.
3. Because adults bring more experience to a learning situation, not only is there a greater need for individualization in teaching but often the "richest resources for learning reside in the adult learners themselves" (p. 57), providing that educators can open up their minds to new approaches.
4. Readiness to learn is as important to adults as to children.
5. Orientation to learning is life centered, that is, task centered or problem centered, not subject centered (e.g., adults learn best when they can perceive application of learning to their daily life).
6. Although adults respond to some external motivators, like money and promotions, the most potent motivation for learning is from internal pressures (e.g., increased job satisfaction, self-esteem, and quality of life).

Knowles advocated such methods as organizing adult learning around needs and interests, life situations (not subjects), analysis of experience, mutual inquiry, and allowing for differences in style, time, place, and pace of learning. In fact, the points he made are compatible with the continuum of supervision. Thus, the continuum is as relevant for the supervisor-in-training as it is for the clinician-in-training.

Knowledge of adult stages of development is also relevant to the preparation of supervisors. Individual differences and needs are factors that should be known. Adult learners are often voluntary participants, which implies sacrifices of time and money (Haverkamp, 1983). On the other hand, they may be meeting mandatory requirements of an organization or a degree requirement, which influences attitudes.

Ethnic, Cultural, and Linguistic Variations

A distinct set of knowledge and skills is identified in ASHA's (2008) Knowledge and Skills Core Area VIII: Diversity (ability, race, ethnicity, gender, age, culture, language, class, experience, and education). While it is beyond the scope of this textbook to comprehensively address how ethnic, cultural, and linguistic differences may potentially impact the supervisory relationship, it is important to recognize the potential challenges that may result from age, disability or ability, ethnicity, gender identity, national origin, race, religion, sex, sexual orientation, and the linguistic variability that may coincide with cultural differences. Recognizing and accommodating differences are essential to developing and maintaining a professional and supportive relationship.

Although sparse, there is some attention in the communication sciences and disorders literature to the influence that gender, sex, race, ethnicity, and age may have on expectations. These variables are important in light of the demographics apparent in ASHA membership. Data indicate that more than 90% of ASHA members are Caucasian women with about 30% in the 34 and younger age bracket, about 28% in the 34 to 44 age range, about 20% in the 45 to 54 year age range, and 23% who are 55 and older (ASHA, 2018). Understanding differences and similarities can lead to more effective outcomes. Furthermore, ethical practice requires that supervisors and supervisees must be able to demonstrate cultural competence as they relate to each other and the diverse populations they serve (ASHA, 2017). CAA added a new section on Professional Practice Competencies with the implementation of standards 3.1.1A (audiology) and 3.1.1B (speech-language pathology) and cultural competence is one of the primary attributes in the new standard (CAA, 2017). Self-understanding as well as an understanding of the impact of cultural and linguistic variables on delivery of care for individuals served, and between those individuals and their caregivers are encompassed in the new standard

Differences in styles of thinking, problem solving, and communicating gained a great deal of popularity in the late 1980s and early 1990s when books such *You Just Don't Understand* (Tannen, 1990), *Talking From 9 to 5* (Tannen, 1994), *Women's Ways of Knowing* (Belenky, Clinchy, Goldberger, & Tarule, 1986), among others became *New York Times* best sellers. These topics emerged at meetings of supervisors in our professions. For example, at the first national Council of Supervisors in Speech-Language Pathology and Audiology (CSSPA) conference, Langellier and Natalle (1987) described the ways in which gender is a profound and pervasive influence on our work and on our self-expressions. Providing facts gleaned from research on gender and interpersonal communication, and integrating facts about the profession of speech-language pathology and the world of academe, Langellier and Natalle offered a number of strategies for analyzing and dealing with differences in conversational styles. Seymour (1992), Larkins (1992), and Pickering (1992) addressed "women's ways of supervising," noting how gender may impact self-esteem, perceptions of roles, the ways we work, and our preferences within our work settings. Pickering (1992) stated, "A woman's way of being in the world, whether the domestic, public, or professional world, is likely to be different from that of a man's" (p. 41).

DeVane (1992) offered multicultural strategies for quality improvement in the management/ supervisory process, stressing the responsibility of supervisors to create a learning and work environment that uses the strengths and expertise of all participants. DeVane described underlying problems that interfere with successful management of diversity in academic and employment settings:

- Maintenance of the homogeneity theory and America as a "melting pot"
- Failure to differentiate between difference and deficit
- Cognitive and behavioral rigidity and ethnocentrism

Understanding is gained by examining what we have in common, how we are alike, and by sharing our values and developing common goals. Empathy and concern for others, evidenced by behaviors such as active listening, asking questions, and honest and open communication are imperative. It is also necessary to recognize the relationship between language and culture, and understand that experiences, concepts, values, beliefs, and attitudes are reflected in how language is used.

Kayser (1993) cited four training issues that are important when supervising Hispanic speech-language students: 1) culture, 2) language proficiency, 3) mentoring, and 4) supervision and clinical management of minority clients. Culture is the knowledge that individuals must have to be functional members of a community and includes rules for interactions, appropriate behaviors, and regulations for interacting with people from different cultures (Saville-Troike, 1986, as cited in Kayser, 1993). Acculturation involves adhering to certain rules for interaction and adopting some values of a second culture while preserving the rules and regulations of one's native culture. Assimilation involves accepting various ideas and values from a second culture but rejecting differing values and expectations of one's native culture. Kayser noted, "bilingual-bicultural graduate students come into graduate programs with differing levels of acculturation and assimilation" (p. 18). The variability within and between ethnic groups and the impact that cognitive, behavioral, and affective differences may have on interactions with peers, supervisors, clients and their families, necessitates self-analysis. The self-awareness that is achieved through self-analysis provides the opportunity to recognize differences in styles and to identify those that enhance clinical effectiveness.

Murray and Owen (1991) defined mentoring as, "a deliberate pairing of a more skilled or experienced person with a lesser skilled or experienced one, with the agreed-upon goal of having the lesser skilled person grow and develop specific competencies" (p. xiv). Mentoring is an unquestionable critical factor in the retention of culturally and linguistically different students. The paucity of persons of color in our professions makes cross racial and cross cultural matches inevitable. Further, it isn't fair to expect the one or few persons of color or ethnicity in an organization to assume the role of "minority in residence" or expert on all issues related to diversity (Brasseur, 1994). Principles of Mentoring constitute Core Area XI in ASHA's (2008) Clinical Supervision Knowledge and Skills policy document.

Since the early 1980s, numerous articles have stressed not only the importance of mentoring, but also have suggested strategies. For example, Murray and Owen (1991) suggested that a mutually developed action plan that includes professional, educational, and personal goals be developed. For each goal, the a) activities, b) skills or knowledge to be achieved, and c) timelines should be detailed. The frequency of regular meetings should be addressed during the planning process. Confidentiality also needs to be addressed. The plan is a contract of sorts, and as such should specify the length of the formal relationship. Murray and Owen call this a "no-fault termination" clause and note that it is similar to a prenuptial agreement in that it provides for a civilized dissolution and a graceful ending. Supervisors who are unfamiliar with the body of literature on mentoring are advised to engage in some self-study to assist in our professions' efforts to recruit and retain diverse professionals. Through its Office of Multicultural Affairs (OMA), ASHA's Student to Empowered Professional Mentoring Program (S.T.E.P.) has been successfully been providing peer and one-to-one mentoring to connect and empower communication sciences and disorders students from underrepresented racial and ethnic groups since 2004. This program offers online resources that would be useful to all who want to learn how to establish an effective mentoring relationship.

In addition, OMA offers a significant array of resources to assist professionals, including:

- *Cultural Competence*: An online program, including a self-assessment, to assist members in developing cultural competence.
- *Faculty*: Information for faculty to aid in recruitment and retention of underrepresented students, infusing multicultural/multilingual issues into the curriculum, etc.

- *Students*: Information for students regarding financial aid, student award programs, identifying academic programs (EDFind), the PRAXIS, etc.
- *Employers and Recruiters*: Resources for the recruitment of bilingual providers.
- *Practice Resources*: Tools and guides to assist in a variety of related practice issues. For example: providing accent modification services, dynamic assessment guide, phonemic inventories across languages, providing transgender voice services, working with internationally adopted children, and so on.

Among the Professional Issues Practice Portals available from ASHA (www.asha.org) are distinct ones for: bilingual service delivery; collaborating with interpreters, transliterators, and translators; cultural competence; and accent modification (ASHA, n.d.-b). The Practice Portal for Clinical Education and Supervision contains sections for students with disabilities, bilingual student clinicians, student clinicians who use nonstandard American English dialects or accented speech, cultural influences on clinical education, and generational differences.

ANXIETY IN THE SUPERVISORY PROCESS

The role of the emotions in the communication process and in the learning process is significant and should be considered in any study of the supervisory process. Gazda (1974), in discussing the emotional tone of the classroom, stated that while it is true that students who are emotionally involved learn best, it is the specific emotion and its intensity that may "either facilitate, distract from, or inhibit learning" (p. 10). Research and experience demonstrate that a little bit of anxiety is motivating and provides incentive for learning. However, too much anxiety can immobilize a learner. Further, "one's values, biases, preconceived notions of how things 'ought to be,'" basic philosophy, roles, etc., influence how a person perceives and interprets the behaviors of others" (Pickering & McCready, 1990, p. 25). Anxiety, fear and confusion are emotions that are experienced by both supervisees and supervisors. A common anxiety for both is the feeling that we ought to know more than we do (Pickering & McCready, 1990).

Anxiety of Supervisees

Weller (1971) said that the initial years of teaching produce great stress, especially for persons who set high standards for themselves. One contributing factor is that the feedback about failures is often more obvious and persistent than feedback about successes. "This may be the first instance of failure for the novice who has had an academic history of success, and such perceptions of failure are frequently taken in an intensely personal way" (p. 8). This is probably equally true for speech-language pathology and audiology supervisees. In fact, the first practicum will probably be the first time the supervisee has had his or her behavior subjected to the type of scrutiny it receives during observations and conferences.

Small wonder, then, that supervisees approach the experience with a broad range of emotions. Anyone who has overheard a conversation between students prior to their first practicum will be aware of the "jitters" that accompany this rite of passage. All professionals probably remember the great amount of anxiety, as well as time, that accompanied the preparation of lesson plans in the early days of their own practicum experience. They also may remember the threat of the unseen, but nevertheless acknowledged, observer on the opposite side of the observation room window or video monitor. Or they may remember the even worse, ever-present possibility of an unplanned interruption in the therapy session by some supervisor. For some, the anxiety produced by observations diminishes only slightly, even with experience.

Possible sources of anxiety for supervisees during their educational program, including off-campus experiences, no matter how good the interpersonal interaction may be, are such factors as evaluations, grades, and recommendations for graduate school or jobs. In the employment setting, anxiety over evaluations relates primarily to retention, promotions, or recommendations for other jobs. Additionally, in the work setting, anxieties are often apparent when supervisors are from another discipline. In every setting, supervisors have some power over supervisees and this can create anxiety.

Openness and the ability to communicate freely will certainly be affected by feelings of anxiety. Such feelings may result in hostility, an inability to think clearly or to be flexible, and will probably increase the amount of "selective listening." People hear what they want to hear or what their emotional state allows them to hear. Some may focus only on the negative; others nay hear only the positive. Supervisors need to do what they can do to decrease the anxiety of supervisees.

The anxiety factor is discussed at length in relation to the colleagueship aspect of the clinical supervision model Cogan (1973) proposed. He said that teachers perceive supervisors as a threat for a variety of reasons, such as: supervisors are searching for weaknesses, supervisors' criteria for good performance are unknown, and supervisees have a low estimation of supervisors' competencies. Energy dissipated through excessive anxiety is energy lost to the task at hand.

Studies of Supervisee Anxiety in Speech-Language Pathology and Audiology

The literature in our professions has addressed the anxieties of supervisees. Rassi (1978) included in her qualifications for audiology supervisors a practical knowledge of human behavior and the ability to deal with supervisees regarding their uncertainty about the future and other concerns. Oratio (1977), on the basis of informal interviews with students, related fear and anxiety experienced by students entering clinical practicum to three sources: anxiety about their inability to attain supervisory standards, the responsibility for the welfare of the client, and the fear that they will be unable to put academic knowledge into practice.

The Sleight Clinician Anxiety Test (SCAT; Sleight, 1985) was developed to rate fears and anxieties of new practicum students. The 40-item scale describes four areas of fears: 1) living up to supervisory standards and relationships between supervisors and supervisees, 2) responsibility for clients, 3) transferring theory into practice, and 4) general feelings about practicum. On the basis of a study in which the test was used with students, Sleight said that during the practicum, students decreased their anxieties and increased their confidence regarding supervisor/clinician interactions and general fears but not regarding client well-being or putting theory into practice. Decreases in anxiety about responsibility to clients was not apparent. This seems to be a continuing source of anxiety, as perhaps it should be. Feelings of confidence increased about their ability to put theory into practice and overall functioning in practicum only after students accrued experience in off-campus settings. Sleight (1985) stated, "It appears that additional experience in the same setting does not affect a student's confidence, but additional experience in a different setting increases confidence in some areas" (p. 41).

Chan, Carter, and McAllister (1994) explored sources of anxiety in 127 students, at different levels in their academic programs and concomitant differences in clinical practicum experience. Five factors contributed to anxiety across all student levels: 1) their ability to fulfill both clinical and academic demands, 2) the amount of preparation required for clinic, 3) the amount of relevant clinical experience they had to date, 4) their ability to apply theory to practice, and 5) high expectations of self. The authors stated that some student anxiety can be eliminated by modifying structural aspects of the training program—for example, rescheduling some courses, modifying the curriculum, and so on. The most significant solution is ongoing dialogue. Students must become skilled in professional and personal communication abilities to enable them to better negotiate their learning experiences with their supervisors.

Although evaluation of clinical performance is only one of the 11 core areas (ASHA, 2008c, sec. VII), it is a task that is evident in every setting in which supervision occurs and one which evokes anxiety for supervisees (Dowling, & Wittkopp, 1982; Larson, Hoag, & Schraeder-Neidenthal, 1987; Pickering, 1981a, 1981b; Russell & Halfond, 1985; Wollman & Conover, 1979). Russell and Halfond (1985) reported that graduate student clinicians perceived practicum grades as anxiety producing, subjective, nonnegotiable, and based on inconsistent standards. Supervisors employ variable criteria and are often influenced by "student's potential," past experience, and level of client difficulty in assigning grades (Russell & Halfond, 1985). A variety of strategies have been proven effective in explicitly defining supervisor expectations for performance and criteria for evaluation, for enhancing objectivity and improving the consistency and specificity of feedback. These include: a contract-based system (Larson et al., 1987; Peaper & Mercaitis, 1989a), competency-based goal setting and evaluation (Rassi, 1987), interactive and joint involvement in the analysis and assessment of clinical performance (Monnin & Peters, 1981; Strike-Roussos, Brasseur, Jimenez, O'Connor, & Boggs, 1991). **Anxiety about evaluation can be diminished or eliminated with early on discussion about how it will be handled and mutual involvement in the assessment process throughout the supervisory experience**.

During the initial supervisory conference, supervisors should share their evaluations procedures and a copy of the evaluation instrument with supervisees to decrease anxiety and facilitate a positive relationship (Brasseur, 1987). Additionally, Hutchinson, Uhl, and Weinrich (1987) demonstrated that "in-depth explanation *prior to the initiation of practicum* of the clinical skills that supervisors expect clinicians to demonstrate, particularly those that will be evaluated, decreases the need for redundant supervisor feedback" (pp. 132-133, emphasis added). Supervisors who are clear and effective communicators increase supervisee satisfaction with the process (Peaper & Mercaitis, 1989b). Discussion about evaluation should continue into the planning phase as certain clinical skills and competencies are transformed into objectives for the supervisee's professional growth (Brasseur, 1987).

Anxieties of Supervisors

One cannot assume that all the anxiety and apprehensions brought into the supervisory experience are brought there by supervisees. Most supervisors have not been prepared for the tasks they must perform as supervisors. Their perceptions of their roles have come from as many different sources as have those of their supervisees. Perhaps they bring even more stereotypes or preconceived notions for they have been supervised even if they have not supervised. In discussing supervisors' anxieties, Pickering and McCready (1990) noted that fear of failure, to varying degrees, and anxiety about being uninformed or being criticized "are simply part of the fabric of supervision" (p. 27).

Anderson (1988) noted that supervisors, in speech-language pathology and audiology at least, do not usually plan to be supervisors—their preparation, their career objectives, and their self-perception as professionals, is that of a clinician. To be suddenly thrust into the new role of supervisor of professional adults, without preparation, may result in a difficult and stressful transition which requires the development of a new and different self-concept. Additionally, supervisors may begin work with little or no organizational assistance or support, that is, job descriptions, models, or opportunity for in-service education to help them learn new skills or define their new role. Indeed, the importance of the role may be downgraded by the casual way in which supervisors are selected and the lack of guidance they receive. Off-campus supervisors, for example, may be provided with very little in the way of guidelines or support from the university for whom they are supervising. Or, the off-campus facility may need to establish policies and procedures for the organization to insure compliance with accreditation standards, regulatory agencies, and relevant laws (e.g., Joint Commission [JCAHO], CAA, Centers for Medicare & Medicaid Services [CMS], Family Educational Rights and Privacy Act [FERPA], Health Insurance Portability and Accountability Act

[HIPPA], Individuals with Disabilities Act [IDEA], etc.) while interns are earning clock hours at the facility. While 2017 CAA Standards 3.9A and 3.9B stipulate that clinical education obtained in external placements must be governed by agreements between the program and external facility and be monitored by program faculty, the reality is that the agreements may address only legal, ethical and regulatory requirements. University supervisors or supervisors in a service delivery setting may receive minimal input about their roles and responsibilities as clinical educators and, thus, may operate autonomously. These are only a few sources of anxieties for supervisors.

Other sources of anxiety for off-campus supervisors may be related to their individual freedom in accepting the responsibility of supervising a graduate student clinician. While many speech-language pathologists are interested in paying back to the profession, they are concerned about the challenge in light of productivity and quality-of-care standards in the workplace. Some administrators state that their staff is too busy to take on the added responsibility of supervision. Lulai and DeRuiter (2012) addressed five concerns of speech-language pathologists in a medical setting who are hesitant to take on the role of supervisor. They provide a set of tools and resources to address the concerns including a progressive "skill of the week" plan for the course of the internship, checklists outlining the required elements in documentation, and documentation worksheets. They suggest involving colleagues as part of the team to develop tools to reflect operating procedures specific to one's facility. Many off-campus supervisors state that support such as some release time for supervisory responsibilities and professional education in supervision or clinical education would diminish anxiety.

Most supervisors recognize the importance of the tasks of supervision, the knowledge and skills required to provide effective supervision, and their lack of preparation. Most are conscientious about fulfilling their roles and responsibilities. Some supervisors' perception of their role is of a professional who must have the answer to every possible clinical question, who must be able to solve every problem or issue that arises. That "heavy" self-perception, along with the inner knowledge that one does not really have that kind of information, skill, or power will surely produce anxiety. This self-concept—that supervisors must have all the answers—has serious consequences in the development of the Collaborative Style. Sometimes the dispelling of this myth comes as a great surprise and a great relief. Every supervisor has the right—and the responsibility—to say, "I don't know."

This initial anxiety about roles may continue. There are very few data in any of the areas where supervision is utilized that supports an exact methodology. Supervisors who want to find hard and fast answers about what they should be doing will search without much result. As with the clinical process, there is no "cookbook" for effective supervision, let alone a recipe for success. Cogan (1973) stated that professional uncertainties have existed for a long time and will probably persist.

As with supervisees, supervisors may experience anxiety about evaluations. In their role as evaluators, supervisors often have to make or participate in life-altering decisions—retention or dismissal from an educational program or job, for promotions, or for tenure. The potential impact of decisions creates an immense responsibility that understandably creates tension and anxiety. While academic programs are required to have policies and procedures for identifying students who need intervention to meet program expectations for acquisition of clinical knowledge and skills (CAA, 2017, sec. 4.3), the process is stressful.

Very little is known about the feelings of supervisors. Pickering and McCready (1983) and Pickering (1984) touched upon it in their studies, especially when they wrote about the use of journal writing by supervisors, as did McCready, Shapiro, and Kennedy (1987). Like most other aspects of the process, supervisor anxiety must be considered as thoughtfully as possible, without the benefit of a great many definitive answers. It is speculated that perhaps the judicial use of a modicum of self-disclosure might contribute to collegiality, encourage better communication and possibly diminish anxieties of both supervisor and supervisee. The image of the supervisor who knows all is difficult to maintain; more reasonable is the image of the supervisor who knows how to problem solve and is willing to enter into this type of activity with the supervisee.

IMPLICATIONS FOR PARTICIPANTS IN THE SUPERVISORY PROCESS

What does all this mean to the supervisor and supervisee facing each other for the first time or the fiftieth time? In implementing the understanding component, supervisors are dealing with two distinct entities. The first is the interpersonal factor; the second a teaching factor, that is, teaching about supervision.

It has already been stated that the interpersonal component of the supervisory process will not be dealt with in great detail here other than to point out the wealth of information on this topic that is available from other sources and the importance of an in-depth knowledge of the interpersonal aspects of human relations. However, this component is one of the places where an understanding of the dynamics of interpersonal interaction is not only relevant but also essential. ASHA's (2008) Knowledge and Skills Core Area II, Interpersonal Communication and the Supervisor-Supervisee Relationship, contains 7 knowledge areas and 10 skills required to ensure competence. This Core Area substantiates the importance of interpersonal communication in the supervisory process.

The very essence of this component is mutual understanding, not only of the mechanics of the process, but of the other person in the interaction. Therefore, supervisors will need to bring to bear all their knowledge, insight, and skills about interpersonal interactions to successfully accomplish the goals of this component. The interpersonal skills that supervisors have learned and taught clinicians to apply to clients are essentially the same ones that are applicable in the supervisory process. In one of their significant articles on preparing clinical personnel, Ward and Webster (1965) stated that clinicians will tend to view others as they have been viewed, to treat others as they have been treated. "They can use knowledge with compassion and meaningfulness or they can apply techniques mechanically" (Ward & Webster, 1965, p. 39). In describing the tasks of supervision, Ulrich (1990) who chaired the committee that drafted the initial ASHA (1985) Position Statement that contained them noted that it was no accident that task 1, establishing and maintaining an effective working relationship with the supervisee, was first on the list and had the most competencies associated with it.

Pickering and McCready (1990) described certain skills as particularly relevant the supervisory process. They advocated that supervisors study and develop at minimum, basic listening, self-disclosure, and conflict management skills. Further, they noted that empathy should be a major component of supervisory interactions because it connotes/denotes accepting or confirming others as individuals. McCrea's (1980) dissertation study, which revealed that empathy occurred at such miniscule levels in supervisory conferences that it could not be measured, suggests that empathy is a skill that supervisors need to be trained to use.

Immediacy

A substantive body of research in the speech communication literature indicates that the notion of immediacy has a positive influence on student-teacher interaction. The basic principle of immediacy is that people are drawn toward persons and things they like, evaluate highly, and prefer (Mehrabian, 1981). Immediacy in communication is defined as the creation of closeness, a sense of togetherness, of oneness between speaker and listener. Immediacy is communicated with both verbal and nonverbal behaviors. Mehrabian (1969a, 1969b) characterized immediacy behaviors as those which reduce physical and psychological distance between interactants. Nonverbal immediacy behaviors may be demonstrated by eye contact, reduced physical distance, appropriate touch, smiling, gesturing, humor, while verbal ones are demonstrated with the use of inclusive language, such as "we" and "us" (Mehrabian, 1981). Later, Gorham (1988) identified the use of personal examples, encouraging students to talk, discussing issues student bring up in class, and using humor as also being important to the demonstration of verbal immediacy of teachers. These behavioral correlates of verbal and nonverbal immediacy are conceptually related to empathy, facilitative genuineness, respect, and concreteness that have been identified in the counseling literature as being foundational to behavior change (Gazda, 1974). Positive relationships have been found between student cognitive achievement and teacher clarity as well as between student affect and teacher immediacy (Powell and Harville, 1990).

Although the term immediacy by itself is a high-inference notion, the behavioral correlates which signify it have been identified via research in education, interpersonal communication and business. This, in turn, means that supervisors can become aware of and manipulate these behaviors in their interactions with students in an effort to enhance them.

Role Discrepancies

Literature on the importance of shared expectations has been reviewed and its application is critical to a positive supervisory experience. A lack of congruence about role expectations may be a major source breakdown in communication and there are many possible scenarios for this type of situation. Consider, for example, supervisees who have had little opportunity in previous family or educational experiences to participate in problem solving and decision making and who have learned to expect authority figures—parent, teacher, employer, and others—to tell them what to do and provide evaluative feedback. Such supervisees will probably expect supervisors to assume the same role. This will cause problems for supervisors who perceive their role as facilitators in joint problem solving and expect supervisees to gradually assume decision-making responsibilities. Supervisors likely expect supervisees to be able to work effectively with increasing levels of independence, but it is essential that supervisors share that expectation with supervisees at the beginning of the relationship to alleviate the probability of frustration and negative experiences.

Managing Discrepancies

If supervisors are to identify the discrepancies that exist between themselves and their supervisees or between expectations and reality, they must take the lead in talking about the supervisory process itself. To do this, they must first raise to a conscious level what it is that they believe about or expect from supervision. They also need to assist their supervisees in developing and ability to discuss their feelings, concerns and expectations.

Further, supervisors must recognize the individuality of their supervisees. Mandel (2015) suggested student preparation for the clinical experience, supervisor training and systematically surveying the expectations of both supervisees and supervisors as ways to manage discrepancies. Mandel noted that conversations about the differences in expectations during conferences "will assist in establishing a positive relationship where constructive feedback and support are the hallmarks of a relationship with open communication" (p. 13).

Some may be tempted to try to deal with potential mismatches of expectations by assigning similar personality types when making clinical assignments. Even if reliable, valid personality metrics existed, supervisory assignments made to avoid discrepancies are not practical for many reasons. Such variables as experience, ability, training needs, and organizational constraints make scheduling difficult enough in most settings as it is. Time, requirements for clinical hours, space, and availability of clients often dictate scheduling in educational programs. In most off-campus assignments, there are only limited numbers of supervisors in each setting and, in the service delivery setting, there is usually only one supervisor available, often for many supervisees. Furthermore, information is not available for making the "perfect" match for the most effective supervision even if it were logistically possible. More important, if supervisees are to grow professionally and move from the evaluation feedback position to the self-supervisory and consultation stage, one cannot assume that the nature of the supervisory experience should be determined by the supervisee's preferences or expectations alone. In other words, the supervisee who prefers or feels a need for guidance and direction from authority figures would not necessarily profit from being matched with a supervisor who will meet that need—very little growth is apt to take place. What supervisees perceive as their needs may not be what is best for their professional growth. Supervisees' preferences for supervisor behavior are not necessarily related to the effectiveness of supervision (Copeland & Atkinson, 1978). Children like and want candy, but it may, after all, produce dental cavities, hyperactivity, and weight gain. What is more consistent with the approach to supervision described in this text is that both participants in the process become aware of the other's role perceptions and expectations, that communication take place about the incongruences that exist and the changes that may be necessary for both the supervisee and supervisor if communication is to be enhanced and professional growth is to occur throughout the experience. Accommodations must be made where there are discrepancies if the interaction is to be successful (Hersey & Blanchard, 1982). This practice is congruent with ASHA (2008) Knowledge and Skill Core Area II, which requires that the supervisor and supervisee evaluate the effectiveness of the ongoing supervisory relationship and address challenges to successful communication interactions.

PREPARING FOR SUPERVISION

As stated previously, most supervisors have not studied the supervisory process. Basic to the approach presented here, however, is some understanding of the dynamics of the process. The first step is for supervisors to prepare themselves for the encounter, learning about themselves as well as the process. This will not only increase their understanding but should allay some of their anxieties as well.

Study of the Process by Supervisors

Although it is true that formal coursework traditionally had not been available to many supervisors, that has changed and there are ways to become more knowledgeable about the process. Speech-language pathologists and audiologists have a professional obligation/ethical responsibility to provide the best services possible to their clients. In shifting roles from clinician to supervisor, the same holds true. The list of 13 tasks and 81 associated competencies in the 1985 ASHA position paper provided a focus for more than 2 decades. This was updated and replaced in 2008 by new ASHA policy documents (e.g., position statement [a], technical report [b], and knowledge and skills [c]). Reading, traditional and online courses, conferences, and presentations at professional meetings are ways to begin. In many organizations or areas, supervisors have formed study groups and blogs. Additionally, self-study is a valuable tool for supervisors who wish to monitor their skills. The ASHA (2013) Ad Hoc Committee on Supervision (AHCS) stated that education should begin early (introduced in graduate curriculum), recommended formal training, and noted that "Effective education for supervision should focus on the unique aspects of knowledge and specialized skills for the supervisory process and should not be limited to regulatory aspects (e.g., observation time, clock hours) of the process" (p. 4). The ASHA (2016) Ad Hoc Committee on Supervision Training (AHCST) developed training goals for the five constituent groups identified by the AHCS and created a set of six "deliverables" to provide a plan and resources for training. In addition to ASHA's Practice Portal for clinical education and supervision, CAPCSD offers free online courses for member programs and their constituents. The bottom line is that a number of opportunities for study exist that are easily accessed at little or no cost. Strategies for accountability and self-study will be detailed in Chapter 8.

Supervisor Self-Knowledge

The admonition to "know thyself" is as important in the approach to the supervisory process as it is in the many other situations in which it is wisely offered as a guideline. Self-knowledge in several categories is critical. Supervisors first must define, or raise to a conscious level, their basic philosophy of what supervision really is. They need to define the purpose of supervision and the principles upon which they determine their supervisory techniques. They must be honest about the supervisory process and values they bring to it.

Anderson (1988) recounted a discussion of supervisory techniques with a supervisor who described her use of indirect behaviors such as questioning and asking supervisees for ideas. These techniques were consistent with the supervisor's philosophy and her beliefs that indirect behaviors would facilitate supervisees' problem solving and independent functioning. She shared, "The supervisee came up with a good idea, so I could go along with it. I don't know what I would have done if I hadn't been comfortable with it." Obviously, there were some discrepancies between what the supervisor really believed and what she perceived she was doing.

Supervisors need to understand their self-perceptions of their own roles. They need to analyze their own behavior to determine if it is consistent with their basic philosophy, and must have a rationale for their behaviors. It is interesting that supervisors expect supervisees to be able to provide rationales for their clinical behaviors—the "whys" to support the strategies and techniques they plan to implement in clinical intervention. Yet, a majority never thinks to ponder the rationales for their own supervisory behaviors. Supervisors must recognize the complexity of the supervisory process and determine if they see it as teaching, evaluation, modeling, collaboration, or a combination of these and many other available models. They need to examine their belief in a scientific approach to observation, data collection, and analysis and their own dedication to maintaining a scientific approach. They must honestly analyze their own philosophical foundation for the practices in which they engage before they can expect to discuss the process with their supervisees.

A further area of self-knowledge is that of personal motivations in relation to supervision. Why do individuals become supervisors? Many would answer the question with noble statements about the professional growth and development of young professionals and the obligations of passing on that which they have learned to new generations thereby contributing to their profession. Those are certainly valid reasons and for the most part, sincere and honest motivations. The reality is, however, that most supervisors became such by accident. Rather than planning to be supervisors, they were in the right place at the right time and, voilà—they became a supervisor. As they continue in this role, however, there is always the specter of the seductiveness of power and authority lurking in the background. Brammer (1985) suggested that many people who are involved in the helping process do so "to meet their own unrecognized needs" (p. 3). This can also be true of supervisors. Supervisors need to be aware of their basic attitude toward people and their worth. If, in their role of supervisor and helper they are going to step back and permit their supervisees to grow, then they must value them as autonomous individuals, believe fully in their ability to think and learn, and recognize these abilities when they are present. If they believe they are responsible for the supervisee's growth and development, if they do not believe that individuals can independently solve problems and formulate solutions to clinical dilemmas, they may become manipulative and self-serving in their supervisory role. They may perceive themselves as "rescuers" and the kinds of satisfactions they obtain from this so-called helping relationship are not likely healthy. Supervisors can determine their values and attitudes only after considerable soul-searching, but it is an essential prerequisite to assuming the role of supervisor.

TEACHING SUPERVISEES ABOUT THE SUPERVISORY PROCESS

Introducing the student to the supervisory process may take several forms and be organizationally or individually based. The approach is analogous to the first experiences students have in observing therapy and in observing therapy in a new, distinct setting. Without guidance, many students look at clinical intervention globally, unable to identify individual behaviors or patterns of behavior, much less understand their significance. The same holds true for the supervisory process.

Based on their research, Mandel (2015) in surveying novice and second semester clinicians and Christodoulou (2016) in her review of speech-language pathology externship clinicians, both recommended preparing students to participate in the supervisory process. Further, the ASHA (2016) AHCST identified educating the supervisee about the supervisory process an essential competency for all five constituent groups identified by the ASHA (2013) AHCS.

In teaching about the clinical process, various methods are used by different programs. In addition to a great amount of coursework related to normal and abnormal speech and language development, the student is introduced to the clinical process through discussion of clinical issues and case studies in academic courses, and clinical process courses (e.g., Introduction to Clinic, Methods of Clinical Practice, etc.). Students are gradually introduced to therapy through observation and participation prior to their first hands-on supervised experience. This important component of the educational process is substantiated by ASHA and CAA curriculum requirements.

Certain techniques are used to teach about the clinical behaviors in the early observations before the student enters the clinical world—joint observations, guided observations, check lists, interaction analysis systems, followed by reports and analysis of observed behaviors. Once the practicum is begun, the focus is on the clinical process in a wide variety of ways.

If students or employed professionals are to be successful as supervisees, it is just as important that they be introduced to the supervisory process in a similar manner. It is imperative that they understand their dual roles and responsibilities as clinician/clinician assistant and supervisee. Ideally, this preparation should begin at the undergraduate level, prior to the first practicum. Subsequently, the supervisory process needs to be examined and analyzed throughout all supervisory experiences, whether in university training programs or professional settings. Because many universities and employment settings do not provide formal training such as courses or in-service workshops, the responsibility for preparing supervisees to participate in the supervisory process usually falls on individual supervisors. The supervisor has the responsibility for setting the stage and directing the supervisory interaction. The supervisor is accountable for preparing the supervisee to participate. In discussing the colleagueship relationship of the clinical supervision model, Cogan (1973) maintained that the supervisor is responsible for structuring the framework of discussion but not the total content of interaction. Supervisors must get the study of the process started while still making it clear that the supervisee has equal responsibility in the relationship.

Preparing supervisees for the supervisory process is expected to contribute to their professional growth and, thus, to facilitate more effective clinical practice and better services for our clients. It should also contribute to more effective clinical supervision. The overarching set of knowledge and skills delineated in the AHCS final report (2013) provide content relative to the initial preparation of supervisees—and certainly provide a structure for the ongoing analysis and discussion of the supervisory process, regardless of the setting in which supervision is occurring or the previous experience of supervisees.

Introducing the Supervisory Process

Topics for supervision training have been provided by ASHA's (2016) AHCST and are a readily available resource on the practice portal. As an introduction to the process, however, each supervisor should take time at the beginning and throughout each interaction to talk about supervision as the situation dictates. The model of supervision to be used, objectives of supervision, roles of the participants, and the components of the process are essential themes regardless of the setting in which supervision is to take place. Topics for discussion at the beginning of the experience might include any of the following, in any order:

1. *Collaborative Models of Supervision.* The model most commonly referenced in Communication Sciences and Disorders and referenced in the 2008 ASHA policy documents is Anderson's

(1988) continuum model, initially described in Anderson's first edition of this text. The lasting appeal of this model is in part a function of its focus on the developmental nature of the process that spans a professional career. It provides a fundamental mindset for professional growth and development for both supervisors and supervisees. It is also congruent with CFCC standards stipulating that "supervision must be commensurate with a student's knowledge, skills and experience" and adjusted upward from the minimum 25% of total contact when warranted.

2. *Components of the Supervisory Process.* This discussion will reflect a content approach to supervision based on the components defined by Anderson (1988) and detailed in this text. It should include both the supervisor's philosophy about supervision and the supervisee's impressions about the process.

3. *Perceptions of Supervisees about Supervision.* Information about the perceptions of roles (i.e., preconceived stereotypes derived from various sources) should be shared. Personal biases, previous experience, theoretical perspectives, information from friends, information derived from the literature and the complexities of the supervisory process itself make many roles available to both supervisors and supervisees. Supervisors will want to know what supervisees' role expectations are for them. Are they perceived as helpers, teachers, counselors, evaluator, trainer, overseer, coach mentor and so on? And, what do these titles means to supervisees? For example, do supervisees perceive the supervisor as the expert? Someone who has all the answers and can provide any and all of the information they might need? Or is the supervisor's role that of evaluator? Someone to tell them what they did right or wrong, point out their weaknesses and then tell them the correct way to do it?

Supervisees' perceptions of their own roles must be discussed. Do they perceive themselves as passive participants in the process? Following directives provided by the supervisor? Do they have insight about their responsibilities in problem solving or for their own professional development? Do they have confidence in their ability to establish objectives for their clients and to devise methods for achieving those objectives?

Techniques we have used to clarify perceived roles for ourselves and our supervisees include the following, done independently and without collaboration.

- ◦ Write your personal definition of supervision.
- ◦ List the characteristics of a "good supervisor."
- ◦ List the characteristics of a "good supervisee."

Share and discuss what you've written.

4. *Goals and Objectives for Supervision.* Setting goals and objectives for the supervisory process will be addressed in Chapter 4. During the introductory phase, supervisees need to know that goals will be established not only for clients, but also for them as supervisees and clinicians, and for supervisors. Goals may be long-term ones, which include overall, broad objectives related to general patterns or short-term ones that are specific to a particular interaction.

5. *Prior Experiences in Supervision.* Supervisors and supervisees need to discuss supervisees' past experiences in supervision, the types of interactions they have had with supervisors, their feelings about supervision, and what they learned about the process. Important questions to pose include: How much previous experience have supervisees had? What was the nature of previous experiences? What positive and negative feelings, likes and dislikes, about supervision does the supervisee have?

6. *Supervisee Style Preference.* It is important to determine whether supervisees prefer a Direct-Active supervisor style which is characterized by a higher proportion of supervisor talk during interactions and involves telling, giving opinions, giving suggestions, critiquing, and so on, or an indirect style which is characterized by supportive supervisor statements, active listening, asking for opinions and suggestions, and reflecting supervisee feelings and ideas (Blumberg, 1974, 1980). Whether supervisees can accurately differentiate behaviors characteristic of these

styles is also important to establish (Brasseur & Anderson, 1983). Further, the consequences of preferred style in relation to supervisee growth and independence needs to be explored. Specifically, how style influences placement and movement on the continuum needs to be discussed. If the preferences of the supervisor and supervisee are not congruent, differences should be examined at the beginning of the relationship.

7. *Supervisee Anxieties.* Cogan (1973) maintained that, during the initial conferences, supervisors need to deal with supervisees' anxieties and uncertainties. This is especially critical for novice supervisees or those working with a new type of client. While a little anxiety is motivating, too much is incapacitating. For some, identifying anxieties and their sources will be a sufficient technique for diffusing them. For others, the process will be more involved. Possible sources of anxiety may include preparing lesson plans, the threat of being continuously observed, the possibility of unplanned interruption or intervention, evaluations, recommendations, grades, inability or lack of confidence regarding one's ability to manage clinical problems, and a host of other concerns. Based on our experience, "fear of the unknown" is often a source of anxiety. Oratio (1977) and Sleight (1985) state that beginning clinicians' anxieties primarily concern their ability to attain supervisory standards; the supervisory relationship itself; responsibility for client welfare; and the ability to apply academic information to the clinical process.

8. *Supervisees' Baseline Needs and Competencies.* The fact that data will be collected should be conveyed in one of the first conferences. Actual data collection procedures and timelines will be thoroughly addressed in the planning stage as supervisors introduce the continuum perspective and the appropriate style of supervision relative to placement on the continuum. Christodoulou (2016) recommends that the first step be "ask specifically what the student needs and expects of the supervisory relationship and then to find a balance between any differences" (p. 45).

Notice that discussion of the client has not yet been suggested. This is appropriate since this is the time for the supervisee to become aware of his or her own feelings and to share expectations with the supervisor. Once preliminary rapport is established, the supervisor and supervisee can move on to the more traditional planning for the client and then for the clinician, supervisee, and supervisor.

Learning How to Talk About Supervision

The discussion described previously may be elicited and enhanced in a variety of ways. First and foremost, the supervisor must be a skilled listener. Scattered throughout the literature on supervisees' expectations are references to the supervisee wanting the supervisor to listen and to take seriously what they say (Kayser, 1993; Larson, 1981; Peaper & Mercaitis, 1989a, 1989b; Russell, 1976; Tihen, 1983). As Anderson (1988) noted, the fact that this is stated at all is significant. Have supervisors communicated to supervisees that they are not taking supervisees seriously? That they do not respect their ideas and abilities? The supervisor who takes time to hear what the supervisee expresses about needs, expectations, and anxieties will learn valuable information and enhance the relationship immeasurably.

Good communication and interpersonal skills, including active listening, are vital supervisor competencies. Specific supervisor behaviors that need to be demonstrated include accepting and using the supervisees' ideas in discussions, reflecting the content and feelings of supervisee utterances, and skilled questioning. Modeling a supportive, collegial communication style may be more important than what is actually said (Anderson, 1988). Both verbal and nonverbal behaviors must be monitored to insure that what a supervisor espouses as her philosophy of supervision is consistent with actual practice.

Getting accurate statements of how supervisees feel at this point may be difficult. They may not know how to express their ideas. The supervisor or the total situation may be so threatening that supervisees' reactions will be inhibited. The supervisor may not be able to resist loaded questions in which the expected answer is obvious. It is sometimes gratifying or easier to hear what one wishes to hear, but it is not productive in the effort to learn supervisees' real feelings. Also, some supervisees may have learned through the grapevine what a particular supervisor likes or expects and may play the game, "Tell the Supervisor What She Wants to Hear." The skill and sensitivity of supervisors in asking questions determines much of the outcome here.

Some supervisors find questionnaires and scales such as Larson's (1981) and Tihen's (1983) scales (Appendixes 3-2 through 3-4) helpful for facilitating honest discussions about supervision. A scale developed and validated by Powell (1987) to measure attitudes toward Cogan's clinical supervision model could also be used at this stage to learn more about the supervisee's ideas and provide a basis for discussion (Appendix 3-6). Indeed, supervisors who have not yet worked out their own personal beliefs about the process might also find it useful. A supervisory conference rating scale developed by Smith (1977; Smith & Anderson, 1982a) and modified by Brasseur (1980a) may also be helpful to obtain specific information about supervisees' perceptions of individual conferences (Appendix 3-7). Both supervisor and supervisees might complete part of Casey's scale (Casey, 1985; Casey, Smith & Ulrich, 1988) to delineate the relative importance of the 13 tasks and 81 associated competencies in ASHA's (1985) Position Statement and discuss their responses (Appendix 3-1). Supervisors and supervisees might modify the *Self-Assessment of Competencies in Supervision* (ASHA, n.d.-a) to independently identify the relative importance of each competency, then rate the skill level and share results as a means to share expectations and identify goals.

Some supervisors ask students to write an informal statement about their feelings at the beginning of the interaction. Others ask students to keep a journal (Laccinole & Shulman, 1985; Lubinsky & Hildebrand, 1996; Maloney, 1994; Pickering & McCready, 1990; Schill & Swanson, 1993) to reflect on or to evaluate their clinical performance throughout a term. This may be difficult for some students so, if the supervisor perceives that a student is somewhat intimidated or is reluctant to share their feelings early on, these writings can be maintained by the supervisee until a climate of trust and openness is firmly established in the relationship. Mormer and Messick (2016) provide guidelines, suggestions and a form for reflective journal writings. These tools provide a structure and guide students in the process of self-reflection. A systematic approach such as this should enable students to learn and become comfortable with reflective writing and thus comply with a new 2017 CAA standard: "the ability to use self-reflection to understand the effects of one's actions and to make changes accordingly" (Std. 3.1.1A and 3.1.1B-Professional Practice Competencies/Accountability).

From the outset, supervisees need to see supervision as a larger issue than "What do I do with my client?" The concept of setting objectives for themselves as a supervisee and as a clinician may never have entered their mind. Even students with prior clinical and supervisory experience, may have had supervisors who focused exclusively on the clinical process and ignored the supervisory process. So, the concept that supervision is not just about and for the client's welfare may be new.

Information from supervisors about what to expect from the situation is helpful in allaying anxieties of supervisees. More of this will be discussed in the planning section, but supervisees deserve to know the organizational requirements, as well as those of the individual supervisor, the format under which they will be operating, and the criteria for success in each experience. Mormer and Messick's (2016) Practicum Expectation Worksheet offers a tool for identifying organizational and supervisor requirements that can be easily formatted for any placement but provides an excellent template for externship supervisors (see Chapter 11, Appendix 11-1). And, as previously noted, Lulai and DeRuiter (2012) developed a set of tools for new supervisors of students in medical settings. Supervisors should not only be cognizant of their biases, quirks, idiosyncrasies, personal operating procedures but they should also share these with supervisees in the first conference.

Because supervisors do evaluate supervisees in every type of supervisory interaction, from university training programs to employment setting, obtaining honest feedback from supervisees during the course of the experience, or after the fact, can be difficult. If supervisors genuinely want it though, they will be able to devise ways to obtain it. To illustrate, common supervisee complaints include: "My supervisor is always late," "My supervisor talks on the phone or texts during our conferences," "My supervisor talks too much during conferences," "I feel like I'm getting mixed messages." Obviously these things are difficult for supervisees to share with their supervisor unless the supervisor has set the stage for receiving feedback, exhibits high-level interpersonal skills that enable supervisees to take risks, and reacts in a nondefensive manner when supervisees provide honest feedback. It will take time to develop the trust and rapport needed to be honest and candid. It is also helpful to teach supervisees some types of communicative behaviors that can decrease the risk of supervisor defensiveness or the possibility of conflict. For example, the use of "I" statements and indirect requests are particularly useful techniques (e.g., "I wonder if it might be possible to turn off phones during our conferences? I have trouble concentrating when interruptions happen," or, "I'm not sure I understand—I think I'm hearing two different things—X and Y—I'm a little confused.")

Although discussion about the general process of supervision is initiated in the first conference, it continues throughout the entire experience. Once objectives have been established for the clinician/supervisee and the supervisor, they must be assessed to see if they are being met, and revised if necessary. A prerequisite to talking about the ongoing interaction is gathering data which will serve as the nucleus of a discussion. Data should include attitudes, perceptions, needs, and actual behaviors. Once collected, data can be analyzed. A data based, analytical focus also facilitates open and honest communication.

The use of some exercises, scales, and other tools, discussed previously, are good ways to set the tone and get the process of talking about supervision established as a norm for the relationship. Formulating goals and strategies for collecting and analyzing data relative to the supervisory process will be discussed in subsequent chapters. We have not provided comprehensive coverage of the topic nor an exhaustive list of techniques for preparing supervisees for the process. However, we hope readers have a better understanding of the importance of preparation, as well as a basic framework for this task. Further, we hope you see how this Understanding, as a component of the supervisory process, will help supervisors achieve the competencies for effective clinical supervision (ASHA, 2008a, 2008b, 2008c).

SUMMARY

The foundation of a productive supervisory relationship is a basic understanding of the supervisory process and effective communication between supervisor and supervisee about philosophies, expectations, perceptions, and objectives. This is more than merely an introduction to the process; it requires ongoing discussion about the continuing interaction.

REFERENCES

American Speech-Language-Hearing Association. (n.d.-a). *Appendix E: Self-assessment of competencies in supervision* [Practice Portal]. Retrieved from https://www.asha.org/uploadedFiles/Self-Assessment-of-Competencies-in-Supervision.pdf

American Speech-Language-Hearing Association. (n.d.-b). *Professional Issues.* Retrieved from https://www.asha.org/Practice-Portal/Professional-Issues/

American Speech-Language-Hearing Association. (1985). *Clinical supervision in speech-language pathology and audiology.* [Position statement]. Retrieved from https://www.asha.org/policy/PS1985-00220/

American-Speech-Language-Hearing Association (2008a). *Knowledge and skills needed by speech-language pathologists providing clinical supervision* [Position statement]. Retrieved from https://www.asha.org/policy/PS2008-00295

American Speech-Language-Hearing Association (2008b). *Knowledge and skills needed by speech-language pathologists providing clinical supervision* [Technical report]. Retrieved from https://www.asha.org/policy/TR2008-00296

American Speech-Language-Hearing Association. (2008c). *Knowledge and skills needed by speech-language pathologists providing clinical supervision* [Knowledge and skills]. Retrieved from https://www.asha.org/policy/KS2008-00294/

American Speech-Language-Hearing Association. (2013, December). *Knowledge, skills and training consideration for individuals serving as supervisors* [Final report of the Ad Hoc Committee on Supervision]. Retrieved from https://www.asha.org/uploadedFiles/Supervisors-Knowledge-Skills-Report.pdf

American Speech-Language-Hearing Association. (2016, May). *A plan for developing resources and training opportunities in clinical supervision* [Final report of the ASHA Ad Hoc Committee on Supervision Training]. Retrieved from https://www.asha.org/uploadedFiles/A-Plan-for-Developing-Resources-and-Training-Opportunities-in-Clinical-Supervision.pdf

American Speech-Language-Hearing Association. (2017). *Issues in ethics: Cultural and linguistic competence.* Retrieved from https://www.asha.org/Practice/ethics/Cultural-and-Linguistic-Competence/

American Speech-Language-Hearing Association. (2018). *ASHA summary membership and affiliation counts, year-end 2017*. Retrieved from https://www.asha.org/uploadedFiles/2017-Member-Counts.pdf

Anderson, J. (1988). *The supervisory process in speech-language pathology and audiology.* Boston, MA: College-Hill.

Belenky, M. F., Clinchy, B. M., Goldberger, N. R., & Tarule, J. M. (1986). *Women's ways of knowing: The development of self, voice, and mind.* New York, NY: Basic Books.

Biddle, B., & Thomas, E. (1966). *Role theory: Concepts and research.* New York, NY: John Wiley and Sons.

Blumberg, A. (1974). *Supervisors and teachers: A private cold war.* Berkeley, CA: McCutchan.

Blumberg, A. (1980). *Supervisors and teachers: A private cold war* (2nd ed.). Berkeley, CA: McCutchan.

Blumberg, A., & Amidon, E. (1965). Teacher perceptions of supervisor-teacher interaction. *Administrator's Notebook, 14,* 1-4.

Blumberg, A., Amidon, E., & Weber, W. (1967). *Supervisor-teacher interaction as seen by supervisors.* Unpublished manuscript, Temple University, Philadelphia, PA.

Brammer, L. (1985). *The helping relationship.* Englewood Cliffs, NJ: Prentice-Hall, Inc.

Brasseur, J. (1980). *The observed differences between direct, indirect, and direct/indirect videotaped supervisory conferences by speech-language pathology supervisors, graduate students, and undergraduate students* (Doctoral dissertation). Retrieved from ProQuest Dissertations & Theses Global. (Accession No. 8029212) http://proxyiub.uits.iu.edu/login?url=https://search.proquest.com/docview/303031314?accountid=11620

Brasseur, J. (1987). Preparation of supervisees for the supervisory process. In S. Farmer (Ed.), *Proceedings of a national conference on supervision—Clinical supervision: A coming of age* (pp. 144-163). Council of University Supervisors of Practicum in Speech-Language Pathology and Audiology, Jekyll Island, GA.

Brasseur, J. (1994). Women and men on top—Getting or being a mentor. In M. Bruce (Ed.), *Proceedings of the 1994 international & interdisciplinary conference on clinical supervision: Toward the 21st century* (pp. 236-243). Cape Cod, MA: Council of Supervisors in Speech-Language Pathology and Audiology.

Brasseur, J., & Anderson, J. (1983). Observed differences between direct, indirect, and direct/indirect videotaped supervisory conferences. *Journal of Speech and Hearing Research, 26,* 349-355.

Broyles, S., McNeice, E., Ishee, J., Ross, S., & Lance, D. (1999). *Influence of selected factors on the perceived effectiveness of various supervision strategies.* Poster session presented at the annual convention of the American Speech-Language-Hearing Association, San Francisco, CA.

Casey, P. (1985). *Supervisory skills self-assessment.* Whitewater, WI: University of Wisconsin-Whitewater.

Casey, P., Smith, K., & Ulrich, S. (1988). *Self supervision: A career tool for audiologists and speech-language pathologists* (Clinical Series No. 10). Rockville, MD: National Student Speech Language Hearing Association.

Chan, J., Carter, S., & McAllister, L. (1994). Anxiety related to clinical education in speech-language pathology students. In M. Bruce (Ed.), *Proceedings of the 1994 International & Interdisciplinary Conference on Clinical Supervision: Toward the 21st Century* (pp. 126-132). Cape Cod, MA: Council of Supervisors in Speech-Language Pathology and Audiology.

Christodoulou, J. (2016). A review of the expectations of speech-language pathology externship student clinicians and their supervisors. *Perspectives in Administration and Supervision, 1*(Part 2). 42-53. doi:10.1044/persp1.SIG11.42

Cogan, M. (1973). Clinical supervision. Boston, MA: Houghton Mifflin.

Copeland, W. (1980). Affective dispositions of teachers in training toward examples of supervisory behavior. *Journal of Educational Research, 74,* 37-42.

Copeland, W. (1982). Student teachers' preference for supervisory approach. *Journal of Teacher Education, 33,* 32-36.

Copeland, W., & Atkinson, D. (1978). Student teachers' perceptions of directive and nondirective supervisory behavior. *Journal of Educational Research, 71,* 123-226.

Council for Clinical Certification in Audiology and Speech-Language Pathology of the American Speech-Language-Hearing Association. (2014). *2014 standards for the certificate of clinical competence in speech-language pathology.* Rev 2016. Retrieved from http://www.asha.org/Certification/2014-Apeech-Language-Pathology-Certification-Standards/

Council of Academic Programs in Communication Sciences and Disorders. (2013). *White paper: Preparation of speech-language pathology clinical educators* [White Paper]. Retrieved from: http://scotthall.dotster.com/capcsd/wp-content/uploads/2014/10/Preparation-of-Clinical-Educators-White-Paper.pdf

Council on Academic Accreditation in Audiology and Speech-Language Pathology. (2017). *Standards for accreditation of graduate education programs in audiology and speech-language pathology.* Retrieved May 21, 2018 from http://caa.asha.org/wp- content/uploads/Accreditation-Standards-for-Graduate-Programs.pdf

Culatta, R., Colucci, S., & Wiggins, E. (1975). Clinical supervisors and trainees: Two views of a process. *Asha, 17,* 152-157.

Culatta, R., & Seltzer, H. (1977). Content and sequence analysis of the supervisory session: A report of clinical use. *Asha, 19,* 523-526.

DeVane, G. (1992). Multicultural strategies for quality improvement in the supervisory process. In S. Dowling (Ed.), *Proceedings of the 1992 National Conference on Supervision—Total quality supervision: Effecting optimal performance* (pp. 150-155). Council of Supervisors in Speech-Language Pathology and Audiology, Nashville, TN.

Dowling, S., & Wittkopp, M. (1982). Students' perceived supervisory needs. *Journal of Communication Disorders, 15,* 319-328.

Edrich, M. (2014). *Effects of online training on off-campus clinical supervisors' knowledge, attitudes and expectations regarding the supervisory process* (Unpublished doctoral dissertation). NOVA Southeastern University, Fort Lauderdale, FL.

Fencel, J. & Mead, J. (2017). A qualitative study describing positive and negative supervisor-student clinician relationships in speech-language pathology. *Perspectives in Administration and Supervision, 2*(Part 1), 17-24. Retrieved from https://doi.org/10.1044/persp2.SIG11.17

Gazda, G. (1974). *Human relations development—A manual for educators.* Boston, MA: Allyn and Bacon.

Gordon-Pershey, M. & Walden, P. (2013). Supervisor and supervisee perceptions of an adult learning model of graduate student supervision. *Perspectives in Administration and Supervision, 23*(1), 12-21. doi:10.1044/aaa23.1.12

Gorham, J. (1988). The relationship between verbal teacher immediacy behaviors and student learning. *Communication Education, 37,* 40-53.

Hatten, J. T. (1965). *A descriptive and analytical investigation of speech therapy supervisors-therapist conferences* (Doctoral dissertation). Retrieved from ProQuest Dissertations and Theses Global. (Accession No. 6513735) http://proxyiub.uits.iu.edu/login?url=https://search.proquest.com/docview/302175416?accountid=11620

Haverkamp, K. (1983). *The orientation experience for the adult learner. In R. Smith (Ed.), Helping adults learn how to learn.* San Francisco, CA: Jossey-Bass.

Hersey, P., & Blanchard, K. (1982). *Management of organizational behavior* (4th ed.). Englewood Cliffs, NJ: Prentice-Hall.

Honey, P. & Mumford, A. (1986). *The learning styles questionnaire.* Retrieved form https://resources.eln.io/honey-mumford-learner-types-1986-questionnaire-online/

Honey, P. & Mumford, A. (1992). *The manual of learning styles* (3rd ed.). London, England: P Honey.

Hutchinson, D., Uhl, S., & Weinrich, B. (1987). A comparative study of student clinician performance under two types of supervisory conditions. In S. Farmer (Ed.), *Proceedings of a national conference on supervision—Clinical supervision: A coming of age* (pp. 131-137). Council of University Supervisors of Practicum in Speech-Language Pathology and Audiology, Jekyll Island, GA.

Kayser, H. (1993). Supervision of the Hispanic speech language pathology graduate student. *The Supervisors' Forum, 1,* 18-23.

Knowles, M. (1984). *Andragogy in action: Applying modern principles of adult learning.* San Francisco, CA: Jossey-Bass.

Kolb, D. (1984). *Experiential Learning.* Upper Saddle River, NJ: Prentice-Hall.

Laccinole, M., & Shulman, B. (1985). Clinical effectiveness for the student clinician. *SUPERvision, 9*(3), 23-26.

Langellier, K. M., & Natalle, E. J. (1987). Gender, interpersonal communication, and supervision. In S. Farmer (Ed.), *Proceedings of A National Conference on Supervision—Clinical supervision: A coming of age* (pp. 14-37). Council of University Supervisors of Practicum in Speech-Language Pathology and Audiology, Jekyll Island, GA.

Larkins, P. (1992). Women's ways of supervising: What's your type? In S. Dowling (Ed.), *Proceedings of the 1992 National Conference on Supervision—Total quality supervision: Effecting optimal performance* (pp. 38-40). Council of Supervisors in Speech-Language Pathology and Audiology, Nashville, TN.

Larson, L. C. (1981). *Perceived supervisory needs and expectations of experienced vs. inexperienced student clinicians* (Doctoral dissertation). Retrieved from ProQuest Dissertations and Theses Global. (Accession No. 8211183) http://proxyiub.uits.iu.edu/login?url=https://search.proquest.com/docview/303157417?accountid=11620

Larson, L., Hoag, L., & Schraeder-Neidenthal, J. (1987). Supervisee satisfaction with a contract-based system for grading practicum. In S. Farmer (Ed.), *Proceedings of A National Conference on Supervision—Clinical supervision: A Coming of age* (pp. 117-124). Council of University Supervisors of Practicum in Speech-Language Pathology and Audiology, Jekyll Island, GA.

Lubinsky, J., & Hildebrand, S. (1996). Journal keeping to help students attain personal goals in practicum. In B. Wagner (Ed.), *Proceedings of the 1996 Conference on Clinical Supervision—Partnerships in supervision: Innovative and effective practices* (pp. 235-242). Council of Supervisors in Speech-Language Pathology and Audiology, Cincinnati, OH.

Lulai, R. & DeRuiter, M. (2012). The new clinical supervisor: Tools for the medical setting. *Perspectives in Administration and Supervision, 22*(3), 85-96. doi:10.1044/aaa22.3.85

Maloney, D. (1994). Client-centered student journaling: A way of reflecting on clinical learning. In M. Bruce (Ed.), *Proceedings of the 1994 International & Interdisciplinary Conference on Clinical Supervision: Toward the 21st century* (pp. 191-195). Council of Supervisors in Speech-Language Pathology and Audiology, Cape Cod, MA.

Mandel, S. (2015). Exploring the differences in expectations between supervisors and supervisees during the initial clinical experience. *Perspectives in Administration and Supervision, 25*(1), 4-15. doi:10.1044/aaa25.1.4

Mastriano, B., Gordon, T., & Gottwald, S. (1999). *Expectations in the supervisory process: An analysis of attitudes II.* Poster session presented at the annual convention of the American Speech-Language-Hearing Association, San Francisco, CA.

McCrea, E. S. (1980). *Supervisee ability to self-explore and four facilitative dimensions of supervisor behavior in individual conferences in speech-language pathology* (Doctoral dissertation). Retrieved from ProQuest Dissertations and Theses Global. (Accession No. 8029239) http://proxyiub.uits.iu.edu/login?url=https://search.proquest.com/docview/303031284?accountid=11620

McCready, V., Shapiro, D., & Kennedy, K. (1987). Identifying hidden dynamics in supervision: Four scenarios. In M. Crago & M. Pickering (Eds.), *Supervision in human communication disorders: Perspectives on a process*. San Diego, CA: College Hill Press.

Mehrabian, A. (1969a). *Methods and designs: Some referents and measures of nonverbal behavior* [Behavioral Research Methods and Instrumentation I].

Mehrabian, A. (1969b). Significance of posture and position in the communication of attitude and status relationships. *Psychological Bulletin, 71*, 359-372.

Mehrabian, A. (1981). *Silent messages: Implicit communication of emotions and attitudes* (2nd ed.). Belmont, CA: Wadsworth.

Mercaitis, P., & Peaper, R. (1989). *Strategies for helping supervisees to participate actively in the supervisory process.* In D. Shapiro (Ed.), Proceedings of the 1989 National Conference on Supervision: Supervision Innovations (pp. 20-28). Council of Supervisors in Speech-Language Pathology and Audiology, Sonoma, CA.

Monnin, L. & Peters, K. (1981). *Clinical practice for speech-pathologists in the schools*. Springfield, IL: Charles C. Thomas.

Mormer, E. & Messick, C. (2016). *Bringing the evidence to clinical education practices.* Pre-Conference workshop presented at the American Speech-Language-Hearing Association Convention in Philadelphia, PA, November 16, 2016.

Murray, M., & Owen, M. (1991). *Beyond the myths and magic of mentoring*. San Francisco, CA: Jossey-Bass.

Myers, F. (1980). Clinician needs in the practicum setting. *SUPERvision, 4*.

Nilsen, J. F. (1983). *Supervisor's use of direct/indirect verbal conference style and alteration of clinical behavior* (Doctoral dissertation). Retrieved from ProQuest Dissertations and Theses Global. (Accession No. 8309991) http://proxyiub.uits.iu.edu/login?url=https://search.proquest.com/docview/303165270?accountid=11620

Oratio, A. (1977). *Supervision in speech pathology: A handbook for supervisors and clinicians*. Baltimore, MD: University Park Press.

Pannbacker, M., Middleton, G., & Lass, N. (1993). Am I a good supervisor? That depends on who's asking! *The Supervisors' Forum, 1*, 57.

Peaper, R., & Mercaitis, P. (1989a). *Satisfactory and unsatisfactory supervisory experiences: Contributing factors.* In D. Shapiro (Ed.), Proceedings of the 1989 National Conference on Supervision: Supervision Innovations (pp. 126-140). Council of Supervisors in Speech-Language Pathology and Audiology, Sonoma, CA.

Peaper, R., & Mercaitis, P. (1989b). Strategies for helping supervisees to participate actively in the supervisory process. In D. Shapiro (Ed.), *Proceedings of the 1989 National Conference on Supervision: Supervision Innovations* (pp. 20-28). Council of Supervisors of Practicum in Speech-Language Pathology and Audiology, Sonoma, CA.

Pickering, M. (1981a). Supervising student teachers: How to provide non-threatening feedback. *Journal of Childhood Communication Disorders, 5*(2), 150-153.

Pickering, M. (1981b). *Supervisory interaction: The subjective side.* Paper presented at the CUSPSPA meeting during the annual convention of the American Speech-Language-Hearing Association, Los Angeles, CA.

Pickering, M. (1984). Interpersonal communication in speech-language pathology supervisory conferences: A qualitative study. *Journal of Speech and Hearing Disorders, 49*, 189-195.

Pickering, M. (1992). A feminist vision for clinical education. In S. Dowling (Ed.), *Proceedings of the 1992 National Conference on Supervision—Total quality supervision: Effecting optimal performance* (pp. 41-45). Council of Supervisors in Speech-Language Pathology and Audiology, Nashville, TN.

Pickering, M., & McCready, V. (1983). Supervisory journals: An "inside" look at supervision. *SUPERvision, 7*, 5-7.

Pickering, M., & McCready, V. (1990). *Interpersonal communication skills: A process in action. In Clinical supervision across settings: Communication and collaboration* (pp. 23-35). Rockville, MD: American Speech-Language-Hearing Association.

Powell, R. G., & Harville, B. (1990). The effects of teacher immediacy and clarity on instructional outcomes: An intercultural assessment. *Communication Education, 39*, 369-379.

Powell, T. (1987). A rating scale for measurement of attitudes toward clinical supervision. *SUPERvision, 11*, 31-34.

Rassi, J. (1978). *Supervision in audiology*. Baltimore, MD: University Park Press.

Rassi, J. (1987). The uniqueness of audiology supervision. In M. Crago & M. Pickering (Eds.), *Supervision in human communication disorders: Perspectives on a process* (pp. 31-54). San Diego, CA: Singular.

Roberts, J., & Smith, K. (1982). Supervisor-supervisee role differences and consistency of behavior in supervisory conferences. *Journal of Speech and Hearing Research, 25,* 428-434.

Russell, L. (1976). *Aspects of supervision.* Unpublished manuscript, Temple University, Philadelphia, PA.

Russell, L., & Engle, B. (1977). *A study of the supervisory process.* Paper presented at the convention of the New Jersey Speech and Hearing Association.

Russell, L., & Halfond, M. (1985). *An expanded view of the evaluative component of clinical supervision.* Paper presented at the annual convention of the American Speech-Language-Hearing Association, Washington, DC.

Schill, M., & Swanson, D. (1993). Use of an audiotaped dialogue journal in the supervisory process: A case study. *The Supervisor's Forum, 33*-35.

Schubert, G. (1978). *Introduction to clinical supervision.* St. Louis, MO: W. H. Green.

Seymour, C. (1992). Women's ways of supervising: Juggling, balancing, and walking a tightrope life under the big top. In S. Dowling (Ed.), *Proceedings of the 1992 National Conference on Supervision—Total quality supervision: Effecting optimal performance* (pp. 32-37). Council of Supervisors in Speech-Language Pathology and Audiology, Nashville, TN.

Shapiro, D. (1985). Clinical supervision: A process in progress. *National Student Speech-Language-Hearing Association Journal.*

Sleight, C. (1985). Confidence and anxiety in student clinicians. *The Clinical Supervisor, 3,* 25-48.

Smith, K. J. (1977). *Identification of perceived effectiveness components in the individual supervisory conference in speech pathology and an evaluation of the relationship between ratings and content in the conference* (Doctoral dissertation). Retrieved from ProQuest Dissertations and Theses Global. (Accession No. 7813175) http://proxyiub. uits.iu.edu/login?url=https://search.proquest.com/docview/302869635?accountid=11620

Smith, K., & Anderson, J. (1982a). Development and validation of an individual supervisory conference rating scale for use in speech-language pathology. *Journal of Speech and Hearing Research, 25,* 252-261.

Smith, K., & Anderson, J. (1982b). Relationship of perceived effectiveness to content in supervisory conferences in speech-language pathology. *Journal of Speech and Hearing Research, 25,* 243-251.

Strike-Roussos, C., Brasseur, J., Jimenez, B., O'Connor, L., & Boggs, T. (1991). *Analysis and evaluation in supervision: An ongoing process.* Presentation at the conference of the California Speech-Language-Hearing Association, Long Beach, CA.

Tannen, D. (1990). *You just don't understand: Women and men in conversation.* New York, NY: William Morrow, Ballatine.

Tannen, D. (1994). *Talking from 9 to 5.* New York, NY: William Morrow.

Tihen, L. D. (1983). *Expectations of student speech/language clinicians during their clinical practicum* (Doctoral dissertation). Retrieved from ProQuest Dissertations and Theses Global. (Accession No. 8401620) http://proxyiub. uits.iu.edu/login?url=https://search.proquest.com/docview/303160597?accountid=11620

Tufts, L. (1983). *A content analysis of supervisory conferences in communicative disorders and the relationship of the content analysis system to the clinical experience of supervisees* (Doctoral dissertation). Retrieved from ProQuest Dissertations and Theses Global. (Accession No. 8401588) http://proxyiub.uits.iu.edu/login?url=https://search. proquest.com/docview/303266850?accountid=11620

Ulrich, S. (1990). The supervisory process: Tasks basic to effective clinical supervision. In *Clinical supervision across settings: Communication and collaboration* (pp. 9-22). Rockville, MD: American Speech-Language-Hearing Association.

Victor, S. (2013). Conflict management and supervision. *Perspectives in Administration and Supervision, 23*(2), 78-81. doi:10.1044/aaa23.2.78

Ward, L., & Webster, E. (1965). The training of clinical personnel: I. Issues in conceptualization. *Asha, 7,* 38-41.

Weller, R. (1971). *Verbal communication in instructional supervision.* New York, NY: Teachers College Press, Columbia University.

Wollman, I. L., & Conover, H. B. (1979). The student clinician's reception of the supervisory process. *Ohio Journal of Speech and Hearing, 14,* 192-201.

 This chapter is a revision of that appearing in the 2003 edition of this book.

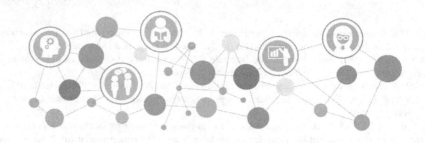

APPENDIX 3-1
CASEY'S SUPERVISORY SKILLS
SELF-ASSESSMENT INSTRUMENT

Instruction

The supervisory skills self-assessment guide contains a number of supervisory TASKS and COMPETENCIES which may or may not be appropriate to your specific working setting. Select the TASK(S) that you want to explore in your supervision development program and complete the self-assessment as follows:

Step 1

For each supervision COMPETENCY within the selected TASK(S) ask "How important is this COMPETENCY for effectiveness in my program?"

0	1	2	3	4	5	6	7	8	9	10
Not important or not applicable			Minimally important		Somewhat important		Rather important		Extremely important	

Insert your rating (0 to 10) under column 1 to the left of each item. Rate each item before going on to Step 2.

Step 2

For each supervision COMPETENCY ask "How satisfied am I with my ability to perform this skill?"

0	1	2	3	4	5	6	7	8	9	10
No experience or training in this area	Not quite satisfied			Moderately satisfied		Well satisfied			Highly satisfied	

Insert your rating (0 to 10) under column 2 to the left of each item. Rate each item before going on to Step 3.

Step 3

Calculate your GAP score for each item by subtracting the number in column 2 from the number in column 1. Insert the GAP score in the column labeled G. Note that some GAP scores will turn up as negative numbers and they should be recorded as such.

Step 4

Record your scores on the scoring sheets. Go on to Step 5 to obtain your Ideal (I) and Present Scores (P) for each TASK. Record these scores on the bottom of each TASK sheet.

Step 5

For each of the targeted TASKS add up the scores in column 1 and place the total on the line marked "Ideal Score" (I) at the bottom of the page.

Add up the scores in column 2 and place the total on the line marked "Present Score" (P) at the bottom of the page.

Divide the Present Score (P) by the Ideal Score (I)

Enter the percentage figure in the space provided at the bottom of page. Ex; P/I = _____%

90% to 100%   = You are satisfied and on top of the demands of TASK area.
80% to 89%   = You are getting by. Develop skill to higher degree.
79% to 79%   = You are struggling, TASK area should become a target for change.
60% to 0%   = You are struggling more than you should. Target change immediately.

Scoring

Step 1

Examine the numbers in the GAP columns for the TASK(S) you selected and circle any score +3 or greater. This suggests a discrepancy exists between the importance of that COMPETENCY and your present performance.

Step 2

Prioritize discrepant COMPETENCIES by listing them (highest point value to lowest point value) on the lines below labeled "ACTION ITEMS."

ACTION ITEMS
Score

_____   _____

_____   _____

_____   _____

_____   _____

_____   _____

_____   _____

_____   _____

Score Interpretation
+6, +7, +8, +9 Needs immediate action, NOW
+4, +5 Needs action sometime soon
+3 Needs action

Step 3

Examine the numbers in the GAP columns for each of the TASK(S) you selected and place an "X" over any score -3 or greater. This means you are "overqualified" in light of your present needs.

Step 4

Prioritize the skills you are most qualified in by listing them on the lines below labeled "AREA OF STRENGTH". Examine the numbers in column 2 for each of the selected TASKS. List all COMPETENCIES for which you scored an 8, 9, or 10.

AREA OF STRENGTH
Score

_____   _____

_____   _____

_____   _____

_____   _____

_____   _____

_____   _____

_____   _____

Interpretation

Congratulations! These are your areas of greatest strength as a supervisor. You should feel qualified to help other supervisors develop skills in these COMPETENCY areas.

1. Establishing and Maintaining an Effective Working Relationship

   1   2   G

   __/__/__   1. Ability to facilitate an understanding of the clinical and supervisory processes.

   __/__/__   2. Ability to organize and provide information regarding the logical sequences of supervisory interaction, e.g., joint setting of goals and objectives, data collection and analysis, evaluation.

   __/__/__   3. Ability to interact from a contemporary perspective with the supervisee in both the clinical and supervisory process.

   __/__/__   4. Ability to apply learning principles in the supervisory process.

   __/__/__   5. Ability to apply skills of interpersonal communication in the supervisory process.

   __/__/__   6. Ability to facilitate independent thinking and problem solving by the supervisee.

   __/__/__   7. Ability to maintain a professional and supportive relationship that allows supervisor and supervisee growth.

   __/__/__   8. Ability to interact with the supervisee objectively.

   __/__/__   9. Ability to establish joint communication regarding expectations and responsibilities in the clinical and supervisory processes.

   __/__/__   10. Ability to evaluate, with the supervisee, the effectiveness of the ongoing supervisory relationship.

   Ideal Score (I)   _____   P/I = _____%
   Present Score (P)   _____

2. Assisting in Developing Clinical Goals and Objectives

   1   2   G

   __/__/__   1. Ability to assist the supervisee in planning effective client goals and objectives.

   __/__/__   2. Ability to plan, with the supervisee, effective goals and objectives for clinical and professional growth.

   __/__/__   3. Ability to assist the supervisee in using observation and assessment in preparation of client goals and objectives.

_/_/_ 4. Ability to assist the supervisee in using self-analysis and previous evaluation in preparation goals and objectives for professional growth.

_/_/_ 5. Ability to assist the supervisee in assigning priorities to clinical goals and objectives.

_/_/_ 6. Ability to assist the supervisee in assigning priorities to goals and objectives for professional growth.

Ideal Score (I)   _____   P/I = _____%
Present Score (P)   _____

3. Assisting in Developing and Refining Assessment Skills

1   2   G

_/_/_ 1. Ability to share current research findings and evaluation procedures in communication disorders.

_/_/_ 2. Ability to facilitate an integration of research findings in client assessment.

_/_/_ 3. Ability to assist the supervisee in providing rationale for assessment procedures.

_/_/_ 4. Ability to assist supervisee in communicating assessment procedures and rationales.

_/_/_ 5. Ability to assist the supervisee in integrating findings and observations to make appropriate recommendations.

_/_/_ 6. Ability to facilitate the supervisee's independent planning of assessment.

Ideal Score (I)   _____   P/I = _____%
Present Score (P)   _____

4. Assisting in Developing and Refining Assessment Skills

1   2   G

_/_/_ 1. Ability to share current research findings and management procedures in communication disorders.

_/_/_ 2. Ability to facilitate an integration of research findings in client management.

_/_/_ 3. Ability to assist the supervisee in providing rationale for treatment procedures.

_/_/_ 4. Ability to assist the supervisee in identifying appropriate sequences for client change.

_/_/_ 5. Ability to assist the supervisee in adjusting steps in the progression toward a goal.

_/_/_ 6. Ability to assist the supervisee in the description and measurement of client and clinician change.

_/_/_ 7. Ability to assist the supervisee in documenting client and clinician change.

_/_/_ 8. Ability to assist the supervisee in integrating documented client and clinician change to evaluate progress and specify future recommendations.

Ideal Score (I)   _____   P/I = _____%
Present Score (P)   _____

5. Demonstrating and Participating in Clinical Process

1   2   G

_/_/_ 1. Ability to determine jointly when demonstration is appropriate.

_/_/_ 2. Ability to demonstrate or participate in an effective client-clinician relationship.

_/_/_ 3. Ability to demonstrate a variety of clinical techniques and participate with the supervisee in clinical management.

__/__/____ 4. Ability to demonstrate and use jointly the specific materials and equipment of the profession.

__/__/____ 5. Ability to demonstrate or participate jointly in counseling of clients or family/guardian of clients.

Ideal Score (I) _____   P/I = _____%
Present Score (P) _____

6. Assisting in Observing and Analyzing Assessment and Treatment

__1__2__G__

__/__/____ 1. Ability to assist the supervisee in learning a variety of data collection procedures.

__/__/____ 2. Ability to assist the supervisee in selecting and executing data collection procedures.

__/__/____ 3. Ability to assist the supervisee in accurately recording data.

__/__/____ 4. Ability to assist the supervisee in analyzing and interpreting data objectively.

__/__/____ 5. Ability to assist the supervisee in revising plans for client management based on data obtained.

Ideal Score (I) _____   P/I = _____%
Present Score (P) _____

7. Maintenance of Clinical and Supervisory Records

__1__2__G__

__/__/____ 1. Ability to assist the supervisee in applying record-keeping systems to supervisory and clinical records.

__/__/____ 2. Ability to assist the supervisee in effectively documenting supervisory and clinically related interactions.

__/__/____ 3. Ability to assist the supervisee in organizing records to facilitate easy retrieval of information concerning clinical and supervisory interactions.

__/__/____ 4. Ability to assist the supervisee to establishing and following policies and procedures to protect the confidentiality of clinical and supervisory records.

__/__/____ 5. Ability to share information regarding documentation requirements of various accrediting and regulatory agencies and third-party funding sources.

Ideal Score (I) _____   P/I = _____%
Present Score (P) _____

8. Planning, Executing, and Analyzing Supervisory Conferences

__1__2__G__

__/__/____ 1. Ability to determine with the supervisee when a conference should be scheduled.

__/__/____ 2. Ability to assist the supervisee in planning a supervisory conference agenda.

__/__/____ 3. Ability to involve the supervisee in jointly establishing a conference agenda.

__/__/____ 4. Ability to involve the supervisee in joint discussion of previously identified clinical or supervisory data or issues.

__/__/____ 5. Ability to interact with the supervisee in a manner that facilitates the supervisee's self-exploration and problem solving.

__/__/____ 6. Ability to adjust conference content based on the supervisee's level of training and experience.

__/__/____ 7. Ability to encourage and maintain supervisee in making commitments or changes in clinical behavior.

___/___/___ 8. Ability to assist the supervisee in making commitments for changes in clinical behavior.

___/___/___ 9. Ability to involve the supervisee in ongoing analysis of supervisory interactions.

Ideal Score (I)   _____   P/I = _____%
Present Score (P)   _____

9. Assisting in Evaluation of Clinical Performance

   1   2   G

___/___/___ 1. Ability to assist the supervisee in the use of clinician evaluation tools.

___/___/___ 2. Ability to assist the supervisee in the description and measurement of his/her progress and achievement.

___/___/___ 3. Ability to assist the supervisee in developing skills of self-evaluation.

___/___/___ 4. Ability to evaluate clinical skills with the supervisee for purposes of grade assignment, completion of Clinical Fellowship Year, professional advancement, and so on.

Ideal Score (I)   _____   P/I = _____%
Present Score (P)   _____

10. Developing Skills of Verbal Reporting, Writing, and Editing

   1   2   G

___/___/___ 1. Ability to assist the supervisee in identifying appropriate information to be included in a verbal or written report.

___/___/___ 2. Ability to assist the supervisee in presenting information in a logical concise and sequential manner.

___/___/___ 3. Ability to assist the supervisee in using appropriate professional terminology and style in verbal and written reporting.

___/___/___ 4. Ability to assist the supervisee in adapting verbal and written reports to the work environment and communication situation.

___/___/___ 5. Ability to alter and edit a report as appropriate while preserving the supervisee's writing style.

Ideal Score (I)   _____   P/I = _____%
Present Score (P)   _____

11. Sharing Ethical, Legal, Regulatory, and Reimbursement Information

   1   2   G

___/___/___ 1. Ability to communicate to the supervisee a knowledge of professional codes of ethics, e.g., ASHA.

___/___/___ 2. Ability to communicate to the supervisee an understanding of legal and regulatory documents and their impact on the practice of the profession (licensure, PL 94-142, Medicare, Medical, and so on).

___/___/___ 3. Ability to communicate to the supervisee an understanding of reimbursement policies and procedures of the work setting.

___/___/___ 4. Ability to communicate a knowledge of supervisee rights and appeal procedures specific to the work setting.

Ideal Score (I)   _____   P/I = _____%
Present Score (P)   _____

12. Modeling and Facilitating Professional Conduct

<u>1   2   G</u>

___/___/___   1. Ability to assumex responsibility.

___/___/___   2. Ability to analyze, evaluate, and modify own behavior.

___/___/___   3. Ability to demonstrate ethical and legal conduct.

___/___/___   4. Ability to meet and respect deadlines.

___/___/___   5. Ability to maintain professional protocols (respect for confidentiality, etc.).

___/___/___   6. Ability to provide current information regarding professional standards (PSB, ESB, licensure, teacher certification, etc.).

___/___/___   7. Ability to communicate information regarding fees, billing procedures, and third-party reimbursement.

___/___/___   8. Ability to demonstrate familiarity with professional issues.

___/___/___   9. Ability to demonstrate continued professional growth.

Ideal Score (I)   _____   P/I = _____%
Present Score (P)   _____

13. Research Skills in Clinical or Supervisory Process

<u>1   2   G</u>

___/___/___   1. Ability to read, interpret and apply clinical and supervisory research.

___/___/___   2. Ability to formulate clinical or supervisory research questions.

___/___/___   3. Ability to investigate clinical or supervisory research questions.

___/___/___   4. Ability to support or refute clinical or supervisory research findings.

___/___/___   5. Ability to report results of clinical or supervisory, research and disseminate as appropriate, e.g., in-service, conference, publications.

Ideal Score (I)   _____   P/I = _____%
Present Score (P)   _____

CASEY'S CLINICIAN/SUPERVISEE SKILLS SELF-ASSESSMENT INSTRUMENT

Instruction

The clinician/supervisee self-assessment guide contains a number of supervisory TASKS and COMPETENCIES which may or may not be appropriate to your specific working setting. Select the TASK(S) that you want to explore in your supervision development program and complete the self-assessment as follows:

Step 1

For each clinician/supervisee COMPETENCY within the selected TASK(S) ask "How important is this COMPETENCY for effectiveness in my program?"

0	1	2	3	4	5	6	7	8	9	10
Not important or not applicable			Minimally important		Somewhat important		Rather important		Extremely important	

Insert your rating (0 to 10) under column 1 to the left of each item. Rate each item before going on to Step 2.

Step 2

For each clinician/supervisee COMPETENCY ask "How satisfied am I with my ability to perform this skill?

0	1	2	3	4	5	6	7	8	9	10
No experience or training in this area		Not quite satisfied		Moderately satisfied		Well satisfied			Highly satisfied	

Insert your rating (0 to 10) under column 2 to the left of each item. Rate each item before going on to Step 3.

Step 3

Calculate your GAP score for each item by subtracting the number in column 2 from the number in column 1. Insert the GAP score in the column labeled G. Note that some GAP scores will turn up as negative numbers and they should be recorded as such.

Step 4

Record your scores on the scoring sheets. Go on to Step 5 to obtain your Ideal (I) and Present Scores (P) for each TASK. Record these scores on the bottom of each TASK sheet.

Step 5

For each of the targeted TASK(S) add up the scores in column 1 and place the total on the line marked "Ideal Score" (I) at the bottom of the page.

Add up the scores in column 2 and place the total on the line marked "Present Score" (P) at the bottom of the page.

Divide the Present Score (P) by the Ideal Score (I)

Enter the percentage figure in the space provided at the bottom of page. Ex; P/I = _____ %

90% to 100%   = You are satisfied and on top of the demands of TASK area.
80% to 89%   = You are getting by. Develop skill to higher degree.
79% to 79%   = You are struggling, TASK area should become a target for change.
60% to 0%   = You are struggling more than you should. Target change immediately.

Scoring

Step 1

Examine the numbers in the GAP columns for the TASK(S) you selected and circle any score +3 or greater. This suggests a discrepancy exists between the importance of that COMPETENCY and your present performance.

Step 2

Prioritize decrepant COMPETENCIES by listing them (highest point value to lowest point value) on the lines below labeled "ACTION ITEMS."

ACTION ITEMS
Score

_____   _____
_____   _____
_____   _____
_____   _____
_____   _____
_____   _____
_____   _____
_____   _____

Score Interpretation
+6, +7, +8, +9 Needs immediate action, NOW
+4, +5 Needs action sometime soon
+3 Needs action

Step 3

Examine the numbers in the GAP columns for each of the TASK(S) you selected and place an "X". over any score -3 or greater. This means you are "overqualified" in light of your present needs.

Step 4

Prioritize the skills you are most qualified in by listing them on the lines below labeled "AREA OF STRENGTH." Examine the numbers in column 2 for each of the selected TASKS. List all COMPETENCIES for which you scored an 8, 9, or 10.

AREA OF STRENGTH
Score

_____   _____
_____   _____
_____   _____
_____   _____
_____   _____
_____   _____
_____   _____
_____   _____

Interpretation

Congratulations! These are your areas of greatest strength as a supervisor. You should feel qualified to help other supervisors develop skills in these COMPETENCY areas.

1. Establishing and Maintaining an Effective Working Relationship

1 2 G

__/__/__ 1. Ability to demonstrate an understanding of the clinical and supervisory processes.

__/__/__ 2. Ability to demonstrate knowledge of the logical sequences of clinical interaction and supervisory interaction, e.g., joint setting of goals and objectives, data collection and analysis, evaluation.

__/__/__ 3. Ability to interact from a contemporary perspective with the supervisor in both the clinical and supervisory process.

___/___/___ 4. Ability to apply learning principles in the clinical process.

___/___/___ 5. Ability to apply skills of interpersonal communication in the clinical and the supervisory process.

___/___/___ 6. Ability to demonstrate independent thinking and problem solving.

___/___/___ 7. Ability to maintain a professional and supportive relationship that allows supervisor and supervisee growth.

___/___/___ 8. Ability to interact with the supervisor objectively.

___/___/___ 9. Ability to demonstrate joint communication regarding expectations and responsibilities in the clinical and supervisory processes.

___/___/___ 10. Ability to evaluate, with the supervisor, the effectiveness of the ongoing supervisory relationship.

Ideal Score (I)   _____   P/I = _____%
Present Score (P)   _____

2. Developing Clinical Goals and Objectives

1   2   G

___/___/___ 1. Ability to plan effective client goals and objectives.

___/___/___ 2. Ability to plan, effective goals and objectives for clinical and professional growth.

___/___/___ 3. Ability to use observation and assessment in preparation of client goals and objectives.

___/___/___ 4. Ability to use self-analysis and previous evaluation in preparation goals and objectives for professional growth.

___/___/___ 5. Ability to assign priorities to clinical goals and objectives.

___/___/___ 6. Ability to assign priorities to goals and objectives for professional growth.

Ideal Score (I)   _____   P/I = _____%
Present Score (P)   _____

3. Developing and Refining Assessment Skills

1   2   G

___/___/___ 1. Ability to share knowledge of current research findings and evaluation procedures in communication disorders.

___/___/___ 2. Ability to integrate and demonstrate knowledge of research findings in client assessment.

___/___/___ 3. Ability to provide a rationale for assessment procedures.

___/___/___ 4. Ability to communicate assessment procedures and rationales.

___/___/___ 5. Ability to integrate findings and observations to make appropriate recommendations.

___/___/___ 6. Ability to demonstrate independent planning of assessment.

Ideal Score (I)   _____   P/I = _____%
Present Score (P)   _____

4. Developing and Refining Assessment Skills

1   2   G

___/___/___ 1. Ability to share current research findings and management procedures in communication disorders.

___/___/___ 2. Ability to demonstrate an integration of research findings in client management.

___/___/___ 3. Ability to provide a rationale for treatment procedures.

___/___/___ 4. Ability to identify appropriate sequences for client change.

___/___/___ 5. Ability to adjust steps in the progression toward a goal.

___/___/___ 6. Ability to describe and measure client and clinician change.

___/___/___ 7. Ability to document client and clinician change.

___/___/___ 8. Ability to integrate documented client and clinician change to evaluate progress and specify future recommendations.

Ideal Score (I)   _____   P/I = _____%
Present Score (P)   _____

5. Interacting in the Clinical Process

__1__2__G__

___/___/___ 1. Ability to determine jointly when demonstration is appropriate.

___/___/___ 2. Ability to demonstrate an effective client-clinician relationship.

___/___/___ 3. Ability to demonstrate the use of a variety of clinical techniques and participate with the supervisor in clinical management.

___/___/___ 4. Ability to demonstrate and use the specific materials and equipment of the profession.

___/___/___ 5. Ability to demonstrate or participate jointly in counseling of clients or family/guardian of clients.

Ideal Score (I)   _____   P/I = _____%
Present Score (P)   _____

6. Observing and Analyzing Assessment and Treatment

__1__2__G__

___/___/___ 1. Ability to demonstrate knowledge of a variety of data collection procedures.

___/___/___ 2. Ability to select and execute data collection procedures.

___/___/___ 3. Ability to accurately record data.

___/___/___ 4. Ability to analyze and interpret data objectively.

___/___/___ 5. Ability to revise plans for client management based on data obtained.

Ideal Score (I)   _____   P/I = _____%
Present Score (P)   _____

7. Developing and Maintaining Clinical and Supervisory Records

__1__2__G__

___/___/___ 1. Ability to apply record-keeping systems to supervisory and clinical records.

___/___/___ 2. Ability to effectively document supervisory and clinically related interactions.

___/___/___ 3. Ability to organize records to facilitate easy retrieval of information concerning clinical and supervisory interactions.

___/___/___ 4. Ability to establish and follow policies and procedures to protect the confidentiality of clinical and supervisory records.

___/___/___ 5. Ability to demonstrate knowledge regarding documentation requirements of various accrediting and regulatory agencies and third-party funding sources.

Ideal Score (I)   _____   P/I = _____%
Present Score (P)   _____

8. Planning, Executing, and Analyzing Supervisory Conferences

<u>1   2   G</u>

___/___/___   1. Ability to determine with the supervisor when a conference should be scheduled.

___/___/___   2. Ability to plan a supervisory conference agenda.

___/___/___   3. Ability to demonstrate involvement in jointly establishing a conference agenda.

___/___/___   4. Ability to jointly discuss with the supervisor previously identified clinical or supervisory data or issues.

___/___/___   5. Ability to demonstrate self-exploration and problem solving.

___/___/___   6. Ability to communicate level of training and experience.

___/___/___   7. Ability to maintain motivation for continued self-growth.

___/___/___   8. Ability to make commitments for changes in clinical behavior.

___/___/___   9. Ability to demonstrate ongoing analysis of supervisory interactions.

Ideal Score (I)   _____   P/I = _____%

Present Score (P)   _____

9. Evaluating Clinical Performance

<u>1   2   G</u>

___/___/___   1. Ability to use clinician evaluation tools.

___/___/___   2. Ability to describe and measure progress and achievement.

___/___/___   3. Ability to develop and demonstrate skills of self-evaluation.

___/___/___   4. Ability to evaluate clinical skills with the supervisor for purposes of grade assignment, completion of Clinical Fellowship Year, professional advancement, and so on.

Ideal Score (I)   _____   P/I = _____%

Present Score (P)   _____

10. Demonstrating Skills of Verbal Reporting, Writing, and Editing

<u>1   2   G</u>

___/___/___   1. Ability to identify appropriate information to be included in a verbal or written report.

___/___/___   2. Ability to present information in a logical concise and sequential manner.

___/___/___   3. Ability to use appropriate professional terminology and style in verbal and written reporting.

___/___/___   4. Ability to adapt verbal and written reports to the work environment and communication situation.

___/___/___   5. Ability to alter and edit a report as appropriate.

Ideal Score (I)   _____   P/I = _____%

Present Score (P)   _____

11. Demonstrating Knowledge of Ethical Legal Regulatory and Reimbursement Information

<u>1   2   G</u>

___/___/___   1. Ability to communicate a knowledge of professional codes of ethics, e.g., ASHA, State Licensure boards, and so on.

___/___/___   2. Ability to communicate an understanding of legal and regulatory documents and their impact on the practice of the profession (licensure, PL 94-142, Medicare, Medical, and so on).

___/___/___ 3. Ability to communicate an understanding of reimbursement policies and procedures of the work setting.

___/___/___ 4. Ability to communicate a knowledge of rights and appeal procedures specific to
the work setting.

Ideal Score (I)   _____   P/I = _____%
Present Score (P)   _____

12. Demonstrating Professional Conduct

1 2 G

___/___/___ 1. Ability to assume responsibility.

___/___/___ 2. Ability to analyze, evaluate, and modify own behavior.

___/___/___ 3. Ability to demonstrate ethical and legal conduct.

___/___/___ 4. Ability to meet and respect deadlines

___/___/___ 5. Ability to maintain professional protocols (respect for confidentiality, etc.).

___/___/___ 6. Ability to demonstrate knowledge of current regarding professional standards
(PSB, ESB, licensure, teacher certification, etc.).

___/___/___ 7. Ability to communicate information regarding fees, billing procedures, and third-
party reimbursement.

___/___/___ 8. Ability to demonstrate familiarity with professional issues.

___/___/___ 9. Ability to demonstrate continued professional growth.

Ideal Score (I)   _____   P/I = _____%
Present Score (P)   _____

13. Demonstrating Research Skills in Clinical Process

1 2 G

___/___/___ 1. Ability to read, interpret, and apply clinical research.

___/___/___ 2. Ability to formulate clinical research questions.

___/___/___ 3. Ability to investigate clinical research questions.

___/___/___ 4. Ability to support or refute clinical research findings.

___/___/___ 5. Ability to report results of clinical research and disseminate as appropriate, e.g.,
in-service, conference, publications.

Ideal Score (I)   _____   P/I = _____%
Present Score (P)   _____

APPENDIX 3-2
LARSON'S EXPECTATIONS RATING SCALE

Please give your assessment of what you expect will happen during your future individual supervisory conferences. Circle the number that best represents the expected level of occurrence of the behaviors suggested by each item. The numbers correspond to the following categories:

1 = to a very little extent
2 = to a little extent
3 = to some extent
4 = to a great extent
5 = to a very great extent

1. Do you expect your supervisors will help you set goals for your client?   1 2 3 4 5

2. Do you expect your supervisors will use conference time to discuss ways to improve materials?   1 2 3 4 5

3. Do you expect your supervisors will motivate you to perform at your highest potential?   1 2 3 4 5

4. Do you expect you will state the objectives of your conferences?   1 2 3 4 5

5. Do you expect your supervisors will pay attention to what you are saying whenever you talk with them?   1 2 3 4 5

6. Do you expect you will ask many questions during your conferences?   1 2 3 4 5

7. Do you expect your supervisors will use your ideas in discussion during conferences?   1 2 3 4 5

8. Do you expect your supervisors will function as teachers who are instructing you?   1 2 3 4 5

9. Do you expect you will inform your supervisors of your needs?   1 2 3 4 5

10. Do you expect your supervisors will tell you the weaknesses in your clinical behavior?   1 2 3 4 5

11. Do you expect you will use conference time to provide information about the clinical session to your supervisors?   1 2 3 4 5

12. Do you expect your supervisors will be willing to listen to your professional problems?   1 2 3 4 5

13. Do you expect your supervisors will be available to talk to you immediately following clinical sessions?   1 2 3 4 5

14. Do you expect your supervisors will be the superiors and you the subordinate in the relationship?   1 2 3 4 5

15. Do you expect you will give value judgments about your clinical behavior?   1 2 3 4 5

16. Do you expect your supervisors will give suggestions on therapy techniques to be used in subsequent clinical sessions?   1 2 3 4 5

17. Do you expect your supervisors will be supportive of you?   1 2 3 4 5

18. Do you expect discussions with your supervisors will be focused on clients' behaviors rather than on your behavior?   1 2 3 4 5

19. Do you expect your supervisors will give a rationale for their statements or suggestions?   1 2 3 4 5

20. Do you expect your supervisors will demonstrate how to improve your performance?   1 2 3 4 5

21. Do you expect your supervisors will give you the opportunity to express your opinions?   1 2 3 4 5

22. Do you expect your supervisors will ask you to think about strategies that might have been done differently or that may be done in the future?   1 2 3 4 5

23. Do you expect your supervisors will be willing to listen to your personal problems?   1 2 3 4 5

24. How often do you expect your supervisors will meet with you for an individual conference?   1 = most expected
    5 = least expected
    _____ weekly throughout practicum   1 2 3 4 5
    _____ weekly at beginning and end of practicum   1 2 3 4 5
    _____ at your request   1 2 3 4 5
    _____ at supervisor's request   1 2 3 4 5

25. What information sources have influenced your responses to the previous questions?   1 = most influential
    5 = least influential

    Please check all applicable sources and then rate only those sources checked according to level of influence.
    _____ peer group (students at same training level)   1 2 3 4 5
    _____ graduate student clinicians (at more advanced level than you)   1 2 3 4 5
    _____ clinical supervisors   1 2 3 4 5
    _____ academic courses   1 2 3 4 5
    _____ training program policies (e.g., practicum manual)   1 2 3 4 5
    _____ other (please specify)   1 2 3 4 5

    _____

26. Do you have any expectations about supervision which have not been covered in the previous questions? If so, please specify in the space below.

    _____
    _____
    _____

Reprinted with permission from Larson, L. C. (1981). *Perceived supervisory needs and expectations of experienced vs. inexperienced student clinicians* (Doctoral dissertation). Retrieved from ProQuest Dissertations and Theses Global. (Accession No. 8211183) http://proxyiub.uits.iu.edu/login?url=https://search.proquest.com/docview/303157417?accountid=11620

APPENDIX 3-3
LARSON'S NEEDS RATING SCALE

Regardless of what you indicated about your expectations, now indicate to what extent you need the same behaviors to occur during your future individual supervisory conferences. Circle the number that best represents the level of occurrence at which the behaviors suggested by each item are needed. The numbers correspond to the following categories:

1 = to a very little extent
2 = to a little extent
3 = to some extent
4 = to a great extent
5 = to a very great extent

1. To what extent do you need your supervisors to give suggestions on therapy techniques to be used in subsequent clinical sessions?   1 2 3 4 5

2. To what extent do you need your supervisors to pay attention to what you are saying whenever you talk with them?   1 2 3 4 5

3. To what extent do you need to inform your supervisors of your needs?   1 2 3 4 5

4. To what extent do you need your supervisors to use your ideas in discussion during conferences?   1 2 3 4 5

5. To what extent do you need your supervisors to be available to talk to you immediately following clinical sessions?   1 2 3 4 5

6. To what extent do you need your supervisors to ask you to think about strategies that might have been done differently or that may be done in the future?   1 2 3 4 5

7. To what extent do you need your supervisors to function teachers who are instructing you?   1 2 3 4 5

8. To what extent do you need to give value judgments about your clinical behavior?   1 2 3 4 5

9. To what extent do you need your supervisors to demonstrate how to improve your performance?   1 2 3 4 5

10. To what extent do you need discussions with your supervisors to be focused on clients' behaviors rather than on your behavior?   1 2 3 4 5

11. To what extent do you need your supervisors to be willing to listen to your professional problems?   1 2 3 4 5

12. To what extent do you need to use conference time to provide information about the clinical session to your supervisors?   1 2 3 4 5

13. To what extent do you need your supervisors to tell you the weaknesses in your clinical behavior?   1 2 3 4 5

14. To what extent do you need to ask many questions during your conferences?   1 2 3 4 5

15. To what extent do you need your supervisors to give a rationale for their statements or suggestions?   1 2 3 4 5

16. To what extent do you need your supervisors to be the superiors   1 2 3 4 5
    and you the subordinate in the relationship?

17. To what extent do you need your supervisors to give you the oppor-   1 2 3 4 5
    tunity to express your opinions?

18. To what extent do you need your supervisors to use conference   1 2 3 4 5
    time to discuss ways to improve materials?

19. To what extent do you need your supervisors to be willing to listen   1 2 3 4 5
    to your personal problems?

20. To what extent do you need to state the objectives of your   1 2 3 4 5
    conferences?

21. To what extent do you need your supervisors to help you set goals   1 2 3 4 5
    for your client?

22. To what extent do you need your supervisors to be supportive of   1 2 3 4 5
    you?

23. To what extent do you need your supervisors to motivate you to   1 2 3 4 5
    perform at your highest potential?

24. How often do you need your supervisors to meet with you for an   1 = most needed
    individual conference?   5 = least needed

    Please check all applicable sources and then rate only those sources
    checked according to level of influence.

    ____ weekly throughout practicum   1 2 3 4 5
    ____ weekly at beginning and end of practicum   1 2 3 4 5
    ____ at your request   1 2 3 4 5
    ____ at supervisor's request   1 2 3 4 5

25. What information sources have influenced your responses to the   1 = most influential
    previous questions?   5 = least influential

    Please check all applicable sources and then rate only those sources
    checked according to level of influence.

    ____ peer group (students at same training level)   1 2 3 4 5
    ____ graduate student clinicians (at more advanced level than you)   1 2 3 4 5
    ____ clinical supervisors   1 2 3 4 5
    ____ academic courses   1 2 3 4 5
    ____ training program policies (e.g., practicum manual)   1 2 3 4 5
    ____ other (please specify)   1 2 3 4 5

    _____

26. Do you have any supervisory needs which have not been covered in the previous questions?
    If so, please specify in the space below.

    _____

    _____

    _____

Reprinted with permission from Larson, L. C. (1981). *Perceived supervisory needs and expectations of experienced vs. inexperienced student clinicians* (Doctoral dissertation). Retrieved from ProQuest Dissertations and Theses Global. (Accession No. 8211183) http://proxyiub.uits.iu.edu/login?url=https://search.proquest.com/docview/303157417?accountid=11620

APPENDIX 3-4
TIHEN'S EXPECTATIONS SCALE

Student:

Please complete both sections of this scale.

Section I contains a number of possible expectations that a student may have of his/her clinical practicum supervisor(s). Each expectation is to receive both a "Student" and "Supervisor" rating. The "Student" rating represents the importance which you, as a student, presently attach to the expectation. The "Supervisor" rating represents the importance which you perceive your clinical supervisor(s), by their actions, as having attached to the expectation. On both the "student" and "supervisor" scales, the relative importance of each expectation is to be rated from one (1) to seven (7), with (1) representing a very unimportant expectation, and seven (7), with representing a very important expectation. A rating of four (4) would represent a neutral rating of the expectation. The following example is provided for clarification purposes.

The supervisor should grade my lesson plans.

(Student)   *Very Unimportant*   1   2   3   4   5   6   7   *Very Important*

(Supervisor)   *Very Unimportant*   1   2   3   4   5   6   7   *Very Important*

In the previous example, the student's circled rating of two (2) on the "student" scale indicated that the student places relatively little importance on having the supervisor grade his/her lesson plans. The student's circled rating of six (6) on the "supervisor" scale indicates that the student perceives his/her supervisor as attaching greater importance to the grading of lesson plans.

Since you will be attaching relative importance to the expectations, with some being more important to you than others, READ ALL OF THE POSSIBLE EXPECTATIONS IN SECTION I, CAREFULLY, BEFORE RATING ANY ITEMS. AFTER READING ALL THE POSSIBLE EXPECTATIONS, RETURN TO ITEM ONE, AND RATE EACH EXPECTATION.

*Students completing Section I who have not yet begun their clinical practicum should provide ratings on the "student" scale ONLY. They would not enter any information on the "supervisor" scale.

Supervisor:

This scale contains a number of possible expectations that a student may have of his/her practicum supervisor(s). Each expectation is to receive both a "student" and "supervisor" rating.

The "supervisor" rating represents the importance which you presently attach to the expectation.

The "student" rating represents the importance which you perceive your student(s), by their actions, as having attached to that expectation.

Since you will be attaching relative importance to the expectations, with some being more important than others, PLEASE READ ALL ITEMS CAREFULLY FIRST, RETURN TO ITEM ONE AND CIRCLE YOUR CHOICES.

Student Expectations of Their Clinical Supervisor(s)

Rating Description

1 = Very Unimportant   5 = Low Importance
2 = Medium Unimportant   6 = Medium Importance
3 = Low Unimportance   7 = Important
4 = Neutral

I expect that:
- The supervisor should provide me with suggestions during the supervisory conference.

(Student)   *Very Unimportant*   1   2   3   4   5   6   7   *Very Important*
(Supervisor)   *Very Unimportant*   1   2   3   4   5   6   7   *Very Important*

- The supervisor should demonstrate behavior modification techniques to control inappropriate behavior by my clients.

(Student)   *Very Unimportant*   1   2   3   4   5   6   7   *Very Important*
(Supervisor)   *Very Unimportant*   1   2   3   4   5   6   7   *Very Important*

- The supervisor should function as a teacher during my clinical practicum.

(Student)   *Very Unimportant*   1   2   3   4   5   6   7   *Very Important*
(Supervisor)   *Very Unimportant*   1   2   3   4   5   6   7   *Very Important*

- The supervisor should relate academic information to therapy situations.

(Student)   *Very Unimportant*   1   2   3   4   5   6   7   *Very Important*
(Supervisor)   *Very Unimportant*   1   2   3   4   5   6   7   *Very Important*

- The supervisor should evaluate my performance during the clinical practicum.

(Student)   *Very Unimportant*   1   2   3   4   5   6   7   *Very Important*
(Supervisor)   *Very Unimportant*   1   2   3   4   5   6   7   *Very Important*

- The supervisor should provide the opportunity for me to express my opinions during supervisory conferences.

(Student)   *Very Unimportant*   1   2   3   4   5   6   7   *Very Important*
(Supervisor)   *Very Unimportant*   1   2   3   4   5   6   7   *Very Important*

- The supervisor should provide the opportunity for me to evaluate my performance during the clinical practicum.

(Student)   *Very Unimportant*   1   2   3   4   5   6   7   *Very Important*
(Supervisor)   *Very Unimportant*   1   2   3   4   5   6   7   *Very Important*

- The supervisor and I should work together in determining the therapy goals and objectives for my clients.

(Student)   *Very Unimportant*   1   2   3   4   5   6   7   *Very Important*
(Supervisor)   *Very Unimportant*   1   2   3   4   5   6   7   *Very Important*

- The supervisor should be patient with me.

(Student)   *Very Unimportant*   1   2   3   4   5   6   7   *Very Important*
(Supervisor)   *Very Unimportant*   1   2   3   4   5   6   7   *Very Important*

- The supervisor should provide the opportunity for me to identify my clinical weaknesses.

(Student)   *Very Unimportant*   1   2   3   4   5   6   7   *Very Important*
(Supervisor)   *Very Unimportant*   1   2   3   4   5   6   7   *Very Important*

- The supervisor should provide the opportunity for me to identify my clinical strengths.

(Student)   *Very Unimportant*   1   2   3   4   5   6   7   *Very Important*
(Supervisor)   *Very Unimportant*   1   2   3   4   5   6   7   *Very Important*

- The supervisor should function as an evaluator during my clinical practicum.

(Student)   *Very Unimportant*   1   2   3   4   5   6   7   *Very Important*
(Supervisor)   *Very Unimportant*   1   2   3   4   5   6   7   *Very Important*

- The supervisor should provide the opportunity for me to regulate my own professional conduct.

(Student)   *Very Unimportant*   1   2   3   4   5   6   7   *Very Important*
(Supervisor)   *Very Unimportant*   1   2   3   4   5   6   7   *Very Important*

- The supervisor should encourage me to discuss my personal feelings about the clinical practicum.

(Student)   *Very Unimportant*   1   2   3   4   5   6   7   *Very Important*
(Supervisor)   *Very Unimportant*   1   2   3   4   5   6   7   *Very Important*

- The supervisor and I should work together in identifying my clinical strengths.

(Student)   *Very Unimportant*   1   2   3   4   5   6   7   *Very Important*
(Supervisor)   *Very Unimportant*   1   2   3   4   5   6   7   *Very Important*

- The supervisor and I should work together in identifying my clinical weaknesses.

(Student)   *Very Unimportant*   1   2   3   4   5   6   7   *Very Important*
(Supervisor)   *Very Unimportant*   1   2   3   4   5   6   7   *Very Important*

- The supervisor should provide the opportunity for me to develop therapy lesson plans.

(Student)   *Very Unimportant*   1   2   3   4   5   6   7   *Very Important*
(Supervisor)   *Very Unimportant*   1   2   3   4   5   6   7   *Very Important*

- The supervisor should evaluate my lesson plans.

(Student)   *Very Unimportant*   1   2   3   4   5   6   7   *Very Important*
(Supervisor)   *Very Unimportant*   1   2   3   4   5   6   7   *Very Important*

- The supervisor should evaluate me primarily for the purpose of making appropriate modifications in my clinical performance.

(Student)   *Very Unimportant*   1   2   3   4   5   6   7   *Very Important*
(Supervisor)   *Very Unimportant*   1   2   3   4   5   6   7   *Very Important*

- The supervisor should keep me informed of my progress throughout the clinical practicum.

(Student)   *Very Unimportant*   1   2   3   4   5   6   7   *Very Important*
(Supervisor)   *Very Unimportant*   1   2   3   4   5   6   7   *Very Important*

- The supervisor and I should work together in the writing of my clients' clinical reports.

(Student)   *Very Unimportant*   1   2   3   4   5   6   7   *Very Important*
(Supervisor)   *Very Unimportant*   1   2   3   4   5   6   7   *Very Important*

- The supervisor should provide me with the clinical techniques/strategies to be used with my clients.

(Student)   *Very Unimportant*   1   2   3   4   5   6   7   *Very Important*
(Supervisor)   *Very Unimportant*   1   2   3   4   5   6   7   *Very Important*

- The supervisor should be a warm, accepting person.

(Student)   *Very Unimportant*   1   2   3   4   5   6   7   *Very Important*
(Supervisor)   *Very Unimportant*   1   2   3   4   5   6   7   *Very Important*

- The supervisor should provide me with well-defined, objective criteria which will be used to determine my success in the clinical practicum.

(Student)   *Very Unimportant*   1   2   3   4   5   6   7   *Very Important*
(Supervisor)   *Very Unimportant*   1   2   3   4   5   6   7   *Very Important*

- The supervisor should provide me the opportunity to determine the therapy goals and objectives for my clients.

(Student)   *Very Unimportant*   1   2   3   4   5   6   7   *Very Important*
(Supervisor)   *Very Unimportant*   1   2   3   4   5   6   7   *Very Important*

- The supervisor and I should work together in developing therapy lesson plans.

(Student)   *Very Unimportant*   1   2   3   4   5   6   7   *Very Important*
(Supervisor)   *Very Unimportant*   1   2   3   4   5   6   7   *Very Important*

- The supervisor's comments and suggestions should be directed to my clinical behavior.

(Student)   *Very Unimportant*   1   2   3   4   5   6   7   *Very Important*
(Supervisor)   *Very Unimportant*   1   2   3   4   5   6   7   *Very Important*

- The supervisor should diagnose the clients' problems/needs.

(Student)   *Very Unimportant*   1   2   3   4   5   6   7   *Very Important*
(Supervisor) *Very Unimportant*   1   2   3   4   5   6   7   *Very Important*

- The supervisor should regulate my professional conduct.

(Student)   *Very Unimportant*   1   2   3   4   5   6   7   *Very Important*
(Supervisor) *Very Unimportant*   1   2   3   4   5   6   7   *Very Important*

- The supervisor should provide the opportunity for us to contribute information during supervisory conferences.

(Student)   *Very Unimportant*   1   2   3   4   5   6   7   *Very Important*
(Supervisor) *Very Unimportant*   1   2   3   4   5   6   7   *Very Important*

- The supervisor should tell me which diagnostic instruments are to be used with my clients.

(Student)   *Very Unimportant*   1   2   3   4   5   6   7   *Very Important*
(Supervisor) *Very Unimportant*   1   2   3   4   5   6   7   *Very Important*

- The supervisor should make positive value judgements about my clinical competence (praise).

(Student)   *Very Unimportant*   1   2   3   4   5   6   7   *Very Important*
(Supervisor) *Very Unimportant*   1   2   3   4   5   6   7   *Very Important*

- The supervisor should provide me behavior modification techniques to control inappropriate behavior by the clients.

(Student)   *Very Unimportant*   1   2   3   4   5   6   7   *Very Important*
(Supervisor) *Very Unimportant*   1   2   3   4   5   6   7   *Very Important*

- The supervisor should evaluate my clinical reports.

(Student)   *Very Unimportant*   1   2   3   4   5   6   7   *Very Important*
(Supervisor) *Very Unimportant*   1   2   3   4   5   6   7   *Very Important*

- The supervisor should have a sense of humor.

(Student)   *Very Unimportant*   1   2   3   4   5   6   7   *Very Important*
(Supervisor) *Very Unimportant*   1   2   3   4   5   6   7   *Very Important*

- The supervisor should provide the opportunity for me to write my clients' clinical reports.

(Student)   *Very Unimportant*   1   2   3   4   5   6   7   *Very Important*
(Supervisor) *Very Unimportant*   1   2   3   4   5   6   7   *Very Important*

- The supervisor should provide the opportunity for me to make suggestions during the supervisory conference.

(Student)   *Very Unimportant*   1   2   3   4   5   6   7   *Very Important*
(Supervisor) *Very Unimportant*   1   2   3   4   5   6   7   *Very Important*

- The supervisor and I should work together in regulating my own professional conduct.

(Student)   *Very Unimportant*   1   2   3   4   5   6   7   *Very Important*
(Supervisor)   *Very Unimportant*   1   2   3   4   5   6   7   *Very Important*

- The supervisor should talk more than me during supervisory conferences.

(Student)   *Very Unimportant*   1   2   3   4   5   6   7   *Very Important*
(Supervisor)   *Very Unimportant*   1   2   3   4   5   6   7   *Very Important*

- The supervisor should demonstrate diagnostic techniques/procedures with my clients.

(Student)   *Very Unimportant*   1   2   3   4   5   6   7   *Very Important*
(Supervisor)   *Very Unimportant*   1   2   3   4   5   6   7   *Very Important*

- The supervisor and I should work together in determining the clinical techniques/strategies to be used with my clients.

(Student)   *Very Unimportant*   1   2   3   4   5   6   7   *Very Important*
(Supervisor)   *Very Unimportant*   1   2   3   4   5   6   7   *Very Important*

- The supervisor should provide the opportunity for me to develop behavior modification procedures to control inappropriate behavior by my clients.

(Student)   *Very Unimportant*   1   2   3   4   5   6   7   *Very Important*
(Supervisor)   *Very Unimportant*   1   2   3   4   5   6   7   *Very Important*

- The supervisor should provide me with therapy goals and objectives for my clients.

(Student)   *Very Unimportant*   1   2   3   4   5   6   7   *Very Important*
(Supervisor)   *Very Unimportant*   1   2   3   4   5   6   7   *Very Important*

- The supervisor should provide the opportunity for me to ask questions during the supervisory conference.

(Student)   *Very Unimportant*   1   2   3   4   5   6   7   *Very Important*
(Supervisor)   *Very Unimportant*   1   2   3   4   5   6   7   *Very Important*

- The supervisor and I should work together in determining which diagnostic instruments are appropriate for use with my clients.

(Student)   *Very Unimportant*   1   2   3   4   5   6   7   *Very Important*
(Supervisor)   *Very Unimportant*   1   2   3   4   5   6   7   *Very Important*

- The supervisor should identify my clinical strengths.

(Student)   *Very Unimportant*   1   2   3   4   5   6   7   *Very Important*
(Supervisor)   *Very Unimportant*   1   2   3   4   5   6   7   *Very Important*

- The supervisor should provide the opportunity for me to determine the clinical techniques/strategies to be used with my clients.

(Student)	*Very Unimportant*	1	2	3	4	5	6	7	*Very Important*
(Supervisor)	*Very Unimportant*	1	2	3	4	5	6	7	*Very Important*

- The supervisor should be an understanding person.

(Student)	*Very Unimportant*	1	2	3	4	5	6	7	*Very Important*
(Supervisor)	*Very Unimportant*	1	2	3	4	5	6	7	*Very Important*

- The supervisor should be considerate of me.

(Student)	*Very Unimportant*	1	2	3	4	5	6	7	*Very Important*
(Supervisor)	*Very Unimportant*	1	2	3	4	5	6	7	*Very Important*

- The supervisor should identify my clinical weaknesses.

(Student)	*Very Unimportant*	1	2	3	4	5	6	7	*Very Important*
(Supervisor)	*Very Unimportant*	1	2	3	4	5	6	7	*Very Important*

- The supervisor should respect my individuality.

(Student)	*Very Unimportant*	1	2	3	4	5	6	7	*Very Important*
(Supervisor)	*Very Unimportant*	1	2	3	4	5	6	7	*Very Important*

- The supervisor should provide supervision that is free of anxiety.

(Student)	*Very Unimportant*	1	2	3	4	5	6	7	*Very Important*
(Supervisor)	*Very Unimportant*	1	2	3	4	5	6	7	*Very Important*

- The supervisor should provide the opportunity for me to diagnose the clients' problems/needs.

(Student)	*Very Unimportant*	1	2	3	4	5	6	7	*Very Important*
(Supervisor)	*Very Unimportant*	1	2	3	4	5	6	7	*Very Important*

- The supervisor should maintain confidentiality about my performance during the clinical practicum.

(Student)	*Very Unimportant*	1	2	3	4	5	6	7	*Very Important*
(Supervisor)	*Very Unimportant*	1	2	3	4	5	6	7	*Very Important*

- The supervisor and I should work together in the application of my academic work to therapy situations.

(Student)	*Very Unimportant*	1	2	3	4	5	6	7	*Very Important*
(Supervisor)	*Very Unimportant*	1	2	3	4	5	6	7	*Very Important*

- The supervisor and I should work together in evaluating my performance during the clinical practicum.

(Student)   *Very Unimportant*   1   2   3   4   5   6   7   *Very Important*
(Supervisor)   *Very Unimportant*   1   2   3   4   5   6   7   *Very Important*

- The supervisor should provide demonstration therapy with my clients.

(Student)   *Very Unimportant*   1   2   3   4   5   6   7   *Very Important*
(Supervisor)   *Very Unimportant*   1   2   3   4   5   6   7   *Very Important*

- The supervisor and I should work together in developing behavior modification procedures to control inappropriate behavior by my clients.

(Student)   *Very Unimportant*   1   2   3   4   5   6   7   *Very Important*
(Supervisor)   *Very Unimportant*   1   2   3   4   5   6   7   *Very Important*

- The supervisor should provide me with therapy lesson plans.

(Student)   *Very Unimportant*   1   2   3   4   5   6   7   *Very Important*
(Supervisor)   *Very Unimportant*   1   2   3   4   5   6   7   *Very Important*

- The supervisor should provide the opportunity for me to select the appropriate diagnostic instruments to use with my clients.

(Student)   *Very Unimportant*   1   2   3   4   5   6   7   *Very Important*
(Supervisor)   *Very Unimportant*   1   2   3   4   5   6   7   *Very Important*

- The supervisor should provide the opportunity for me to relate my academic work to therapy situations.

(Student)   *Very Unimportant*   1   2   3   4   5   6   7   *Very Important*
(Supervisor)   *Very Unimportant*   1   2   3   4   5   6   7   *Very Important*

- The supervisor should provide me with information during supervisory conferences.

(Student)   *Very Unimportant*   1   2   3   4   5   6   7   *Very Important*
(Supervisor)   *Very Unimportant*   1   2   3   4   5   6   7   *Very Important*

APPENDIX 3-5
BROYLE ET AL.'S PERCEIVED EFFECTIVENESS TOOLS

Clinical Supervisor Survey I: Perceived Effectiveness of Various Supervision Strategies

The following is a list of supervision strategies obtained through reviewing the literature and interviewing supervisors and student clinicians. Please rate each strategy according to its perceived effectiveness in facilitating student clinician's clinical and professional growth. If a strategy is not familiar to you please rate it according to how effective you perceive it would be. For supervision strategies you have used, rate to the left, for supervision strategies you have not used, rate to the right.

Rating Scale

5 = Highly Effective	4 = Effective	3 = Moderately Effective	2 = Minimally Effective	1 = Not Effective

Perceived Effectiveness of Strategies I HAVE USED in Supervision	Strategy	Perceived Effectiveness of Strategies I HAVE NOT USED in Supervision
5　4　3　2　1		5　4　3　2　1
☐ ☐ ☐ ☐ ☐	Provide reading material (e.g., articles, journals, student manual, previously completed paperwork) as examples	☐ ☐ ☐ ☐ ☐
☐ ☐ ☐ ☐ ☐	Provide information regarding legal and ethical issues	☐ ☐ ☐ ☐ ☐
☐ ☐ ☐ ☐ ☐	Model professional behavior	☐ ☐ ☐ ☐ ☐
☐ ☐ ☐ ☐ ☐	Assist in the development of goals and objectives	☐ ☐ ☐ ☐ ☐
☐ ☐ ☐ ☐ ☐	Request information from clinician to test retention of given information	☐ ☐ ☐ ☐ ☐
☐ ☐ ☐ ☐ ☐	Provide specific guidelines to adhere to (e.g., time constraints, dress code, paperwork format)	☐ ☐ ☐ ☐ ☐
☐ ☐ ☐ ☐ ☐	Adhere to specific guidelines/timelines as a supervisor	☐ ☐ ☐ ☐ ☐
☐ ☐ ☐ ☐ ☐	Create an atmosphere of mutual respect and sharing of attitudes, feelings, beliefs, and philosophies	☐ ☐ ☐ ☐ ☐
☐ ☐ ☐ ☐ ☐	Demonstrate/model clinical techniques during conference (role play)	☐ ☐ ☐ ☐ ☐
☐ ☐ ☐ ☐ ☐	Demonstrate/model clinical techniques during session with client	☐ ☐ ☐ ☐ ☐

☐ ☐ ☐ ☐ ☐   Focus on student clinician's overall clinical performance (e.g., clinical strengths/weaknesses)   ☐ ☐ ☐ ☐ ☐

☐ ☐ ☐ ☐ ☐   Focus on client behaviors as opposed to clinician behaviors   ☐ ☐ ☐ ☐ ☐

☐ ☐ ☐ ☐ ☐   Give gestural guidance, cues using gestures (e.g., head nod, hand motion) during a session   ☐ ☐ ☐ ☐ ☐

☐ ☐ ☐ ☐ ☐   Give verbal guidance during a session   ☐ ☐ ☐ ☐ ☐

☐ ☐ ☐ ☐ ☐   Review session plans before each session   ☐ ☐ ☐ ☐ ☐

☐ ☐ ☐ ☐ ☐   Make general suggestions for revisions in paperwork   ☐ ☐ ☐ ☐ ☐

☐ ☐ ☐ ☐ ☐   Make specific written corrections on paperwork for revisions   ☐ ☐ ☐ ☐ ☐

☐ ☐ ☐ ☐ ☐   Encourage student clinician to express opinions and ideas   ☐ ☐ ☐ ☐ ☐

☐ ☐ ☐ ☐ ☐   Turn most of the responsibility for the client over to the student clinician   ☐ ☐ ☐ ☐ ☐

☐ ☐ ☐ ☐ ☐   Observe in therapy room (actually inside the room or sitting outside with doors slightly open)   ☐ ☐ ☐ ☐ ☐

Clinical Supervisor Survey II: Perceived Effectiveness of Various Supervision Strategies

Rating Scale

5 = Highly Effective	4 = Effective	3 = Moderately Effective	2 = Minimally Effective	1 = Not Effective

Perceived Effectiveness of Strategies I HAVE USED in Supervision	Strategy	Perceived Effectiveness of Strategies I HAVE NOT USED in Supervision
5 4 3 2 1		5 4 3 2 1
☐ ☐ ☐ ☐ ☐	Observe through a two-way mirror	☐ ☐ ☐ ☐ ☐
☐ ☐ ☐ ☐ ☐	Observe through a closed-circuit television monitor	☐ ☐ ☐ ☐ ☐
☐ ☐ ☐ ☐ ☐	Observe by viewing a video/audio recorded session	☐ ☐ ☐ ☐ ☐
☐ ☐ ☐ ☐ ☐	Require joint-analysis of video/audio recorded sessions	☐ ☐ ☐ ☐ ☐
☐ ☐ ☐ ☐ ☐	Require a written agreement to ensure follow through after suggestions have been given	☐ ☐ ☐ ☐ ☐

☐ ☐ ☐ ☐ ☐ Hold regularly scheduled individual confer- ☐ ☐ ☐ ☐ ☐
ences (e.g., weekly)

☐ ☐ ☐ ☐ ☐ Hold regularly scheduled group supervi- ☐ ☐ ☐ ☐ ☐
sion conferences

☐ ☐ ☐ ☐ ☐ Hold supervision conferences upon clini- ☐ ☐ ☐ ☐ ☐
cian request

☐ ☐ ☐ ☐ ☐ Interact with the supervisee in planning, ☐ ☐ ☐ ☐ ☐
executing, and analyzing assessment and
treatment sessions.

☐ ☐ ☐ ☐ ☐ Give written rating in numerical form ☐ ☐ ☐ ☐ ☐
immediately after a session

☐ ☐ ☐ ☐ ☐ Give written feedback in narrative form ☐ ☐ ☐ ☐ ☐
immediately after a session

☐ ☐ ☐ ☐ ☐ Give oral feedback immediately after a ☐ ☐ ☐ ☐ ☐
session

☐ ☐ ☐ ☐ ☐ Give a summary rating sheet within 1 ☐ ☐ ☐ ☐ ☐
week of a session

☐ ☐ ☐ ☐ ☐ Give written feedback during conference ☐ ☐ ☐ ☐ ☐

☐ ☐ ☐ ☐ ☐ Give oral feedback during conference ☐ ☐ ☐ ☐ ☐

☐ ☐ ☐ ☐ ☐ Ensures confidentiality when clinical feed- ☐ ☐ ☐ ☐ ☐
back is provided

☐ ☐ ☐ ☐ ☐ Uses subjective evaluations ☐ ☐ ☐ ☐ ☐

☐ ☐ ☐ ☐ ☐ Uses a comprehensive evaluation system ☐ ☐ ☐ ☐ ☐
which takes into account clinicians' level of
experience.

☐ ☐ ☐ ☐ ☐ Gives rationale for statements and ☐ ☐ ☐ ☐ ☐
suggestions

☐ ☐ ☐ ☐ ☐ Requires student to rate their own perfor- ☐ ☐ ☐ ☐ ☐
mance during a clinical session

☐ ☐ ☐ ☐ ☐ Requires student to self-evaluate with ☐ ☐ ☐ ☐ ☐
video/audio recording

☐ ☐ ☐ ☐ ☐ Requires student to evaluate supervisor ☐ ☐ ☐ ☐ ☐
performance

Please indicate your total years of experience as a clinical supervisor: _____

Graduate Student Supervision Survey I: Perceived Effectiveness of Various Supervision Strategies

The following is a list of supervision strategies obtained through reviewing the literature and interviewing supervisors and student clinicians. Please rate each strategy according to its perceived effectiveness in facilitating student clinicians' clinical and professional growth. If a strategy is not familiar to you please rate it according to how effective you perceive it would be. For supervision strategies your supervisors used, rate to the left, for supervision strategies your supervisors have not used, rate to the right.

Rating Scale

5 = Highly Effective	4 = Effective	3 = Moderately Effective	2 = Minimally Effective	1 = Not Effective

Perceived Effectiveness of Strategies I HAVE USED in Supervision	Strategy	Perceived Effectiveness of Strategies I HAVE NOT USED in Supervision
5 4 3 2 1		5 4 3 2 1
☐ ☐ ☐ ☐ ☐	Provides reading material (e.g., articles, journals, student manual, previously completed paperwork as examples)	☐ ☐ ☐ ☐ ☐
☐ ☐ ☐ ☐ ☐	Provides information regarding legal and ethical issue	☐ ☐ ☐ ☐ ☐
☐ ☐ ☐ ☐ ☐	Models professional behavior	☐ ☐ ☐ ☐ ☐
☐ ☐ ☐ ☐ ☐	Assists in the development of goals and objectives	☐ ☐ ☐ ☐ ☐
☐ ☐ ☐ ☐ ☐	Requests information from clinician to test retention of given information	☐ ☐ ☐ ☐ ☐
☐ ☐ ☐ ☐ ☐	Provides specific guidelines to adhere to (e.g., time constraints, dress code, paperwork format)	☐ ☐ ☐ ☐ ☐
☐ ☐ ☐ ☐ ☐	Adheres to specific guidelines/timelines as a supervisor	☐ ☐ ☐ ☐ ☐
☐ ☐ ☐ ☐ ☐	Creates an atmosphere of mutual respect and sharing of attitudes, feelings, beliefs, and philosophies	☐ ☐ ☐ ☐ ☐
☐ ☐ ☐ ☐ ☐	Demonstrates/models clinical techniques during conference (role play)	☐ ☐ ☐ ☐ ☐
☐ ☐ ☐ ☐ ☐	Demonstrates/models clinical techniques during a therapy session with client	☐ ☐ ☐ ☐ ☐
☐ ☐ ☐ ☐ ☐	Focuses on student clinician's overall clinical performance (e.g., clinical strengths/weaknesses)	☐ ☐ ☐ ☐ ☐
☐ ☐ ☐ ☐ ☐	Focuses on client behaviors as opposed to clinician behaviors	☐ ☐ ☐ ☐ ☐
☐ ☐ ☐ ☐ ☐	Gives gestural guidance, cues using gestures (e.g., head nod, hand motion) during a session	☐ ☐ ☐ ☐ ☐
☐ ☐ ☐ ☐ ☐	Gives verbal guidance during a session	☐ ☐ ☐ ☐ ☐
☐ ☐ ☐ ☐ ☐	Reviews session plans before each session	☐ ☐ ☐ ☐ ☐
☐ ☐ ☐ ☐ ☐	Makes general suggestions for revisions in paperwork	☐ ☐ ☐ ☐ ☐
☐ ☐ ☐ ☐ ☐	Makes specific written corrections on paperwork for revisions	☐ ☐ ☐ ☐ ☐

❏ ❏ ❏ ❏ ❏	Encourages student clinician to express opinions and ideas	❏ ❏ ❏ ❏ ❏
❏ ❏ ❏ ❏ ❏	Turns most of the responsibility for the client over to the student clinician	❏ ❏ ❏ ❏ ❏
❏ ❏ ❏ ❏ ❏	Observes in therapy room (actually inside the room or sitting outside with door slightly open)	❏ ❏ ❏ ❏ ❏

Graduate Student Supervision Survey II: Perceived Effectiveness of Various Supervision Strategies

Rating Scale

5 = Highly Effective	4 = Effective	3 = Moderately Effective	2 = Minimally Effective	1 = Not Effective

Perceived Effectiveness of Strategies I HAVE USED in Supervision	Strategy	Perceived Effectiveness of Strategies I HAVE NOT USED in Supervision
5 4 3 2 1		5 4 3 2 1
❏ ❏ ❏ ❏ ❏	Observes through a two-way mirror	❏ ❏ ❏ ❏ ❏
❏ ❏ ❏ ❏ ❏	Observes through a closed-circuit television monitor	❏ ❏ ❏ ❏ ❏
❏ ❏ ❏ ❏ ❏	Observes by viewing a video/audio recorded session	❏ ❏ ❏ ❏ ❏
❏ ❏ ❏ ❏ ❏	Requires joint-analysis of video/audio recorded sessions	❏ ❏ ❏ ❏ ❏
❏ ❏ ❏ ❏ ❏	Requires a written agreement to ensure follow through after suggestions have been given	❏ ❏ ❏ ❏ ❏
❏ ❏ ❏ ❏ ❏	Holds regularly scheduled individual conferences (e.g., weekly)	❏ ❏ ❏ ❏ ❏
❏ ❏ ❏ ❏ ❏	Holds regularly scheduled group supervision conferences	❏ ❏ ❏ ❏ ❏
❏ ❏ ❏ ❏ ❏	Holds supervision conferences upon clinician request	❏ ❏ ❏ ❏ ❏
❏ ❏ ❏ ❏ ❏	Interacts with the supervisee in planning, executing, and analyzing assessment and treatment sessions.	❏ ❏ ❏ ❏ ❏
❏ ❏ ❏ ❏ ❏	Gives written rating in numerical form immediately after a session	❏ ❏ ❏ ❏ ❏
❏ ❏ ❏ ❏ ❏	Gives written feedback in narrative form immediately after a session	❏ ❏ ❏ ❏ ❏

☐ ☐ ☐ ☐ ☐	Gives oral feedback immediately after a session	☐ ☐ ☐ ☐ ☐
☐ ☐ ☐ ☐ ☐	Gives a summary rating sheet within 1 week of a session	☐ ☐ ☐ ☐ ☐
☐ ☐ ☐ ☐ ☐	Gives written feedback during conference	☐ ☐ ☐ ☐ ☐
☐ ☐ ☐ ☐ ☐	Gives oral feedback during conference	☐ ☐ ☐ ☐ ☐
☐ ☐ ☐ ☐ ☐	Ensures confidentiality when clinical feedback is provided	☐ ☐ ☐ ☐ ☐
☐ ☐ ☐ ☐ ☐	Uses subjective evaluations	☐ ☐ ☐ ☐ ☐
☐ ☐ ☐ ☐ ☐	Uses a comprehensive evaluation system which takes into account clinicians' level of experience.	☐ ☐ ☐ ☐ ☐
☐ ☐ ☐ ☐ ☐	Gives rationale for statements and suggestions	☐ ☐ ☐ ☐ ☐
☐ ☐ ☐ ☐ ☐	Requires student to rate their own performance during a clinical session	☐ ☐ ☐ ☐ ☐
☐ ☐ ☐ ☐ ☐	Requires student to self-evaluate with video/audio recording	☐ ☐ ☐ ☐ ☐
☐ ☐ ☐ ☐ ☐	Requires student to evaluate supervisor performance	☐ ☐ ☐ ☐ ☐

Please indicate your total number of clinical clock hours completed to date: _____

Reprinted with permission from Broyles, S., McNeice, E., Ishee, J., Ross, S., & Lance, D. (1999). *Influence of selected factors on the perceived effectiveness of various supervision strategies.* Poster session presented at the annual convention of the American Speech-Language-Hearing Association, San Francisco, CA.

APPENDIX 3-6
POWELL'S ATTITUDES TOWARD CLINICAL SUPERVISION

This scale is designed to measure attitudes toward clinical supervision. Please read each item carefully and circle the response which best describes your attitude for that item.

SA = strongly agree
A = agree
U = undecided
D = disagree
SD = strongly disagree

1. Supervisees should analyze their own behavior.   SA A U D SD

2. The supervisor and the supervisee should strive for a collegial relationship rather than a superior-subordinate relationship.   SA A U D SD

3. The supervisor should be more responsible for the client than the supervisee.   SA A U D SD

4. Supervisees should play an active role in the supervisory process.   SA A U D SD

5. The supervisee should be subordinate to the supervisor.   SA A U D SD

6. The supervisee should be more responsible for the client than the supervisor.   SA A U D SD

7. Written feedback should consist of the supervisor's opinions.   SA A U D SD

8. The supervisor and the supervisee should plan jointly for the supervisory conference.   SA A U D SD

9. Self-analysis by the supervisee is more important than the supervisor's analysis of the supervisee.   SA A U D SD

10. The supervisor should dominate the supervisory conference.   SA A U D SD

11. The supervisory conference should focus on the supervisee rather than on the client.   SA A U D SD

12. The supervisory conference should focus on the client's behavior.   SA A U D SD

13. The supervisor should select goals for the supervisee.   SA A U D SD

14. Problems in therapy should be solved by the supervisor.   SA A U D SD

15. Supervisee's ideas are less important than the supervisor's ideas.   SA A U D SD

Directions for Administration and Scoring of the Clinical Supervision Attitude Scale

1. Respondents should be asked to read each item and mark whether they strongly agree, agree, are undecided, disagree, or strongly disagree with the statement.

2. For positively worded items (e.g., items 1, 2, 4, 6, 8, 9, 11), assign values as follows:
   - ◦ 5 points: strongly agree
   - ◦ 4 points: agree
   - ◦ 3 points: undecided
   - ◦ 2 points: disagree
   - ◦ 1 point: strongly disagree

3. For negatively worded items (e.g., items 3, 5, 7, 10, 12, 13, 14, 15), assign values as follows:
   - ◦ 1 point: strongly agree
   - ◦ 2 points: agree
   - ◦ 3 points: undecided
   - ◦ 4 points: disagree
   - ◦ 5 points: strongly disagree

4. Once point values have been assigned to each item, sum the points across all 15 items. The total should be between 15 (lowest possible score corresponding to one point per item) and 75 (highest possible score corresponding to five points per item).

Reprinted with permission from Powell, T. (1987). A rating scale for measurement of attitudes toward clinical supervision. *SUPERvision, 11*, 31-34.

APPENDIX 3-7
BRASSEUR'S ADAPTED
SUPERVISORY CONFERENCE RATING SCALE

Your Name: _____   Date: _____

Name of Supervisor or Supervisee: _____

Circle one: Individual   Client   Group

Circle one: Individual   Individual conference   Group   (N =   )

Directions: Please give your assessment of what happened in the conference just completed by rating the following items. Circle the number that best represents the level of occurrence of the activity suggested by each item. You can rate each item anywhere from one to seven.

Please do not confer with the other participants while you are completing this task.

	Definitely No		Neutral			Definitely Yes	
1. The supervisee asks many questions.	1	2	3	4	5	6	7
2. The supervisor provides justification for statements or suggestions.	1	2	3	4	5	6	7
3. The supervisor uses conference time to discuss ways to improve materials.	1	2	3	4	5	6	7
4. The supervisor offers suggestions on therapy techniques during the conference.	1	2	3	4	5	6	7
5. The supervisor uses the supervisee's ideas in discussion during the conference.	1	2	3	4	5	6	7
6. The supervisor responds to statements, questions, or problems presented by the supervisee.	1	2	3	4	5	6	7
7. The supervisee uses the conference time to provide feedback to the supervisor about the clinical session.	1	2	3	4	5	6	7
8. The supervisor and supervisee participate in a teacher-student relationship.	1	2	3	4	5	6	7
9. The supervisor uses a supportive style.	1	2	3	4	5	6	7
10. The supervisor helps the supervisee set realistic goals for the clients.	1	2	3	4	5	6	7
11. The supervisee verbalizes needs.	1	2	3	4	5	6	7
12. The supervisor uses conference time to discuss weaknesses in the supervisee's clinical behavior.	1	2	3	4	5	6	7
13. The supervisor presents value judgements about the supervisee's clinical behavior.	1	2	3	4	5	6	7
14. During the conference, the supervisee requests a written copy of the supervisor's behavioral observations.	1	2	3	4	5	6	7

15. The supervisor and supervisee participate in a superior-subordinate relationship.   1 2 3 4 5 6 7

16. The supervisor states the objectives of the conference.   1 2 3 4 5 6 7

17. The supervisor asks the supervisee to analyze or evaluate something that has occurred or may occur in the clinical sessions.   1 2 3 4 5 6 7

18. The supervisor asks the supervisee to think about strategies that might have been done differently, or that may be done in the future.   1 2 3 4 5 6 7

Reprinted with permission from Brasseur, J., & Anderson, J. (1983). Observed differences between direct, indirect, and direct/indirect videotaped supervisory conferences. *Journal of Speech and Hearing Research, 26*, 349-355 and adapted from Smith, K., & Anderson, J. (1982). Relationship of perceived effectiveness to content in supervisory conferences in speech-language pathology. *Journal of Speech and Hearing Research, 25*, 243-251.

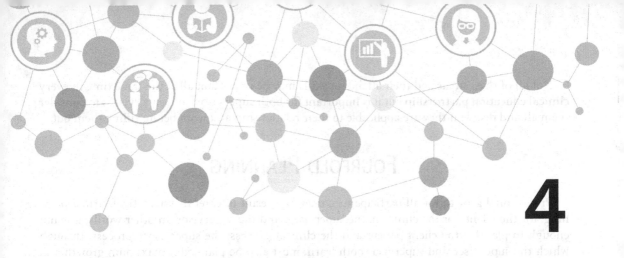

4

Planning in the Supervisory Process

Elizabeth S. McCrea, PhD, CCC-SLP, F-ASHA and
Judith A. Brasseur, PhD, CCC-SLP, F-ASHA

Planning in one form or another has long been a fundamental task of professionals in audiology and speech-language pathology. Historically, the main emphasis in planning has been in support of client service delivery, for example individualized education programs and SOAP (i.e., subjective, objective, assessment, and plan) notes. Reflection on the complexity of the needs and expectations of the supervisory dyad as they are overlaid onto the clinical process, however, leads to the conclusion that, if all participants in the supervisory process are to grow and develop professionally, clinical teaching cannot take place haphazardly or spontaneously. Every facet of it must be thoughtfully considered and planned.

Several Core Areas from the Knowledge and Skills to Provide Clinical Supervision (American Speech-Language-Hearing Association [ASHA], 2008) are important to the planning stage. These areas include:

- I. Preparation for the Supervisory Process
- II. Interpersonal Communication and Supervisor-Supervisee Relationship
- III. Development of Supervisee's Critical Thinking and Problem-Solving Skills
- IV. Development of Supervisee's Clinical Competence in Assessment
- V. Development of Supervisee's Clinical Competence in Intervention
- VI. Supervisory Conferences and Meetings of Clinical Teaching Teams
- VII. Evaluating the Growth of the Supervisee both as a Clinician and as a Professional
- VIII. Diversity

McCrea, E. S., & Brasseur, J. A. *The Clinical Education and Supervisory Process in Speech–Language Pathology and Audiology* (pp 107-166). © 2020 Taylor & Francis Group.

Not all of these areas and their attendant skills may be important all at the same time in every clinical education partnership but it is important for both supervisors and supervisees to consider them all and decide if they are applicable to their relationship and work before ruling them out.

FOURFOLD PLANNING

Professional growth for all participants comes as a result of careful systematic, fourfold planning: for the client, for the clinician, the supervisee, and the supervisor. In other words, it is not enough to plan for the client-patient and the clinical process; the supervisory process, through which the supervisee and supervisor both learn, must also be planned if maximum growth and professional development is to be achieved. The importance of planning can be fully appreciated in a review of the scope of the knowledge and skills identified in the report of the Ad Hoc Committee on Supervision (ASHA, 2008) which identifies 11 knowledge domains and their associated skills important in the provision of clinical supervision to students. Seven of the 11 knowledge domains directly reference the supervisee; the verbs often used in the identification of individual skills within these knowledge domains are "assist" or "facilitate"; however, it is the premise of this chapter that no matter what verb is used, none of that action can happen in a meaningful and productive way without appropriate planning.

Fourfold planning needs to be seen as the very foundation upon which the supervisory process is built. All future action in the process and the evaluation of it is based on what is done during the planning component. All activities for all participants are planned—not only clinical activities but also observation, data collection, methods of self-analysis and reflection, and evaluation. Planning, then, is a continuous process from the first interaction between supervisor and supervisee to the last. It should always be integrated with data collection and analysis. Predictions are made on the basis of the data about what will and will not work; the accuracy of these predictions will form the basis for further activity or action in each set of plans coming out of the data from previously planned activities. Furthermore, this component is considered necessary in all settings (e.g., educational settings, external practicum sites, and service delivery settings); however, the focus, procedures, and intensity of planning activities may differ in each.

Importance of Planning

Planning is a basic and important activity of all supervisors; however, the focus on planning has most often been on the client and has been frequently discussed in the literature (Flower, 1984; Goldberg, 1997; Hegde & Davis, 1995; Irwin et al., 1961; Kleffner, 1964; Knight, Hahn, Ervin, & McIssac, 1961; Miner, 1967; Prather, 1967; Van Riper, 1965; Villareal, 1964). All of these authors recognized the importance of planning for appropriate service delivery to clients; however, their discussions did not mention the importance of also planning for the clinician, supervisee, and supervisor.

Cogan (1973) talked about joint lesson planning for the teacher and took a long-range view of planning in which the daily lesson plan is only one element of the continuum of planning. He believed that the daily lesson plan produces episodic, discontinuous supervision and preferred to take a long view while at the same time checking to see that the daily plan is "in tune" with the larger objectives. Planning for supervision of teachers was presented by Goldhammer, Anderson, and Krajewski (1980) as the preobservation conference. They stressed the importance of mutual understanding of the plans and how each participant was to function. This collaborative phase of the process includes goal setting, developing rationales for instruction, and deciding on instructional methods with an emphasis on teacher behavior.

Planning was so important to Acheson and Gall (1980) that they differentiated between planning conferences and feedback conferences. The planning conference, the first phase of supervision their framework, includes:

- Identifying the teacher's concerns about instruction
- Translating these concerns into observable behaviors
- Identifying procedures for improving instruction
- Assisting teachers in setting self-improvement goals
- Arranging details of the observation (e.g., time, observational instruments, behaviors to be recorded, context in which behaviors will be recorded)

Although Cogan (1973), Goldhammer and colleagues (1980), and Acheson and Gall (1980) all were writing about supervision of teachers working in schools, their ideas are directly applicable to supervision in speech-language pathology and audiology.

Perceptions About Planning

As long ago as 1965, Anderson and Milisen (1965) and then Culatta, Colucci, and Wiggins (1975) documented discrepancies between supervisors' perception of the value of planning via lesson plans and the value placed on this activity by their supervisees. Eighty-eight percent of the supervisors ranked the preparation of lesson plans as important, but only 60% of their supervisees reported that their plans were ever returned to them.

Peaper and Wener (1984) collected extensive early data in speech-language pathology about the frequency and perceived value of various types of planning required in educational programs and professional settings. They administered a 55-item questionnaire to 219 clinical supervisors, students, and working professionals. Not surprisingly, differences in perceptions were found between educational and professional settings and between supervisors and supervisees. In summarizing their results, Peaper and Wener reported that their analysis indicated that all types of written planning need to be included in the educational process, especially written long-term goals, and they suggested an alternative to daily lesson planning: first-year students might be required to write fairly detailed weekly lesson plans to develop skills in identifying short-term goals and accompanying procedures. Second-year students might eliminate the weekly lesson plan after the projected treatment plan has been submitted, with a brief lesson plan being required when goals and procedures are revised. Based on the continuum proposed in this book, it is more appropriate to base planning requirements on individual competencies of supervisees and their place on the continuum. Emphasis should also be placed on projected treatment plans and logs with special attention to writing long-term goals because many aspects of professional documentation require them such as individualized education programs and SOAP notes. Despite what has seemed to be a trend toward the writing of comprehensive long-term intervention programs in service delivery settings, this study reflected an opinion held by many supervisors in educational programs that the detailed writing of treatment plans is a necessary phase of the preparation of students for the future planning they will need to do (i.e., an initial step in the ability to formulate comprehensive long-term service plans).

Planning as a Joint Process

The principle that all direction and input in the supervisory process should not come from the supervisor is tested more vigorously in the planning stage. Planning begins as soon as the supervisor, presumably the more knowledgeable of the dyad, has introduced the supervisee to the supervisory process or has provided the opportunity for discussion of the process. The supervisor is responsible for operationalizing the planning process and for involving the supervisee at whatever stage of the continuum she/he is able to participate. In addition, it is the major responsibility of the supervisor to help the supervisee increase the amount of participation in planning over time in a manner that reflects the supervisee's capabilities. In addition, it is the major responsibility of the supervisor to help the supervisee increase the level of their participation in planning over time in a manner that reflects his or her growing competence. The planning component is particularly important in encouraging and assisting students to develop a sense of ownership of and responsibility for their own clinical and professional behavior as well as for the outcomes achieved with a client/patient. Planning should be approached as a joint effort by supervisor and supervisee to determine what is best for the client as well as themselves to ensure continued professional growth.

The early part of the planning component is the place to begin avoiding situations that encourage a supervisees dependence on the supervisor. It is a time for encouraging and accepting supervisee's ideas, being sensitive to their feelings of insecurity, sometimes threat, and fostering a sense of responsibility. Here, as in the previous component, is another place where the supervisor models the communication style that is appropriate given the supervisee's needs and which will probably become the standard for subsequent interactions.

Perhaps the process is equally, if not more important, than the product at this point. The manner in which planning is carried out lets supervisees know that supervisor's really mean it when they talk about supervisee's participation, that supervisors are planning with them, not for them (Cogan, 1973). It is a time when supervisors can demonstrate to their supervisees that it is possible for them to hold back in the conference and welcome their supervisee's full participation.

ASSESSMENT OF SUPERVISEES

References have been made elsewhere to analogies between the clinical and supervisory processes, but nowhere is that analogy clearer than it is in this early stage, which might be thought of as the assessment phase of supervision. Audiologists and speech-language pathologists respect the essential role that a thorough assessment plays in planning appropriate treatment procedures for every individual client's specific needs. Why, then, when they become supervisors, do they neglect to apply the same principle of assessment to supervisees and, subsequently, assume that one style of supervision can meet the needs of all supervisees.

Part of the planning process, basic to successful implementation of the supervisory methodology presented here, is the accurate determination of the point on the continuum at which the supervisee is capable of functioning and the appropriate supervisory style to be used at each point. This aspect of the planning process takes on even greater importance in light of the revision of the Council on Accreditation of Graduate Programs in Audiology and Speech-Language Pathology (CAA; 2017) standards for accreditation of academic programs and, ultimately, for certification in either audiology or speech-language pathology. Standards 3.7A and 3.7B specifically state that the "type and structure of clinical education are commensurate with the development of the knowledge and skill of each student" (pp. 16 and 24). Several issues need to be resolved in making this determination:

- The supervisee's ability to actively problem solve
- The degree of dependency and independency of the supervisee as a clinician and supervisee
- The ability of the supervisee to engage in self-observation, self-analysis, and reflection
- The supervisor's flexibility in adapting his or her style to supervisee's level of development

Fourfold planning cannot be accomplished until these issues are resolved. Only then can the supervisor and supervisee break away from the traditional patterns revealed in the data and place themselves properly on the continuum.

This expanded need for planning adds a new dimension to what is probably the most traditional procedure in which the supervisor spends some time at the beginning of the interaction obtaining information about the clinical experience of the supervisee. This new dimension makes it necessary for the supervisor to learn what kinds of supervisory experiences the supervisee has had. Rockman (1977) supported an assessment approach to the supervisory process when she pointed out that the parallels between the clinical and the supervisory processes and emphasized the importance of the assessment of clinical skills of the supervisee prior to the beginning of the treatment program and supervision. She continued to say that the supervisor must rely on questionnaires, personal interview and direct observation for this entry-level evaluation. She further suggested "exploration of academic background, prior clinical experiences, personal experiences and work history" (p. 3) and stressed the importance of early observation in obtaining information about basic clinical skills. Although directed mainly toward clinical skills, this procedure can be extended to obtain information about the student as a supervisee.

Obtaining Information About Supervisees

Assuming that the supervisor and supervisee have engaged in some preliminary discussion of the supervisory process, each supervisory interaction will begin with an assessment process, as does every clinical interaction. The following outline is a brief overview, certainly not exhaustive, of information needed before the point on the continuum can be determined. Some supervisors may want to explore additional aspects of a student's experience that are important to unique settings and/or patients/clients. As soon as this information is collected, planning can begin.

1. Clinician information
   o General clinical experience
   o Experience with clients with same presenting communication disorder
   o Academic background in the disorder area
   o Other experiences relevant to client or disorder
   o Clinician's perception of strengths and needs in terms of the client
   o Anxieties about this client or disorder
   o Understanding the concomitant needs of the client

2. Supervisee information
   o Nature of supervisory interactions previously experienced
   o Perception of self in terms of dependence/independence in general and in relation to client
   o Prior responsibility for data collection and analysis of client behavior
   o Experience in data collection and analysis of own clinical behavior prior to conferences
   o Perception of responsibility for bringing data and questions to the conference, assisting in problem solving and decision making
   o Expectations for learning or modification of clinical skill from current status
   o Perception of need for feedback (e.g., amount, timing, type)

3. Supervisor information
   o General clinical and supervisory experience
   o Experience with type of client and disorder
   o Theoretical and practical approach to the disorder as compared to that of supervisee
   o Preferred or customary supervisory style
   o Clarification of expectations for the supervisee as a clinician and as a supervisee
   o Clarification of expectations for the supervisory interaction
   o Perception of own role

Determining Dependence and Independence

Phillips (2009) acknowledged the importance of determining a supervisee's level of independence prior to the initiation of practicum, to enable supervisors to adjust style and provide the level of support an individual student will need. Results of this qualitative study revealed that 8 of 11 supervisors, asked their supervisees to present their client. The presentation included case history, previous treatment and communication needs; the supervisors then evaluated the manner, organization, accuracy and completeness to estimate the supervisee's level of understanding of the disorder and knowledge of treatment. Level of clinical independence was then confirmed or modified based on supervisee performance in the initial treatment session.

Shriberg and colleagues (1974, 1975) developed a valuable instrument for making decisions about a supervisee's dependence or independence. Over several years, Shriberg and several members of the clinical staff at the University of Wisconsin-Madison developed and validated the Wisconsin Procedure for Appraisal of Clinical Competence (W-PACC; Appendix 4-1). This appraisal form will be discussed again under the topic of evaluation, but it is relevant here because of its basic approach. Rather than using client or clinician change as the criterion for effectiveness, this instrument "appraises the extent to which effectiveness is dependent upon continued supervisory input" (Shriberg et al., 1975, p. 160). This instrument is concerned, not just with the fact that a supervisee is able to competently demonstrate a range of clinical skills but also, with the amount and degree of supervisory support that was required to achieve that competence. The instrument provides for clinicians to be identified as operating at one of four levels at the beginning of the supervisory interaction, understanding that this identification may vary across settings/clients. The criteria for assigning levels, as suggested by Shriberg and colleagues, are hours of experience, number of clients, experience with the disorder area or management approach, and the supervisor's judgment of supervisee's academic preparation. Although these criteria are more relevant to the clinical process than to the items suggested previously for the supervisory assessment, the part of the W-PACC relevant to diagnosing the needs or skills of supervisees is the scale used to identify the level of dependence or independence the supervisee. The scale consists of the following levels of scoring:

- Score 1: Specific direction from the supervisor, does not alter unsatisfactory performance and is unable to make changes
- Score 2-3-4: Needs specific direction or demonstration from supervisor to perform effectively
- Score 5-6-7: Needs general direction from supervisor to perform effectively
- Score 8-9-10: Demonstrates independence by taking initiative, making changes when appropriate and is effective

Each of the 10 interpersonal skills and 28 professional-technical skills that comprise the instrument is scored using this scale.

The listed scales are mainly directed toward the clinician-client interaction but a few are related to the action of the clinician as a supervisor. For example, item 6 (listens, asks questions, participates with supervisor in therapy and/or client-related discussions—is not defensive) and item 7 (requests assistance from supervisor or other professionals when appropriate), along with item 6, is focused on behavior important to the supervisory process.

Indiana University developed a tool (Appendix 4-2) for evaluating supervisees' progress in practicum that is similar to the W-PACC in that the basis for the evaluation is the dependence-independence demonstrated by the supervisee in accomplishing the 64 items encompassed by it. It is procedurally less complex than the W-PACC and only considers student experience as a diagnostic variable.

In a similar vein, Solomon-Rice and Robinson (2015) developed an evaluation tool that focused on clinical skills across three levels of student clinical performance. They further refined the evaluation process by arranging skills in a hierarchy such that beginning students are evaluated on 25 skills, intermediate student clinicians on the beginning plus 5 additional skills (40 total), and advanced students on all 51 skills. Five areas of knowledge and skill are assessed: evaluation (9), intervention (13), documentation and report writing (11), professional and personal qualities (12), and response to supervisor (51).

When completing evaluations of clinical performance, Zylla-Jones (2006) suggested that students' performance on the continuum may fluctuate depending on their comfort level with any given case. She maintained that involving students in analyzing and evaluating their clinical skills should increase their independence. Encouraging students to identify not only clinical strengths and challenges, but also to indicate their comfort level with particular tasks will enable supervisors to better understand placement on the continuum. The following scale was developed to accompany evaluation of clinical tasks: 0 = not comfortable, requires maximum assistance and/ or supervisor demonstration; 1 = uncomfortable, requires moderate assistance; 2 = comfortable, requires minimal assistance; 3 = very comfortable, is independent.

In addition to the maturity and demonstrated independence of a supervisee's technical skill, Whalen (2001) suggests that there are other aspects of behavior that are equally as important to their education and training. She describes the results of a study conducted at the University of Wisconsin physical therapy training program (May et al., 1995) which identified 10 "generic abilities" and 4 levels of behavioral criteria that define them (Appendix 4-3) Although demonstrated independence is not specifically identified as part of the levels of these behavioral criteria, it is implied by them. Generic abilities are behaviors, attributes, or characteristics that are not explicitly part of a profession's core of knowledge and technical skill but nevertheless are required for success in the profession. These abilities include:

- *Commitment to learning*: the ability to self-assess, self-correct, and self-direct and to identify needs and sources of learning and to continually seek new knowledge and understanding
- *Interpersonal skills*: the ability to interact effectively with patients, families, colleagues, other health care professionals, and the community to deal effectively with cultural and clinic diversity issues
- *Communication skills*: the ability to communicate effectively (e.g., speaking, body language, reading, writing listening) for varied audiences and purposes
- *Effective use of time and resources*: the ability to obtain the maximum benefit from a minimum investment of time and resources
- *Use of constructive feedback*: the ability to identify sources of and seek out feedback and to effectively use and provide feedback for improving personal interaction
- *Problem solving*: the ability to recognize and define problems, analyze data, develop and implement solutions, and evaluate outcomes
- *Professionalism*: the ability to exhibit appropriate professional conduct and to represent the profession effectively
- *Responsibility*: the ability to fulfill commitments and to be accountable for actions and outcomes
- *Critical thinking*: the ability to question logically, to identify, generate, and evaluate elements of logical argument; to recognize and differentiate facts, illusions, assumptions, and hidden assumptions; and to distinguish relevant and irrelevant information
- *Stress management*: the ability to identify sources of stress and to develop effective coping behaviors (May et al., 1995)

According to Whalen (2001), mastery of this repertoire of generic abilities facilitates the entry-level (beginning graduate practicum) supervisee's ability to:

- Generalize from one context to another
- Integrate information from different sources
- Successfully apply knowledge and skills in practice settings
- Synthesize cognitive, affective, and psychomotor behaviors
- Interact effectively with clients, families, the community and other professionals

Whalen (2001) also describes a process in the University of Cincinnati Physical Therapy Training Program in which each physical therapy student assesses him or herself according to the 10 generic abilities along with a simultaneous assessment by a member of the faculty. If the student demonstrates skills that are not at the developing level, an action plan that contains goals, timelines, benchmarks, and consequences is implemented by the student in consultation and collaboration with their supervisors to address the deficiencies, often before the student can begin practicum. These abilities continue to be monitored for sustained growth by both the student and his or her supervisors throughout the student's training. If at any time, they are found to be deficient, an action plan is again implemented that requires active involvement of both student and supervisors in engaging these behaviors in the context of their professional training experiences.

It is important, not only during student training but in professional settings as well, to document continued development, through self-assessment, peer review, and performance review by administrators of these generic abilities in and among staff members. Accordingly, Henri (2001), as early as almost 2 decades ago, incorporated aspects of Goldman's (1995) emotional intelligence competence framework in performance reviews for staff for whom he had responsibility. This framework, although organized differently than the 10 generic abilities, contains many of the same aspects of an individual's behavior. This framework includes:

- *Self-awareness*: knowing one's internal states, preferences, resources, intuitions
- *Self-regulation*: managing one's internal states, impulses, resources
- *Motivation*: emotional tendencies that guide and facilitate reaching goals
- *Empathy*: awareness of others' feelings and concerns
- *Social skills*: adeptness of inducing desirable responses in others

All of these instruments are of value in several ways. They can be used as assessment tools to determine level of student dependence. They can be used by supervisees at any level of training or professional practice as a self-appraisal of their perception of their own independence and professional maturity as well as a means to define their own goals. They can be used by the supervisor and supervisee together, in total or in part, for the same purpose. Furthermore, if all supervisors in an organization used them, and could maintain agreement, appraisals from previous semesters or employment periods could provide a ready basis for determining the stage of dependence and independence and, therefore, the need for an action plan to address areas of need. These notions, such as longitudinal tracking along with independent and competent skill documented through formative assessment, are foundational to the CAA (2017) standards that require training programs to ensure training is commensurate with the knowledge and skill of the student. Finally, continued use of instruments such as these could help both supervisors and supervisees focus on the over-arching goal of clinician or supervisee independence and professional maturity as a primary facilitator of client behavior change, rather than the client alone. This shared focus is necessary to progress along the continuum of supervision at any level of practice.

IMPLEMENTING THE PLANNING COMPONENT

Supervisors must orchestrate all the various aspects of fourfold planning in collaboration with the supervisee. Fourfold planning expands the basic planning responsibility to a shared responsibility between supervisor and supervisee to plan for all participants. Methodologies for planning for each will be discussed in this section. Because planning for the client is discussed first, each additional method will be treated in somewhat greater detail in its own section. It should be remembered, however, that any planning method described for clients can also be applied to planning for other participants as an extension of the planning for the client. For example, goals and objectives should be set for all participants and written plans, programs, or contracts should include planning for more than the client.

Influence of Behavioral Objectives

Whatever the format, it seems that nearly all planning has been strongly influenced by a movement that has come from business management, education, and psychology—the setting of behavior objectives (BO). "A behavioral objective is any educational objective which is stated in terms of behaviors which can be observed and measured" (Mowrer, 1977, p. 146). This approach has been treated generously in the literature in several fields, particularly education, where the value of setting behavioral objectives has been stressed repeatedly (Baker & Popham, 1973; Mager, 1962; Mager & Pipe, 1970; Popham & Baker, 1970). Fundamentally, a BO will identify who will achieve a behavior/action, in what context will it be achieved, how will it be achieved, and how well must it be achieved; they are learner focused and specify behavior, conditions, and criteria.

SMART objectives (SO) (Doran, 1981) are a derivative of the BO movement and process and emerged from business and project management initiatives as well as performance management and personal development. An SO has five criteria: it must be specific; it must be measurable; it must be assignable; it must be realistic/attainable; and it must be time-bound. While SOs have different descriptors, they are conceptually consistent with BOs and utilization of either objective setting process is important in achieving thoughtful and productive behavior change.

Utilization of such goal- and objective-setting processes have become standard in planning for clients in rehabilitative audiology and speech-language pathology. Although the principles for their use are often included in clinical coursework, supervisors are usually responsible for implementing their use during practicum. Andrews (1971) described their importance to the student in clinical practicum, not in measuring progress, but also in learning to rely on something other than intuition and subjective impression. "Among the advantages," he said, "are that both the student and the supervisor know exactly the purpose of each therapy session and whether or not the purpose has been accomplished" (p. 387). This intentional approach in planning treatment and intervention services for clients/patients can be directly adapted in support of the supervisory process and the professional development of both the supervisor and the supervisee.

Written Plans

Traditionally, supervisors in audiology and speech-language pathology have worked from the assumption that written plans are important and indeed necessary for the adequate preparation of students and for appropriately meeting the needs of clients (Peaper & Wener, 1984). These written plans, however, can become an ordeal for students, sometimes requiring much more time in their preparation than in their execution. Supervisors need to balance the intensity of their feedback on such plans and the semantics with which it is provided with the need to allow students their own initiative and perhaps, even the dubious pleasure of learning through their mistakes. Intensive and directive feedback from supervisors does not facilitate the assumption of responsibility for appropriate planning because "my supervisor will change it anyway." The nature of feedback to students about their written plans should be determined by their place on the continuum.

The practice of students writing plans that are revised and altered by supervisors also does not encourage the joint participation advocated for all phases of the supervisory process. A more desirable approach would be to allow time for joint planning during the conference when there is input from both supervisor and supervisee based on data collected in previous therapy sessions and analyzed by either or both of the participants. This approach was supported by Peaper and Wener (1984). Verbal planning can be formalized into a written plan if it is needed for the clinician's guidance during the next session. Verbal planning (as well as written) also provides the foundation for the observation and analysis phases. At some point on the continuum it may also lead to setting long- and short-term objectives or to the use of other methods instead of detailed written plans. With the availability of secure electronic communication and messaging systems, it is likely that the documentation associated with the planning phase, can be accomplished much more efficiently for both supervisor and supervisee, understanding that protection of the patient or client's personal information is consistent with standards in the Health Insurance Portability and Accountability Act (U.S. Department of Health & Human Services).

Contracts

Joint discussion and joint planning lend themselves to another form of written plans—contracts, which are mentioned frequently in the literature on supervision in other professions. Goldhammer and colleagues (1980) stressed the importance of agreement between supervisor and supervisee on the plans that have been discussed in the preobservation conference and suggested a supervisory contract is a good way to reach such agreement, assuming that both are willing to modify the contract at a later time if it should become necessary. The contract, as they perceive it, is an agreement between the teacher and the supervisor that includes objectives of the lesson and their relationship to the overall learning program, activities to be observed, possible changes to which supervisor and supervisee may agree, feedback desired by the teacher, and methods of evaluation. The contract may be short-term for a specific task or lesson or long-term covering a specific period of time. This type of contract can easily be modified to include planning in the other three aspects of fourfold planning.

Contracts based on goals are seen as a powerful tool for supervision in social work by Fox (1983). It is performance oriented, goes beyond "tell me what to do" to mobilize the resources of the worker in self-directed activity and enlists the worker's cooperation in identifying and, to a significant degree, the shape of supervision. "Furthermore, the goal oriented contract for supervision provides a concrete and objective means for measuring and documenting progress and performance" (p. 37).

Christadoulou (2016) cited research by Sweeney, Webley, and Treacher (2001a, 2001b) in occupational therapy that recommended that contracts be developed to determine practicum objectives, evaluation and feedback methods, and to identify expectations of both supervisor and supervisee. Such a contract clarifies roles and responsibilities and enhances the relationship. Further, it allowed participants in their study to develop and grow during the experience by stating clear goals, reviewing them regularly and revising as needed. Furthermore, both supervisors and supervisees valued the time set aside to participate in feedback, reflection and evaluation which led to an effective relationship.

Three studies in speech-language pathology have studied the use of contracts to structure the practicum experiences of students. Shapiro (1985) addressed the effectiveness of written commitments, essentially in the form of a contract between supervisor and supervisee. He classified commitments into five types: clinical procedures, clinical process administration, supervisory procedures, supervisory process administration, and academic information. The greatest number of commitments involved planning, analysis, and evaluation of the clinical process with a particular focus on the behavior of the client (47%) with the second most frequent being commitments related to specific treatment or diagnostic techniques, again focusing on the behavior of the client (39%). Shapiro contrasted two types of commitments made by supervisees: verbal (reached through discussion in the conference) and written (again reached through discussion but agreed on in writing by supervisor and supervisee), in essence a contract. The documentation also included specification of the observable behaviors that the supervisees needed to demonstrate to indicate follow through of each commitment. Data analysis indicated that inexperienced clinicians completed more commitments when written documentation was required and experienced clinicians completed more when no written documentation was required. This study indicated the value of structured written documentation as a productive supervisory methodology, especially for beginning clinicians (e.g., those in the Evaluation-Feedback Stage, Dreyfus's novice stage, and the D1-2 stages of the SQF Model of Supervision [Chapter 2]) and for the early stages of the supervisory dyad as well.

Larson, Hoag, and Schrader-Niedenthal (1987) investigated both supervisor and supervisee satisfaction with a contract-based system for grading practicum. The data indicated that there were positive impressions about objectivity, explicitness, and clarity of expectations as well as consistency of feedback for most of the student participants, which led to supervisees understanding the relationship between contract objectives and expectations of performance. This enabled supervisees to understand the relationship between contract objectives and expectations for performance.

Peaper and Mercaitis (1989) used a variation of Fox's (1983) work. They developed a process for participation by both the supervisor and supervisee in determining baseline levels of behavior, for identification of goals, priorities, roles of both supervisor and supervisee, and establishment of measurement criteria. In a rank order of 16 factors contributing to a satisfactory supervisory experience, the item ranked as most important by the participating students was "their input is encouraged and valued." Peaper and Mercaitis noted that "the contract is an excellent vehicle to encourage student input and participation" (p. 27).

A contract or written agreement between supervisor and supervisee will vary in its content depending upon the situation, but if it is approached as a plan that will be followed to help both participants have a clear understanding of their goals and the procedures that will be followed to meet those goals, it is a natural way to approach collaborative supervision. The process of agreeing on specifics of the contract forces discussion. If goals and objectives are mutually written and agreed on, there should be much less opportunity for incongruence between the expectations of both supervisor and supervisee. There will also be direction for the supervisory process that may not otherwise exist.

Planning for the Client

Planning for clients is one of the activities that most beginning clinicians spend considerable amounts of time and energy completing. Every practicing clinician is familiar with Individualized Educational Plans or Section 504 Plans in school settings or Medicare Plan of Care (POC) documentation in adult settings. The early literature on this aspect of the clinical process was heavily influenced by Skinner (1954). Programmed instruction as it was then called, went through a period of evolution before being adapted to speech-language pathology and audiology. Costello (1977) defined it as a "systematically designed remediation plan which specifies a priori the teaching and learning behaviors required of both the teacher and the learner" (p. 3). She presented principles and procedures that would enable clinicians and (researchers) to develop their own programmed instruction and in doing so, contributed a resource to enable clinicians to design and evaluate the success of their treatment services for their clients.

Whatever form the planning and documentation takes, it results in improved accountability for clients and payer sources, better communication between supervisor and supervisee, and continuity of service to clients, as well as increased ability of students to draft effective treatment objectives and develop a professional writing style (Lemmer & Drake, 1983). Students develop a clearer understanding of the therapeutic process and clinical expectations. Here, as in traditional lesson planning, the dependence or independence of the supervisee may determine the supervisor's style and intensity of participation.

Planning for the Clinician

The previous discussion of planning objectives and activities for the client is only one component of the planning needed for the fourfold approach to supervision. Similar documentation and planning of objectives and procedures for the clinician are equally as important.

Plans for the clinician must include the planning of specific clinician behaviors that are needed to modify client behavior across disorder areas. This may seem as if the obvious is being stated; however, student clinicians often say, "My supervisor never talks about my behavior, just the client's." Although this may be the result of student misperception, it is often their reality; the analyses of historical conference content have repeatedly established that the client, not the clinician, is the focus of most discussion (Culatta & Seltzer, 1976; McCrea, 1980; Pickering, 1979, 1984; Roberts & Smith, 1982; Shapiro, 1985; Shapiro, 1984; Tufts, 1983). Some studies (Blumberg, 1980; Culatta & Seltzer, 1977; Roberts & Smith, 1982; Tufts, 1983) have also indicated that evaluation is not frequently included in the content of regular conference interaction.

Lack of specific discussion of clinician behavior probably had its beginning in the traditional concept of planning as it is reflected in the literature: plans are for clients, not the clinician, and goals are set for clients. This is particularly incongruous when several points are considered: 1) supervisee expectations for supervision, 2) the types of evaluation forms used by supervisors that focus on clinician behavior and skill, and 3) the notion that clinical education is more than just evaluation of clinicians in their work with clients.

Planning as Related to Expectations

Expectations of supervisees are initially related to their own needs. Supervisees in Russell's (1976) study, for example, indicated that they wanted fair treatment in terms of their evaluation. Similar studies have consistently indicated a desire by supervisees not only to learn what to do with clients, but also for feedback about their own behavior, that is, to know if they are doing what they should be doing (Larson, 1981; Tihen, 1983). Although these expectations will have been addressed during the first component (interpreting and facilitating the supervisee's understanding of the supervisory process), such expectations are important in planning activities as well. If specific behavioral objectives are set for clinician activities, if data are collected, clinicians will be able to determine more clearly the progress they have made and whether their expectations and intentions have been met. If the approach to supervision presented here is to become reality, specific attention must be given to the behavior, needs, and growth of the clinician in the clinical process, as well as to clients. Indeed, it is this attention that begins to develop the self-awareness on the part of clinicians that lays the foundation for their growth and increasing independence.

Planning as Related to Evaluation

Although not the topic of this chapter, evaluation must be considered here in terms of setting objectives. Historically, evaluation forms often had a significant portion of their content predicated on client behavior (Dopheide et al., 1974; Klevans & Volz, 1974; Shriberg et al., 1975). Consequently, if significant portions of supervisory conferences are about the client's behavior but if evaluation is based on clinician behavior, where is the bridge between the two? Planning should evidence a fundamental balance within evaluation protocols and tools between clinical competencies for student clinicians and supervisory competencies for supervisees. Certainly clinicians/supervisees should be aware of the criteria for themselves as it is reflected in the content of any evaluation form. Most importantly, student clinicians/supervisees should be involved in whatever planning takes place surrounding the use of evaluation protocols and tools.

Over 40 years ago, Rockman (1977) cited the need for identifying both short- and long-term range goals for student clinician behavior. Objectives may be as specific as improving the accuracy of phoneme judgments or learning to administer a specific test battery or as general as "the ability to plan treatment," "the ability to analyze treatment interaction," or "the ability to analyze my behavior." Obviously, the more specific the objective, the easier it is to document the achievement of that objective. Basically, we have to ask ourselves the same questions we ask the clinician in regard to their client: are the objectives that are selected clear, unambiguous, reasonable, appropriate, and capable of being achieved (Rockman, 1977)?

The importance of planning the role of the clinician was also stressed by Hunt and Kauzlarich (1979) in an ASHA presentation in which they affirmed that the fundamental relationship in the supervisory triad (supervisor-supervisee-client) is between the supervisor and supervisee rather than the client and the supervisee or clinician. They also stressed the importance of objectively defining the competencies of supervisees and clinicians which forms the basis for their evaluation. Further support for the need to attend to more than client behavior is also found in the knowledge and skills for clinical supervision (ASHA, 2008) which places a major focus on assisting supervisees to develop certain clinical and supervisory process skills and abilities.

Lulai and DeRuiter (2012) offered a systematic plan for new clinical supervisors in medical settings. With the general end goal that student interns will be clinical fellowship ready, they suggested formulating a weekly agenda of important topics and skills, which they provide, and focus on a "skill of the week" (p. 86; Appendix A). Their suggested approach provides clear expectations, tools to facilitate supervisor-supervisee communication, and an approach that facilitates problem solving and critical thinking.

This setting of objectives for the supervisee/clinician is related to subsequent steps in the supervisor process of observation, analysis and reflection, further planning, and evaluation. These components will be more fully developed if they are based on stated objectives and procedures. Supervisee/clinician progress can only be adequately measured if clear objectives have been set and behaviors relating to those behaviors quantified.

Long-Term Planning

Generalization of clinician behavior to a variety of situations should receive fully as much attention as does the generalization of client behavior. Generalization is considered by Elbert and Gierut (1986) to be the "hallmark of a 'successful' remediation program" and is defined as the "accurate production and use of trained target sounds in other untrained contexts or environments" (p. 121). This generalization is dependent on a comprehensive and informed planning process and is necessary for the total professional development of independent, analytical, problem solving, self-evaluating, and reflective clinicians who are ready to enter independent professional practice which is the goal of a a revised CAA (2017) standards.

Supervisees' ability to objectively observe, to analyze their own behavior, to reflect on its consequences, to problem solve, and to set objectives for themselves is what will enable them to generalize across situations and to be increasingly effective. The ability to problem solve, to devise solutions/techniques for changing situations, and to determine what may or may not have produced change is as important and probably more far reaching in terms of professional development than direct instruction from the supervisor.

Supervisors need to be aware of their broader responsibility beyond simply session-to-session planning. They should assist clinicians and supervisees in setting objectives for ongoing professional growth. Moreover, when general professional development is considered as the overriding purpose of the total supervisory process, short-term objectives must be seen as fitting into this larger perspective of total professional growth. In the educational program, where interaction may be fragmented because of short-term assignments, it can be easy to lose sight of general long-term professional development. Supervisees, too, may not see the relationship between today's events and tomorrow's professional responsibilities unless they see the day-to-day activities against a framework of long-range goals.

The site where supervision takes place may have a major impact on this issue. In all service delivery settings, the first and foremost responsibility is to the client. Immediate concerns about delivery of service to clients may make the urgency of the moment seem more important that the growth of the clinician. In the educational program, however, or in clinical fellowship settings, supervisors have a dual responsibility: preparation of clinicians and service delivery to clients/patients. They must learn to balance the needs of supervisees with the needs of clients. Awareness by both the supervisor and supervisee of the status of the supervisee's overall professional competence and goals in support of them will make it easier to coordinate them with patient and client needs. These dynamics and challenges are best dealt with in all settings during the planning component. Setting short- and long-term goals and objectives for client, clinician/supervisee, and supervisor makes it clear throughout the interaction what each person's responsibility will be.

Clinicians who have been involved in the planning of their own goals and objectives and who have learned reflective self-analysis and self-evaluation skills should be able to carry their long-term objectives from one client to another, from one practicum site to another, and then into employment settings where professional development will continue. Such multi-focused planning with clinicians/supervisees is not a separate and additional activity that necessarily requires more time. It is not a different process, but rather an extension of customary planning with its patient/client focus and becomes included naturally as a counterbalance to planning for the client.

Short-Term Planning

Short-term planning focuses on the current session-to-session interaction between the clinician and the client. It includes a) identification of clinician competencies or needs related to specific clinical sessions, the current client, or specific clinical challenges; b) determining how a baseline of clinician behaviors related to those competencies will be obtained; c) identifying clinician strategies to be used to modify the client's behavior; and d) planning observation, including identification of behavioral data to be collected and by whom, planning the logistics of the observation, and the identification of date collections methods.

Identification of Clinician Skill and Need

In educational programs and professional settings, supervisors may be familiar with clinicians' skills from previous supervisory situations or from evaluations of previous experiences. The emphasis on the Collaborative and Consultative Style embodied in the continuum model of supervision mandates that clinicians themselves demonstrate increasing responsibility for identifying their own strengths and weaknesses. This is a more positive approach than the philosophy in which the supervisor attends only to the weaknesses of the clinician and is underscored by clinicians who almost beg for "balanced feedback and evaluation."

The challenge of the CAA (2017) standards to provide supervision that is "structured to be consistent with the knowledge and skills of each student" will require supervisors to develop a methodology for determining this level of consistency. What factors should be considered in making this determination-number of client contact hours, previous grades in practicum, supervisor's standard practice? Is it the supervisor alone or in collaboration with the student who will make this determination? Should the intensity of supervision along with supervisory strategy change over the course of a practicum experience? All of these questions, and probably others, need to be asked and answered during this planning phase.

Areas of competency and need can be identified in three primary ways. Some may be identified during the first conference as the supervisor and clinician progress through the understanding component. Phillips (2009) reported on a study in which supervisors asked their supervisees to present their client during their first practicum meeting; based on that presentation, supervisors evaluated the manner, organization, accuracy, and completeness of the presentation and, subsequently, made decisions about the supervisees' level of independence. Supervisory style and level of support were then adjusted to meet the needs of the supervisee. The use of items from evaluation forms has already been discussed and may help clinicians who are unsure of their areas of competency and need. But not all competencies and needs can be identified prior to beginning the clinical experience. Others will be identified after clinical interactions have begun through observation, data collection and analysis of clinical sessions. As part of the planning process, supervisor and supervisee will need to decide what data will be collected about the clinician; these then will be studied during the analysis phase and areas of competency and need confirmed.

Determining Baselines of Clinician Behavior

The same procedures used for determining baselines of client behavior are relevant for determining baselines for clinician behavior. The evaluation systems for practicum previously described, clinician-stated needs or preferences, and information obtained from interaction analysis systems (see Chapter 5) are all sources of baseline data about clinician behavior that may need modification. Methods of obtaining baselines on clinical behaviors described by Brookshire (1967) would also be helpful to clinicians and supervisors at this stage.

Identification of Clinician Strategies for Modifying Client Behavior

Clinicians need different amounts of assistance in planning strategies for clinical sessions. It is tempting for supervisors, however, to provide too much from their own experience at this point and, thus, discourage creative participation by the clinician in the planning of clinical activities.

This is a crucial point in the process of supervision and the point at which the role of the clinical educator can by fully realized. It is where supervisors must use all of their skills in assisting the clinician to develop clinical strategies, in allowing the clinician to try and succeed or fail, to assume responsibility for the results of their plans and subsequent behavior, and, most importantly, to be a participant in the discussion of why the strategy succeeded or failed. This is the point at which clinicians can begin to become participants in the supervisory process and not just receivers of information. Certainly supervisor input is necessary during this period, but it should not dominate the process unless the supervisee exhibits major inadequacies and clients are disadvantaged.

Setting Clinical Development Objectives

An example of clinician planning has been contributed by the second author (McCrea & Brasseur, 2003, pp. 119-120):

After my clinicians have completed baseline testing on the client (usually two or three sessions) and three therapy sessions, I require them to complete the W-PACC (Shriberg et al., 1974). This independent self-evaluation enables me to see how they perceive their own strengths and weaknesses. They are also required to write three personal goals on the back of the W-PACC at the same time. During our next conference we discuss and refine these goals to ensure that they are measurable and attainable (i.e., reasonable expectations for the semester).

Some typical first-time goals may be: a) to feel more comfortable with my client and not feel nervous in my session; b) to make sure I have enough things to do to keep my client interested and involved for the entire session; c) to help my client improve, and d) to be an effective clinician. When I get this type of goal, we talk so I can identify sources of anxiety and get more specificity. For example, related to the first goal, the comfort factor may involve: a) identifying appropriate short- and long-term goals; b) developing and searching for activities that are motivating and productive and that lead to goal attainment; c) overplanning or trying to ensure that they don't run out of activities; d) developing branching steps for each step of the program in case the client is unable to perform the planned tasks; and e) the fear of making mistakes, for example incorrectly evaluating client responses. Just as client objectives are planned together, based on baseline data, so are clinician objectives. Based on the general goals previously stated, specific goals might be:

- The clinician will incorporate at least X number (usually one or two) of new activities or materials into therapy session weekly.
- The clinician will plan at least X number of activities for each session.
- The clinician will use at least X number of activities for each session goal. Appropriateness will be judged by his or her subjective evaluation of client interest and objectively by number of elicited responses (number to be determined in the planning process).
- The clinician will develop X branch steps for each major/primary step. A branch step will be implemented when the client's level of success is below 60% in X number of consecutive responses.

- The clinician and supervisor (this then also becomes a supervisor objective) will independently evaluate and record client responses for selected 10-min portions of each therapy session until a 90% or more point-by-point interrater agreement is achieved for three consecutive sessions. (We mutually decide to do this live, by recorded replay or a combination of both.)

These examples are predicated on a highly structured therapy sequence, presumably at the beginning of both the clinician's clinical experience and the client's participation in the therapy process. It illustrates, however, the process of targeting specific aspects of behavior and skill, which are implied by more general statements about behavior and which can be measured and observed. This same approach can be adapted across disorders, levels of clinician experience, and across settings to help clinicians actively and objectively engage their own behavior, to understand it, and gain control over it. It is this process of learning to understand how behavior can be objectified and measured that is foundational to becoming reflective, independent, competent, and problem-solving clinicians. Khami (1995) advocated specific planning for the professional growth of clinicians, including setting goals and developing plans to achieve them. Supervisors intentional mediation of planning and formulating clinical development goals with clinicians/supervisees is pivotal to the clinical education process and in implementing the continuum model of supervision.

Planning the Observation

The essential factor in the ongoing identification of competencies and needs is in the collection of appropriate data and their interpretation. The next chapter will detail the principles and operationalizing strategies for observation, but what needs to be emphatically stated here is the need to plan the observation. Traditionally, supervisors have decided what data will be collected, but often this decision is made after the observation has begun and it is often based on the supervisor's own "square boxes." Clinicians then have no opportunity to participate in the decision or have their concerns considered. Bernthal and Beukelman (1975) stressed the importance of providing specific information to clinicians about their own behaviors. The list of behaviors on which data may be collected is limitless—statements of instruction or direction, use of client cues, on-task behaviors, talk behavior of all types, and types of questions. In order for this information to be most beneficial to clinicians and to ensure that it addresses their clinical development needs, it must come directly out of the collaborative planning and goal-setting process.

Basically, the purpose of planning the observation is to allow input form clinicians; to ensure that observation time is spent profitably; and that appropriate data are collected that will make it possible for clinicians to begin to understand their behavior and competency. Whatever form the planning takes—written plans, contracts, programs, verbal agreements—it should include clearly understood objectives for the clinician, and perhaps the supervisor. In addition to "The client will _____," a portion of the plan should always include "The clinician will _____"; and, as appropriate, "The supervisor will _____." Such statements give clinicians more direction for self-observation, data collection, self-analysis and reflection, and modification of their own behavior. They also clearly identify the supervisor's contribution to the clinician's clinical education. They are measurable, if appropriately written, and are much more meaningful than a subjective statement from either clinician or supervisor that "it went better today."

PLANNING FOR THE SUPERVISORY PROCESS

The Supervisee

This is the point in the process at which clinicians begin to change roles. In terms of a superior-subordinate paradigm, they shift from a superior role with the client in which they are "in charge" to the subordinate role of the supervisee. This is the point in the process that will be defined and redefined as they develop and demonstrate skill and competency. In the Direct-Active Style of the

Evaluation-Feedback Stage, supervisees will play mainly a respondent role and will need assistance in planning and assuming expanded roles in conferences and the supervisory process. In the Collaborative and Consultative Styles, however, they will be much more directly involved. If the understanding component has been developed thoroughly, supervisees will understand their role in supervision and the purpose of planning their participation in it.

The literature from education provides a range of suggestions concerning the importance of involving supervisees in planning for the supervisory process: "The lesson planning is not complete until the teacher has been prepared for the role he will take in the supervisory conference to follow" (Cogan, 1973, p. 130). Maintaining the collegial role, as implied in the clinical supervision model, requires that supervisees understand their role as active participants in the conference, that they are not just passive respondents to supervisors' input, that they do not abdicate responsibility for joint problem solving, which is important in any type of cooperative supervision, including group supervision initiatives. The historical literature indicates that supervisees are not active in conferences; they do not ask questions or ask only factual, information seeking questions and only provide raw data while supervisors provide strategies and suggestions. One can conjecture about the reasons for this. Perhaps, they are overwhelmed by their clinical experience in general. Perhaps, supervisees do not know how to engage the process and be active even though expectancy studies indicated that they want to be. Perhaps, supervisors are too overwhelming and do not set the stage appropriately for them to be active and participative. Whatever the reason, there is often a discrepancy between what supervisors say they want to accomplish in the conference and what actually happens (Tihen, 1983). This solution to these dynamics is likely in the planning stage.

Planning the role of the supervisee will include: 1) setting the objectives for the supervisory process, 2) planning the data to be collected from the conference by the supervisee, 3) planning the self-analysis of the conference data by the supervisee, 4) planning what the supervisee will bring into the conference on the basis of those data, and 5) planning the role of each participant in the conference (e.g., planning an agenda for the conference).

Planning for the supervisee will become clearer in the subsequent chapters of the book. For now, overall long-term goals for supervisees might include: 1) more active participation in planning, data collection, and analysis; 2) modifying their own verbal behavior in the conference so that it is clear, specific and concrete; 3) participating in reflection and problem solving of their own clinical performance rather than expecting solutions from the supervisor; and 4) other goals that will make the supervisory process more productive and unique to the supervisee. The long-term goals can then be broken down and stated behaviorally in short-term objectives. Bartlett (2001) developed a tool, the Supervisory Action Plan (Appendix 4-4), which she used to plan with the supervisee and which includes the identification of specific objectives for both supervisor and supervisee in regard to increasing participation and independence of the supervisee within the supervisory process. O'Sullivan, Peaper-Fillyaw, Plante, and Gottwald (2014) and Walden and Gordon-Pershey (2013) both present approaches to planning that involve collaboration between supervisor and supervisee and suggest tools that support their processes as part of their discussion. Such planning for and with the supervisees should diminish the domination of the supervisor by specifically stating what the supervisee will do as they move along the continuum to independence (proficiency, conscious competency, reflective learning) and self-supervision.

The Supervisor

Planning for the supervisor is the component of the proposal made in this book that is probably the farthest from the traditional model of supervision. Such planning is based on the thesis that joint participation by supervisor and supervisee in the process produces not only independence in the clinician but satisfaction and growth in the supervisor as well. Planning for specific supervisory activity contributes to the process of continuous improvement and is consistent with the philosophy of lifelong learning for supervisors. In addition, with the need of supervisors to adapt their strategies and style of supervision to meet the specific needs of individual supervisees, the need for planning is increased to avoid the "one size (style)" fits all syndrome that has been identified by the descriptive supervisory style data in the literature and which is clearly inconsistent with CAA standards.

Fundamentally, supervisors must be aware of their own behavior. The importance of self-knowledge and self-study for supervisors is discussed in other places in this book. Behaviors must be identified that make up patterns in the supervisor's behavior and that may need to be modified or strengthened overall, or enhanced in relation to a specific supervisory interaction. A total plan for the supervisory process should then include objectives and procedures for the supervisor, as well as the client and the clinician/'supervisee. Because procedures for the supervisor will be fully addressed later, this section focuses on the planning aspect of supervisor objectives.

Supervisor objectives, like those of other participants in the clinical and supervisory processes, may be short- or long-term in nature; for example, broad objectives may be related to the supervisor's general patterns of behavior or specific to certain interactions with specific supervisees. The setting of such objectives assumes ongoing self-study by supervisors and supervisees of their interactions. This may come as the result of listening to and analyzing audio-recordings or viewing video recordings; from evaluations by supervisees, analysis with their peers or program administrators; and in the best of all experiences, from open discussion with supervisees about whether what is happening is congruent with their perceived needs and expectations and with the objectives that have been set. Mormer and Messick (2016) citing Palomo, Beinhart and Cooper (2010) suggested The Supervisory Relationship Questionnaire (Appendix 4-5) as a tool to gather information directly from the supervisee about the nature of their supervisory experience; this information can then be used by the supervisor to understand her or his supervisory interaction and as a consequence, make adjustments to it to better meet the needs of the supervisee. The list of knowledge and skills (ASHA, 2008) and Appendix E of the report of the Ad Hoc Committee on Supervision Training (ASHA, 2016) both provide support for supervisors (and supervisees) in formulating objectives, especially for those just beginning to analyze and modify their practice. Examples of objectives might be such general ones as reducing verbal behavior in the conference or providing less information. Other supervisor objectives might be supervisee specific as in the instance of a supervisee having difficulty in engaging the problem-solving process with regard to their own behavior with a client; in this case, the supervisor may pay special attention to their question-asking strategies with the supervisee to ensure that they are posing questions that require divergent, critical-thinking responses. Participation by supervisees in planning the supervisor's goals and objectives reinforces the collaborative nature of not only the planning phase but the entire supervisory process as well.

Planning for supervisors should provide direction for the supervisory process with respect to setting objectives and procedures for observation, data collection and analysis. If objectives are set appropriately, the control of the process by the supervisor should be reduced and along with that, supervisee anxiety. Activities should be planned so that supervisees know what to expect and be confident that their needs will be reflected in the supervisor's objectives as well as their own. Just as importantly, their involvement in this planning augments their understanding of the supervisory process and will help eliminate unpredictable supervisory activity.

REALITIES OF PLANNING

The immediate reaction of many supervisors and clinician/supervisees to this discussion of planning may well be, "How can I find time to do one more thing?" In the real world where supervisors can be assigned too many supervisees and service providers, too many patients and clients, and where there are more demands for increased productivity, this is not an unrealistic reaction or question. Rather than thinking of this process as additional work, however, it seems more profitable to think of it, instead, as doing the same things but in a different way. It would require a shift in focus away from the client as the primary consideration of planning to the adoption of a shared, more structured approach to supervision.

When the supervisory process is engaged, it is assumed that some time will be spent in face-to-face interactions between supervisor and supervisee, usually a conference. If not, it cannot be considered supervision and nothing that has been said applies. In educational programs, time is usually planned for regular conferences, although occasionally there are reports of programs where conferences are arranged on an as needed basis for support and assistance to the student clinician. This is appropriate for the Self-Supervision Stage of the continuum but cannot be considered adequate supervision, particularly for those students who may not know how to identify their own training needs. But, even when this is the case, the principles presented here are directly applicable for the times that face-to-face conferences are held.

How can the fourfold planning described here be operationalized? The setting of client clinical objectives and supervisee objectives is basically a matter of broadening one's thinking about the nature of planning. Decisions about what the clinician will do to support the client in attaining his or her stated objectives is the first level of planning. Fourfold planning only suggests that objectives for the other participants in the process which will, in most cases be derivative of or will certainly be related to the client's objectives, be stated clearly and behaviorally. If planning is extended in this way, clinician behaviors can be observed, data collected, and analyzed concurrently with the data documenting client performance. Occasionally, a supervisee might present with unique needs and challenges and when this occurs, the time spent in planning and subsequent follow-through on activities in support of the supervisee may increase. If, however, we are to meet the challenge of the CAA (2017) standard requiring clinical education be appropriately structured to meet the knowledge and skills of each student, ultimately moving them to readiness for independent professional practice, it is time supervisors must be prepared to spend. The full implementation of the planning phase of the continuum model is one way to fulfill this responsibility and in the experience of the authors, one way which will save time later in the process of developing independent clinicians and supervisees.

REFERENCES

Acheson, K., & Gall, M. (1980). *Techniques in the clinical supervision of teachers.* New York, NY: Longman.

American Speech-Language-Hearing Association. (2008). *Knowledge and skills needed by speech-language pathologists providing clinical supervision* [Knowledge and skills]. Retrieved from https://www.asha.org/policy/KS2008-00294/

American Speech-Language-Hearing Association. (2016, May). *A plan for developing resources and training opportunities in clinical supervision.* [Final Report of the Ad Hoc Committee on Supervision]. Retrieved from https://www.asha.org/uploadedFiles/A-Plan-for-Developing-Resources-and-Training-Opportunities-in-Clinical-Supervision.pdf

Anderson, J., & Milisen, R. (1965). *Report on pilot project in student teaching in speech and hearing.* Bloomington, IN: Indiana University.

Andrews, J. (1971). Operationally written therapy goals in supervised clinical practicum. *Asha, 13,* 385-387.

Baker, E., & Popham, W. J. (1973). *Expanding dimensions of instructional objectives.* Englewood Cliffs, NJ: Prentice-Hall.

Barlett, S. (2001). Supervisory action plan. Presented in Supervision 102: Short Course conducted with J. Brasseur, E. McCrea, W. Newmann, J. Rassi, B. Solomon, & B. Weinrich at the annual convention of the Speech-Language-Hearing Association, Washington, DC.

Bernthal, J., & Beukelman, D. (1975). Self-evaluation by the student clinician. *National Student Speech and Hearing Association Journal,* 39-44.

Blumberg, A. (1980). *Supervisors and teachers: A private cold war* (2nd ed.). Berkeley, CA: McCutchan.

Brookshire, R. (1967). Speech pathology and the experimental analysis of behavior. *Journal of Speech and Hearing Disorders, 32,* 215-227.

Christodoulou, J. (2016). A review of expectations of speech-language pathology externship student clinicians and their supervisors. *Perspectives on Administration and Supervision, 1*(Part 2), 45-53. doi: 10:1044perspl.SIG11.42.

Cogan, M. (1973). *Clinical supervision.* Boston, MA: Houghton Mifflin Co.

Costello, J. (1977). Programmed instruction. *Journal of Speech and Hearing Disorders, 42,* 3-28.

Council on Accreditation of Graduate Programs in Audiology and Speech-Language Pathology. (2017). *Standards for accreditation of graduate programs in audiology and speech-language pathology.* Retrieved from https://caa.asha/ org/wp-content/uploads/Accred-Standards-for-Grad-Programs.pdf/

Culatta, R., Colucci, S., & Wiggins, E. (1975). Clinical supervisors and trainees: Two views of a process. *Asha, 17,* 152-157.

Culatta, R., & Seltzer, H. (1976). Content and sequence analysis of the supervisory session. *Asha, 18,* 8-12.

Culatta, R., & Seltzer, H. (1977). Content and sequence analysis of the supervisory session: A report of clinical use. *Asha, 19,* 523-526.

Dopheide, W., Thornton, B., & McCready, V. (1984). *A preliminary validation of a practicum performance assessment scale.* Paper presented at the annual convention of the American Speech-Language-Hearing Association. San Francisco, CA.

Doran, G.T. (1981). There's a S.M.A.R.T. way to write Management goals and objectives. *Management Review, 11,* 35-36.

Dospheide, W., Thorton, B., & McCready, V. (1984). *A preliminary validation of a practicum performance assessment scale.* Paper presented at the annual convention of the American Speech-Language-Hearing Association. San Francisco, CA.

Elbert, M., & Geirut, J. (1986). *Handbook of clinical phonology.* San Diego, CA: College-Hill.

Flower, R. (1984). *Delivery of speech-language pathology and audiology services.* Baltimore, MD: Williams and Wilkins.

Fox, R. (1983). Contracting in supervision: A goal oriented process. *The Clinical Supervisor, 1,* 37-49.

Goldberg, S. (1997). *Clinical skills for speech-language pathologists.* San Diego, CA: Singular.

Goldhammer, R., Anderson, R., & Krajewski, R. (1980). *Clinical supervision* (2nd ed.). New York: Holt, Rinehart and Winston.

Goldman, D. (1995). *Emotional intelligence.* New York, NY: Bantam.

Hegde, M., & Davis, D. (1995). *Clinical methods and practicum in speech-language pathology* (2nd ed.). San Diego, CA: Singular.

Henri, B. (2001, June). *Performance review and emotional intelligence: A necessary synthesis.* Paper presented at ASHA Special Interest Division 11 Leadership Conference: Power Tools for Leadership and Supervision, Chicago, IL.

Hunt, J., & Kauzlarich, M. (1979). *Enhancing the effectiveness of the supervisory process.* Paper presented at the annual convention of the American Speech-Language-Hearing Association, Atlanta, GA.

Irwin, R., Van Riper, C., Breakey, M., & Fitzsimmons, R. (1961). Professional standards in training [monograph]. *Journal of Speech and Hearing Disorders, 8.*

Khami, A. (1995). Defining, developing, and teaching clinical expertise. *The Supervisor's Forum, 2,* 30-35.

Kleffner, F. (Ed.). (1964). *Seminar on guidelines for the internship year.* Washington, DC: American Speech and Hearing Association.

Klevans, D., & Volz, H. (1974). Development of a clinical evaluation tool. *Asha, 16,* 489-491.

Knight, H., Hahn, E., Ervin, J., & McIsaac, G. (1961). The public school clinician: Professional definition and relationships [Monograph]. *Journal of Speech and Hearing Disorders, 8,*

Larson, L. C. (1981). *Perceived supervisory needs and expectations of experienced vs. inexperienced student clinicians* (Doctoral dissertation). Retrieved from ProQuest Dissertations and Theses Global. (Accession No. 8211183) http://proxyiub.uits.iu.edu/login?url=https://search.proquest.com/docview/303157417?accountid=11620

Larson, L., Hoag, L., & Schraeder-Neidenthal, J. (1987). Supervisee satisfaction with a contract-based system for grading practicum. In S. Farmer (Ed.), *Proceedings of A National Conference on Supervision—Clinical supervision: A coming of age* (pp. 117-124). Council of University Supervisors of Practicum in Speech-Language Pathology and Audiology, Jekyll Island, GA.

Lemmer, E., & Drake, M. (1983). Client management and professional development. *Asha, 25,* 33-39.

Mager, R. (1962). *Preparing instructional objectives.* Palo Alto, CA: Fearon.

Mager, R., & Pipe, P. (1970). *Analyzing performance problems.* Belmont, CA: Fearon.

May, W.T., Morgan, B. J., Lemke, J.C., Kurst, G.M. & Stone, H.L. (1995). Model of ability-based assessment in physical therapy educations.*Journal of Physical Therapy Education, 9*(1), 3-6.

McCrea, E. S. (1980). *Supervisee ability to self-explore and four facilitative dimensions of supervisor behavior in individual conferences in speech-language pathology* (Doctoral dissertation). Retrieved from ProQuest Dissertations and Theses Global. (Accession no. 8029239) http://proxyiub.uits.iu.edu/login?url=https://search.proquest.com/docview/303031284?accountid=11620

McCrea, E. & Brasseur, J. (2003). *The supervisory process in speech-language pathology and audiology.* Boston, MA: Pearson.

Miner, A. (1967). A symposium: Improving supervision of clinical practicum. *Asha, 9,* 471-482.

Mormer, E., & Messick, C. (2016, November 16). *Bringing the evidence to clinical education practices.* Pre-conference workshop presented at the American Speech-Language-Hearing Association Convention in Philadelphia, PA.

Mowrer, D. (1977). *Methods of modifying speech behaviors.* Columbus, OH: Charles E. Merrill.

O'Sullivan, J., Peaper-Fillyaw, R., Plante, A., & Gottwald, S. (2014). On the road to self-supervision. *Perspectives in Administration and Supervision, 24,* 44-50. doi:10.1044/aas24.2.44

Palomo, M., Beinart, H., & Cooper, J. (2010, June). Development and validation the Supervisory Relationship Questionnaire (SRQ) in UK trainee clinical psychologists. *British Journal Clinical Psychology, 45*(2), 131-149.

Peaper, R., & Mercaitis, P. (1989). *Strategies for helping supervisees to participate actively in the supervisory process.* In D. Shapiro (Ed.), Proceedings of the 1989 National Conference on Supervision: Supervision Innovations (pp. 20-28). Council of Supervisors of Practicum in Speech-Language Pathology and Audiology, Sonoma, CA.

Peaper, R., & Wener, D. (1984). A comparison of perceptions of written clinical plans and reports. *Asha, 26,* 37-41.

Phillips, D. (2009). Supervisory practices in speech-language pathology: Pre-practicum assessment of clinicians in graduate training programs. *Perspectives on Administration and Supervision, 2009,* (19), 107-113. doi: 10.1044 aas/19.3.107.

Pickering, M. (1979). *Interpersonal communication in speech-language pathology clinical practicum: A descriptive humanistic perspective* (Doctoral dissertation). Retrieved from ProQuest Dissertations and Theses Global. (Accession No. 7923892) http://proxyiub.uits.iu.edu/login?url=https://search.proquest.com/docview/303001992?accountid=11620

Pickering, M. (1984). Interpersonal communication in speech-language pathology supervisory conferences: A qualitative study. *Journal of Speech and Hearing Disorders, 49,* 189-195.

Popham, W. J., & Baker, E. (1970). *Establishing instructional goals.* Englewood Cliffs, NJ: Prentice-Hall.

Prather, E. (1967). An approach to clinical supervision. In A. Miner, A symposium: Improving supervision of clinical practicum. *Asha, 9,* 471-482.

Roberts, J., & Smith, K. (1982). Supervisor-supervisee role differences and consistency of behavior in supervisory conferences. *Journal of Speech and Hearing Research, 25,* 428-434.

Rockman, B. (1977). *Supervisor as clinician: A point of view.* Paper presented at the annual convention of the American Speech and Hearing Association, Chicago, IL.

Russell, L. (1976). *Aspects of supervision.* Unpublished manuscript, Temple University, Philadelphia, PA.

Shapiro, D. (1985). Clinical supervision: A process in progress. *National Student Speech-Language-Hearing Association Journal.*

Shapiro, D. A. (1984). *An experimental and descriptive analysis of supervisees' commitments and follow-through behaviors as one measure of supervisory effectiveness in speech-language pathology and audiology* (Doctoral dissertation). Retrieved from ProQuest Dissertations and Theses Global. (Accession No. 8426682) http://proxyiub.uits.iu.edu/login?url=https://search.proquest.com/docview/303311796?accountid=11620

Shriberg, L., Filley, F., Hayes, D., Kwiatkowski, J., Shatz, J., Simmons, K., & Smith, M. (1974). *The Wisconsin procedure for appraisal of clinical competence (W-PACC).* Madison, WI: Department of Communicative Disorders, University of Wisconsin-Madison.

Shriberg, L., Filley, F., Hayes, D., Kwiatkowski, J., Shatz, J., Simmons, K., & Smith, M. (1975). The Wisconsin procedure for appraisal of clinical competence (W-PACC): Model and data. *Asha, 17,* 158-165.

Skinner, B. F. (1954). The science of learning and the art of teaching. *Harvard Educational Review, 24,* 86-97.

Solomon-Rice, P. & Robinson, N. (2015). Clinical supervision in the use of a three-tiered hierarchial approach to evaluate student performance. *Perspectives on Administration and Supervision, 25* (1), 31-41. doi 10:.1044/aas25.1.31.

Sweeney, G., Webley, P., & Treacher, A. (2001a). Supervision in occupational therapy: Part 2: The supervisor's dilemma. *British Journal of Occupational Therapy, 64*(8), 380-386. doi:10-1177/030802260106400802.

Sweeny, G., Webely, P. & Treacher, A., (2001b). Supervision in occupational therapy: part 3; Accommodating the supervisor and supervisee. *British Journal of Occupational Therapy, 64*(9), 426-431. doi: 10.1077/03082260106400902.

Tihen, L. D. (1983). *Expectations of student speech/language clinicians during their clinical practicum* (Doctoral dissertation). Retrieved from ProQuest Dissertations and Theses Global. (Accession No. 8401620) http://proxyiub. uits.iu.edu/login?url=https://search.proquest.com/docview/303160597?accountid=11620

Tufts, L. (1983). *A content analysis of supervisory conferences in communicative disorders and the relationship of the content analysis system to the clinical experience of supervisees* (Doctoral dissertation). Retrieved from ProQuest Dissertations and Theses Global. (Accession No. 8401588) http://proxyiub.uits.iu.edu/login?url=https://search. proquest.com/docview/303266850?accountid=11620

U.S. Department of Health & Human Services. *Health Information Privacy.* Retrieved from https://www.hhs.gov/hipaa/index.html.

Van Riper, C. (1965). Supervision of clinical practice. *Asha, 3,* 75-77.

Villareal, J. (Ed.). (1964). *Seminar on guidelines for supervision of clinical practicum.* Washington, DC: American Speech and Hearing Association.

Walden, P., & Gordon-Pershey, M. (2013). Applying adult experiential learning theory to clinical supervision: A practical guide for supervisors and supervisees. *Perspectives in Administration and Supervision, 23,* 121-144. doi:10.1044/aas.23.3.121

Whalen, T. (2001, June). *Incorporating professional behavior expectations into performance appraisals.* Paper presented at ASHA Special Interest Division 11 Leadership Conference: Power Tools for Leadership and Supervision, Chicago, IL.

Zylla-Jones, E., (2006). Supervison: Using mid-semester student self-evaluations to improve clinical performance. *Perspectives on Administration and Supervision, 16,* 8-12. 8-doi:10.1044/aas16.1.8.

 This chapter is a revision of that appearing in the 2003 edition of this book.

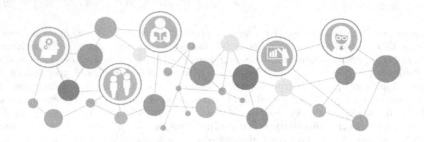

Appendix 4-1
The Wisconsin Procedure for Appraisal of Clinical Competence

In 1971, the clinical staff of the Department of Communicative Disorders, University of Wisconsin-Madison assigned themselves an in-house research project: to make explicit the processes by which students in clinical practicum are appraised and graded. In serial studies over 3 years, this research has yielded information in three areas: 1) a working conception of clinical supervision and the appraisal process, 2) a procedure for summative appraisal of clinical competence, and 3) an aggregate of descriptive information on correlates of supervisory processes and clinical competence.

The purpose of this applications manual is to train potential users in the summative appraisal procedure titled, The Wisconsin Procedure for Appraisal of Clinical Competence (W-PACC). Information on both the conception of supervision underlying this procedure and reliability and validity data are presented in detail elsewhere. However, the following section is a brief summary of critical assumptions underlying application of W-PACC.

Assumptions About Clinical Supervision and Appraisal

Figure 1 is a conception of basic elements in the supervisory process and appraisal. Subsequent sections of this manual will clarify terms and concepts expressed in Figure 1 and those which are incompletely developed here. Essentially, W-PACC is based on the following three working assumptions:

1. In its fullest sense, clinical practicum competence is currently assessable only through the individual "filters" of a supervisor. This is comparable to the academic freedom given to faculty in the classroom situation. "Objective" competency criteria for the full range of clinical skills and professional behaviors have not been (and may never be) universally adopted by working professionals.

2. Assessment of clinical skills involves two types of judgments. Is the clinician effective in a given skill? To what extent is effectiveness independent of the need for supervisory input?

3. Several factors may delimit the effective and independence scores achieved during any term of supervision; however, an adjustment for both entry characteristics and "process" characteristics (i.e., rate of clinician's learning and nature and quantity of a supervisor's input efforts can be made when assigning a grade).

In W-PACC, each supervisor is given both the right and the responsibility to appraise the output "product" (e.g., clinician effectiveness during the last 20% of a semester, quarter, etc.) of his or her "supervisory-cycle" efforts. Summative product appraisal then is based on the extent to which effectiveness is demonstrated to be independent of supervisory input, and grades can be assigned from normative or criterion-referenced product score tables which adjust for the entrance characteristics of each trainee.

FIGURE 1			
A CONCEPTION OF CLINICAL SUPERVISION AND APPRAISAL			
ENTRY CONSIDERATIONS	**CYCLE OF SUPERVISION**	**SUMMATIVE APPRAISAL**	**GRADE ASSIGNMENT**
Client Type and extent of disorder Other behavioral characteristics	**Supervisory Input** Conferences Demonstration Formative appraisal	**Product** Interpersonal skills Professional- Technical skills	Norm-referenced Or Criterion-referenced **Process** Personal qualities Formative appraisal
Clinician Academic and clinical experience • General • With client's disorder • With supervisor's approach	**Supervisor's Standards** Desired (Output) Product		**Entry Considerations** Clinician qualifications
Supervisor Experience with client's disorder Management approach Style of supervision	**Clinician Input** Conduct of management Conference behavior Reports, etc		Difficulty of Task **Grade**
Initial Conference	Period of Client Contact <u>Final 20%</u> Report Writing		Final Conference

Overview of the Wisconsin Procedure for Appraisal of Clinical Competence

Subsequent pages of this manual are organized as a series of Guidelines that roughly correspond to the chronology of application of W-PACC. Following the assumptions just reviewed, W-PACC is a quantitative framework for appraisal of clinical trainees. Importantly, it allows the flexibility needed to accommodate individual differences across supervisors, practicums, and clinicians. Hence, the Guidelines include choice points for the supervisor. The chronology of W-PACC administration is as follows:

STEP PROCEDURES	W-PACC MANUAL REFERENCE
1. During the initial conference(s) the supervisor assigns the clinician to a level	Figure 1 (entry considerations) Guideline I

2. During the initial conference(s) with the clinician, the supervisor reviews all pertinent information in this manual, including item descriptors for the practicum. The clinician should be fully aware of the basis for appraisal and grading.	Figure 1 All Guidelines All Appendices
3. Supervision proceeds in the customary mode for the practicum, including use of formative appraisal instruments, observational analyses, etc. Filling out a Clinician Appraisal Form (CAF) at mid-term is optional.	Figure 1 (Cycle of Supervision)
4. At the completion of the term the supervisor fills out a CAF, based on the clinician's performance during the last 20% of the term, e.g., appraisal of the "product" of supervision.	Figure 1 (appraisal) Guidelines II, III, IV, V
5. Supervisor calculates Interpersonal Skills, Professional-Technical Skills and "Average" Scale scores on CAF.	Figure 1 Guideline VI
6. Supervisor assigns a grade.	Guideline VII

Guideline I. Assignment of Clinician to Level

Rationale

As indicated in Figure 1, a clinician's entrance characteristics for a practicum experience should be taken into account at the end-of-term grade assignment. To accomplish this, entry considerations have been formalized to four clinician levels (Level I, II, III, IV; Figure 2). Each level accounts for a) the clinician's academic and clinical background relative to the practicum needs and expectations (e.g., client, task, supervisor) and b) the total number of supervised clinical clock hours the clinician has accumulated. On this latter criterion, the assumption is that basic principles of and experience in clinical management are summative and generalizable.

When to Assign Level

At the *beginning* of the practicum assignment, the clinician and the supervisor should review the clinician's previous experiences (as below) and circle the appropriate level on the Clinician Appraisal Form (CAF).

How to Assign Level (Refer to Figure 2)

1. Under the column titled "Experience," find the level at which the clinician meets the total number of supervised therapy clock hours criteria (do not include observation hours).
2. Inspect the other criteria at that level:
   a. If the clinician meets all of the criteria for the Level as required under the column titled "Requirements," assign the clinician to that level.
   b. If the clinician does not meet the required criteria, move back one level only and assign the clinician to this level (even though some of the requirements will be exceeded). Note that if the clinician does not meet the criteria listed under "Academic or Equivalent Information" listed for Level III and Level IV, move back *only one level*.

LEVEL	REQUIREMENTS	EXPERIENCE	NUMBER OF CLIENTS	IMMEDIATE PRACTICUM	ACADEMIC OR EQUIVALENT INFO
		FIGURE 2			

FIGURE 2

CRITERIA FOR ASSIGNMENT OF CLINICIAN LEVEL

LEVEL	REQUIREMENTS	EXPERIENCE	NUMBER OF CLIENTS	IMMEDIATE PRACTICUM	ACADEMIC OR EQUIVALENT INFO
I	Student clinician must meet two or more criteria	Less than 20 clock hours of practicum	None previously or first semester of practicum	Past experiences, number of clients, or clinical preparation is insufficient in supervisor's judgement	Is or is not prepared, in supervisor's judgement
II	Student clinician must meet or exceed all criteria	At least 30 to 40 hours of practicum	At least two clients or the equivalent of a semester's therapy experience	First client with this problem	Has or is currently receiving, in supervisor's judgement
III	Student clinician must meet or exceed all criteria	At least 90 to 100 hours of practicum	At least five to six clients or a student teaching experience	First client with this problem or first experience with this specific management approach	*Has or is currently receiving, in supervisor's judgement
IV	Student clinician must meet or exceed all criteria	At least 150 to 200 hours of practicum	At least 8 to 10 clients	Approximately the same management approach used with at least one other client	*Has or is currently receiving, in supervisor's judgement

*If the student clinician does not meet this criterion, move back only one level.

Guideline II. Structure of the Clinician Appraisal Form

The CAF (see pp. 138-143) consists of: a) the face sheet for summarizing pertinent information; b) an Interpersonal Skills Scale (10 items); c) a Professional-Technical Skills Scale (28 items);

d) a Personal Qualities Scale (10 items). Completion of face sheet information (see p. 138) is self-explanatory; calculation of scale scores is discussed in Guideline VI.

Interpersonal Skills Scale

The 10 items in this scale appraise the clinician's ability to relate to and interact with the client, the client's family, and other professionals in a manner which is conducive to effective management.

Professional-Technical Skills Scale

The 28 items in this scale are nominally divided into four subdomains:

1. Developing and Planning (8 items): the clinician's approach to the task
2. Teaching (9 items): the clinician's ability to modify behavior
3. Assessment (7 items): the clinician's ability to assess behavior and make recommendations
4. Reporting (4 items): the clinician's ability to formulate oral and written reports

Personal Qualities

The 10 items of this scale provide additional information about the clinicians' general responsibility in clinical tasks. Clinicians' scores on this scale have been found to be statistically unrelated to effectiveness decisions. However, this information is available for grading decisions (see Guideline VII).

Guideline III. Interpretation of Clinician Appraisal Form Items

Background

The following statements about interpretation of items on each Scale (Interpersonal Skills, Professional-Technical Skills) on the CAF are important to an understanding of the appraisal procedure:

1. At first inspection, some items on the CAF may appear to be appraising similar behaviors. In part, this is due to the necessary brevity of description for each item. Each of the items is meant to tap a *different* subskill within a scale domain or subskill domain.
2. In keeping with the conception of supervision described, some items are interpreted differently by different supervisors—or the same supervisor may need to interpret an item differently for different practicum sites. Hence, explicit "Item Descriptors" are needed.
3. Sample Item Descriptors are contained on pages 144 to 148. These descriptors should both *clarify item wording* and indicate *item flexibility*; they are suggestive rather than exhaustive.

Recommendation

Each supervisor who uses the CAF should derive his or her own descriptors for CAF items, using the descriptors presented on pages 144 to 148 only as possible guidelines. This suggestion is critical because:

1. Preparing descriptors for items will force an explicit understanding of how each item relates to the Scale domain (and for Professional-Technical Skills items, to subskill domains).
2. Items that initially seem similar can be differentiated.
3. Different practicums may warrant different descriptors for the same item.
4. Both test-retest stability and consistency in scoring items across students will be enhanced.
5. Supervisors have found such pre-determined descriptors to be extremely helpful in conferencing with students—both as initial Guidelines to appraisal domains and for end-of-term feedback (see Overview of W-PACC, Step 1).

FIGURE 3			
A DESCRIPTIVE/QUALITATIVE SCHEME FOR MATCHING CLINICIAN BEHAVIORS TO NUMERICAL VALUES			
FIRST DECISION			
Which column heading describes clinician behavior for 70% of the time or occasions during final 20% of the supervisory term?			
Specific direction from supervisor does not alter unsatisfactory performance and inability to make changes	*Needs specific directions and/or demonstration from supervisor to perform effectively*	*Needs general direction from supervisor to perform effectively*	*Demonstrates independence by taking initiative; makes changes when appropriate; and is effective*
1	2 - 3 - 4	5 - 6 - 7	8 - 9 - 10
SECOND DECISION			
Which Number to Circle?			
1.	2. Needs specific direction and demonstration with the client*	5. Needs general direction consisting of direct discussion with repetition and further clarification of ideas immediately or in succeeding discussions	8. 80% of the time operates independently
	3. Needs specific direction and role-played demonstration where supervisor and clinician verbalize client-clinician interaction	6. Needs general direction with no repetition or further clarification	9. 90% of the time operates independently
	4. Needs specific direction but no demonstration	7. Via limited general direction the student can be led to problem solve	10. 100% of the time operates independently
*Specific directions: step-by-step review of every aspect of the problem			

Guideline IV. Matching Clinician Behaviors to Numerical Values

Supervisors should adopt some explicit scheme for matching clinician behaviors to numerical values—that is, the "decision" process. Scoring a CAF requires that a number from 1 to 10 be circled for each item (or "does not apply" can be used for any of a number of reasons). Data (available elsewhere) indicate that supervisors can use this 10-point system reliably. Each of the following two schemes has been used successfully. *Scheme 2 may be particularly useful when a supervisee has more than one client.*

Scheme 1. A Descriptive/Quantitative Scheme

Figure 3 contains the information and the sequence of decisions used in application of this scheme. For each item on the CAF, essentially two sequential decisions are made:

1. *First decision*: Referring to the column headings on the CAF (as reproduced in Figure 3) the supervisor first decides which of the four column headings best matches the clinician's behavior for 70% of the time or occasions. Recall that this decision is made on the "product" of supervision, that is, clinician behavior during the last 20% of the supervisory term. If clinician behaviors appear to warrant placement between either of two column headings, select the number next to the boundary which best quantifies the level of assistance needed—and no second-level decision is necessary.

2. *Second decision*: The decision as to which of the numbers within a column heading best matches clinician behavior is next made by applying the descriptors listed under each column heading (Figure 3).

Scheme 2. A Proportional/Quantitative Scheme

Figure 4 is an alternative scheme for matching clinician behaviors to a numerical value. This scheme accounts for the "proportion" of time or occurrences which a clinician needs assistance from the supervisor. It assumes that clinicians will need varying amounts of assistance only in adjacent column headings. To use this procedure:

1. For each CAF item, decide the proportion of time or occurrences for which a clinician requires the type of assistance described by the four column headings.

2. Then, using the conversion values in Figure 4, circle the number on the CAF that corresponds to that proportion.

Guideline V. Maximizing Reliable Scoring

Completing a CAF should average 20 minutes per student. The following suggestions, which are based on experience and extensive discussion, are recommended for the "mechanics" of completing the forms at the conclusion of each semester:

1. Keep notes on supervisory observations, conferences, lesson plans, and formative appraisals. This is endorsed as the most important aid to making valid and reliable judgments for each item.

2. Complete the forms as soon as possible after the term of therapy has ended. Furthermore, try to complete all appraisals within a relatively short space of time, that is, try to avoid spacing the task over more than a few days.

3. Organize the total of clinicians to be appraised according to some subgroup commonality. The following organizing principles, listed here in decreasing order of endorsed value, have been employed:

FIGURE 4

A PROPORTIONAL/QUALITATIVE SCHEME FOR MATCHING CLINICIAN BEHAVIORS TO NUMERICAL VALUES

What proportion of the time or occurrences does clinician behavior "match" each category?

Specific direction from supervisor does not alter unsatisfactory performance and inability to make changes	*Needs specific direction and/or demonstration from supervisor to perform effectively*	*Needs general direction from supervisor to perform effectively*	*Demonstrates independence by taking initiative; makes changes when appropriate; and is effective*	**ASSIGN NUMERICAL VALUE**
70%	30%			1
	70%	30%		2
	60%	40%		3
	50%	50%		4
		60%	40%	5
		50%	50%	6
		40%	60%	7
		30%	70%	8
		15%	85%	9
		0% to 5%	95% to 100%	10

A combination of these grouping principles may be most useful, with one principle being used for the first organization into subgroups, and a second principle for further sequencing of clinicians for scoring within each group. The important recommendation is for supervisors to adopt some organizing principle for scoring a group of clinicians, rather than filling out CAFs in a non-specified or chance sequence.

GROUPING PRINCIPLE	COMMENTS
1. Group clinicians by practicum site	This is by far the most useful principle; students practicum site from similar sites are grouped and scored sequentially.
2. Group clinicians by similar client disorders	This may or may not result in a grouping similar client to the above, e.g. group all clinicians who worked disorders with stuttering, etc.
3. Group clinicians with clinicians of similar levels	Grouping by Level, e.g., all Level I clinicians, similar levels then all Level II etc. may at first appear logical. However, supervisors have found the two principles above to be more useful, although for some supervisory situations this principle is preferred.
4. Group clinicians by similarity in overall clinical skills	Some supervisors prefer to appraise their "best" similarity in overall clinicians first, regardless of level, etc. clinical skills

Guideline VI. Computational Procedures for Deriving Skill Scale Percentages

After circling values for each item chosen for appraisal, the supervisor can calculate scale scores on Interpersonal Skills, Professional-Technical Skills, and an average of these two scales. These values, expressed as percentages (to adjust for unscored items) are entered in the appropriate boxes on the face sheet of the CAF (Appendix 4-1). For each scale, completing the following procedure will yield the scale percentage:

1. Add the values circles for each item used. This total becomes the NUMERATOR.

    Example: If a student received five 7s and three 8s on the Interpersonal Skills Scale (two items were not scored) the total equals:

    35 + 24 = 59

2. Multiply only the number of items actually used by 10. This product becomes the DENOMINATOR.

    Example: For the student above, only eight items were used, hence:

    8 x 10 = 80

3. Divide the NUMERATOR by the DENOMINATOR; move the decimal point two places to the right; round to a whole number (move any decimal .5 or above to the next highest whole number)

    Example: As above 59/80   = .7375

    = 73.75

    = 74%

4. Record each of the percentages obtained, Interpersonal Skills and Professional-Technical Skills, in the appropriate boxes on the face sheet. An average of these two scores (i.e., the sum of the two scores divided by two) is also entered in the appropriate box on the face sheet.

Guideline VII. Suggestions for Grade Assignments

Discussion

A conception of the elements of grade assignment is presented in Figure 1 (see Summative Appraisal and Grade Assignment). The working assumption is that a grade can be derived from a three-way weighting of "product" information, "process" information, and "entry characteristics" considerations. Both the function of "clinical" grades and the contingencies for receiving a specific grade in a particular setting should influence weighting and grading decisions. For example, grades can be used 1) to certify skill, 2) to predict success, 3) to suggest entry points for subsequent practicums, 4) as feedback to clinicians, 5) to compare the outcomes of different groups, and 6) to allow continuation in a clinical program (the customary academic contingency). Functional differences among grades of A, AB, B, BC, C, D, for example, might vary according to the purposes above for which a set of grades is used. As with previous Guidelines, the suggestion is that some explicit framework for grade assignment must be developed by a supervisory team. Three suggestions for grade assignment are presented here.

Suggestions for Grade Assignment

Procedure 1: Nonspecified

Some supervisors or supervisory groups may prefer to use the CAF skill scores (Interpersonal, Professional-Technical, and Average) and Personal Qualities Summary solely as advisory input to grading decisions. Some supervisors prefer to avoid unwarranted use of "numbers" to characterize clinician competence. Following this procedure, which might be closest to a *subjective approach to grading*, the supervisor weighs 1) the CAF skill scores, 2) the "process" information, and 3) the student's level and difficulty of the client—and in some nonspecified fashion, determines an appropriate grade. Such procedures are defensible to the extent that grading decisions obtain the same validity, on any of the six purposes for grading listed above, as that obtained by supervisors using more explicit quantitative procedures.

Procedure 2: Individual-Supervisory Norms

Procedures 2 and 3 are each in turn, subdivided into two options. These options refer to two possible ways of converting Interpersonal Skills or Professional-Technical Skills scores (or the average) to tentative letter grades.

Option A—Normative-Referenced

- Step 1. Each supervisor plots the distributions of scale scores[1] obtained by his/her supervisees at each level (or each level by practicum site), for the current term and cumulatively over several terms.

- Step 2. A tentative letter-grade is assigned based on a clinician's performance in comparison with peers. Either natural "breaks" in the distribution or frequency percentages can be used, similar to grading practices in some large academic courses.

- Step 3. The final grade assignment may be derived by weighting the tentative letter grade derived above against information on "process" characteristics, personal qualities, and difficulty of task (other than as already adjusted for by level assignment—see Figure 1, Grade Assignment).

Comment: Such norm-referenced grading generally promotes competition rather than cooperation among clinicians and is counter to the objectives of skills competency training.

Option B—Criterion-Referenced[2]

- Step 1. In criterion-referencing grading, the distribution of scores is not used for grade assignments. Rather, each supervisor has a particular CAF score in mind which corresponds to a specific letter grade. (For example, in one practicum a supervisor may decide that a Level II clinician will need to obtain a CAF Professional-Technical Skills score of 88 or above to be considered for an A. In normative-referenced grading, a clinician's grade depends on how well the other clinicians in the practicum performed; in criterion-referenced grading such comparisons are *not* relevant.) These decisions may not be possible to make until a supervisor has had several terms of experience with W-PACC and CAF data.

- Step 2. Grades may again be weighed against "process" information, personal qualities summary, and difficulty of task—final grading may be adjusted up or down accordingly.

Procedure 3: Group Supervisory Norms

The steps to apply each of the two options in Procedure 3 are essentially the same as those reviewed for Procedure 2 above. However, In Procedure 3, grouped supervisory CAF scores are used for all clinicians, rather than each supervisor's individual distribution of scores.

Option A—Normative Referenced

- Step 1. The CAF skill scores (Interpersonal, Professional-Technical, and Average) from all clinicians in a training program are arranged in distributions for each Level or Level by Practicum Site.

- Step 2. Based on this frequency distribution, the supervisory group determines which scores will be considered for As, which scores will be considered for Bs, etc.

---

[1] Pages 148-149 present sample grade assignments aggregated over several supervisors. As evident in the assumptions about supervision and appraisal reviewed, Option B has been of greatest interest to the authors of this manual.
[2] Of the three scores, Interpersonal, Professional-Technical, and Average, Professional-Technical appears to correlate highest with subjective grades.

- Step 3. Each supervisor may adjust these tentative grades of the clinician she supervised up or down, according to "process" information, personal qualities summary, and difficulty of task considerations.

Option B—Criterion-Referenced

- Step 1. The supervisory group determines the CAF score that is required for each tentative letter grade at each Level or Level by Practicum Site.
- Step 2. Each clinician is assigned a tentative letter grade, according to the CAF skill scores obtained.
- Step 3. Each supervisor adjusts grades by the other three considerations previously mentioned.

Clinician Appraisal Form

CLINICIAN'S NAME _____   DATE _____

CIRCLE:

Clinician Level   1   2   3   4

Class Standing: JR. 1st. Sem.   JR. 2nd Sem.   SR. 1st Sem.   SR. 2nd Sem.

GRAD. 1st Sem.   GRAD. 2nd Sem. GRAD. 3rd Sem.

OTHER _____

TYPE(S) OF PROBLEM(S) _____

_____

PROBLEMS IN ADDITION TO COMMUNICATION _____

AGE(S) OF CLIENTS(S) _____

TOTAL NUMBER OF THERAPY SESSIONS _____

SUPERVISOR _____

INTERPERSONAL SKILLS SCALE ---------------------------------- /____/   COMMENTS:

PROFESSIONAL-TECHNICAL SKILLS SCALE -------------------- /____/

AVERAGE (IS   +   PTS) = ---------------------------------- /____/

           2

PERSONAL QUALITIES SUMMARY

No. of "SATISFACTORY" items --- /____/

No. of "INCONSISTENT" items -- /____/

No. of "UNSATISFACTORY" items --- /____/

No. of "LACK INFORMATION" items --------------------------------------- /____/

No. of "DOES NOT APPLY" items -- /____/

      (total should = 10)

% SCORE =   ___ SUM OF SCORED ITEMS ___
          NUMBER OF ITEMS SCORED X 10

INTERPERSONAL SKILLS	Does not apply	Specific direction from supervisor does not alter unsatisfactory performance and inability to make changes	Needs specific direction and/ or demonstration from supervisor to perform effectively	Needs general direction from supervisor to perform effectively	Demonstrates independence by taking initiative; makes changes when appropriate; and is effective
1. Accepts, empathizes, shows genuine concern for the client as a person and understands the client's problems, needs, and stresses		1	2 – 3 – 4	5 – 6 – 7	8 – 9 – 10
2. Perceives verbal and nonverbal cues which indicate the client is not understanding the task; is unable to perform all or part of the task; or when emotional stress interferes with performance of the task		1	2 – 3 – 4	5 – 6 – 7	8 – 9 – 10
3. Creates an atmosphere based on honesty and trust; enables client to express his/her feelings and concerns		1	2 – 3 – 4	5 – 6 – 7	8 – 9 – 10
4. Conveys to the client in a nonthreatening manner what the standards of behavior and performance are		1	2 – 3 – 4	5 – 6 – 7	8 – 9 – 10
5. Develops understanding of teaching goals and procedures with client		1	2 – 3 – 4	5 – 6 – 7	8 – 9 – 10
6. Listens, asks questions, participates with supervisor in therapy and/or client related discussions; is not defensive		1	2 – 3 – 4	5 – 6 – 7	8 – 9 – 10
7. Requests assistance form supervisor and/or other professionals when appropriate		1	2 – 3 – 4	5 – 6 – 7	8 – 9 – 10
8. Creates an atmosphere based on honesty and trust enabling family members to express their feelings and concerns		1	2 – 3 – 4	5 – 6 – 7	8 – 9 – 10

	Does not apply	Specific direction from supervisor does not alter unsatisfactory performance and inability to make changes	Needs specific direction and/or demonstration from supervisor to perform effectively	Needs general direction from supervisor to perform effectively	Demonstrates independence by taking initiative; makes changes when appropriate; and is effective
9. Develops understanding of teaching goals and procedures with family members		1	2 - 3 - 4	5 - 6 - 7	8 - 9 - 10
10. Communicates with other disciplines on a professional level		1	2 - 3 - 4	5 - 6 - 7	8 - 9 - 10
PROFESSIONAL-TECHNICAL SKILLS					
Developing and Planning					
1. Applies academic information to the clinical process		1	2 - 3 - 4	5 - 6 - 7	8 - 9 - 10
2. Researches problems and obtains pertinent information form supplemental reading and/or observing other clients with similar problems		1	2 - 3 - 4	5 - 6 - 7	8 - 9 - 10
3. Develops a semester management program (conceptualized or written) appropriate to the client's needs		1	2 - 3 - 4	5 - 6 - 7	8 - 9 - 10
4. On the basis of assessment and measurement can appropriately determine measurable teaching objectives		1	2 - 3 - 4	5 - 6 - 7	8 - 9 - 10
5. Plans appropriate teaching procedures		1	2 - 3 - 4	5 - 6 - 7	8 - 9 - 10
6. Selects appropriate stimulus materials (age and ability level of client)		1	2 - 3 - 4	5 - 6 - 7	8 - 9 - 10
7. Sequences teaching tasks to implement designated program objectives		1	2 - 3 - 4	5 - 6 - 7	8 - 9 - 10

	1	2 - 3 - 4	5 - 6 - 7	8 - 9 - 10
8. Plans strategies for maintaining on-task behavior (including structuring the teaching environment and setting behavioral limits)		2 - 3 - 4	5 - 6 - 7	8 - 9 - 10
Teaching				
9. Gives clear, concise instructions in presenting materials and/or techniques in management and assessments	1	2 - 3 - 4	5 - 6 - 7	8 - 9 - 10
10. Modifies level of language according to the needs of the client	1	2 - 3 - 4	5 - 6 - 7	8 - 9 - 10
11. Utilizes planned teaching procedures	1	2 - 3 - 4	5 - 6 - 7	8 - 9 - 10
12. Adaptability–makes modifications in the teaching strategy such as shifting materials and/or techniques when the client is not understanding or performing the task	1	2 - 3 - 4	5 - 6 - 7	8 - 9 - 10
13. Uses feedback and/or reinforcement which is consistent, discriminating, and meaningful to the client	1	2 - 3 - 4	5 - 6 - 7	8 - 9 - 10
14. Selects pertinent information to convey to the client	1	2 - 3 - 4	5 - 6 - 7	8 - 9 - 10
15. Maintains on-task behavior	1	2 - 3 - 4	5 - 6 - 7	8 - 9 - 10
16. Prepares clinical setting to meet individual client and observer needs	1	2 - 3 - 4	5 - 6 - 7	8 - 9 - 10
17. If mistakes are made in the therapy situation, is able to generate ideas of what might have improved the situation	1	2 - 3 - 4	5 - 6 - 7	8 - 9 - 10

Assessment

	1	2 – 3 – 4	5 – 6 – 7	8 – 9 – 10
18. Continues to assess client throughout the course of therapy using observational recording, standardized and nonstandardized measurement procedures and techniques	1	2 – 3 – 4	5 – 6 – 7	8 – 9 – 10
19. Administers diagnostic tests according to standardization criterion	1	2 – 3 – 4	5 – 6 – 7	8 – 9 – 10
20. Prepares prior to administering diagnostic tests by: (a) having appropriate materials available and (b) familiarity with testing procedures	1	2 – 3 – 4	5 – 6 – 7	8 – 9 – 10
21. Scores diagnostic tests accurately	1	2 – 3 – 4	5 – 6 – 7	8 – 9 – 10
22. Interprets results of diagnostic testing accurately	1	2 – 3 – 4	5 – 6 – 7	8 – 9 – 10
23. Interprets accurately results of diagnostic testing in light of other available information to form an impression	1	2 – 3 – 4	5 – 6 – 7	8 – 9 – 10
24. Makes appropriate recommendations and/or referrals based on information obtained form the assessment or teaching process	1	2 – 3 – 4	5 – 6 – 7	8 – 9 – 10

Reporting

	1	2 – 3 – 4	5 – 6 – 7	8 – 9 – 10
25. Reports information in written form that is pertinent and accurate	1	2 – 3 – 4	5 – 6 – 7	8 – 9 – 10
26. Writes in an organized, concise, clear, and grammatically correct style	1	2 – 3 – 4	5 – 6 – 7	8 – 9 – 10
27. Selects pertinent information to convey to family members	1	2 – 3 – 4	5 – 6 – 7	8 – 9 – 10

	Does not apply	1 — Lack Information	2 - 3 - 4 — Unsatisfactory	5 - 6 - 7 — Inconsistent	8 - 9 - 10 — Satisfactory
28. Selects pertinent information to convey to other professionals (including all nonwritten communications such as phone calls and conferences)					
PERSONAL QUALITIES					
1. Is punctual for client appointments					
2. Cancels client appointments when necessary					
3. Keeps appointments with supervisor or cancels appointments when necessary					
4. Turns in lesson plans on time					
5. Meets deadlines for reports					
6. Turns in attendance sheets on time					
7. Respects confidentiality of all professional activities					
8. Uses socially acceptable voice, speech and language					
9. Personal appearance is appropriate for clinical setting and maintaining credibility					
10. Appears to recognize own professional limitations and stays within boundaries of training					

Sample Item Descriptors

(See Guideline III for perspective on these descriptors.)

Interpersonal Items

1. Accepts, empathizes, shows genuine concern for the client as a person and understands the client's problems, needs, and stresses.

   The clinician demonstrates openness, acceptance, supportiveness, and honesty through verbal and nonverbal language. The clinician does not make parent-like statements or reassurances such as "Don't feel that way"; "Don't worry"; "Everything will be all right"; "You should…"; "You shouldn't…" etc.

   During the session, the clinician demonstrates acceptance, empathy and concern for the client. During conferences with the supervisor the clinician discusses the client, reflects these feelings and understanding of the client. Thoughtful preparation for session is one indication of concern.

2. Perceives verbal and nonverbal cues which indicate the client is not understanding the task; is unable to perform all or part of the task; or when emotional stress interferes with performance of the task.

   The clinician demonstrates this by 1) making attempts to alter the task or terminating the task, and 2) using language which indicates that he or she is aware the client is unable to perform the task. (This statement is made either to the client or to the supervisor, or to both.)

   The clinician's behavior indicates an awareness of the client's difficulty although he or she may not have the professional-technical skills to make the most appropriate and effective changes during the session.

3. Creates an atmosphere based on honesty and trust; enables client to express his/her feelings and concerns.

   Verbal and nonverbal responses of the client are included. The clinician does not "turn off" client questions, knows limits of knowledge and can say, "I don't know," and listens to client.

   Look to the behavior of the client to measure the clinician's interpersonal skill. Does the client feel the clinician is accepting, interested, concerned for the client as a person, and understanding of the client's needs, problems, and stressors.

   The client's behavior is interpreted as a reflection of the atmosphere created by the clinician.

4. Conveys to the client in a nonthreatening manner what the standards of behavior and performance are.

   In a positive manner the clinician indicates acceptable behavioral limits, verbally and nonverbally by manner and facial expression.

   The language of the clinician reflects a willingness to confront undesirable behavior and talk about it objectively and constructively.

   The clinician is able to state expectations in a positive manner, and to handle unacceptable behaviors in such a way that the client feels that a positive relationship with the clinician is not in jeopardy.

   Applies only to interactions which occur after the client has performed inappropriately.

5. Develops understanding of teaching goals and procedures with client.

   The clinician informs the client of immediate and long range goals, explains the sequencing of tasks and procedures, and questions the client for his ideas regarding teaching objectives and therapy procedures.

   The client is made aware of his purpose in therapy to the extent to which it is appropriate at any point in time. He or she is led to understand the goals and procedures and recognize them as something he can accomplish.

6. Listens, asks questions, participates with supervisor in therapy and/or client-related discussions; is not defensive.

   The clinician contributes to discussion at a level commensurate with academic background and clinical experience and "teams" for problem solving with the supervisor.

   The clinician is candid with the supervisor. The clinician discusses successes and failures and attempts to look for alternatives to deal with problems about teaching objectives and related clinical issues.

7. Requests assistance from supervisor and/or other professionals when appropriate.

   The clinician recognizes when he or she needs assistance. The clinician indicates when he or she is unsure about teaching tasks or behavioral expectations and checks with the supervisor regarding any changes made on the lesson plans.

   The clinician is willing to ask for assistance as soon as possible to ensure that teaching is continuously effective.

8. Creates an atmosphere based on honesty and trust enabling family members to express their feelings and concerns.

   Look to the behavior of the parents to measure the clinician's interpersonal skills. Do the parents feel that the clinician is accepting of and concerned for their child and for them? Can the parents openly discuss their feelings and concerns without feeling defensive?

9. Develops understanding of teaching goals and procedures with family members.

   The clinician's manner is straightforward and self-assured. The clinician respects the desire of family members "to know."

   The clinician clarifies goals and procedures without being judgmental. The clinician encourages and rewards parent involvement.

10. Communicates with specialists in other disciplines on a professional level.

    The clinician exhibits professional self-confidence. The clinician attempts to understand the background of other professionals involved and adapts his or her language accordingly.

    The clinician respects the integrity of specialists in other disciplines when there is an exchange of information.

Professional–Technical Items

1. Applies academic information to the clinical process:

   This item includes the application of classroom information as well as supervisory information given during the current assignment.

   As a result of attending class, group meetings, and discussions with supervisors, the clinician demonstrates an understanding of 1) the psychology of fear, 2) use of the CAF, 3) use of problem solving, and 4) stuttering behavior (these are only some examples).

2. Researches problems and obtains pertinent information from supplemental reading and observing other clients with similar problems:

   The clinician actively seeks additional information. The clinician reads and evaluates materials recommended by other sources including the clinical supervisor.

3. Develops a semester therapy program (conceptualized or written) appropriate to the client's needs:

   The development of a therapy program is an ongoing procedure which extends throughout the clinicians' assignment with the client.

   Within the first half of the semester the clinician defines short- and long-range goals.

4. On the basis of assessment and measurement, can determine measurable teaching objectives:

   The clinician uses information obtained through formal and informal assessment procedures to determine appropriate teaching objectives.

As a result of analyzing the client's speaking behavior and expressed feelings and attitudes, the clinician can identify the problems and determine appropriate objectives to alleviate these problems.

The clinician can delineate which aspects of behavior on which to keep data.

5. Plans appropriate teaching procedures:

Teaching procedures reflect knowledge of what the client might be able to do and at what level he is functioning.

6. Selects appropriate stimulus materials (age and ability level of client):

The clinicians makes good use of commercial materials; altering them if necessary to meet the client's needs, and creatively devises his or her own materials.

The clinician respects limits imposed by motor development and interest.

7. Sequences teaching tasks to implement designated program objectives:

The clinician knows baseline behaviors for task requirements and places the client's ability along the continuum.

The clinician teaches various tasks using a hierarchy of difficulty format. He or she does not start with a difficult level of performance before client demonstrates ability to perform at a lower level.

8. Plans strategies for maintaining on-task behavior (including structuring the teaching environment and setting behavioral limits):

The clinician explores alternate teaching environments and strategies for maintaining on-task behavior in order to provide structure for the client's progress.

The clinician knows when it is important to keep the client on task and when it is important to deal with something else. The clinician helps define criteria for acceptable or successful speech behavior at a particular stage.

The clinician can deal effectively with client behaviors such as inattentiveness, hyperactivity or distractibility

9. Gives clear concise instructions in presenting materials and techniques in therapy and assessment:

The clinician demonstrates adequate preparation, which eliminates the need to reword instructions or redesign materials during the session.

The clinician uses language that is clear, specific, and concise and is not redundant when giving direction or explanations.

10. Modifies level of language according to the needs of the client:

The clinician uses active rather than passive language. The clinician uses "doer" language ("You are pressing your lips together"), and descriptive language rather than labels such as pullouts, cancellations, and such.

By use of his or her words, the clinician indicates his or her understanding of the concept of the "total child," that is, does not talk down to the child yet uses words which can be understood.

The clinician provides a verbal model which is within the client's comprehension and modifies his or her speaking behavior so that the client's fluency is not adversely affected.

11. Utilizes planned teaching procedures:

The clinician knows in advance the planned teaching procedures. He or she does not have to refer extensively to written lesson plan.

The clinician demonstrates knowledge and purpose of the teaching procedure. The clinician uses this knowledge to: a) identify and describe those behaviors which facilitate the client's use of the procedure; b) monitor the client's behavior as it relates to achieving the objective.

12. Remains adaptable and makes modifications in the teaching strategy such as shifting materials and techniques when the client is not understanding or performing the task:

    The clinician overplans by having alternate procedures and materials available in case they may be needed. He or she knows baseline behaviors and can spontaneously return to these or to more advanced behaviors as appropriate with the session.

    This item deals with how the clinician reacts in one particular session, for example, ability to see that, for that particular day, the material is too complex and is therefore able to modify the material; ability to modify a particular technique that is not effective (change from pullouts to cancellations, change from modifying real blocks to faked blocks, etc.).

13. Uses feedback and reinforcement which is consistent, discriminating, and meaningful to the client:

    The clinician's own verbal and nonverbal behaviors are used as reinforcement for desired verbal and nonverbal client behaviors.

    The clinician positively reinforces on-target behavior. The clinician positively reinforces attitudes and feelings that the client verbalizes that are conducive to progress.

14. Selects pertinent information to convey to the client:

    The clinician includes information related to the client's problems with communication and knows when to extend the information. The clinician keeps the client informed of progress during each session.

    The clinician demonstrates the ability to give information that is relevant to the client's problems, questions, and so on.

    The clinician explains teaching strategies and expectations for progress to the client, that is, this item may be particularly applicable to school age and adult clients.

15. Maintains on-task behavior:

    The clinician is consistent in maintaining set behavioral standards.

    The clinician facilitates client concentration or attentiveness to task.

16. Prepares clinical setting to meet individual client and observer needs:

    The clinician uses appropriate furniture for the client and places chairs so observers can see the client's face; arranges supplies including personal notes and books so they are available, but not cluttered; and respects the client's wishes regarding observers.

    Setting is interpreted to include not only physical elements (furniture, materials) but people as well. When teaching in a group situation, the clinician prepares seating arrangements, which recognize the needs of individual children in relationship to the needs and behavior of other children.

17. If mistakes are made in the therapy situation, is able to generate ideas of what might have improved the situation:

    In conferences with the supervisor the clinician indicates an understanding of his or her mistakes and can creatively plan alternate procedures to meet problems which were unsuccessfully dealt with during the session.

    The clinician can independently verbalize future modifications in the therapy format.

18. Continues to assess client throughout the course of therapy using observational recording, standardized and non-standardized measurement procedures and techniques:

    The clinician recognizes goal achievement and moves the client through a systematic progression of designated objectives.

    The clinician recognizes when the client should add another goal, or when a particular goal needs to be emphasized (e.g., desensitization procedures, identification of stresses, etc.).

    The clinician keeps systematic data on measurable aspects of behavior.

19. Administers diagnostic tests according to standardization criterion:

    (no descriptors)

20. Prepares prior to administering diagnostic tests by a) having appropriate materials available, b) becoming familiar with testing procedures:

    The clinician knows how to administer various diagnostic tests. He or she does not become overly absorbed in test materials and procedures and so miss interpersonal contact with the client.

21. Scores diagnostic tests accurately:

    (no descriptors)

22. Interprets results of diagnostic testing accurately:

    (no descriptors)

23. Interprets results of diagnostic testing accurately in light of other available information to form an impression:

    (no descriptors)

24. Makes appropriate recommendations and referrals based on information obtained from the assessment or teaching process:

    (no descriptors)

25. Reports information in written form that is pertinent and accurate:

    The clinician includes information that enables the reader to understand goals and procedures. The clinician effectively summarizes the information rather than detailing it.

    The clinician's first draft of the final report reflects a knowledge of client's behavior, teaching objectives, and clinical procedures.

26. Writes in an organized, concise, clear, and grammatically correct style:

    The clinician is able to write, using language which will be meaningful and useful to people outside the speech and hearing clinic.

27. Selects pertinent information to convey to family members:

    The clinician selects relevant facts from therapy sessions or other observable aspects of behavior to share with family members.

28. Selects pertinent information to convey to other professionals (including all nonwritten communications such as phone calls and conferences):

    The clinician selects relevant facts from therapy sessions or other observable aspects of behavior to share with allied professionals. The clinician knows when to initiate contact with these professionals.

Sample Grade Assignments

The following table summarizes the correspondence between the "product" scores and grade assignments obtained over one group of supervisors ($n \geq 400$ appraisals). Briefly, the values for each scale represent the mean value obtained by clinicians who would subjectively have been given the corresponding letter grade. Obviously, no claim is intended or should be inferred that these values are the recommended norms for grade assignments. Recall that the authors of this manual have been most interested in developing criterion-referenced norms at the individual supervisory level (again, the values below have been aggregated over several supervisors solely for the purposes of summary inspection). Moreover, in addition to reflecting "product" or scale scores, an individual grade can be adjusted up or down by a supervisor in consideration of a) "process" information (up or down), b) personal qualities summary information (usually down), or c) "difficulty of task" information (usually up).

LEVEL	GRADE	INTERPERSONAL SKILLS	PROFESSIONAL-TECHNICAL SKILLS	"AVERAGE"
1	A	92	85	88
	AB	81	72	76
	B	78	65	72
	BC	--	--	--
	C	48	41	45
2	A	94	88	90
	AB	88	81	84
	B	76	67	72
	BC	--	--	--
	C	--	--	--
3	A	96	93	95
	AB	92	86	89
	B	80	76	78
	BC	--	--	--
	C	81	61	71
4	A	98	96	97
	AB	96	89	93
	B	92	87	89
	BC	98	66	82
	C	--	--	--

Reprinted with permission from Shriberg, L., Filley, F., Hayes, D., Kwiatkowski, J., Schatz, J., Simmons, K., & Smith, M. (1974). *The Wisconsin procedure for appraisal of clinical competence (W-PACC)*. Madison, WI: Department of Communicative Disorders, University of Wisconsin-Madison.

APPENDIX 4-2
INDIANA UNIVERSITY EVALUATION OF
SPEECH-LANGUAGE PATHOLOGY STUDENT PRACTICUM

Student: _____   Midterm Date: _____   Final Date: _____

Clock hours this report: _____   Client initials/disorder: _____

7 - Independent/Excellent

6 - Minimal or occasional assistance/Very good

5 - Performed well with guidance/Good

4 - Attempted, required specific guidance some demonstration or modeling/Average

3 - Attempted, but frequently required specific direction or modeling/Below average

2 - Relied on supervisor to direct each aspect

1 - Performance unacceptable

First and Second Semester Clinician:
A+ = 6.0-5.8   A = 5.7-5.4   A- = 5.3-5.0
B+ = 4.9-4.5   B = 4.4-3.5   B- = 3.4-3.1
C = 2.6-3.0

Third Semester Clinician:
A+ = 6.5-6.3   A = 6.2-5.9   A- = 5.8-5.5
B+ = 5.4-5.0   B = 4.9-4.1   B- = 4.0-3.6
C = 3.1-3.5

Fourth Semester Clinician:
A+ = 7.0-6.8   A = 6.7-6.4   A- = 6.3-6.0
B+ = 5.4-5.0   B = 4.9-4.1   B- = 4.0-3.6
C = 3.6-4.0

Section	Total Score		Grade Equivalent		Contract Required	
	M	F	M	F	M	F
I. Beginning Program Preparation	___	___	___	___	___	___
II. Initial Documentation	___	___	___	___	___	___
III. Program Development	___	___	___	___	___	___
IV. Documentation/Lesson Plan	___	___	___	___	___	___
V. Documentation/SOAP	___	___	___	___	___	___
VI. Program Implementation	___	___	___	___	___	___
VII. Treatment Process: Feedback/ Reinforcement	___	___	___	___	___	___
VIII. Treatment Process: Data	___	___	___	___	___	___
IX. Treatment Process: Interaction Skills	___	___	___	___	___	___
X. Documentation/Report Writing	___	___	___	___	___	___
XI. Response to Supervision	___	___	___	___	___	___
XII. Professional Behavior	___	___	___	___	___	___

(M = Midterm grade / F = Final grade)

(Any section with grade below B average will be identified as requiring clinical contract)

Mean Score ____ (M) ____ (F)   Clinical Practicum Total Grade ____ (M) ____ (F)

Supervisor _____   Date _____

Graduate Clinician _____   Date _____

Indiana University Evaluation of Student Practicum

Student: _____   Date: _____

I. Beginning Program Preparation

____ ____ Researched client disorder (class notes, textbooks, articles)

____ ____ Demonstrated ability to read file and gather critical information re: client's communication

____ ____ Extracted pertinent information from client file

____ ____ Demonstrated understanding of client's communication level and disorder

____ ____ Demonstrated ability to analyze client's program/communication for appropriateness/Additional need area(s)

____ ____ Attended and participated in supervision meetings/conferences

____ ____ **Total score for section/Grade equivalent**

____ ____ **Clinical contract required**

II. Initial Documentation

____ ____ Developed appropriate initial session plan to obtain pertinent information (tests, probes)

____ ____ Administered and scored standardized tests accurately

____ ____ Interpretation and analysis of standardized tests done appropriately

____ ____ Reported test data accurately

____ ____ Administered appropriate probes/baseline

____ ____ Obtained accurate initial baseline data

____ ____ Interpreted/analyzed baseline data appropriately

____ ____ Observed time-lines to submit initial plans/revisions

____ ____ **Total score for section/Grade equivalent**

____ ____ **Clinical contract required**

III. Program Development

____ ____ Clinician demonstrated adequate application of clinical knowledge/theory to develop appropriate treatment program

____ ____ Developed goals and objectives that were a logical outgrowth of gathered information and testing

____ ____ Lesson activities planned supported client treatment goals

____ ____ Materials and activities were appropriate to client's age, needs, abilities

____ ____ Demonstrated appropriate modifications for treatment materials and activities

____ ____ Clinician demonstrated the ability to appropriately modify the program for the client as necessary

____ ____ **Total score for section/Grade equivalent**

____ ____ **Clinical contract required**

IV. Documentation/Lesson Plan

____ ____ Goals and objectives were written in behavioral terms

____ ____ Goals and objectives encompassed appropriate treatment areas

____ ____ Demonstrated ability to break down goals into appropriate steps (task analysis skills)

____ ____ Lesson plan written with appropriate teaching techniques/materials
____ ____ Lesson plan written with appropriate verbal script
____ ____ Lesson plan written with appropriate criteria
____ ____ Lesson plan written with appropriate cueing levels
____ ____ Lesson plan written with appropriate reinforcement and feedback
____ ____ Clinician made appropriate edits based on supervisor comments in a timely manner
____ ____ Observed time-lines to submit initial plans, lessons and revisions

____ ____ **Total score for section/Grade equivalent**
____ ____ **Clinical contract required**

V. Documentation/SOAP

____ ____ Accurately completed SOAP with information in appropriate sections
____ ____ Accurately and appropriately reported data in session notes
____ ____ Interpreted data and session appropriately
____ ____ Note writing was clear, well-organized
____ ____ Indicated when objective had been met with revision of plan timely and appropriately
____ ____ SOAPs were edited with attention to supervisory comments
____ ____ Observed time-lines to submit notes/revisions and utilized suggestions to modify notes

____ ____ **Total for section/Grade equivalent**
____ ____ **Clinical contract required**

VI. Program Implementation

____ ____ Level of treatment was appropriate for the client
____ ____ Clinician implemented treatment activities which supported client treatment goals
____ ____ Clinician used materials and activities appropriately for client's age, needs, abilities
____ ____ Clinician used teaching techniques to maximize client performance
____ ____ Clinician used teaching techniques to maximize client cooperation and motivation
____ ____ Clinician effectively used instruction to support the client's success
____ ____ Clinician effectively used demonstration with instruction to support the client's success
____ ____ Clinician demonstrated ability to modify session during treatment to meet client's needs
____ ____ Clinician effectively modeled/shaped the desired response
____ ____ Clinician effectively obtained responses with a variety of stimuli
____ ____ Clinician efficiently obtained adequate number (N) of responses
____ ____ Clinician followed through on supervisor suggestions

____ ____ **Total score for section/Grade required**
____ ____ **Clinical contract required**

VII. Treatment Process: Feedback/Reinforcement

A. Feedback

____ ____   Accurate, corrective feedback was used to support client progress
____ ____   Feedback was contingent upon client responses
____ ____   Schedule of feedback was planned and consistently observed
____ ____   Type of feedback was appropriate for the client
____ ____   Feedback produced continued effort on the part of the client

B. Reinforcement

____ ____   Reinforcement was used appropriately
____ ____   Reinforcement was contingent upon client responses
____ ____   Schedule of reinforcement was planned and consistently observed
____ ____   Type of reinforcement was appropriate for the client
____ ____   Reinforcement produced continued effort on the part of the client

____ ____   **Total score for section/Grade required**
____ ____   **Clinical contract equivalent**

VIII. Treatment Process: Data

____ ____   Data was consistently taken
____ ____   Data was accurate and reliable
____ ____   Data was collected on-line quickly and discreetly
____ ____   Analysis and evaluation of data was accurate and comprehensive
____ ____   Data was used for on-going case management (changes in program)
____ ____   Data was accurately reported in the SOAP

____ ____   **Total score for section/Grade required**
____ ____   **Clinical contract equivalent**

IX. Treatment Process: Interaction Skills

____ ____   Clinician clearly set and consistently enforced behavioral limits
____ ____   Clinician employed behavior management techniques that were appropriate for client
____ ____   Clinician's pace of session allowed for maximum use of time
____ ____   Clinician recognized communicative intent of nonverbal/challenging behaviors and responded appropriately
____ ____   Clinician conducted session in an organized and sequenced manner that reflected preplanning
____ ____   Clinician demonstrated warmth, ease, and sensitivity to the client or family's feelings
____ ____   Clinician recognized the impact of communication style/speaking style on success of client and made appropriate adjustment
____ ____   Clinician recognized impact of eye contact/other nonverbal behaviors on the performance of client
____ ____   Clinician employed appropriate conference/counseling skills with client/family
____ ____   Clinician conducted appropriate parent in-service on an ongoing basis
____ ____   Clinician encouraged client and/or family responsibility in management

____ ____   **Total score for section/Grade equivalent**
____ ____   **Clinical contract required**

X. Documentation/Report Writing

_____ _____ Included all pertinent information in client report
_____ _____ Reported information accurately
_____ _____ Demonstrated appropriate writing skills (spelling, grammar, and sentence construction)
_____ _____ Used professional writing style
_____ _____ Report was understandable for client or parent/caregiver
_____ _____ Report was well organized
_____ _____ Test, results, interpretation written accurately and appropriately
_____ _____ Report discussion of procedures and progress written accurately
_____ _____ Report summary written comprehensively with synthesis and integration of information
_____ _____ Made appropriate recommendations
_____ _____ Observed time-lines to submit drafts, revisions

_____ _____ **Total score for section/Grade equivalent**
_____ _____ **Clinical contract required**

XI. Response to Supervision

_____ _____ Considered supervisory suggestions and openly discussed differences in ideas
_____ _____ Demonstrated reflective practice and engaged in self-supervision to discover areas of strength and those which needed improvement
_____ _____ Suggested ways to enhance clinical performance
_____ _____ Developed increasing confidence about own performance and professional growth
_____ _____ Positively dealt with own frustrations in treatment and/or supervision
_____ _____ Discussed supervisory analysis and evaluation in a positive manner

_____ _____ **Total score for section/Grade equivalent**
_____ _____ **Clinical contract required**

XII. Professional Behavior (+/-)

A. General

_____ _____ Demonstrated cooperation and teamwork
_____ _____ Kept verbal commitments
_____ _____ Never had an unexcused clinical or supervisory absence
_____ _____ Observed legal mandates, most especially client privacy and confidentiality policies
_____ _____ Dressed for activities with respect for observers, clients, and the professional setting
_____ _____ Was punctual in beginning and ending clinical sessions
_____ _____ Encouraged client and/or family responsibility in management
_____ _____ Written and/or verbal communication is free from judgmental statements

B. Public Health Precautions (+/-)

_____ _____ Demonstrated care and concern for general well-being of client
_____ _____ Adhered to standards of health practices for clinical materials
_____ _____ Adhered to standards of sanitary conditions for room space and equipment

_____ _____   Understand and observed the health precaution information provided by the setting

_____ _____   Other (_____)

_____ _____   **Clinical contract required**

MIDTERM COMMENTS:

_____
_____
_____
_____
_____
_____
_____
_____

RECOMMENDATIONS FOR CONTINUED CLINICAL AND PROFESSIONAL GROWTH:

_____
_____
_____
_____
_____
_____
_____
_____

FINAL COMMENTS:

_____
_____
_____
_____
_____
_____

RECOMMENDATIONS FOR CONTINUED CLINICAL AND PROFESSIONAL GROWTH:

_____
_____
_____
_____
_____
_____
_____
_____

Reprinted with permission from: Department of Speech and Hearing Sciences, Indiana University, Bloomington, IN. In-house document. 1996.

APPENDIX 4-3
10 GENERIC ABILITIES SCALE FROM UNIVERSITY OF WISCONSIN-MADISON

STUDENT GENERIC ABILITIES SELF-ASSESSMENT
Physical Therapy Program
University of Wisconsin-Madison

Student - Clinical Experiences

General Instructions - Student

1.   Read description and definitions of Generic Abilities - page 2.

2.   Become familiar with behavioral criteria for each level - pages 3 & 4.

3.   **Self-assess your performance**. At mid-term and upon completion of your clinical, *highlight (or underline) the sample behaviors you feel you have consistently performed.*

4.   Based upon your self-assessment, complete page 5 of the Generic Abilities. Rank each GA along the visual analog scale and provide a brief example of the highest sample behavior you have demonstrated thus far in the clinical experience.

5.   Ask your Clinical Instructor to review and discuss your self-assessment, then sign page 5, signifying that they agree with your assessment.

6.   Return entire packet to ACCE, University of Wisconsin-Madison upon completion of this experience.

PLEASE NOTE:

1.   The criteria provide **examples** of behaviors required for competence at a given level.

2.   **It is NOT necessary for the student to demonstrate all of the criteria to be considered competent at a given level. However, if a behavior is not highlighted because it is a problem area, comments are required on page 5.**

Student _____
                    (Please Print)

Clinical Instructor _____
                                (Please Print)

Facility _____ **City/State** _____

PT Program _____ **Rotation (# or type)** _____

Generic Abilities*

Generic abilities are attributes, characteristics or behaviors that are not explicitly part of the profession's core of knowledge and technical skills but are nevertheless required for success in the profession. Ten generic abilities were identified through a study conducted at UW-Madison in 1991-92. The ten abilities and definitions developed are:

Generic Ability	Definition
1. Commitment to Learning	The ability to self-assess, self-correct, and self-direct; to identify needs and sources of learning; and to continually seek new knowledge and understanding.
2. Interpersonal Skills	The ability to interact effectively with patients, families, colleagues, other health care professionals, and the community and to deal effectively with cultural and ethnic diversity issues.
3. Communication Skills	The ability to communicate effectively (i.e., speaking, body language, reading, writing, listening) for varied audiences and purposes.
4. Effective Use of Time and Resources	The ability to obtain the maximum benefit from a minimum investment of time and resources.
5. Use of Constructive Feedback	The ability to identify sources of and seek out feedback and to effectively use and provide feedback for improving personal interaction.
6. Problem-Solving	The ability to recognize and define problems, analyze data, develop and implement solutions, and evaluate outcomes.
7. Professionalism	The ability to exhibit appropriate professional conduct and to represent the profession effectively.
8. Responsibility	The ability to fulfill commitments and to be accountable for actions and outcomes.
9. Critical Thinking	The ability to question logically; to identify, generate, and evaluate elements of logical argument; to recognize and differentiate facts, illusions, assumptions, and hidden assumptions; and to distinguish the relevant from the irrelevant.
10. Stress Management	The ability to identify sources of stress and to develop effective coping behaviors.

* *Developed by the Physical Therapy Program, University of Wisconsin-Madison, May, W., et al. Journal of Physical Therapy Education. 9:1, Spring 1995.*

Generic Abilities	Beginning Level Behavioral Criteria	Developing Level Behavioral Criteria	Entry Level Behavioral Criteria
1. Commitment to Learning	Identifies problems; formulates appropriate questions; identifies and locates appropriate resources; demonstrates a positive attitude (motivation) toward learning; offers own thoughts and ideas; identifies need for further information	Prioritizes information needs; analyzes and subdivides large questions into components; seeks out professional literature; sets personal and professional goals; identifies own learning needs based on previous experiences; plans and presents an in-service, or research or case studies; welcomes and/or seeks new learning opportunities	Applies new information and re-evaluates performance; accepts that there may be more than one answer to a problem; recognizes the need to and is able to verify solutions to problems; reads articles critically and understands the limits of application to professional practice; researches and studies areas where knowledge base is lacking
2. Interpersonal Skills	Maintains professional demeanor in all clinical interactions; demonstrates interest in patients as individuals; respects cultural and personal differences of others; is non-judgmental about patients' lifestyles; communicates with others in a respectful, confident manner; respects personal space of patients and others; maintains confidentiality in all clinical interactions; demonstrates acceptance of limited knowledge and experience	Recognizes impact of non-verbal communication and modifies accordingly; assumes responsibility for own actions; motivates others to achieve; establishes trust; seeks to gain knowledge and input from others; respects role of support staff	Listens to patient but reflects back to original concern; works effectively with challenging patients; responds effectively to unexpected experiences; talks about difficult issues with sensitivity and objectivity; delegates to others as needed; approaches others to discuss differences in opinion; accommodates differences in learning styles
3. Communication Skills	Demonstrates understanding of basic English (verbal and written): uses correct grammar, accurate spelling and expression; writes legibly; recognizes impact of non-verbal communication: listens actively; maintains eye contact	Utilizes non-verbal communication to augment verbal message; restates, reflects and clarifies message; collects necessary information from the patient interview	Modifies communication (verbal and written) to meet needs of different audiences; presents verbal or written messages with logical organization and sequencing; maintains open and constructive communication; utilizes communication technology effectively; dictates clearly and concisely
4. Effective Use of Time and Resources	Focuses on tasks at hand without dwelling on past mistakes; recognizes own resource limitations; uses existing resources effectively; uses unscheduled time efficiently; completes assignments in timely fashion	Sets up own schedule; coordinates schedule with others; demonstrates flexibility; plans ahead	Sets priorities and reorganizes when needed; considers patient's goals in context of patient, clinic and third party resources; has ability to say "No"; performs multiple tasks simultaneously and delegates when appropriate; uses scheduled time with each patient efficiently

Instructions: Highlight all criteria that describes the student's performance

5. Use of Constructive Feedback	Demonstrates active listening skills; actively seeks feedback and help; demonstrates a positive attitude toward feedback; critiques own performance; maintains two-way information	Assesses own performance accurately; utilizes feedback when establishing pre-professional goals; provides constructive and timely feedback when establishing pre-professional goals; develops plan of action in response to feedback	Seeks feedback from clients; modifies feedback given to clients according to their learning styles; reconciles differences with sensitivity; considers multiple approaches when responding to feedback
6. Problem-Solving	Recognizes problems; states problems clearly; describes known solutions to problem; identifies resources needed to develop solutions; begins to examine multiple solutions to problems	Prioritizes problems; identifies contributors to problem; considers consequences of possible solutions; consults with others to clarify problem	Implements solutions; reassesses solutions; evaluates outcomes; updates solutions to problems based on current research; accepts responsibility for implementing of solutions
7. Professionalism	Abides by APTA Code of Ethics; demonstrates awareness of state licensure regulations; abides by facility policies and procedures; projects professional image; attends professional meetings; demonstrates honesty, compassion, courage and continuous regard for all	Identifies positive professional role models; discusses societal expectations of the profession; acts on moral commitment; involves other health care professionals in decision-making; seeks informed consent from patients	Demonstrates accountability for professional decisions; treats patients within scope of expertise; discusses role of physical therapy in health care; keeps patient as priority
8. Responsibility	Demonstrates dependability; demonstrates punctuality; follows through on commitments; recognizes own limits	Accepts responsibility for actions and outcomes; provides safe and secure environment for patients; offers and accepts help; completes projects without prompting	Directs patients to other health care professionals when needed; delegates as needed; encourages patient accountability
9. Critical Thinking	Raises relevant questions; considers all available information; states the results of scientific literature; recognizes holes in knowledge base; articulates ideas	Feels challenged to examine ideas; understands scientific method; formulates new ideas; seeks alternative ideas; formulates alternative hypotheses; critiques hypotheses and ideas	Exhibits openness to contradictory ideas; assess issues raised by contradictory ideas; justifies solutions selected; determines effectiveness of applied solutions
10. Stress Management	Recognizes own stressors or problems; recognizes distress or problems in others; seeks assistance as needed; maintains professional demeanor in all situations	Maintains balance between professional and personal life; demonstrates effective affective responses in all situations; accepts constructive feedback; establishes outlets to cope with stressors	Prioritizes multiple commitments; responds calmly to urgent situations; tolerates inconsistencies in health care environment

Behavioral Criteria Refined 11/96

Instructions: Highlight all criteria that describes the student's performance

Generic Abilities
Mid-term and Final Assessment

Instructions: Assess each ability based on your self-assessment (highlighted areas - page 3 & 4) by circling appropriate level. Mark the scale to reflect your **mid-term** and **final** assessment. Examples are required to justify level marked. Please sign and date the assessment.
B=Beginning Level   **D**=Developing Level   **E**=Entry Level

1. **Commitment to Learning**   B   D   E
   Comments & Examples: _____

2. **Interpersonal Skills**   B   D   E
   Comments & Examples: _____

3. **Communication Skills**   B   D   E
   Comments & Examples: _____

4. **Effective Use of Time & Resources**   B   D   E
   Comments & Examples: _____

5. **Use of Constructive Feedback**   B   D   E
   Comments & Examples: _____

6. **Problem Solving**   B   D   E
   Comments & Examples: _____

7. **Professionalism**   B   D   E
   Comments & Examples: _____

8. **Responsibility**   B   D   E
   Comments & Examples: _____

9. **Critical Thinking**   B   D   E
   Comments & Examples: _____

10. **Stress Management**   B   D   E
    Comments & Examples: _____

Facility _____ Rotation (# or type) _____

Mid-term
Student _____ Date _____
                        (Signature)
Clinical Instructor _____ Date _____
                        (Signature)
Final
Student _____ Date _____
                        (Signature)
Clinical Instructor _____ Date _____
                        (Signature)

APPENDIX 4-4
BARTLETT'S SUPERVISORY ACTION PLAN

Supervisory Action Plan

Date of Plan _____

Supervisee _____
Supervisor _____

Site/Setting _____
Assignment Period _____

ANALYSIS AND EVALUATION		SUPERVISOR SEE RELATIONSHIP		ACTION PLAN	
Supervisee's strengths/ weaknesses	*Effect(s) on supervision*	*Expected outcome*	*Behaviors/ skills to modify*	*Techniques and strategies*	*Results*
Should include documented evidence of Supervisee's skills and behaviors	Is the effect positive or negative? Is there a problem?	What is the desired end result? What will happen with planned change?	What changes need to be made by supervisee/ supervisor	Who will do what?	Date and document what occurred.

Action Plan Case Study

Jessica is a third semester graduate student in speech-language pathology assigned to a practicum in an elementary school that uses a collaborative approach to service delivery. Her caseload consists of preschool and K-3 students with moderate to severe communication disorders who are enrolled in inclusive classrooms. Several of the children also receive special education and related services in the context of daily school activities.

Jessica has previously completed 175 hours of clinical practicum in the university's clinic and in an acute care facility; in both places she worked with clients individually. The assignment to the school is her fourth practicum experience after having completed a full academic year and an 8-week intensive summer experience. She has a strong academic background for normal and disordered communication and a solid grasp of theoretical concepts to support her assessment and intervention activities. Previous supervisors have rated her clinical skills as good to excellent. She is skilled in using computers for clinical and search applications and she routinely familiarizes herself with resources that are available for clinical implementation. Using the university's checklist for clinical skills—a formative tool for assessing progress in developing skills and competencies—at the conclusion of her third practicum assignment, Jessica's strengths were in the areas of: behavior management, data collection, preparation for treatment and assessment, and professionalism. She independently seeks out opportunities to solicit and share relevant information with families, teachers, and other for the purpose of identifying functional outcomes. She is conscientious about submitting lesson plans, progress summaries, and evaluation reports on time.

In the school setting, she has used spare time to conduct classroom observations, meet with teachers, and review records.

Skills in self-evaluation and modifying objectives are rated as emerging. One supervisor reported that if an objective or procedure is not successful, Jessica is likely to omit them from her plans, rather than to analyze the session and to alter them for a future session. She remains dependent on the supervisor for support in this area. While Jessica's observation and evaluation of the client's behaviors are usually accurate and insightful, she has expressed her lack of confidence at evaluating her own clinical performance. Her written and verbal summaries of test findings and of clients' progress are areas that have been identified as weak. A sample from a recent conference with a parent illustrates this observation:

> "Max's speech is problematic. At this point in time, it is apparent that there is some evidence of residual phonological processes; coalescence, voicing of unvoiced consonants, devoicing consonants that should be voiced, metathesis, and syllable reduction. Vowel distortions are present in nasalized contexts."

Postsession entries in the chart notes are usually one half to one quarter of a page and Jessica has difficulty with separating subjective from objective data in reporting the outcomes of her sessions. She needs to refine her skills in presenting information succinctly.

The supervisor reviews Jessica's lesson plans and other written work pertaining to her client and to her own clinical growth on a weekly basis. Direct observation of her management sessions occurs 75% of the time and verbal and written feedback are provided following each observation. Jessica has not consistently negotiated the focus of subsequent supervision or evaluated her own progress over time, and she has not proposed changes to the frequency or type of feedback. She has been asked to complete a questionnaire that will assist her with developing a supervisory plan.

Supervisory Action Plan

Date of Plan _____

Supervisee _____
Supervisor _____

Site/Setting _____
Assignment Period _____

ANALYSIS AND EVALUATION		SUPERVISOR SEE RELATIONSHIP		ACTION PLAN	
Supervisee's strengths/ weaknesses	*Effect(s) on supervision*	*Expected outcome*	*Behaviors/skills to modify*	*Techniques and strategies*	*Results*
Include documented evidence of Supervisee's skills and behaviors	Is the effect positive or negative? Is there a problem?	What is the desired end result? What will happen with planned change?	What changes need to be made by supervisee/supervisor?	Who will do what?	Date and document what occurred.
e.g., Strengths • Thorough preparation • Accurate data collection • Initiates contact with family and education team • Solid theory • Meets deadlines • Uses time efficiently Weaknesses • Overuse of professional jargon • Lengthy documentation	• Alter use of supervisory time for direct observation • Supervisee is a reliable and valued resource • Moving toward collaboration model on continuum • Not considered a problem to supervision	Supervisor: • Collaborative role Supervisee: • Self-evaluation • Independence	Supervisor: • Amount of feedback • Direct feedback • Daily review of lesson plans Supervisee: • Initiate focus of supervision • Propose changes to supervision • Efficiency of documentation	Supervisor: • Conference 1x/wk and reduce frequency to bi-weekly • Audio recording analysis of conference • 25% direct observation of treatment Supervisee: • Self evaluation with video recording • Use of analysis tool • Use of personal journal for self reflection • Set personal goals • Review a variety of documentation formats	

Reprinted with permission from Barlett, S. (2001). Supervisory action plan. Presented in *Supervision 102: Short course* [conducted with J. Brasseur, E. McCrea, W. Newmann, J. Rassi, B. Solomon & B. Weinrich] at annual convention of the American Speech-Language-Hearing Association, Washington, DC: November 16, 2000.

APPENDIX 4-5
THE SUPERVISORY RELATIONSHIP QUESTIONNAIRE

THE SUPERVISORY RELATIONSHIP QUESTIONNAIRE (SRQ)
Developed by Marina Palomo (supervised by Helen Beinart) Copyright SRQ.
Reproduce freely but please acknowledge source

The following statements describe some of the ways a person may feel about his/her supervisor.

To what extent do you agree or disagree with each of the following statements about your relationship with your supervisor? Please tick the column which matches your opinion most closely.

	Strongly Disagree	Disagree	Slightly Disagree	Neither Agree nor Disagree	Slightly Agree	Agree	Strongly Agree
SAFE BASE SUBSCALE							
1. My Supervisor was respectful of my views and ideas							
2. My supervisor and I were equal partners in supervision							
3. My supervisor had a collaborative approach in supervision							
4. I felt safe in my supervision sessions							
5. My supervisor was non-judgemental in supervision							
6. My supervisor treated me with respect							
7. My supervisor was open-minded in supervision							
8. Feedback on my performance from my supervisor felt like criticism							
9. The advice I received from my supervisor was prescriptive rather than collaborative							
10. I felt able to discuss my concerns with my supervisor openly							
11. Supervision felt like an exchange of ideas							
12. My supervisor gave feedback in a way that felt safe							
13. My supervisor treated me like an adult							
14. I was able to be open with my supervisor							
15. I felt if I discussed my feelings openly with my supervisor, I would be negatively evaluated							
STRUCTURE SUBSCALE							
16. My supervision sessions took place regularly							
17. Supervision sessions were structured							
18. My supervisor made sure that our supervision sessions were kept free from interruptions							
19. Supervision sessions were regularly cut short by my supervisor							
20. Supervision sessions were focused							
21. My supervision sessions were disorganised							
22. My supervision sessions were arranged in advance							
23. My supervisor and I both drew up an agenda for supervision together							
COMMITMENT SUBSCALE							
24. My supervisor was enthusiastic about supervising me							

25. My supervisor appeared interested in supervising me								
26. My supervisor appeared uninterested in me								
27. My supervisor appeared interested in me as a person								
28. My supervisor appeared to like supervising								
29. I felt like a burden to my supervisor								
30. My supervisor was approachable								
31. My supervisor was available to me								
32. My supervisor paid attention to my spoken feelings and anxieties								
33. My supervisor appeared interested in my development as a professional								
REFLECTIVE EDUCATION SUBSCALE								
34. My supervisor drew from a number of theoretical models								
35. My supervisor drew from a number of theoretical models flexibly								
36. My supervisor gave me the opportunity to learn about a range of models								
37. My supervisor encouraged me to reflect on my practice								
38. My supervisor linked theory and clinical practice well								
39. My supervisor paid close attention to the process of supervision								
40. My supervisor acknowledged the power differential between supervisor and supervisee								
41. My relationship with my supervisor allowed me to learn by experimenting with different therapeutic techniques								
42. My supervisor paid attention to my unspoken feelings and anxieties								
43. My supervisor facilitated interesting and informative discussions in supervision								
44. I learnt a great deal from observing my supervisor								
ROLE MODEL SUBSCALE								
45. My supervisor was knowledgeable								
46. My supervisor was an experienced clinician								
47. I respected my supervisor's skills								
48. My supervisor was knowledgeable about the organisational system in which they worked								
49. Colleagues appeared to respect my supervisor's views								
50. I respected my supervisor as a professional								
51. My supervisor gave me practical support								
52. I respected my supervisor as a clinician								
53. My supervisor was respectful of clients								
54. I respected my supervisor as a person								
55. My supervisor appeared uninterested in his / her clients								
56. My supervisor treated his / her colleagues with respect								

FORMATIVE FEEDBACK SUBSCALE

57. My supervisor gave me helpful negative feedback on my performance						
58. My supervisor was able to balance negative feedback on my performance with praise						
59. My supervisor gave me positive feedback on my performance						
60. My supervisor's feedback on my performance was constructive						
61. My supervisor paid attention to my level of competence						
62. My supervisor helped me identify my own learning needs						
63. My supervisor did not consider the impact of my previous skills and experience on my learning needs						
64. My supervisor thought about my training needs						
65. My supervisor gave me regular feedback on my performance						
66. As my skills and confidence grew, my supervisor adapted supervision to take this into account						
67. My supervisor tailored supervision to my level of competence						

Scoring Key

Scored 1 (Strongly Disagree) to 7 (Strongly Agree)

Reverse Scoring
Scored 7 (Strongly Disagree) to 1 (Strongly Agree)

References:
Palomo, M. (2004). Development and validation of a questionnaire measure of the supervisory relationship. Unpublished DClinPsych Thesis, Oxford University.

Palomo, M., Beinart, H. & Cooper, M. (June, 2010). Development and validation of the Supervisory Relationship Questionnaire (SRQ) in UK trainee clinical psychologists. *British Journal of Clinical Psychology, 45* (2), 131-149.

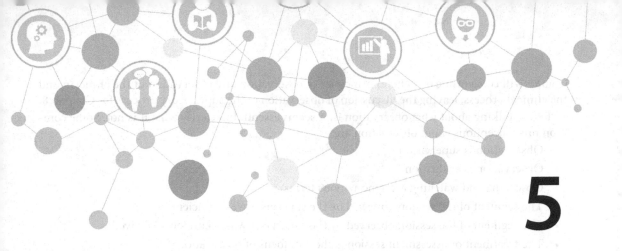

5

Observing in the Supervisory Process

Judith A. Brasseur, PhD, CCC-SLP, F-ASHA and
Elizabeth S. McCrea, PhD, CCC-SLP, F-ASHA

Core Areas I, III, V, VI, and VII in American Speech-Language-Hearing Association's (ASHA; 2008) Clinical Supervision Knowledge and Skills policy document are directly related to observing, the third component of the supervisory process.

- I. Preparation for the Supervisory Experience
  - ○ Skill 4: Adapt or develop observational formats that facilitate objective data collection.
- III. Development of the Supervisee's Critical and Problem-Solving Skills
  - ○ Skill 1: Assist the supervisee in using a variety of data collection procedures.
- V. Development of the Supervisee's Clinical Competence in Intervention
  - ○ Skill 4: Demonstrate the use of a variety of data collection procedures appropriate to the specific clinical situation.
- VI. Supervisory Conferences of Meetings of Clinical Teaching Teams
  - ○ Skill 7: Use data collection to analyze the extent to which the content and dynamics of the conference are facilitation goal achievement, desired outcomes, and planned changes.
- VII. Evaluating the Growth of the Supervisee Both as a Clinician and as a Professional
  - ○ Skill 1: Use data collection methods that will assist in analyzing the relationship between client [and] supervisee behaviors and specific clinical outcomes.

As with the other components of the supervisory process, observation is a fourfold activity; each participant becomes the object of some type of observation at various times during the process. Further, the assumption in the Collaborative and the Consultative Styles is that clinicians, supervisees, and supervisors will all be involved in self-observation followed by self-analysis. This

McCrea, E. S., & Brasseur, J. A. *The Clinical Education and Supervisory Process in Speech–Language Pathology and Audiology* (pp 167-204).
© 2020 Taylor & Francis Group.

chapter will concentrate on general principles of observation and observation of the clinician and the clinical process, leaving the discussion of observation of the supervisory process for Chapter 8.

Before talking about what observation is, it seems essential to clarify what it is not. Some common misconceptions about observation are:

- Observation is supervision
- Observation is evaluation
- Observing and watching are synonymous terms
- The segment of the session observed by the supervisor was sufficient
- The segment of the session observed by the supervisor was accurately perceived
- The treatment or assessment session is the sole focus of observation

Although these misconceptions may be evident in a variety of behaviors, the following examples illustrate some of the more frequent ones we have observed.

MISCONCEPTION	EXAMPLE
Observation is supervision	"I'm supervising between 2:00 and 5:00 o'clock today"—meaning, I'm observing between 2:00 and 5:00 o'clock today.
Observation is evaluation	Immediately after an observation, the supervisor says to the supervisee: "You did a great job of discriminating correct-incorrect responses. Now you need to work on eliciting more responses."
Observing and watching are synonymous terms	Supervisor looks at interaction but no writing or audio or video recording takes place during the time he or she is attending.
The segment observed was sufficient	During an hour, the supervisor is observing two supervisees. After the session, one supervisee sees the supervisor and asks, "Were you watching when…?"
The segment observed was accurately perceived	The supervisor records only those client-clinician behaviors that she feels characterize "good" therapy. Client and clinician goals are minimally included.
The treatment or assessment session is the sole focus of observation	No data on written reports and records, verbal and written communication with families and other professionals are collected throughout the term.

PURPOSES OF OBSERVATION

Before delving into the "how to," it seems pertinent to first address the purposes of observation. In educational programs, one obvious purpose is to meet the requirements stipulated by the ASHA's Council for Clinical Certification in Audiology and Speech-Language Pathology (CFCC). The CFCC 2014 Standards, revised 2016, for speech-language pathologists stipulate: "The amount of direct supervision must be commensurate with the student's knowledge, skills, and experience, must not be less than 25% of the student's total contact with each client/patient, and must take place periodically throughout practicum. Supervision must be sufficient to ensure the welfare of the client/patient." This minimum of 25% for any clinical activity must be in real time. Observation requirements are apparent in other settings. For example, in some service delivery programs, supervisors are required to perform a certain number of observations before a formal evaluation of an employee is written.

In examining the skills associated with Core Areas I, III, V, VI, and VII, it is obvious that an essential purpose is to collect data. Goldhammer, Anderson, and Krajewski (1980) considered observation synonymous with data gathering and stated, "Observation is the activity through which a supervisor becomes aware of the events, interactions, physical elements, and other phenomena in a particular place…during a particular time" (p. 70). Anderson (1988) stressed, "observation without data collection is a waste of time" (p. 123). According to Goldhammer (1969), the principal purpose of observation is to collect objective and comprehensive data in such a way that each session can be reconstructed validly enough to analyze it. He emphasized that the observer should write what he sees, not how he feels about what he sees. That instruction along with the following straightforward guideline should probably be posted in every room where observation takes place, and on the front of every supervisor's notebook: *Perceptions—not inferences; description—not commentary!*

Specific purposes will be related to the goals established for the clinical and supervisory processes. Content and procedures will depend on the exact purpose. Harris (1975) noted that an observation will focus on the learner when our purpose is to gather evidence on learning, will focus on the instructor when our purpose is to gather evidence about the instructor's behaviors and competencies, and will focus on the interaction among the learner-instructor-and things when we attempt to gather evidence about the teaching-learning process. Observers need to have a clear concept of their purpose, a focus, before they begin an observation. For example, are they attempting to collect baseline data? Monitor to assure quality services? Measure progress toward therapy objectives? Or to identify patterns of clinician behaviors that facilitate/impede the clinical process?

In reality, there may be multiple purposes. Surely, the subsequent analysis of the clinical or diagnostic process will be more productive and the conference more meaningful if it is assumed that the fundamental purpose of the observation is to collect data. Further, the data should be collected in a manner that will enable the observer, or someone else, to relate the behavior of the clinician to the consequences of that behavior in the client. Later, in the case of the observation of the conference, the importance of relating the behavior of the supervisor to consequences of that behavior on the supervisee will be considered. In other words, does the action of the clinician or supervisor appear to make a difference, positive or negative, in what the client or supervisee achieves? Can inferences or assumptions be made about the situation that has been observed? What data have been collected to support the inferences or assumptions about those behaviors?

CHARACTERISTICS OF OBSERVATION

Two main characteristics of observation are of importance. One is its scientific nature; the other is the fact that, to be of value, observation must be an active process.

Observation Is Scientific

Anderson (1988) stressed that the observation component is the point at which supervision begins to move from the realm of a somewhat undefined art to a scientific endeavor. It is the objective collection of data in the observation that changes supervision from being solely an art to more closely approximating science. Principles can be borrowed from the behavioral sciences, as Cogan (1973) suggested. "Supervisors need to apply the intellectual rigor and discipline of science" and "to internalize the standards of evidence and proof that are characteristic of science" (pp. 18-19). In regard to assessment, Emerich and Hatten (1979) noted that the scientific approach leads to, among other factors, "more rigorous adherence to standardized procedures" and "objectivity, quantifiability and structure" (pp. 12-13). The artistic approach, on the other hand, depends more upon "casual and non-structured scrutiny…the hunch, or clinical intuition." Emerich and Hatten stated further that "diagnosis is a unique blending of science and art" (pp. 12-13). Blending science and art in supervision is precisely what Anderson (1988) advocated.

It is in the observation component that supervision assumes an objective approach, where quantifying procedures begin to be utilized, where data are collected which will be submitted to much the same type of analysis required for research projects. Researchers describe data as numerical and verbal descriptions of attributes and events (Silverman, 1998), not a new concept to supervisors. Data from the observation provide the raw material for the conference. If they are not accurate, objective, and reliable, all subsequent stages of the process will be distorted or ineffectual. Without behavioral data as a foundation, the conference will become a potpourri of supervisee reports about what happened in the assessment or treatment session, supervisor attempts to recall the events, general discussion of treatment or assessment principles, guesses about the direction to take in future sessions, and subjective evaluations by the supervisor.

A clear distinction must be made between *data collection*, *analysis*, and *evaluation*. The purpose of the observation in the Collaborative and Consultative Styles is not "instant evaluation," but rather, to collect data. Inferences will be made from these data which will lead to interpretation, to further planning, and eventually to evaluation. The inferences are determined jointly to provide an opportunity for learning by the supervisee.

Many supervisors may find it difficult to resist writing instant evaluations during the observation. The fallacy of instant evaluations can be recognized by supervisors who recall how many times, in the darkness of the observation room or in the corner of the room where they were observing, have written an evaluative statement on the basis of one event or a few behaviors, only to erase the statement later, when subsequent events invalidated the previously written evaluation. In teaching courses or conducting workshops on supervision, it is obvious that eliminating instant evaluations from observation reports is a difficult habit to eliminate for many supervisors. Research substantiates that written comments tend to be highly evaluative. For example, Runyan and Seal (1985) reported that 46% of comments written by supervisors during an observation were evaluative. Peaper and Mercaitis (1987) reported a 40% rate in their investigation of written feedback provided to students. This propensity toward evaluation suggests that many supervisors perceive evaluation as their primary role. While this supervisor as evaluator role is consistent with the Direct-Active Style, it is incongruent with the Collaborative and Consultative Styles.

Observation Is Active

Observation is more than just looking at what is occurring, and to be done well, it demands attention, practice, and precision. Observation is an active, systematic process. It may be done by supervisors during the actual assessment or treatment session within the room, through an observation window, via a video monitoring system, or after the session by listening to an audio recording or viewing a video recording. Data may also be tabulated by clinicians themselves during sessions or subsequently by audio or video recorded observations. Observation may include data gathering by colleagues in the case of team therapy (Wegner, 1999), the teaching clinic (Dowling, 1983a, 1983b, 2001), or peer review. Whatever the circumstances, the observer will be actively involved in careful tabulation of events. As indicated in the planning session, the data to be collected will have been identified based on the objectives that have been set, and the method of data collection will have been determined. Planning provides guidance for the activities of the supervisor during the observation, or for the supervisee during self-observation. The end product, then, is a set of carefully recorded data which can be utilized for a variety of purposes during the analysis and evaluation processes.

IMPORTANCE OF OBSERVATION

Systematic observation of supervisees is crucial in the process of supervision. Observational techniques formulate the data that provide the foundation for feedback which leads to change in the supervisee. It is an essential activity, upon which the effectiveness and accuracy of the remainder of the supervisory process are dependent.

In speech-language pathology and audiology, the clinician's ability to observe the client has always been of concern, as evidenced by the inclusion of items related to observation on evaluation forms. Probably no existing evaluation forms are without items that assess observation and data collection skills in clinicians. Teaching these skills has been one of the responsibilities of supervisors, a fact substantiated by ASHA's (2008) Knowledge and Skills (see Core Areas and Skills on the first page of this chapter).

Skills related to the observation of the client have received greater emphasis than has observation of the clinician in the literature in speech-language pathology and audiology. Discussion of the techniques and skills of observation of clients have historically been available in various texts on evaluation of communication disorders (Darley & Spriestersbach, 1978; Emerich & Hatten, 1979; Johnson, Darley, & Spriestersbach, 1963; Shipley & McAfee, 2016).

Mowrer (1977) devoted several chapters to an in-depth treatment of observation and behavioral assessment of speech behaviors and stated, "*How* we observe, *what* we observe, *where* we observe, and *when* we observe, and what we do with the observations is, as you will discover, a very complex process" (p. 46).

Skilled observation of communicative behavior is the basis of all effective efforts in evaluation and treatment of disorders, according to Kunze (1967), who stated that "techniques in the observation of communicative behavior should be systematically taught as the first step in our clinical training program and the student should have obtained observational skill before he faces his first practicum assignment" (p. 473). As supervisors in university settings know, completing 25 hours of observation prior to enrollment in practicum has been standard practice for decades. However, with the new standards for Certificate of Clinical Competence (CCC) in speech-language pathology (effective 2014/revised 2016), the 25 hours of observation are no longer a prerequisite to beginning direct patient or client contact. Rather, implementation of Council for Clinical Certification in Audiology and Speech-Language Pathology (CFCC) Standard V-C notes "guided observation hours generally precede direct contact with clients/patients" (p. 6). In off-campus practicum, students typically complete a period of observation, shadowing their master clinician, before beginning any service delivery to clients.

The scientific approach to case management, the need to validate techniques and strategies for learning, and the current emphasis on evidence-based practice in CFCC certification (CCC/speech-language pathologyIV-F) and Council on Academic Accreditation in Audiology and Speech-Language Pathology (CAA) accreditation standards (3.5A, 3.5B) implicitly mandate the systematic collection of data. The need for the supervisor to teach the supervisee techniques of scientific observation and data collection is apparent. In addition, supervisors have a responsibility to model this kind of approach in their observations of the clinical process.

There are many sources of information about collecting and utilizing data on client behavior that the supervisor can use in assisting supervisees and themselves to attain or improve observational skills. These sources also provide a basis for competent evaluation and treatment (Hedge & Davis, 2010; Lund & Duchan, 1993; Moon Meyer, 2004; Mowrer 1969, 1972; Shipley, 1997; Shipley & McAfee, 2016). Supervision research substantiates the need to "calibrate" observers in order to effect reliable, valid data (Cascia, 2013; Filter, Brandell, Smith, & Kopin, 1989; Runyan & Seal, 1985; Sbaschnig & Williams, 1983). Further, the similarity between the research and supervisory processes should be clear here; that is, training for researchers has always emphasized the importance of precise data collection and we know that is achieved by training prior to and monitoring during an experiment (McReynolds & Kearns, 1983; Orlikoff, Schiavetti, & Metz, 2015; Silverman, 1998).

Objectivity

An individual's perceptual sets, biases, and predispositions about what is seen pose a threat to objectivity. Total objectivity is a myth (Goldhammer et al., 1980). Perceivers attend to different aspect of situations and behavior. Their needs, values, purposes, and past experiences affect their categorization and coding of events or the way they describe them. Additionally, physical, cultural, and social contexts influence the perceiver's interpretation of behaviors and determine the kinds of inferences drawn from their observations (Schneider, Hastorf, & Ellsworth, 1979). Andersen (1981) found biases in supervisor ratings based on prior information about the supervisee. Familiarity with the supervisee was hypothesized to be a source of bias in Blodgett, Schmidtt, and Scudder's (1987) study of supervisor ratings. Hatten, Bell, and Strand (1983) and Runyan and Seal (1985) found lack of agreement among speech-language pathologists viewing the same clinical session. That perceptions, biases and preconceived notions affect observations is readily apparent when witnesses report differently at an accident scene, or when jurors render different decisions after hearing the same testimonies and seeing the same pieces of evidence in a trial.

Another problem in relation to objectivity and accuracy of data collection is that of reactivity. In research, subjects may behave differently simply because they know they are participants in a study (the "Hawthorne effect"). The very presence of observers, change in routine, the setting itself or attention the subject receives may change a subject's behaviors (Campbell & Stanley, 1963; Orlikoff, Schiavetti, & Metz, 2015). In addition, certain measures may yield reactive effects; tests, inventories, rating scales, video recordings, audio recordings, computers, iPads and tablets, smartphones, or other equipment may produce changes in the phenomenon being studied. "The more novel and motivating the test device, the more reactive one can expect it to be" (Campbell & Stanley, 1963, p. 9). In attempting to become more scientific in their techniques, supervisors should assume that the risks to objectivity and the basic facts on reactivity are as valid for supervision as they are for research.

One way to manage problems associated with reactivity is to apply the principles of desensitization. Anyone who has observed a new client's initial attention to a recorder on a table and watched it become as unobtrusive as piece of paper over time knows that reactivity can be diminished.

There are several ways to manage the risks to objectivity. One is training. In addition to some of the training resources cited previously, self-knowledge is an integral part of training to enhance objectivity. Awareness is the first step in the change process. All individuals have what Cogan (1973) termed "square boxes" or "inferential sets," our biases and preconceived notions of "the way things ought to be." Not all of these may be bad. The important thing is to bring them to a level of consciousness, understand them and test their validity. One technique to identify inferential sets is to pay attention to "gut feelings." If an urge to make an instant evaluation or to intervene in a session being observed is experienced, the supervisor should pause, write the feeling down, and carefully examine it after the observation.

Consider this example from the second author. Early in her career as an untrained supervisor, she felt that enthusiasm was an important variable for the clinical process and thought that it was manifested by exuberant, "peppy," lively clinician behavior. If a clinician's style was more subdued, more calm and quiet than she thought it ought to be, she'd pop into a session, demonstrate and instruct the clinician to follow her model. After being introduced to the concept of "square boxes," she refrained from commenting or interrupting the session of a calm clinician working with an active preschooler. Over the period of a few weeks, the data collected substantiated that the clinician's style was equally as effective as hers, as evidence by client response rate, success, time on task, and such. She learned the first of many valuable lessons.

PLANNING THE OBSERVATION

Observation should not "just happen." Given the vast amount of behavior available to supervisor and supervisee in the clinical session, and the variability in recording methods, some selection must be made to make the observation manageable and the subsequent analysis meaningful. Like all other activities, the planning should be done jointly by the participants. At the Evaluation-Feedback Stage, the bulk of decision making about observation will probably be done by the supervisor. As the participants move away from this stage, there will be more participation by the supervisee in deciding what behaviors are important enough for data collection. This moves the interaction away from the traditional style, where behaviors to be observed are selected by the supervisor, possibly after entering the observation situation. It is essential to limit the extent of data collection by deciding which behaviors will be the focus of the observation, how the observation will be conducted, and how and by whom the data will be recorded.

Planning for observation will take place at different times during the term of supervision. It certainly will occur at the beginning when long-range plans are being worked out and also throughout the supervision sequence as plans are being made for subsequent therapy sessions or conferences.

Early Planning for Observation

When supervisees begin their clinical experiences, they may need specific assistance from the supervisor in data collection methods not only for their clients but also for themselves. Although novice supervisees will have had limited experience with data collection as part of their experience in observing all or part 25 hours of therapy, it is different when you are on the inside looking out vs. the outside looking in. Assisting the supervisee in learning a variety of data collection procedures (Core Area III.1) and in selecting data collection procedures to be used in sessions (Core Area V.4) are likely to be among the first tasks the supervisor performs. Variety is important. Although clinicians need to learn that certain observation tools exist for their use, they should not view such tools as the exclusive approach to data collection.

At the beginning planning stages, certain general principles about observation should be discussed as required by each supervisee. This discussion will cover such topics as the purpose and importance of data collection; the supervisee's past experiences and skills in recording data; potential methodologies for recording both client and clinician data and the possible reasons for selecting one or another of those methodologies; the responsibilities of the supervisor for observation; the responsibility of clinicians for data collection on the client and on themselves; and the preferences, biases, or feelings of each participant about observation. A thorough, rational, objective discussion of the purposes of observation at this point will encourage efficient and effective data collection; it may also relieve some of the anxieties of the supervisees if they know what is to be recorded.

Clinicians must be helped to see at a very early point in their education that, without complete, accurate, ongoing data collection on their clients, as well as their own behaviors, there is no measurement, no accountability. They must learn that they, as well as the supervisor, have responsibilities for data collection that will benefit them and the client.

Data collection may seem to be a given, but supervisors often have to be vigilant in determining that it is actually done. Many clinicians, and indeed supervisors, resist data collection. It is sometimes hard work, and often tedious. It requires concentration and purpose. Clinicians often take great pains to collect objective data on the client during the diagnostic period but then do not continue the collection of the same kind of objective data to measure progress during therapy. Rather, comments about therapy may be subjective and evaluative (Turton, 1973b). For this reason, some supervisors instruct supervisees to take the "S" out of SOAP (subjective, objective, assessment, and plan) notes. Long-range planning for observation of the clinical session makes it more meaningful to clinicians and results in a greater commitment to the task. A clear, specific intent to collect certain data will make the clinical process not only more purposeful, but more interesting. Tangible evidence of change is much more reinforcing than subjective guesses about results of therapy. Clinicians also need to understand that responsibility for data collection does not end with the receipt of their degree—it continues into the job setting, wherever it may be.

There are advantages for the supervisor, too, in planning the data collection. Tangible evidence of progress in their supervisees is rewarding. Definite goals for data collection keep the observation more interesting. Any supervisor who has ever nodded off momentarily in the dark shadows of the observation room will probably welcome structure and direction in the data collection task. Supervisors also report that data collection makes them feel more fair and impartial later, when they evaluate the supervisee's clinical performance.

Who Does the Data Collection?

Supervisors and supervisees will have different responsibilities for data collection, depending upon the situation. Basically, there is a natural division of labor between them. The supervisee collects client data as a part of treatment or assessment session or later via audio or video recordings. The supervisor usually collects data on the clinician or the interaction between clinician and client. There will be times when supervisors, to be truly collaborative, also will collect data on clients for certain purposes, for example, to check the reliability of the clinician's observation, to gather data about behaviors that cannot be collected by the clinician during the session, to identify behaviors not perceived by the clinician, or to record the unexpected. Particularly at the beginning of the interaction, both will want to collect baseline on the clinician for purposes of establishing objectives, parallel to the process used for clients.

At some point, clinicians will need to be responsible for collecting data on their own behavior, as well as that of the client. For some time, we have known that clinicians can develop an awareness of their own abilities through analysis of their own audio or video recordings (Boone & Stech, 1970). Some clinicians may reach the stage where they can collect data on their behaviors during rather than after the clinical session. This is one of the areas where supervisees must be involved if a true collaborative relationship is to develop and if they are going to learn the process of self-analysis and self-evaluation.

Ongoing Planning of Observation

A portion of every conference should be used for dual planning of the details of the observation of the next clinical session. Just as selection of client data to be collected depends upon the stated objectives, so does the collection of clinician data. Progress of clinicians toward their objectives must be measured just as client behavior is measured. Once again there is blending of one component of the supervisory process into another. Establishing the relationship and determining needs lead to planning and setting of objectives. Data collections planning comes directly out of those objectives—with space left for serendipity (Goldhammer et al., 1980).

Leaving space for serendipity is an important point. Despite the stress placed here on planning the observation, supervisors and supervisees must allow for the unexpected. Cogan (1973) described the importance of capturing "critical incidents," those unanticipated events that have a profound impact on learning. The impact may be positive or negative. For example, a child who volunteers to answer a question in class and whose answer is followed by laughter may quickly learn not to answer questions.

Observation that is not planned but left to the supervisor's choice, however, is subject to bias. What supervisors will see and choose to record as they observe without planning will depend to a great extent on their theoretical base, their own mood or feelings at the time, and the importance that their own professional experience or expertise places on certain aspects of the clinical session such as direction giving, stimulation, reinforcement, modeling, client participation, expansion, and feedback (Roberts & Naremore, 1983). Unplanned, subjective observations also make it difficult to document change or to provide feedback other than evaluative judgments based on impressions.

Ongoing, joint planning includes planning what behaviors will be observed, how they will be operationalized, what kinds of data will be collected, how it will be recorded (e.g., tallies, observations systems, verbatim written notes, etc.), the physical aspects of the observation (e.g., in-room, observation room, video monitor, etc.), who will collect what behaviors, and when the data will be collected. Comparable planning for observations of the supervisory process will need to be competed and will be discussed in Chapter 8.

Checklist for Observation Planning

- Observation and data collection have been jointly planned
- There is a rationale for data collection
- Data to be collected are consistent with short- and long-term goals for the client and clinician
- Data come out of the needs, concerns, or self-identified strengths or weaknesses of the supervisee, and from the experience and impressions of the supervisor
- Options for supervisor selection of behaviors not in the plan have been discussed
- Plans are detailed sufficiently and mutually understood
- Data collection methods will facilitate effective analysis
- The plan allows for variance such as interruptions, mood of the client, unexpected client learning, and so on
- The amount of data to be collected is sufficient for drawing inferences
- The plan includes data collection by the clinician of his or her own behavior
- The plan has accounted for changes necessitated from previous observation plans and outcomes

All supervisors have experienced the frustration of losing some important observation while madly trying to synthesize previous ones to support a point—or, at times, not being able to substantiate a point because of insufficient data. Data collection on clinician behavior is so important that each supervisor must make a great effort to perfect systems for recording that they can use easily and efficiently. Anyone who has had a problem supervisee understands this even more. A word of caution seems warranted here. To avoid litigation, it is essential to be able to demonstrate that all supervisees are being treated the same and being treated fairly. Thus, a supervisor must use the same general procedures for planning, observing, collecting data, and keeping records for all of his or her supervisees; that is, while individual variation between supervisors is to be expected, individuals should strive for a reasonable degree of internal consistency.

STRATEGIES FOR OBSERVATION

Selection of the method of observation depends on a number of variables, including:

- Setting
- Philosophy or personal preference of the participants
- Objectives for the observation
- Availability of equipment
- Time
- Training and experience of the supervisor and supervisee

Concurrent Observation

Probably the most frequently used form of observation is recording in real time. Observations may be done with the clinician and the client in the room, in an adjacent observation room, or from a remote location (Dudding & Justice, 2004).

Based on the previous discussion of reactivity, it is apparent that observers in the same room with the clinician and client will have some effect on them. At the same time, clinicians and clients are usually conscious of the ever-present possibility of a live body on the other side of the window or at a video monitor. The self-consciousness of being observed may influence the behaviors of the individuals being observed, and it is important for observers to be sensitive to this possibility.

Audio or Video Recording

Speech-language pathologists and audiologists have used audio and video equipment to enhance the learning process with clients and clinicians for decades, but there is a paucity of research to demonstrate the usefulness of recording or to support any specific methodology.

The most extensive study of the use of video in the preparation of speech-language pathologists was conducted by Boone and Stech (1970). They reported that both audio and video confrontation, listening, or viewing, were useful in changing the behavior of clinicians. They also indicated that mere listening or viewing was not as powerful as when accompanied by the use of an analysis matrix on which clinicians notated their behavior. Further, Boone and Stech found audio recording and behavioral scoring to be as effective in changing verbal behaviors as video confrontation because 80% to 95% of the therapy process occurs at the verbal level. They added that this does not imply that video confrontation is not more effective in studying therapy. Rather, viewers of video should concentrate more on the nonverbal level—facial expressions and gestural cues, attending to the client, and behaviors used to punctuate therapy interaction.

Video recording as a teaching device in speech-language pathology was investigated by Hall (1970), Irwin (1972, 1975, 1981a, 1981b), Irwin and Hall (1973), and Schubert and Gudmundson (1976). Most of their studies incorporated the microteaching techniques developed in education by Ivey (1971) and used in preparing teachers and counselors (Kagan, 1970). This technique varies in its use but essentially follows this pattern: a short microlesson is conducted and video recorded, the recording is observed by the clinician and supervisor, behaviors to be modified are identified, the lesson is redone and video recorded, another observation and analysis by supervisor and clinician is conducted to determine if behaviors have changed. Irwin (1981a) recommended this method for speech-language pathology and audiology education and made a case for further study of its use.

Schubert (1978) advocated the use of video recording for teaching, demonstration, and for self-analysis. He stated clearly that the video recording should not become a substitute for live, in real time observation. The quantification of behaviors from video provides an invaluable method of analyzing change in the clinical process.

The use of audio or video recordings in observation and self-observation provide a powerful teaching tool. As with any type of observation, these techniques are only as useful as the data that are collected and analyzed. To maximize the effectiveness of audio or video recordings, users have to learn methods for collecting and analyzing data (Camarata, 1992; Farmer, 1987; Farmer & Farmer, 1989; Schill, 1992). Merely listening or watching is likely a waste of time.

Live Supervision

The term *live supervision* appears to have its origin in counseling and psychotherapy. As practiced in those disciplines, it involves simultaneous observation and feedback. The supervisor is in the room and participates with the supervisee in the session. Rassi (2001) reports this type of supervision in audiology practice. Speech-language pathology programs which use an apprenticeship model to train their students also use live supervision (Gillam, 1999; Messick, 1999). Another form of live supervision is the "bug-in-the-ear" (BIE) technique. This technique has newfound popularity not only in speech-language pathology but also in related disciplines as a "bug-in-the-ear technology" Google search will reveal. Using online and mobile technology, the BIE system includes one transmitting microphone and a separate receiving headpiece. The supervisor or peer coach who is out of the room coaches the clinician in real time while a session is occurring. Used in the early 1950s in training counselors (Korner & Brown, 1952), it has also been used in speech-language pathology (Brooks & Hannah, 1966; Engoth, 1973; Hagler, 1986; Hagler and Holdgrapher, 1987; Simons, 2014). This will be discussed further in Chapter 7 in the section on feedback.

DEVELOPMENT OF OBSERVATIONAL TECHNIQUES

The techniques of observation are a part of scientific heritage and have long been the tools of scientists who have studied behavior in a variety of disciplines. The behavior modification movement of the 1960s had a strong influence on approaches to observation in education and in our professions. Structured observation systems proliferated in the 1970s (Simon and Boyer, 1970a, 1970b, 1974) and had a powerful impact on the study of many types of interactions. Naturalistic or qualitative research suggests other strategies for observation (Lincoln & Guba, 1985; Pickering, 1980). In the 1980s, the explosion in technology and the advent of the personal computer in particular, have further expanded approaches to observation and data collection.

Methods of Data Collection

The understanding and appropriate use of systematic observation and data collection methods by supervisors is important for establishing supervision as a thoughtful, scientific, and validated process. Supervisors need to be skilled observers, but more than that, they must also develop efficient, practical procedures for recording their observations for later use. The following methods have been used in our professions, some more than others. Readers are encouraged to try some they have not used to expand their personal repertoire and to become proficient in using a variety of procedures.

Recording Evaluative Statements

The most traditional procedure, and perhaps the method of least effort or the most expediency for supervisors, is to simply write evaluative statements reflecting their perceptions of the appropriateness of the behaviors in the treatment or assessment session as they view it; for example, "Your directions were too difficult for the client," or "You did a good job of motivating him today." Such action is consistent with the Direct-Active Style of the Evaluation-Feedback Stage. This procedure may be expanded slightly as supervisors record behavioral data selected to support their judgments or to illustrate to the clinician what they perceived as good or poor clinical practice. This methodology is neither appropriate nor inappropriate per se. It may be decided during the planning component that there is a need for such direct evaluative procedures, if not in the entire session, at least in certain parts of it.

If it has been determined that there is a need for such judgments at certain times, however, the aim of supervisors and supervisees should be to reduce their numbers as rapidly as possible and to involve the supervisee in more self-evaluation. The caution here should not be against occasional, but rather against habitual, use of the instant evaluation without rationale. Furthermore, regardless of intent, supervisors written comments tend to be highly evaluative (Peaper & Mercaitis, 1987; Runyan & Seal, 1985). As stated previously, it is these active, direct behaviors of the supervisor that do not encourage, in fact probably discourage, self-analysis and creative thinking on the part of supervisees.

Tallies of Behaviors

Collection of baseline data or recording of data on clinician behaviors selected during the joint planning session may be done by a simple tallying by supervisor and supervisee—exactly the type of tallying and charting completed for clients. For example, if the clinician is working on a simple, straightforward goal such as decreasing the number of utterances of "OK," a simple tally by the supervisor over a period of time will measure progress toward that goal. Certain reinforcement techniques, accurately or inaccurately evaluated target sounds, responses to clients, or other specific behaviors can be tallied in this manner. As clinicians gain more experience, they can tally their own behavior. Dowling (2001) provided a number of innovative examples for collecting data using a tally technique. The Kansas Inventory of Self-Supervision (KISS) developed by Mawdsley (1985) contains seven clinician behaviors: overuse of "OK," corrective feedback, response rate, group management rotation rates, positive reinforcement, clinician response to client social comments, and clinician vs. client talk-time. The system provides an easy technique for supervisors to tally one of the target behaviors during observations (see Appendix 5-1). Because of its simplicity, it is good tool for supervisees to use as they begin to observe and analyze their own behaviors.

In developing this skill, it is usually easier to tally behaviors from an audio or video recording before attempting to do so live in an actual session. It may appear gratuitous to discuss this method since most supervisors and supervisees do this at some time. The important point for the Collaborative or Consultative Styles is that the data collection for clinician behaviors be jointly planned, that both parties be involved in some portions of the record keeping, and that it is done systematically, not at the whim of the supervisor.

Rating Scales

Rating scales may be used in observation when behaviors to be observed are known ahead of time and there is a need for qualitative data. In such instruments, behaviors or events are listed and value judgments are made as to the quality of the behaviors, that is, the degree to which the rater perceives that the behavior has been performed adequately or inadequately, appropriately or inappropriately. Degree is typically assessed using a Likert scale. Rosenshine (1970) called rating scales "high-inference systems" because they call for inference and judgment on the part of the observer, as opposed to analysis systems, which he labeled "low inference" because of their relatively more objective nature. Many rating scales are of very poor quality, reflect the bias of those who constructed them, and have no validity or reliability.

Rating scales that have been developed to evaluate clinical competencies (e.g., Wisconsin Procedure for Appraisal of Clinical Competence) are usually not appropriate for tallying behaviors in the clinical sessions although they may sometimes be used in that way. If the descriptors are specific and are stated behaviorally they might be modified for data collection, which would then feed into analysis and subsequent evaluation. Generally, however, rating forms used for evaluation are not useful for data collection because of the global nature of the items and the inherent judgmental factor that is built in. These types of instruments are, however, useful for making summative assessments about clinical performance over time, provided that ratings are based on data collected over time.

Verbatim Recording

Goldhammer (1969) dismissed all methods of data collection except verbatim transcripts, which contain everything done or spoken during a session. The transcripts are then examined in the analysis stage. Goldhammer's reasoning is sound—analysis systems or rating scales force behaviors into a priori categories, record supervisors' interpretations or perceptions, usually are not reliable or valid, and may miss important behaviors. Audio or video recordings are unmanageable unless submitted to extensive analysis. Operationalizing Goldhammer's approach is more easily discussed than accomplished. Recording everything that happens during an observation, writing comments and questions in the margin, recording descriptions of nonverbal behaviors, and diagramming clinician and client positions requires practice and the skills of a stenographer;

that is, one must be adept in taking notes, using symbols, abbreviations, diagrams and some type of shorthand to complete verbatim transcripts. Realistically, most supervisors and supervisees need to prepare transcripts from recordings.

Despite the drawbacks, Goldhammer's (1969) discussion of the need for totality in recording the activities observed is important. Verbatim recordings are particularly useful for obtaining baseline data with a new supervisee. They are also an excellent technique for making problem behaviors salient. For example, if a supervisee is having difficulty with accurate auditory discrimination of /r, ɝ/and centering diphthongs, the supervisor can complete a verbatim transcript, employing narrow transcription. The power of seeing antecedent events; the kind of stimuli that evoke correct, incorrect, and close approximations of the desired behavior; and the precise verbalizations and events used to consequate client responses enables a clinician to carefully analyze the clinical interactions and figure out what needs to be done differently to increase the client's success.

The amount of time required to complete a verbatim transcript of an entire 30- or 50-minute session makes it impractical for most supervisors and supervisees. In practice, it is likely more viable to select a segment of interest and completed a transcript on that portion of a session. Even a 5-minute segment of a session provides compelling, robust data for analysis.

Selected Verbatim

An alternative to Goldhammer's (1969) method involves narrowing the scope and making a verbatim transcript only of certain events or categories of events selected during the planning stage by the supervisor and supervisee. Such recording may be done concurrently with the session or from a recording. Acheson and Gall (1980) list the advantages of selective verbatim recordings:

- The supervisee becomes sensitized to the verbal process in teaching
- The supervisee does not have to respond to all aspects of the teaching-learning process, only those that have been selected
- An objective, noninterpretive record of behavior that can be analyzed is constructed
- It is a simple procedure

These advantages may also be problems, according to Acheson and Gall. The supervisee, knowing what is to be recorded, may become self-conscious in using the behaviors or may use them more often during the observation period only. There is also the possibility of bias in the selection of behaviors and the way they are analyzed and interpreted, the possibility of selecting trivial behaviors, and the difficulty in keeping up with verbal behaviors.

Selective verbatim transcripts are a useful tool for self-analysis. Nothing reveals the inaccuracies, monotonies, ambiguities, and irregularities in a person's own verbosity as quickly as a written script. Although time consuming, it is a potent tool for behavior change. For example, some clinicians have difficulty providing clear directions to their clients. Rather than a supervisor providing an evaluation after a session such as, "Your directions were too complex/confusing/ambiguous," he or she could instruct the supervisee to complete a self-analysis; that is, the supervisee would be instructed to record the session, then make verbatim transcriptions of each direction used during the session. These would be examined relative to how the client responded after each direction and the supervisee would identify those that caused confusion for the client. These would be rewritten to simplify and clarify the direction, discussed with the supervisor to refine if needed, and the supervisee would use the revised directions in the next session. The process would be repeated until the objective of clear directions is achieved.

Block (1982) developed an innovative method called the Pre-Conference Observation System (PCOS), which is a kind of selective verbatim method. It used a coding system for recording some client and clinician behaviors such as giving directions, models, responses and verbal reinforcement. She also used a standard set of symbols, initials, abbreviations, and placements on a page to enable objective, systematic data collection to be completed. Supervisors may find it helpful to develop a similar technique, using their own personal shorthand. Following are some examples of Block's system:

Notation

+	clinician thought the response was good
•	clinician thought the response was bad
IM	immediate model
DM	delayed model
X	model repeated
(+)	supervisor evaluated response as correct
⊖	supervisor evaluated response as incorrect

} these symbols used when Supervisor and Supervisee disagree

Clinician vs. client talk can be distinguished by differential placement on the page; for example, clinician talk can always be started at the margin and client talk can always be indented.

Example

book-X-X+

Explanation

Clinician said "book"

Response was incorrect [-]

Clinician repeated model [X]

Second attempt was incorrect [-]

Clinician repeated model again [X]

Third response was correct [+]

Interaction Analysis Systems

The most structured form of recording observations is the interaction analysis systems that have been used in education, counseling, and psychotherapy for years (Amidon & Flanders, 1967; Bales, 1950; Pelton, 2010; Simon & Boyer, 1970a, 1970b, 1974). Systems are constructed so that interactions between events can be analyzed and patterns identified. They have been developed by taking the behaviors that occur in teaching or in clinical sessions and categorizing them into sets that are distinguishable from each other, relevant to the purpose of the observation, and mutually exclusive, that is, all behaviors with common characteristics are placed in a category. They enable users to examine the relationship between events and to correlate interactional patterns with outcomes.

The use of interaction analysis systems by supervisors or in self-study by the supervisee is based on the assumption that the supervisee will change behavior as a result of feedback. These systems are very useful but should not been seen as a panacea.

A few systems have been developed in speech-language pathology and audiology. They may be used in supervision, research, and self-study to focus observations and structure data collection. Before discussing specific systems, the advantages and disadvantages of their use will be presented. (Several interaction analysis systems for use with the supervisory conference are available and will be discussed in Chapter 8. The advantages and disadvantages of the systems listed here also apply to those used for the conference.)

Advantages of Interaction Analysis Systems

There are many advantages in the use interaction analysis systems. The quantity of behaviors generated in most observations is so great that it must be structured in some way that enables the observer to analyze the total. Some people may be able to do this without observation systems, but certainly they make such analysis quicker, easier, and relatively more reliable. The systems also help establish a baseline and a record of progress for included behaviors. Analysis systems are helpful for training individuals in the observation process—to sort individual behaviors out of the mass of new behaviors they may be encountering as they take on clinical or supervisory tasks (Golper, McMahon, & Gordon, 1976). They help observers focus their attention. They allow comparisons between sessions and simplify both the recording of data and the feedback. They also provide the "grist" for the analysis component. When used by clinicians themselves, analysis systems help them become aware of components of clinical sessions as well as their own behaviors—this self-recognition and self-analysis is perhaps one of the best uses. They may contribute to clearer communication between supervisors and supervisees about clinical sessions. They are more objective in their classification and identification of behaviors because behaviors are operationalized and ground rules are usually provided for categorizing ambiguous behaviors. Certainly, they reduce a large amount of the opinion, judgment, some of the inaccuracies, impressions, misinterpretations, and poor memory that may go into less structured observations.

Disadvantages of Interaction Analysis Systems

The disadvantages of interaction analysis systems may be found in their construction, their use, or their interpretation. The assumption that they are completely "objective" is a dangerous one. It is true that they do force a certain amount of objectivity onto the observer because the behaviors are preselected and defined. However, that very selection may reflect the bias of the authors or a specific theoretical approach. Additionally, the possibility of subjectivity in the form of interpretation, selection of one category over another, or perceptual errors is ever present.

Some interaction analysis systems focus on the clinical process but not on the content, giving incomplete information. Thus, a question may be checked as a question but nothing is known about the type of question or appropriateness without additional analysis. Further, systems usually do not relate to the efficacy of treatment. What happened is identified and quantified, but its effectiveness is still open to the judgment of the observer. Additionally, most systems do not account for nonverbal behavior.

The volume of behavior included in the system may be so great that it is not only difficult to record all of it, even with the system, but it may also then be impossible to manipulate it to make it meaningful. At the same time, the types of behaviors are limited; therefore, many important behaviors may be missed.

Supervisors or clinicians may become too dependent on such systems, limiting their ability to examine the "large picture." Many systems are poorly constructed and have no established reliability or validity. But perhaps the greatest sin against analysis systems is when they are equated as evaluation systems, which they are not, nor were ever intended to be. Anderson (1988) reported that she often heard the content and sequence analysis system devised by Boone and Prescott (1972) referred to as "the Boone evaluation form" or heard supervisors say, "I evaluated her on the Boone." This misconception and misuse is a distinct disadvantage.

Despite the negatives, interaction analysis systems are invaluable tools in the supervisory process when chosen well and used properly. The next section will provide guidelines for choice and evaluation of the instruments.

Selection and Use

Certain guidelines must be followed in choosing and using interaction analysis systems. Individuals must know what data they wish to collect and select the system accordingly. In addition, users must be cognizant of the strengths and weaknesses of a particular system. Preparation and practice with a system is crucial for effective use. A valuable outline of criteria for developers and users of interaction analysis systems has been provided by Herbert and Attridge (1975), which includes three categories of criteria: identifying, validity, and practicality.

Identifying criteria are those which enable users to select the instrument that is correct for their purpose and application. These include such items as appropriateness of the title to the system's purpose, the rationale or theoretical support, the specificity of its uses, and the behaviors included.

Validating criteria include characteristics such as clarity, lack of ambiguity, and consistency with theory. Under this heading, Herbert and Attridge (1975) suggested questioning whether the items are exhaustive (i.e., include all behaviors of the kind being examined, even if it is labeled "other"), are representative of the dimensions of the behavior being studied (related to sampling and generalizability), and are mutually exclusive (i.e., behaviors can only be categorized into a single category). They also stated that in addition to procedures for use, ground rules should be provided to assist the coder in making individual decisions about borderline or unusual behaviors. Other aspects of validity include the nature and degree of inference to be made from items, context, observer effect, reliability, and validity measures.

Practicality criteria include relevance or items, method of coding, qualifications and training for users, and provisions made for collection and recording of data.

Unfortunately, no known system meets all the standards of Herbert and Attridge (1975). Nevertheless, users who are knowledgeable about the criteria will be able to identify the strengths and weaknesses of systems they use and make adjustments accordingly. Anyone wishing to use interaction analysis systems for research should become familiar with the Herbert and Attridge criteria.

ANALYSIS SYSTEMS IN
SPEECH-LANGUAGE PATHOLOGY AND AUDIOLOGY

Although interaction analysis systems have not proliferated in our disciplines as they have in some others, there was a surge of interest in this methodology during the late 1960s and early 1970s, coming out of the behavioral paradigm originally described by B. F. Skinner (Johnson, 1971). Systems for use in studying the clinical process were developed by Boone and Prescott (1972), Brookshire, Nicholas, Kruger, and Redmond (1978), Conover (1979), Deidrich (1969, 1971), Johnson (1969), Johnson (1971), and Schubert, Miner, & Till (1973). Other systems for studying behaviors in interviews have been developed (Farmer, 1980; Molyneaux & Lane, 1982; Shipley, 1997). Based on citations in the literature, the systems developed by Boone and Prescott (1972) and Schubert et al. (1973) are the most frequently used by speech-language pathologists and are two that have withstood the test of time. These systems will be discussed and examples presented.

Content and Sequence Analysis of Speech and Hearing Therapy (Boone and Prescott)

The Content and Sequence Analysis of Speech and Hearing Therapy (Boone, 1970; Boone & Prescott, 1972; Boone & Stech, 1970; Prescott, 1971), based on an operant model, provides a method of quantifying certain behaviors of clinicians and clients. Clinician behaviors include: (1) explain, describe; 2) model, instruction; 3) good evaluative; 4) bad evaluative; and 5) neutral-social. Client behaviors include: 6) correct response; 7) incorrect response; 8) inappropriate/social; 9) good self-evaluative; and 10) bad self-evaluative. All behaviors are recorded on a matrix and a summary form is available for analysis of the data. The system and an example are contained in Appendix 5-2.

The publication of the system had a major impact on supervisors and clinicians. It was probably the first time that an instrument had so clearly "dissected" the clinical process. University supervisors found it useful in preparing students to observe and identify components of the clinical process, to quantify the behaviors included in the system, to keep records of changes in those behaviors, to identify patterns of interactions and a multitude of other clinical activities.

The system meets many of the criteria delineated by Herbert and Attridge (1975), but not all. Users of the system, particularly for research, might wish to evaluate it more thoroughly on the basis of these criteria. It is useful for collecting data on client/clinician interactions, is easily learned, practical, and quantifies the 10 behaviors contained in the system. Given the limited number of categories, it is important not to overuse it—keeping in mind that other behaviors are important in the therapeutic process. Furthermore, as previously stated, it is not intended as an evaluation tool. The data generated by the system are quantitative and although inferences and assumptions can be made after data are analyzed, the system does not include qualitative ratings that are inherent in evaluation measures.

Analysis of Behavior of Clinicians System

The Analysis of Behavior of Clinicians (ABC) system (Schubert, 1978; Schubert et al., 1973) is identical in purpose to Boone and Prescott's system (1972): to quantify behaviors in the clinical session so that supervisors and clinicians can more accurately recognize, recall, and analyze the behaviors and sequential patterns. The systems differ in that the ABC is a time-based system. Behaviors are recorded at 3-second intervals or when a behavior changes within a 3-second interval, by writing down the number assigned to a particular behavior.

The ABC categories are derived from the categories of the original Flanders (1970) system, which was based on behaviors of teachers and children in the classroom. Clinician categories include: (1) observing and modifying lesson appropriately, 2) instruction and demonstration, 3) auditory and/or visual stimulation, 4) auditory and/or visual positive reinforcement of client's correct response, 5) punishment, 6) auditory and/or visual positive reinforcement of client's incorrect response, 7) clinician relating irrelevant information or asking irrelevant questions, 8) using authority or demonstrating disapproval. Client categories include: 9) client responds correctly, 10) client responds incorrectly, 11) client relating irrelevant information or asking irrelevant questions. Category 12 is silence. The system and an example are contained in Appendix 5-3.

In a comparison of the Boone and Prescott and ABC systems, Schubert and Glick (1974) found that the two systems obtain essentially the same information when therapy consists mainly of stimuli- response—reinforcement. However, in a long occurrence of one behavior, such as reading a story in a language lesson, the ABC naturally provides a clearer indication of the length of time spent on a particular behavior. They concluded that both systems provide useful, objective information about the clinical session.

The ABC should also be evaluated against the Herbert and Attridge (1975) criteria to determine its appropriateness for the situation in which it is to be used. The same statements can be made about the ABC that were made about the Boone and Prescott system, that the behaviors are limited and the same opportunities for misuse exist.

Observing Nonverbal Behavior

The tendency to concentrate on verbal behavior makes it easy to forget the importance of nonverbal behavior, especially as it relates to affective components of interaction. Certainly, interaction between persons cannot be discussed without acknowledging the importance of nonverbal behavior in communicating meaning either through facial expressions, body positions, or gestures. Nonverbal behavior is assumed to be less consciously controlled than verbal behavior. Nonverbal behavior may support, contradict, substitute for, complement, accent, or relate and regulate verbal behavior. Where there are inconsistencies between the two, the listener is more likely to believe the nonverbal (Condon, 1977).

Unfortunately, popular literature in the past several years has encouraged an overemphasis on and overinterpretation of nonverbal behavior. Many of the "how to" books related to interpersonal interaction, communication, or success in life, careers, and social life have oversimplified the meaning of nonverbal communication. It is tempting to move ahead of complex scientific analysis and speculate about such behavior. "If we are at all serious about understanding our nonverbal expressiveness in interpersonal communication, we must be somewhat cautious. There is a great difference between reading and reading into the expressions of others" (Condon, 1977, p. 106).

This is a particularly important warning for the supervisor. It is difficult, if not impossible, for individuals to interpret most of the nonverbal cues directed at them. How much more difficult it is to interpret as an observer! Not everyone reacts in the same way to nonverbal cues. Much interpretation is dependent upon the context as well as the observer's own perceptual processes, attitudes, beliefs, and expectations (Stewart & D'Angelo, 1975). Gender, cultural, and age factors may also account for differences in nonverbal behaviors, which lead to misunderstanding. Therefore, for the supervisor to interpret the meaning of the clinician's behavior to a client or its effect on the client, or vice versa, is folly.

Nevertheless, such behaviors are an important part of clinical interaction and, no doubt, are frequently recorded by supervisors, whether or not they can be interpreted accurately. Often they are obviously distracting; at other times the effect on the client can be observed in backing away from a clinician, facial expression, or other movement. Goldberg (1997) provided some basic information that gives clinicians and supervisors an introduction to the influence that nonverbal behaviors may have on the clinical process. Shipley (1997) addressed the influence of some nonverbal behaviors on interviewing and counseling in communicative disorders. Those interested in a more in-depth study of nonverbal behaviors may refer to counseling and interpersonal communication texts.

Where Have all the Systems Gone?

Methodology for collecting data is a crucial variable in the supervisory chain of events, particularly in moving it toward the realm of the scientific. In actuality, the efforts to approach observation of the clinical process, and therefore, its assessment, more scientifically through the development of interaction analysis systems, seem to have had a brief history and limited attention in speech-language pathology and audiology. Most of the systems were never published; others have been abandoned by the developers for reasons such as loss of interest, complexity of the task, cessation of funding, or higher priority of other interests. Other disciplines, particularly education, have continued to examine the teaching-learning process through the development and use of interaction analysis systems (Evertson & Green, 1986).

Anderson (1988) raised several questions about the infrequent use of interaction analysis systems:

- Is this a reflection of the lack of concern in the profession about the clinical and supervisory processes resulting in a modicum of research on or with analysis systems?
- Does the minimal use of these systems reflect supervisors' lack of interest in using a structured form of data collection?
- Do the systems seem to involve too much work?
- Did the systems fail to tap important dimensions of the clinical process?
- Are they perceived not to be useful?
- Are researchers or supervisors any worse off for not having more validated ways of observing and recording those observations?
- Are they viewed only as another form of tallying, albeit more structured, providing more information, and slightly more objective?

Anderson believed that the possibilities of interaction analysis systems in our professions were never fully explored because so few were published and thus, not well known to many supervisors. They have great utility for supervisors, particularly if used carefully with full knowledge of their limitations. They certainly provide a method for exploring and obtaining information about important variables in the clinical process. Even though categories in the systems reflect the biases of developers, and users must make some subjective analyses of data, Anderson maintained this is no different than what occurs in the assessment process; that is, no matter how many tests are given, it is still necessary to subjectively integrate and interpret information.

Obviously, there is still much to be learned about the clinical process and the efficacy of various treatments. According to Kendall and Norton-Ford (1982), treatment efficacy is a term the encompasses effectiveness, efficiency, and effects. Treatment effectiveness evaluates the causal relationship between a particular treatment and documented changes in client behavior. Treatment efficiency compares two or more treatments to assess if one method is superior to another, or more cost-effective than another (Olswang, 1990). Treatment effects investigations examine which behaviors change in relationship to each other as an outcome of treatment (Olswang, 1990). These latter studies obviously necessitate a dependent variable that can measure relationships between certain clinician-client behaviors. It seems then that the time is ripe for the resurrection, refinement, and development of interaction analysis systems that can be used to examine the intricacies of the clinical process.

Other Methods of Recording Observations

Traditional approaches to clinical intervention and assessment techniques are being modified rapidly with the advent of new knowledge and technologies. Without question, the proliferation of the personal computer, iPads, smartphones, and easy internet access have influenced the clinical process for both clinicians and clients. One of ASHA's three focused initiatives for 2001 was related to the use of web-based and advanced technologies and in particular, the use of telepractices in the delivery of clinical services. Part of the ASHA initiative provided a plan for generating technical reports, position statements, and guidelines that consider reimbursement systems; provision of services to rural and underserved populations; and ethical, privacy, legal, licensing, and credentialing issues. Another part of the initiative addressed "the application of current and emerging technology to deliver services in a manner that will: reduce barriers to access and/or specialized expertise, be cost effective, enhance provider productivity and/or effectiveness, and create additional value/benefits for the health care provider and/or the consumer" (Bernthal, 2001, p. 23). These goals were achieved. Fast forward to today. Telepractice has a practice portal (ASHA, n.d.-b) and a Special Interest Group (SIG 18). The Telepractice Practice Portal defines it as using telecommunication technology to deliver speech-language pathology and audiology professional services at a distance by linking clinician to client or clinician to clinician for assessment, intervention, and consultation. It describes the types: synchronous, asynchronous and hybrid. This portal also addresses key issues and provides resources and references for professionals who engage or want to engage this distance service delivery. Supervision, mentoring, pre-service instruction, and continuing education are other activities that may be conducted using technology and are found on the Practice Portal for Clinical Education and Supervision (ASHA, n.d.-a).

Dudding and Justice (2004) pioneered the use of videoconferencing for distance supervision in speech-language pathology. Telesupervision or e-supervision in our profession has also been addressed and explored by Carlin (2012), Carlin, Boarman, Carlin, and Inselmann (2013), and Laughlin and Sackett (2015). In addition to real-time synchronous videoconferencing, telesupervision or e-supervision can also include asynchronous technologies such as e-mail, texting, instant messaging, and web-based resources. These researchers describe some obvious benefits including convenience and flexibility in scheduling observations and conferences, decreasing or eliminating supervisor travel time, the ability to serve a greater number of supervisees in a term, facilitating placements in remote and "hard-to-fill" sites and increased supervisee autonomy. Disadvantages include technology glitches or failures, transmission problems, limited ability to observe in broader environments such as an entire classroom or meetings with other professionals (e.g., meetings for individualized education programs [IEPs], case staffings) and a "different" kind of interpersonal relationship between supervisor and supervisee.

Computer-based scoring for standardized tests is increasingly more available in speech-language assessment. It allows clinicians to input client data and raw scores and then view a variety of derived scores such as quotients, percentile ranks, means, and standard deviations. This is an asset when scoring is complicated and thus, time-consuming and subject to error. In-depth individual client profiles and normative comparisons that would be labor intensive to complete by hand are easily generated. Advances in quantifying aspects of respiration, vocal intensity, fundamental frequency, resonance, and various aspects of vocal quality (e.g., jitter, shimmer, etc.) continue to improve with technological advances.

Various types of software can be used for speech-language intervention:

- Dedicated software: Commercial software designed to assist in the remediation of specific problem areas (e.g., vocabulary, phonological processes, grammatical structures etc.)
- Educational software: Programs designed for use by teachers to assist in the instruction of reading, writing, spelling that can be modified by clinicians to meet individual client needs
- Entertainment software: Computer books and games that can be used in a similar fashion to the traditional toys, books, and other materials to elicit target behaviors in therapy
- Productivity software: Word processing, e-mail, spreadsheets, calendar software, and the like, can facilitate the program management aspects of service delivery
- Instrument-based biofeedback: Computer instrumentation that provides immediate performance information on various aspects of speech production

A perusal of Pinterest will yield a plethora of ideas, tools, and diagnostic and therapy materials generated by very creative speech-language pathologists and audiologists that are useful in a wide array of practice settings. In addition, there are a number of education applications available for the iPad, iPhone, or computer that can be adapted for use in clinical education. For example, with a school account, *Teacher Evaluator* (Rediker Software; https://www.rediker.com/solutions/evaluations-walkthroughs) streamlines observation and data collection. Observations are able to be framed from a teacher's self-improvement goals; then the notes, videos, and pictures recorded during observations are used to track goal achievement. *iAspire* (https://iaspireapp.com/) provides forms for IEP compliance audit, evaluation rubric, and an observation form that includes categories for: teacher engagement, student-centered instruction, student-engagement, skills, instruction, type of instruction teacher-student responsibility, questioning, learning objectives, content reading, and other additional comments. Photos, videos, and voice recordings can be used to supplement written notes. *Insight: Observation Timer* (Logan Radoff; https://itunes.apple.com/us/app/insight-observation-timer/id1212950867?mt=8) allows users to tabulate behaviors, save, and compile individual data, and keep records. *Catalyst Client* (Data Finch Technologies; https://www.datafinch.com/), designed for behavior analysts, can collect and track a number of types of data, such as frequency, fluency and rate, duration, discrete trials, task analysis, and percentages; it also can create SOAP notes. These latter two are but a few of many tools that clinical educators could use in training students to collect client data. Walz Garrett (2013) notes that practitioners "must consider the needs of the client, pros and cons of the app, cost and other available options before using any app for data collection and management" (p. 12). She also cautions that ethical data storage and security of identifying information in electronic formats must be considered when using technology to support data collection and monitor progress.

ASHA (www.asha.org) provides a wealth of information for the public, students, and ASHA members, such as links to directories, practice management resources including a number of practice portals, access to all of ASHA publications, and continuing education opportunities. The most up to date information regarding technology resources is available at this site. Every aspect of speech-language pathologists' and audiologists' professional lives, as well as those of our consumers, will change drastically in the next decades. What the future holds is uncertain but it will require a commitment to maintaining an awareness of impending improvements and changes, adjustment, flexibility, and innovation on the part of supervisors.

SUMMARY

Observation is a required task in the supervisory process and competence in observation necessitates skill in using a variety of data collection procedures. Verbatim or selected verbatim recordings, tallies of behaviors, and the use of interaction analysis systems are among the more objective data collection techniques, whereas rating scales and checklists are evaluative and subjective. To be effective, observations must be scientific in nature and observers must be actively involved in systematically collecting data. This scientific, active approach necessitates mutual planning and involvement in observing the clinical or supervisory process.

REFERENCES

Acheson, K., & Gall, M. (1980). *Techniques in the clinical supervision of teachers.* New York, NY: LongmanFKendall.

American Speech-Language-Hearing Association. (n.d.-a). *Practice portal: Clinical education and supervision.* Retrieved from https://www.asha.org/Practice-Portal/Professional-Issues/Clinical-Education-and-Supervision/

American Speech-Language-Hearing Association. (n.d.-b). *Practice portal: Telepractice.* Retrieved from https://www.asha.org/Practice-Portal/Professional-Issues/Telepractice/

American Speech-Language-Hearing Association. (2008). *Knowledge and skills needed by speech-language pathologists providing clinical supervision* [Knowledge and skills]. Retrieved from https://www.asha.org/policy/KS2008-00294/

Amidon, E., & Flanders, N. (1967). *The role of the teacher in the classroom.* Minneapolis, MN: Association for Productive Teaching.

Andersen, C. F. (1981). *The effect of supervisor bias on the evaluation of student clinicians in speech/language pathology and audiology* (Doctoral Dissertation). Retrieved from ProQuest Dissertations & Theses Global. (Accession No. 8112499) http://proxyiub.uits.iu.edu/login?url=https://search.proquest.com/docview/303153045?accountid=11620

Anderson, J. (1988). *The supervisory process in speech-language pathology and audiology.* Boston, MA: College-Hill.

Bales, R. (1950). *Interaction process analysis: A method for the study of small groups.* Reading, MA: Addison-Wesley.

Bernthal, J. (2001). Focused initiative on web-based and advanced technology. *The ASHA Leader, 6*(4), 23.

Block, F. (1982). The preconference observation system: Supervisor's point of view. *SUPERvision, 6,* 1-6.

Blodgett, E., Schmitt, J., & Scudder, R. (1987). Clinical session evaluation: The effect of familiarity with the supervisee. *The Clinical Supervisor, 5,* 33-43.

Boone, D. (1970). A close look at the clinical process. In J. Anderson (Ed.), *Proceedings of conference on supervision of speech and hearing programs in the schools.* Bloomington, IN: Indiana University.

Boone, D., & Prescott, T. (1972). Content and sequence analysis of speech and hearing therapy. *Asha, 14,* 58-62.

Boone, D., & Stech, E. (1970). *The development of clinical skills in speech pathology by audiotape and videotape self-confrontation* [Final Report. Project No. 1381—Grant No. OEG-9-071318-2814]. Washington, DC: U.S. Department of Health, Education, and Welfare.

Brooks, R., & Hannah, E. (1966). A tool for clinical supervision. *Journal of Speech and Hearing Disorders, 31,* 383-387.

Brookshire, R., Nicholas, L., Krueger, K., & Redmond, K. (1978). The clinical interaction analysis system: A system for observational recording of aphasia treatment. *Journal of Speech and Hearing Disorders, 43,* 437-447.

Camarata, M. (1992). Facilitating self-analysis of videotaped treatment: A generalization effect. In S. Dowling (Ed.), *Proceedings of the 1992 National Conference on Supervision—Total Quality supervision: Effecting optimal performance* (pp. 46-52). Council of Supervisors in Speech-Language Pathology and Audiology, Nashville, TN.

Campbell, D., & Stanley, J. (1963). *Experimental and quasi-experimental designs for research.* Chicago, IL: Rand McNally.

Carlin, C. H. (2012). E-supervision of graduate students in speech-language pathology: Preliminary research findings. *Perspectives in Telepractice, 2*(1), 26-30.

Carlin, C. H., Boarman, K., Carlin, E., & Inselmann, K. (2013). The use of e-supervision to support speech-language pathology graduate students during student teaching practica. *International Journal of Telerehabilitation, 5*(2), 21-31.

Cascia, J. (2013). Analysis of clinical supervisor feedback in speech-language pathology. *Perspectives in Administration and Supervision, 23*(2), 39-58. doi:10.1044/aaa23.2.39

Cogan, M. (1973). *Clinical supervision.* Boston, MA: Houghton Mifflin.

Condon, J. (1977). *Interpersonal communication.* New York, NY: Macmillan.

Conover, H. (1979). *Conover analysis system.* Unpublished manuscript, Ohio University, Athens, OH.

Council for Clinical Certification in Audiology and Speech-Language Pathology of the American Speech-Language-Hearing Association. (2014). *2014 standards for the certificate of clinical competence in speech-language pathology.* Rev 2016. Retrieved from http://www.asha.org/Certification/2014-Speech-Language-Pathology-Certification-Standards/

Council on Academic Accreditation in Audiology and Speech-Language Pathology. (2017). *Standards for accreditation of graduate education programs in audiology and speech-language pathology.* Retrieved from http://caa.asha.org/reporting/standards/2017-standards/

Darley, F., & Spriestersbach, D. C. (1978). *Diagnostic methods in speech pathology* (2nd ed.). New York, NY: Harper and Row.

Diedrich, W. (1969). Assessment of the clinical process. *Journal of Kansas Speech and Hearing Association.*

Diedrich, W. (1971). Functional description of therapy and revised multidimensional scoring system. In T. Johnson (Ed.), *Clinical interaction and its measurement.* Logan, UT: Utah State University.

Dowling, S. (1983a). An analysis of conventional and teaching clinic supervision. *The Clinical Supervisor, 1,* 15-29.

Dowling, S. (1983b). Teaching clinic conference participant interactions. *Journal of Communication Disorders, 16,* 385-397.

Dowling, S. (2001). *Supervision: Strategies for successful outcomes and productivity.* Boston, MA: Allyn & Bacon.

Dudding, C., & Justice, L. (2004). An e-supervision model: Videoconferencing as a clinical training tool. *Communication Disorders Quarterly, 25*(3), 145-151.

Emerich, L., & Hatten, J. (1979). *Diagnosis and evaluation in speech pathology.* Englewood Cliffs, NJ: Prentice-Hall.

Engnoth, G. L. (1973). *A comparison of three approaches to supervision of speech clinicians in training* (Doctoral dissertation). Retrieved from ProQuest Dissertations and Theses Global. (Accession No. 7412552) http://proxyiub.uits.iu.edu/login?url=https://search.proquest.com/docview/302670407?accountid=11620

Evertson, C., & Green, J. (1986). Observation as inquiry and method. In M. Wittrock (Ed.), *Handbook of research on teaching.* New York, NY: Macmillan.

Farmer, S. (1980). *Interview analysis system.* Paper presented at the annual convention of the American Speech-Language-Hearing Association, Detroit, MI.

Farmer, S. (Ed.). (1987). *Clinical supervision: A coming of age.* Proceedings of a conference held at Jekyll Island, GA. Las Cruces, NM, New Mexico State University.

Farmer, S., & Farmer, J. (1989). *Supervision in communication disorders.* Columbus, OH: Merrill.

Filter, M., Brandell, M., Smith, J., & Kopin, M. (1989). Reliability of counting supervisee responses/errors during a treatment session. In D. Shapiro (Ed.), *Proceedings of the 1989 National Conference on Supervision: Supervision innovations* (pp. 84-86). Council of Supervisors in Speech-Language Pathology and Audiology. Sonoma, CA.

Flanders, N. (1970). *Analyzing teacher behavior.* Reading, MA: Addison-Wesley.

Gillam, R. (1999). ISSUE III: Models of clinical instruction. Adopting an integrated apprenticeship model in a university clinic. In P. Murphy (Ed.), *Council of Academic Programs in Communication Sciences and Disorders— Proceedings of the Annual Conference on Graduate Education* (pp. 97-99). Council of Academic Programs in Communication Sciences and Disorders, Minneapolis, MN.

Goldberg, S. (1997). *Clinical skills for speech-language pathologists.* San Diego, CA: Singular.

Golper, L., McMahon, J., & Gordon, M. (1976). *The use of interaction analysis for training in observation.* Paper presented at the annual convention of the American Speech-Language-Hearing Association, Houston, TX.

Goldhammer, R. (1969). *Clinical supervision.* New York, NY: Holt, Rinehart and Winston.

Goldhammer, R., Anderson, R., & Krajewski, R. (1980). *Clinical supervision* (2nd ed.). New York, NY: Holt, Rinehart and Winston.

Hagler, P. H. (1986). *Effects of verbal directives, data, and contingent social praise on amount of supervisor talk during speech-language pathology supervision conferencing* (Doctoral dissertation). Retrieved from ProQuest Dissertations and Theses Global. (Accession No. 303410764) http://proxyiub.uits.iu.edu/login?url=https://search.proquest.com/docview/303410764?accountid=11620

Hagler, P., & Holdgrafer, G. (1987). Effects of supervisory feedback on clinician and client discourse participation. In S. Farmer (Ed.), *Proceedings of A National Conference on Supervision—Clinical supervision: A coming of age* (pp. 106-111). Council of University Supervisors of Practicum in Speech-Language Pathology and Audiology, Jekyll Island, GA.

Hall, A. S. (1970). *The effectiveness of videotape recordings as an adjunct to supervision of clinical practicum by speech pathologists* (Doctoral dissertation). Retrieved from ProQuest Dissertations and Theses Global. (Accession No. 7118014) http://proxyiub.uits.iu.edu/login?url=https://search.proquest.com/docview/302574772?accountid=11620

Harris, B. (1975). *Supervisory behavior in education.* Englewood Cliffs, NJ: Prentice-Hall.

Hatten, J., Bell, J., & Strand, J. (1983). *A comparative study of supervisor evaluation of a clinical session.* Paper presented at the annual convention of the American Speech-Language-Hearing Association, Washington, DC.

Hegde, M.N., & Davis, D. (2010). *Clinical methods and practicum in speech-language pathology* (5th ed.). Clifton Park, NJ: Cengage.

Herbert, J., & Attridge, C. (1975). A guide for developers and users of observation systems and manuals. *American Educational Research Journal, 12,* 1-20.

Irwin, R. (1972). *Microsupervision—A study of the behaviors of supervisors of speech clinicians.* Unpublished manuscript, Ohio State University, Columbus, OH.

Irwin, R. (1975). Microcounseling interview skills of supervisors of speech clinicians. *Human Communication, 4,* 5-9.

Irwin, R. (1981a). Training speech pathologists through microtherapy. *Journal of Communication Disorders, 14,* 93-103.

Irwin, R. (1981b). Video self-confrontation on speech pathology. *Journal of Communication Disorders, 14,* 235-243.

Irwin, R., & Hall, A. (1973). Microtherapy—A study of the behaviors of speech clinicians. *Central States Speech Journal, 24,* 297-303.

Ivey, A. E. (1971). *Microcounseling.* Springfield, IL: Charles C. Thomas.

Johnson, T. (Ed.). (1971). *Clinical interaction and its measurement.* Logan, UT: Utah State University, Department of Communicative Disorders.

Johnson, T. S. (1969). *The development of a multidimensional scoring system for observing the clinical process in speech pathology* (Doctoral dissertation). Retrieved from ProQuest Dissertations and Theses Global. (Accession No. 7011036) http://proxyiub.uits.iu.edu/login?url=https://search.proquest.com/docview/302422014?accountid=11620

Johnson, W., Darley, F., & Spriestersbach, D. (1963). *Diagnostic methods in speech pathology.* New York, NY: Harper and Row.

Kagan, N. (1970). Human relationships in supervision. In J. Anderson (Ed.), *Conference on Supervision of Speech and Hearing Programs in the Schools.* Bloomington, IN: Indiana University.

Kendall, P. C., & Norton-Ford, J. D. (1982). *Scientific and professional dimensions.* New York, NY: Wiley.

Korner, I., & Brown, W. (1952). The mechanical third ear. *Journal of Consulting Psychology, 16,* 81-84.

Kunze, L. (1967). Program for training in behavioral observation. In A. Miner, A symposium: Improving supervision of clinical practicum. *Asha, 9,* 473-497.

Laughlin, L., & Sackett, J. (2015). Telesupervision and ASHA's tasks of supervision. *Perspectives on Telepractice, 5,* 4-13. doi:10.1044/tele5.1.4

Lincoln, Y., & Guba, E. (1985). *Naturalistic inquiry.* Beverly Hills, CA: Sage.

Lund, N., & Duchan, J. (1993). *Assessing children's language in naturalistic contexts* (3rd ed.). Englewood Cliffs, NJ: Prentice-Hall.

Mawdsley, B. (1985). *Kansas inventory of self-supervision.* Paper presented at the annual convention of the American Speech-Language-Hearing Association, Washington, DC.

McReynolds, L., & Kearns, K. (1983). *Single-subject experimental designs in communicative disorders.* Baltimore, MD: University Park Press.

Messick, C. (1999). ISSUE III: Models of clinical instruction. Clinical network: The challenges of establishing a new training model. In P. Murphy (Ed.), *Council of Academic Programs in Communication Sciences and Disorders Proceedings of the Annual Conference on Graduate Education* (pp. 90-96). Minneapolis, MN: Council of Academic Programs in Communication Sciences and Disorders.

Molyneaux, D., & Lane, V. (1982). *Effective interviewing: Techniques and analysis.* Boston, MA: Allyn and Bacon.

Moon Meyer, S. (2004). *Survival guide for the beginning speech-language clinician* (2nd ed).. Austin, TX: Pro Ed.

Mowrer, D. (1969). Evaluating speech therapy through precision recording. *Journal of Speech and Hearing Disorders, 34,* 239-245.

Mowrer, D. (1972). Accountability and speech therapy. *Asha, 14,* 111-115.

Mowrer, D. (1977). *Methods of modifying speech behaviors.* Columbus, OH: Merrill.

Olswang, L. (1990). Treatment efficacy research, a path to quality assurance. *Asha, 32,* 45-47.

Orlikoff, R., Schiavetti, N., & Metz, D. (2015). *Evaluating research in communication disorders* (7th ed.). Upper Saddle River, NJ: Pearson.

Peaper, R., & Mercaitis, P. (1987). The nature of narrative written feedback provided to student clinicians: A descriptive study. In S. Farmer (Ed.), *Clinical supervision: A Coming of Age.* Proceedings of a conference held at Jekyll Island, GA. Las Cruces, NM: New Mexico State University.

Pelton, R. P. (Ed.). (2010). *Making classroom inquiry work: Techniques for effective action research.* Lanham, MD: Rowman & Littlefield

Pickering, M. (1980). *Introduction to qualitative research methodology: purpose, characteristics, procedures, examples.* Paper presented at the annual convention of the American Speech-Language-Hearing Association, Detroit, MI.

Prescott, T. (1971). The development of a methodology for describing speech therapy. In T. Johnson (Ed.), *Clinical interaction and its measurement.* Logan, UT: Utah State University.

Rassi, J. (2001, June/July). A comparison of supervision practices in audiology and speech-language pathology. *California Speech-Language-Hearing Association (CSHA) Magazine, 30*(1), 12-13.

Roberts, J., & Naremore, R. (1983). An attributional model of supervisors' decision-making behavior in speech-language pathology. *Journal of Speech and Hearing Research, 26,* 537-549.

Rosenshine, B. (1970). Evaluation of classroom instruction. *Review of Educational Research, 40,* 282.

Runyan, S., & Seal, B. (1985). A comparison of supervisors' ratings while observing a language remediation session. *The Clinical Supervisor, 3,* 61-75.

Sbaschnig, K., & Williams, C. (1983). *A reliability audit for supervisors.* Paper presented at the annual meeting of the American Speech-Language-Hearing Association, Cincinnati, OH.

Schill, M. (1992). Quality supervision: Beginning with observation. In S. Dowling (Ed.), *Proceedings of the 1992 National Conference on Supervision—Total quality supervision: Effecting optimal performance* (pp. 53-57). Council of Supervisors in Speech-Language Pathology and Audiology, Nashville, TN.

Schneider, D., Hastorf, A., & Ellsworth, P. (1979). *Person perception.* Reading, MA: Addison-Wesley.

Schubert, G. (1978). *Introduction to clinical supervision.* St. Louis, MO: W. H. Green.

Schubert, G., & Glick, A. (1974). A comparison of two methods of recording and analyzing student clinician-client interaction: ABC system and the "Boone" system. *Acta Symbolica, 5,* 39-56.

Schubert, G., & Gudmundson, P. (1976, November). *Effects of videotape feedback and interaction upon nonverbal behavior of student clinicians.* Paper presented at the annual convention of the American Speech-Language-Hearing Association, Houston, TX.

Schubert, G., Miner, A., & Till, J. (1973). *The analysis of behavior of clinicians (ABC) system.* Unpublished manuscript. University of North Dakota, Grand Forks, ND.

Shipley, K. (1997). *Interviewing and counseling in communicative disorders—Principles and procedures* (2nd ed.). Boston, MA: Allyn & Bacon.

Shipley, K., & McAfee, J. (2016). *Assessment in speech-language pathology: A resource manual* (5th ed.). Boston, MA: Cenage.

Silverman, F. (1998). *Research design and evaluation in speech-language pathology and audiology.* Boston, MA: Allyn & Bacon.

Simons, E. (2014). *Merge of behavior analysis procedures into a speech-language pathology autism clinic. Unpublished master's thesis.* James Madison University, Harrisonburg, VA. Retrieved from http://commons.lib.jmu.edu/master2019/327

Simon, A., & Boyer, E. (Eds.). (1970a). *Mirrors for behavior: An anthology of classroom observation instruments* (Vol. A). Philadelphia, PA: Research for Better Schools.

Simon, A., & Boyer, E. (Eds.). (1970b). *Mirrors for behavior: An anthology of classroom observation instruments* (Vol. B). Philadelphia, PA: Research for Better Schools.

Simon, A., & Boyer, E. G. (1974). *Mirrors for behavior III: An anthology of observation instruments.* Wyncote, PA: Communication Materials Center in cooperation with Humanizing Learning Program Research for Better Schools.

Stewart, J., & D'Angelo, G. (1975). *Together: Communicating interpersonally.* Reading, MA: Addison-Wesley.

Turton, L. (Ed.). (1973). *Proceedings of a workshop on supervision in speech pathology.* Ann Arbor, MI: University of Michigan, Institute for the Study of Mental Retardation and Related Disabilities.

Walz Garrett, J. (2013). Technology to support data collection and management in the public schools. *SIG 16 Perspectives on School-Based Issues, 14*(1), 10-14. doi:10.1044/sbi 14.1.10

Wegner, J. (1999). K-TEAM: Empowering students. In P. Murphy (Ed.), *Proceedings of the Annual Conference on Graduate Education—New horizons* (pp. 100-106). Council of Academic Programs in Communication Sciences and Disorders, Minneapolis, MN.

 This chapter is a revision of that appearing in the 2003 edition of this book.

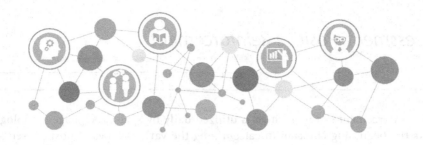

APPENDIX 5-1
KANSAS INVENTORY OF SELF-SUPERVISION (KISS)

Brenda L. Mawdsley

Self-Assessment: Overuse of "OK"

Clinician _____

Date _____

When supervising beginning students in speech-language pathology, it becomes apparent that many tend to say "OK" an excessive number of times during the management session. Four main types of "OK" responses seem to be the ones overused. They are "OK" used as (1) a filler, (2) a positive reinforcer, (3) corrective feedback, and (4) tag question. The definitions are as follows:

- "OK" as a filler: This happens when the clinician says "OK" for no reason throughout the session. For example "OK, now let's turn to the back page."
- "OK" as a positive reinforcer: This is used after the client has given a correct response. Used in this manner, it can often appear as if clinicians are really not committing themselves to the client's production.
- "OK" as corrective feedback: This often occurs when beginning clinicians are afraid to commit as to the correctness or incorrectness of a response. After an error the clinician would say "OK" instead of giving a rich descriptive feedback.
- "OK" as a tag question: An example of this is "Pull your tongue up and back, OK?" or "Let's get out our speech books, OK?" The addition of "OK" makes a statement into a nonassertive request.

During a 20-minute session, count the number of times each of the following types of "OK" are spoken by the clinician.

TYPE	DATA
"OK" used a filler	
"OK" as positive reinforcer	
"OK" as corrective feedback	
"OK" as a tag question	
Total number of "OK"s _____	

After listening to the recording, set a realistic goal for reducing the incidence of "OK." Audio or video sessions weekly until the goal is met up.

Self-Assessment: Positive Reinforcement

Clinician _____

Date _____

Positive reinforcement is a tool which is utilized daily by speech-language pathologists. This form assists the beginning clinician in categorizing the various types of positive reinforcement used, and in examining sequences of positive reinforcement. For example, the clinician might say, "Good talking," then smile at the client, then give him a token. Three types of positive reinforcement have been utilized and now can be categorized and counted. The clinician can analyze the type and amount of reinforcement being used, examine the amount of progress the client is making and adjust the reinforcement sequences accordingly.

Utilizing the coding system below, tally the type of positive reinforcement given the client after a correct response in the blank matrix, placing only one code per box. (Note: For a young client who needs maximum reinforcement, one may chart type of positive reinforcement used after any responses.)

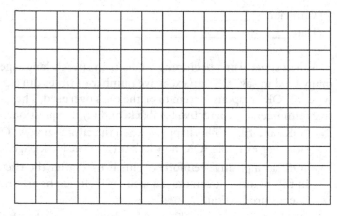

RESPONSE CODE
C = correct response
I = incorrect response

FEEDBACK CODE
PV = positive verbal
NVP = nonverbal positive (smiling, nodding, leaning)
PT = positive touch
T = token reinforcement
E = edible reinforcement

Total number of responses (C+I) = _____

Percentage of correct responses $\dfrac{C}{C+I}$ = _____

Examine the matrix and circle the sequences of positive reinforcement used. For example, a correct response followed by a smile, positive touch and a token would have a sequence code of C/NVP/PT/T. (Slashes indicate "followed by" in sequence counts). List the sequences and the number of times that sequences is used during the session.

SEQUENCE COUNTS

Sequence	# of Events
C/PV	
C/NVP	
C/T	
C/E	
C/PV/NVP	
C/PV/NVP/PT/T	
Etc.	

Self-Assessment: Corrective Feedback

Clinician _____

Date _____

Corrective feedback is defined as the type of corrective measures the clinician will utilize after the client has made as incorrect response. Beginning clinicians have historically demonstrated difficulty in this area by (1) using ambiguous feedback resulting in confusion for the client as to whether the response was correct or incorrect and (2) using feedback lacing descriptive qualities such as modeling, phonetic placement and motokinesthetic techniques. This critique form looks at types and sequences of corrective feedback used, then asks the clinician to review the percentage of correct responses to determine if the corrective feedback techniques utilized resulted in maximum gain by the client.

Utilizing the coding system below, tally the type of corrective feedback given the client after an incorrect or approximated response. Place the code for each event in one box of the matrix working left to right.

RESPONSE CODE

I = incorrect response

A = approximated response

C = correct response

FEEDBACK CODE

NR = no response from clinician

VN = verbal negative, e.g. "No, try again."

M = model

VC = visual clue

PP = phonetic placement e.g. "Put your tongue up and back."

MC = motokinesthetic cue, e.g., giving tactile cues.

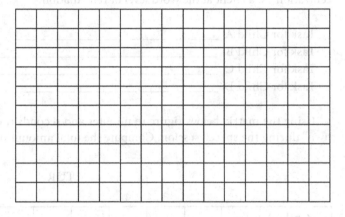

Total number of responses (I + A + C) = _____

Percentage of correct responses $\dfrac{C}{I + A + C}$ = _____

Examine the matrix and circle the sequences of corrective feedback. In the space below, list the sequences and the number of times each sequence occurred in the session. The slash indicates "followed by" in sequence counts.

SEQUENCE COUNTS

Sequence	# of Events
I/NR	
I/VN	
I/VN/PP/M	
I/MC/PP/M	

Self-Assessment: Group Management Rotation Rates

Clinician _____

Date _____

Group management is not the norm in most practicum sites for speech-language pathology. Therefore, when the beginning student is faced with teaching two or more children at the same time, he often does not understand how to rotate from child to child quickly in order to keep all children as involved as possible and behavior problems at a minimum. With this self-assessment form student clinicians can assess, in minutes and seconds, the amount of time spent with each child in a group management session. This not only given information regarding how quickly the speech-language pathologist rotates from child to child, but this count will also yield a total amount of time spent with each individual child so the clinician can note if more time is being spent with one client than the others.

Below, write out the session task for each child. This will help in the analysis since, for example, in articulation management more time may appropriately be spent with a client at the level of concentration vs. a client at the word level of remediation.

Task for Child A _____

Task for Child B _____

Task for Child C _____

Task for Child D _____

Using the matrix below, figure in minutes and seconds the time spent with each child for "his turn" during the speech session. Compute the total amount of time spent with each child.

TURN

	1	2	3	4	5	6	7	8	9	10	11	12
Child A												
Child B												
Child C												
Child D												

Total time spent with   Child A _____

Child B _____

Child C _____

Child D _____

$$\frac{\text{Total time with all children}}{\text{Total number of turns}} = \text{Mean length of each turn} = \underline{\hspace{2cm}}$$

Self-Assessment: Response Rate

Clinician _____

Date _____

The response rate form was developed so the clinician can self-assess how many responses per minute are being elicited from the client. When a supervisor says that the pace of the session is too slow, the supervisee can count responses to see if this is an area which needs to be improved. The clinician can accumulate baseline data and attempt to improve number of responses per minute until the supervisor and supervisee agree the number of responses per session appropriate.

To figure response rate, add together correct and incorrect responses and divide by number of minutes of direct management. For example, if in an individual management session the client had 37 correct and 24 incorrect responses, add these scores together for a total of 61. Then divide by the time involved in direct drill, e.g., 20 minutes. The response rate for the session would be:

$$\frac{61 \text{ total responses}}{20 \text{ min. direct drill}} = 3.05 \text{ responses per minute}$$

An example of figuring group response rates would be:
- Child A has 12 correct and 43 incorrect for a total of 55
- Child B has 29 correct and 12 incorrect for a total of 41
- Child C has 42 correct and 9 incorrect for a total of 51

Add these totals together to find a total number of responses for the session. In this example the total equals 147. Next, divide total number of responses in the session by the time involved in direct drill, 23 minutes.

$$\frac{147 \text{ responses}}{23 \text{ min. direct drill}} = 6.4 \text{ responses per minute}$$

Client	Task	# Correct	# Incorrect	Minutes of Drill	Responses per Minute

Comments:

Self-Assessment: Clinician Response to Client Social Comments

Clinician _____

Task _____

Date _____

As you listen to the audio or video, after each social comment from the client note the category of the clinician's next remark by placing a checkmark in the appropriate space. Next note the effect your behavior had on the child in the column marked "Consequence." Indicate the topic of the "Client Social" by paraphrasing the comment in a few words, e.g., "recess fight."

CLIENT SOCIAL (COMMENT)	CLINICIAN			CONSEQUENCES
	Social	Bad Evaluation	Return to Task	
Example 1. "Mary hit Tom" recess fight				Client returned
2.				
3.				
4.				
5.				
6.				
7.				
8.				
9.				

Comments regarding the data: _____

_____

_____

_____

_____

_____

_____

_____

Self-Assessment: Clinician Versus Client Talk-Time

Clinician _____

Task _____

Date _____

For this self-analysis, you will need to have two stopwatches. As you listen to the audio or video, measure the clinician's talk-time with one stopwatch and the client's talk-time with the other.

Talk-time of the clinician   _____

Talk-time of the client   _____

Total talk-time for session   _____

Percentage of the clinician talk-time   _____

(Clinician talk-time / total talk = % clinician talk-time)

Comments regarding the data: _____

_____

_____

_____

_____

_____

_____

Reprinted with permission from: Mawdsley, B. (1985). *Kansas inventory of self-supervision*. Paper presented at the annual convention of the American Speech-Language-Hearing Association.

APPENDIX 5-2A
BOONE AND PRESCOTT 10-CATEGORY SYSTEM

Category Numbers and Definitions

Category	Definition
1. Explain/Describe	Clinician describes and explains the specific goals or procedures of the session.
2. Model/Instruction	Clinician specifies client behavior by direct modeling or by specific request.
3. Good Evaluation	Clinician evaluates client response and indicates a verbal or nonverbal approval.
4. Bad Evaluation	Clinician evaluates client response as incorrect and gives verbal or nonverbal disapproval.
5. Neutral/Social	Clinician engages in behavior which is not therapy-goal oriented.
6. Correct Response	Client makes a response which is correct for clinician instruction or model.
7. Incorrect Response	Client makes incorrect response to clinician instruction or model.
8. Inappropriate/Social	Client makes response which is not appropriate for session goals.
9. Good Self-Evaluative	Client indicates awareness of his own correct response.
10. Bad Self-Evaluative	Client indicates awareness of his own incorrect response.

Procedures for Using Boone and Prescott 10-Category System

1. The clinician records the middle 20 minutes of his or her therapy, using an audio or video recorder. Experience and investigation using these confrontation devices have found that the first 5 minutes and the last 5 minutes of a half-hour therapy session are not particularly representative of the whole session. Our investigations (Boone & Goldberg, 1969) have also found that a 5-minute segment, selected either randomly or specifically because the clinician wishes to study a particular part of his therapy, will offer about as much information as scoring the total 20-minute segment. In any case, record approximately 20 minutes of therapy.

2. Select for playback and study about a 5-minute segment from the total 20-minute recording. This segment should be studied as soon as the session is completed as possible, particularly in self-confrontation. Whenever possible, playback should not be deferred more than one day from taping.

3. The clinician views or hears the total 5-minute segment first with no attempt to score what she or he sees or hears. She or he then plays back the 5-minute segment and scores the segment using a 10-category system analysis. An experienced scorer can do this with a minimum of stop-starting of the playback. Scoring a typical 5-minute segment takes a total of about 7 to 8 minutes.

4. The total number of events scored in the session and the particular sequences of events are then summarized on the speech and hearing therapy session scoring form. This permits the clinician to determine, for example, how many of the therapy events he did, how many the clients did, and client's percentage of correct responses. By computing a few ratios with his total number of events in particular categories he can find such information as the ratio of his good evaluative reinforcements, bad evaluative responses, and socialization within session. The average time for determining the summary data on the session scoring form is also about 7 or 8 minutes.

5. The total time required for playback, scoring, and summary tabulation should not exceed 20 minutes.

APPENDIX 5-2B
BOONE AND PRESCOTT SCORING FORM

Clinician _____ Date:

Client _____

Goal

1. Explain/Describe	1
2. Model, Instruction	2
3. Good Evaluation	3
4. Bad Evaluation	4
5. Neutral/Social	5

6. Correct Response	6
7. Incorrect Response	7
8. Inappropriate/Social	8
9. Good Self-Evaluative	9
10. Bad Self-Evaluative	10

1. Explain/Describe	1
2. Model, Instruction	2
3. Good Evaluation	3
4. Bad Evaluation	4
5. Neutral/Social	5

6. Correct Response	6
7. Incorrect Response	7
8. Inappropriate/Social	8
9. Good Self-Evaluative	9
10. Bad Self-Evaluative	10

1. Explain/Describe	1
2. Model, Instruction	2
3. Good Evaluation	3
4. Bad Evaluation	4
5. Neutral/Social	5

6. Correct Response	6
7. Incorrect Response	7
8. Inappropriate/Social	8
9. Good Self-Evaluative	9
10. Bad Self-Evaluative	10

APPENDIX 5-2C
BOONE AND PRESCOTT SESSION ANALYSIS FORM

Clinician _____

Client _____

Date _____

Session Goal: _____

_____

Category	No. of Events	% of Total		Category	No. of Events	% of Total
1				6		
2				7		
3				8		
4				9		
5				10		

Clinician Total: _____   Clinician Total: _____   Total # Interactions: _____

% of Session: _____   % of Session: _____

Sequence Counts	**Ratio Scoring**

Sequence No. of Events

Correct Response $\dfrac{6}{6+7}$ _____%

Incorrect Response $\dfrac{7}{6+7}$ _____%

6/3 (6 followed by 3)

Good Evaluation Ratio $\dfrac{6/3}{6}$ _____%

7/4 (7 followed by 4)

Bad Evaluation Ratio $\dfrac{7/4}{7}$ _____%

Inappropriate Response $\dfrac{8}{6+7+8}$ _____%

8/1,2 (8 followed by 1 or 2)

Direct Control $\dfrac{8/1,2}{8}$ _____%

Socialization $\dfrac{5+8}{\text{Total \#}}$ _____%

Reprinted with permission from Boone, D., & Prescott, T. (1972). Content and sequence analysis of speech and hearing therapy, *Asha, 14*, 58-62.

Appendix 5-3A
Analysis of Behavior of Clinicians (ABC) System

George Schubert, Ada Miner, and James Till

Categories and Definitions

Category	Definition
1. Observing and modifying lesson appropriately	Using response or action of the client to adjust goals and/or strategies
2. Instruction and demonstration	Process of giving instruction or demonstrating the procedures to be used
3. Auditory and/or visual stimulation	Questions, cues, and models intended to elicit a response
4. Auditory and/or visual positive reinforcement of client's correct response	Process of giving any positive response to correct client response
5. Auditory and/or visual negative reinforcement of client's incorrect response	Process of giving any negative response to an incorrect client response
6. Auditory and/or visual positive reinforcement of client's incorrect response	Process of giving any positive response to an incorrect client response
7. Clinician relating irrelevant information and/or asking irrelevant question	Talking and/or responding in a manner unrelated to changing speech patterns
8. Using authority or demonstrating disapproval	Changing social behavior from unacceptable to acceptable behavior
9. Client responds correctly	Client responds appropriately, meets expected level
10. Client responds incorrectly	Client apparently tries to respond appropriately but response is below expected level
11. Client relating irrelevant information and/or asking irrelevant questions	Talking and/or responding in a manner unrelated to changing speech patterns
12. Silence	Absence of verbal and relevant motor behavior

Recording Procedures

Raw data is collected by recording a number on the "Raw Data Collection Sheet" every 3 seconds. This number corresponds with the clinician-client interaction occurring at the time of the observation. Therefore, a number is placed on the raw data collection sheet every 3 seconds.

The following basic steps are suggested for learning the recording procedures:

1. *Learn the categories* so you can identify a behavior by number. A cue word list may help you recall the behavior quickly. Make yourself a cue card using the suggested list or one of your own choosing.

Behavioral Categories

1. Modifies	7. Clinician Irrelevant
2. Instructs	8. Authority
3. Stimulus	9. C/R—Correct Response
4. P/R—Positive Reinforcer	10. I/R—Incorrect Response
5. N/R—Negative Reinforcer	11. Irrelevant response
6. R/Inc.—Reinforcement Incorrect	12. Silence

It will also help if you remember that categories 1 through 8 are clinician's behavior; categories 8 through 11 are client behavior; and 12 is silence.

2. *Learn the time unit!* Categories are identified and recorded at 3-second intervals. Form the habit of observing and then writing the number which identifies the behavior.

3. *Record the behavior* (write the numbers) in the squares shown on the raw data collection.

4. *Analyze the data.* The data can be analyzed by completing either or both of the data analysis forms. The two forms are: Quick Analysis Form and the ABC Analysis Form.

APPENDIX 5-3B
RAW DATA COLLECTION SHEET—ABC FORM

Clinician _____

Client _____

Date _____

Session Goal:

Appendix 5-3C
ABC Quick Analysis Form

Clinician _____

Client _____

Date _____

Time _____

Category	Number of Occurrences	% of Total
1. Modifies		
2. Instructs		
3. Stimulus		
4. P/R		
5. N/R		
6. R/Inc		
7. Irrelevant		
8. Authority		
Subtotal—All clinician behaviors		
9. Correct Response		
10. Incorrect Response		
11. Irrelevant		
Subtotal—All client behaviors		
12. Silence		

Reprinted with permission from Schubert, G., Miner, A., & Till, J. (1973). *The analysis of behavior of clinicians (ABC) system* and McCrea, E. & Brasseur, J. (2003). The Supervisory Process in Speech-Language Pathology and Audiology. Boston, MA: Allyn & Bacon.

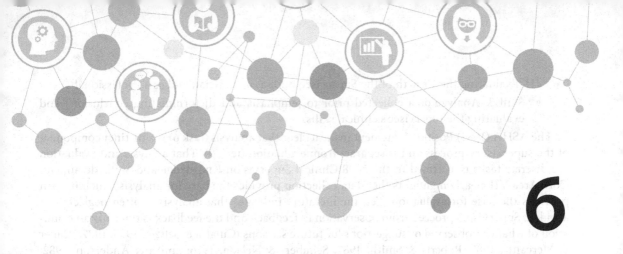

6

Analyzing the Supervisory Process

Judith A. Brasseur, PhD, CCC-SLP, F-ASHA and
Elizabeth S. McCrea, PhD, CCC-SLP, F-ASHA

Core Areas I, III, V, VI, and VII in the American Speech-Language-Hearing Association's (ASHA; 2008) Clinical Supervision Knowledge and Skills policy document are directly related to analyzing, the fourth component of the supervisory process.

- I. Preparation for the Supervisory Experience
  - ○ Skill 7: Be able to analyze the data collected to facilitate the supervisee's clinical skill development and professional growth.
- III. Development of the Supervisee's Critical and Problem-Solving Skills
  - ○ Skill 2: Assist the supervisee in objectively analyzing and interpreting the data obtained and in understanding how to use it for modification of intervention plans.
  - ○ Skill 3: Assist the supervisee in identifying salient patterns in either clinician or client behavior that facilitate or hinder learning.
  - ○ Skill 5: Assist the supervisee in determining whether the objectives for the client and/or the supervisory experience have been met.
- V. Development of the Supervisee's Clinical Competence in Intervention
  - ○ Skill 5: Assist the supervisee in analyzing the data collected in order to reformulate goals, treatment plans, procedures, and techniques.
- VI. Supervisory Conferences or Meetings of Clinical Teaching Teams
  - ○ Skill 7: Use data collection to analyze the extent to which the content and dynamics of the conference are facilitating goal achievement, desired outcomes, and planned changes.

McCrea, E. S., & Brasseur, J. A. *The Clinical Education and Supervisory Process in Speech-Language Pathology and Audiology* (pp 205-218).

- VII. Evaluating the Growth of the Supervisee Both as a Clinician and as a Professional
  - Skill 3: Analyze data collected prior to [emphasis added] formulating conclusions and evaluating the supervisee's clinical skills.

The ASHA (1985) Position Statement made it clear that analysis (task 6) is a distinct component of the supervisory process and is separate from evaluation (task 9). That analysis and evaluation are discrete tasks is affirmed in the 2008 Clinical Supervision Knowledge and Skills document; Core Area VII clearly highlights that data collection provides the base for analysis which in turn provides the base for evaluation. Yet, the literature indicates that analysis is often neglected or avoided. Supervisors proceed from observation to feedback and the feedback is typically an evaluation of what was observed or suggestions for future sessions (Culatta & Seltzer, 1976, 1977; Peaper & Mercaitis, 1987; Roberts & Smith, 1982; Schubert & Nelson, 1976; Smith & Anderson, 1982; Tufts, 1983). Analysis should not be equated with evaluation; rather it should be the bridge between observation and evaluation. It is the time when the supervisor's "square box" is put on the shelf. It is also the time when the clinician/supervisee begins looking at her or his clinical activities with an objective eye.

Analysis is the process of making sense of the data that have been collected. As in research, analysis is driven by the questions formulated before data collection occurred—questions formulated from the goals/purposes of the project. It is the time when the behaviors of the clinician are related to the behaviors of the client and the behaviors of the supervisor are related to those of the supervisee (i.e., the search for relationships or a logical way to account for significant differences).

Professional growth for all participants comes as a result of careful, systematic, fourfold planning, observing and analyzing: for the client, the clinician, the supervisee, and the supervisor. To reiterate, it is not enough to plan, observe, and analyze the clinical process, the process through which the client learns; the supervisory process, through which the supervisor and supervisee learn, must also be examined if maximum professional growth is to be achieved. The focus of this chapter will be on analysis of the clinical process to facilitate the supervisee's clinical skill development and professional growth. Analysis of the supervisory process will be addressed in Chapter 8. Readers are reminded that the basic principles of analysis are applicable to both clinical sessions and supervisory conference.

SCIENTIFIC ASPECTS OF ANALYSIS

In clinical endeavors, as in research, scientific procedures must be used for answering questions—not only the large, global questions, of which there are many, but the day-by-day, session-by-session, conference-by-conference needs for information. After goals have been established and data collected, scientific principles are used to analyze the data. Then, conclusions can be drawn, and inferences can be made. This scientific approach to supervision underscores the importance of analysis to the total process. In research, it would be ludicrous to formulate conclusions and make recommendations for the future immediately after collecting data. It is equally ludicrous to do in the clinical or supervisory processes. Analysis counteracts the superior role of supervisors solely as *evaluators* or *overseers* and highlights their role as scientific coinvestigator.

Ventry and Schiavetti (1980) stated, "We see the practitioner as an applied scientist or a clinical scientist who uses the clinic or school as a laboratory for the application of the scientific method toward the end of providing the best clinical services possible. The scientific method, we think, is at the heart of clinical enterprise" (p. 14). Orlikoff, Schiavetti, and Metz (2015) emphasized the need to eliminate the gap between clinician and researcher. They affirm that the search for knowledge depends on the use of a systematic method, commonly called *scientific method*. The scientific method includes identifying a problem that can be studied objectively, collecting data via observation or experiment, and drawing conclusions based on the analysis of the data that have been gathered (Orlikoff et al., 2015).

In a discussion of the "clinician-investigator," Silverman (1998) stressed that the most compelling reason for functioning as a clinical scientist is to comply with the ASHA (2016) Code of Ethics, which stipulates that individuals who hold a Certificate of Clinical Competence shall evaluate the effectiveness of services provided, technology employed, and products dispensed (I-K). This requires systematic evaluation of the impacts of services rendered. Silverman described several benefits for the clinician who functions as researcher:

- It would "probably make one's job more stimulating, less routine, and would probably increase the possibilities for positive reinforcement" (p. 12).

- It would help satisfy an employer's requirements for accountability (Olswang, 1990).

- It would likely help an individual become a more effective clinician because it would enable a clinician to answer questions relevant to managing one's caseload, to compare the effectiveness of current approaches to new ones, to establish the reliability of nonstandardized diagnostic measures, and to provide documentation for the efficacy of new clinical services being offered which in term could improve funding.

With this approach, supervisors and supervisees are asking questions that are "answerable" and stating hypotheses that are "testable." Analyzing data for a research project may be more extensive or more formal than analyzing data from a clinical session or supervisory conference, but the process is the same. Relevant data have to be summarized, organized and categorized in a manner that is meaningful to the users of the results.

Careful adherence to the scientific method in analysis will ensure a greater degree of supervisor objectivity. In addition, the organization and quantification of observable behaviors and events, inherent in a systematic approach, enhances accountability. This kind of approach forces supervisors and supervisees to test their hunches, rather than use "gut instincts" exclusively when making judgements. The scientific approach does not automatically guarantee objectivity—supervisors and supervisees have to be vigilant in their quest for nonbiased practice. They must constantly be conscious of their own "square boxes," because it would be very easy to look for patterns or categories of behaviors and draw conclusions that support a hypothesis or bias.

IMPORTANCE OF ANALYSIS

It is at the point where supervisors and supervisees begin to use analysis techniques that their supervision style probably differs most from what has previously been called *traditional supervision* or an apprenticeship model of supervision. Developing analytical skills may well be the most important step in producing thoughtful, self-analytical professionals.

If supervisors are serious about what often seems to be platitudinous voicing of the goal of producing "self-supervising" clinicians, this is a crucial point in the development of that ability. If clinicians are to become unconsciously competent, independent functioning professionals, they must develop expertise in self-analysis. It is essential that clinicians be cognizant of their behaviors and the effect of those behaviors on their clients if they are to modify or strengthen those behaviors. The analysis process enables clinicians to extract from a mass of behaviors a design—a configuration—from which they can begin to see what is happening, to draw some inferences, to construct some hypotheses about what was effective and what was not, to test those hypotheses, and then to plan for the future on the basis of their findings.

Organizing raw data on both clinician and client so that it becomes coherent and usable sets up the supervisor and supervisee for a more meaningful and efficient conference. Also, when supervisors analyze clinician behavior they are modeling an approach that is transferable to the clinician's analysis of client behavior. Later, as they study behaviors in the supervisory interaction, they will find the same techniques applicable. Such analysis shows supervisees a method for functioning within the supervisory process. They are learning how to use the scientific approach, observing that it applies to both the clinical and supervisory processes and acquiring a valuable self-analysis technique.

Analysis—particularly joint analysis—should contribute in a major way to meeting the expectations of supervisees for fair and rational feedback and evaluation, because evaluation will be derived from objective data and supervisees will be involved in analyzing and evaluating their own behavior.

When analysis is done jointly, it offers supervisees some protection from the subjective judgements made by supervisors, emphasizing behavior rather than the person. As a result, there may be less defensiveness, which, in turn, enhances communication. Supervisees' also participate in measuring progress toward their objectives. If well planned and executed, the analysis will enable supervisees to function as colleagues in the conference (Andersen, 1981).

Reconstructing or rehashing the clinical session during conferences is the antithesis of analysis. Note this statement from a recording of an actual conference:

> Well, one thing—he got out of his chair and then I couldn't get him to do anything. He was OK while he was sitting. So I was waiting for him to sit down. I said, "OK, I'll wait." He asked me something about my glasses and I answered him. I shouldn't have done that. Then he started talking about his mother's glasses. Finally, I asked him again to sit down. So, he sat down but when I asked him to make his sound he just sat.

If this behavior had been what Cogan (1973) labeled a critical incident, that is, a onetime occurrence that affected the child's learning, it might have been appropriate to report this lengthy rehash of the client's behavior. In this particular conference, however, a similar monologue continued in excruciating detail for over half the conference, occupying nearly half as much time as the actual events. The supervisor's followed it, "Well why don't you…next time." This exemplifies Culatta and Seltzer's (1976, 1977) findings. They found that 61% of all strategy statements were made by supervisors following provision of observation and information (i.e., reconstruction of the clinical session) by the supervisee. The pointlessness of the discussion in this example is underscored by the fact that the supervisor had observed the entire session and was aware of what had happened! Had the session been submitted to some type of organized data collection and analysis, the supervisor and supervisee could have quantified the data on the basis of certain patterns and interactions. The provision of a solution to the problem by the supervisor deprived the supervisee of the opportunity to problem-solve and draw inferences from the data.

If the analysis component is not taken seriously or, worse yet, not understood by supervisors who proceed directly to feedback, conferences will likely continue to consist of a mass of raw data or anecdotal reports used essentially to unnecessarily reconstruct the clinical session, evaluations communicated directly to the supervisee, or a collection of trivial items that have no importance in the learning process.

PURPOSES OF ANALYSIS IN SUPERVISION

The major purposes of analysis are rooted in the works of Cogan (1973), Goldhammer (1969), Goldhammer, Anderson, and Krajewski (1980), and Acheson and Gall (1980), who were the first to verbalize the concept of analysis as an essential part of the supervisory process. One purpose is to distill the raw data to a point where it becomes coherent, manageable, and usable for the feedback component. Another is to organize the observational data in such a way that it can be used to draw conclusions and make rational judgements about what happened in the teaching-learning process. It then becomes the basis for further planning.

In discussing analysis of data collected on the behaviors or teachers and students in the classroom, Cogan (1973) lists the objectives of analysis:

1. Determining if objectives have been met

2. Identifying salient patterns in the teacher's behavior

3. Identifying unanticipated learnings by the student

4. Identifying critical incidents in the interaction (teacher behaviors that occur once but that appear to significantly affect the learning that takes place or the relationship between teacher and student)

5. Organizing the data to determine what was learned

6. Determining if what was planned really was carried out

7. Developing a database for the rest of the supervision program

Cogan urged careful examination of interactions between the behaviors of students and teachers. In addition, he discussed the identification of process learning, which he identified as "learning how to learn." Goldhammer (1969) and Goldhammer et al. (1980) concentrated on the notion that all human behavior is patterned and stressed the point that it is the cumulative effects of those patterns that are important to the learning that occurs. Therefore, supervisors should concentrate on identifying salient patterns, not unusual or incidental variables. The aim of supervision, they said, is to strengthen, extinguish, or modify the salient behaviors.

METHODS OF ANALYSIS

Analysis may be performed by the supervisor, the supervisee, or cooperatively by the two (Cogan, 1973). Each fulfills a need at various times along the continuum of supervision. The Council on Academic Accreditation in Audiology and Speech-Language (CAA) (2017) Standard 5.2 mandates a combination of formative and summative assessments of knowledge and skills. Formative assessment is ongoing measurement throughout the educational program to monitor acquisition of knowledge and skills and improve student learning. Summative assessment involves the comprehensive evaluation of learning outcomes, including knowledge and skills, at the culmination of an educational experience. Comprehensive clinical education experiences must encompass the breadth of the current scope of practice and be sufficient for competent entry-level practice. Formative assessment of clinical knowledge and skills necessitates observations, analyses and evaluations of an individual's clinical competencies by all supervisors of that student. Students must also have analytical abilities. Specifically, they must be able to *analyze* [emphasis added], synthesize and evaluate information about prevention, evaluation, and intervention over the range of differences and disorders specified in the Council for Clinical Certification in Audiology and Speech-Language Pathology (CFCC; 2014) current standards.

Analysis by Supervisors

At the beginning of the supervisory experience, the supervisee's clinical repertoire may be a blank slate to the supervisor. If the supervisor is to determine the salient features of this repertoire, it will require a broad look at data and a dedicated effort to determine baseline. Supervisors must be cautious and avoid looking solely for patterns that fit their personal prejudices or pet assumptions. They must constantly strive to keep in mind that they are concerned about the documented effect of the behaviors. Initially, then, the task of the supervisor is to examine the data carefully, looking for patterns, critical incidents, behaviors related to session objectives or plans, the interactions between clinician and client, and the visible learning effects. This is not a time for judgements. Evaluation will come later after conclusions are drawn and inferences made. For supervisors who have been accustomed to providing direct evaluation this will require a great amount of restraint at first.

At the Evaluation-Feedback Stage, little or no analysis is done; supervisors provide evaluations based on their perceptions and judgements. This is the prominent characteristic of the style used at this stage—judgmental statements from the supervisor's "square box." As supervisees move into the Transitional Stage, a Collaborative Style is apparent. Questions posed prior to and after the observation by supervisees and supervisors serve as the basis for quantifying and categorizing behaviors and interactions. For example, consider that data collected by the clinician during a session revealed 40% correct responses, 15% close approximations, and 45% incorrect responses. The supervisor's data revealed that correct responses and close approximations were intermittently followed by verbal praise; incorrect responses were consistently followed by "OK" and a subsequent model. Depending on client and clinician goals, a number of additional questions would be formulated to guide analysis. For example:

1. How many times did the clinician model, expand, instruct?
2. What clinician behaviors preceded correct responses, close approximations, incorrect responses?
3. What was the nature of the tasks used to elicit responses?
4. What was the client's response rate (number of responses per minute)?
5. What was the content of the directions and instructions?
6. What client behaviors followed certain clinician behaviors?

Once additional analysis is completed, supervisors and supervisees can begin to draw some conclusions, make some inferences and formulate hypotheses to be tested in future sessions.

Introducing Analysis to Supervisees

It is imperative that the supervisee be involved in analysis as soon as possible. Initially, supervisors will likely need to teach these skills. Clinicians are trained to observe client behavior but are rarely taught to extend this observation to their own behaviors. Teaching procedures will depend upon the supervisee's competence level. Supervisees may be asked to read certain material about data collection and analysis (e.g., Brookshire, 1967; Ingram, Bunta, & Ingram, 2004; Mowrer, 1969; Olswang & Bain, 1994; Walz Garrett, 2013). Practice using a particular method or system for coding clinical behaviors and interactions is essential (Boone & Prescott, 1972; Camarata & Rassi, 1991; Lougeay-Mottiger, Harris, & Stillman, 1987; Schubert, Miner, & Till, 1973). Supervisors may opt to demonstrate the analysis procedure after the observation by doing it alone at first and presenting the analyzed data as feedback during the conference. At some point, supervisees must be involved. The supervisor may present data recorded during an observation to the clinician prior to the conference so that the clinician can do the analysis and bring the information to the conference. A supervisor may choose to perform the analysis with the supervisee, again modeling the behaviors that contribute to the analysis. Gillam, Stike-Roussos, and Anderson (1990) demonstrated that joint analysis effected positive changes in supervisees' clinical behaviors. Supervisors may use, or suggest that the supervisee use, interaction analysis systems and their summary forms to learn how to identify categories and patterns of clinical behavior (Brasseur & Jimenez, 1994, Francis, 1993). In a study of two supervisees with more than 200 clock hours, who prior to the study had not self-analyzed, Camarata (1992) concluded that "there was something inherent in observing and analyzing their own work that allows for more productive evaluation and change" (p. 48).

The literature reveals that an initial client-centered focus is typical of beginning clinicians and that they must develop adequate clinical skills and a certain level of comfort in interactions with their clients before they will be able to be involved in data collection and analysis (Brasseur & Jimenez, 1994; Dowling, 2001; Francis, 1993). Beginning clinicians are focused on planning appropriate activities for therapy sessions, finding adequate materials, writing progress notes, and just making it through a session. This is likely to be the case for any supervisee in a new assignment who has neither learned how to self-analyze nor the importance of analyzing prior to evaluating one's behaviors. They are not ready to be active participants in the supervisory process. In addition, there may need to be some sort of contingency for completing assigned analyses (Dowling, Sbaschnig, & Williams, 1991) or a period of time when commitments are written (Shapiro & Anderson, 1988). The supervisor may need to be direct and establish professional development goals for the novice supervisee (Dowling, 2001; Lubinsky & Hildebrand, 1996). Yet, it appears that there must be some method for facilitating ownership and a commitment to change before novice supervisees will care about setting goals, and collecting and analyzing data (Brasseur & Jimenez, 1994, 1996). The supervisor also must provide timely feedback for the supervisee about their performance in self-analysis (Freeman, 1982; Maloney, 1994).

Beginning supervisees need to learn that there is a core of categories of clinical behaviors that are important to most clinical interactions—recording and charting client behaviors, determining types and schedules of reinforcement, giving instructions, establishing types of cues and feedback provided to clients, staying on task, and other behaviors appropriate to the specific client. Goldberg (1997) described two types of foundation skills, technical and process, which "should be learned by new clinicians, preferably before they begin therapy" (p. 93). Hegde and Davis (2010) and Dwight (2014) provided a number of methods that are vital to effective therapy in speech-language pathology and could operationalize important categories for supervisees. Roth and Worthington (2016) detail "basic skills for good therapy" that could provide a structure for data collection and analysis. Whatever framework is selected, the supervisor and supervisee will need to establish the supervisee's baseline relative to selected categories. Mawdsley's (1985) self-assessment instrument, the Kansas Inventory of Self-Supervision (KISS), discussed in Chapter 5, is a useful tool for beginning clinicians because of its simplicity. It is helpful for learning to assign behaviors to certain categories. A quick Google search of "data collection methods in special education" produces an assortment of instructions, forms, and templates that can provide a focus for analysis of selected target behaviors. From here, the analysis proceeds to a less-structured search for other patterns that affect the clinical interaction.

If interaction analysis systems such as the Boone and Prescott (1972) system or Analysis of Behavior of Clinicians system (Schubert, Miner, & Till, 1973) have been used, the summary forms that accompany them facilitate analysis. If other systems are used that do not have summary forms, they can easily be constructed. As previously noted, interaction analysis systems do not cover all possible categories, interactions, or behaviors, thus supervisors must identify categories for other data they have collected.

Whatever strategy is selected to initiate the supervisee to analysis, the supervisor's objective should always be increased responsibility on the part of the supervisee for self-analysis. If supervisees are involved initially with their supervisors and then gradually assume responsibility for themselves, they will develop skills with which they can continue to be self-analytical even when they are working alone or with no supervision. Supervisors who do all the analysis for supervisees inhibit and prevent their learning. Similarly, the supervisor who uses the analyzed data to develop all the conclusions and inferences and, even worse, to evaluate and provide the strategies, is abrogating the responsibilities of supervision. As they move along the continuum, the balance of supervisor-supervisee responsibility for analysis should progress toward increased supervisee participation.

Research

Some research has been completed that has examined the impact of joint analysis and self-analysis of therapy on supervisee's clinical behaviors. Results reveal that clinicians can develop an awareness of their abilities through the analysis of their own audio or video recordings (Boone & Stech, 1970; Schubert & Gudmundson, 1976). Studies of inexperienced student clinicians have demonstrated that they are able to learn to systematically score audio or video recordings of their sessions after a few hours of training (Brasseur & Jimenez, 1994; Camarata, 1992; Camarata & Rassi, 1991; Francis, 1993; Lougeay-Mottiger, Harris, & Stillman, 1987) but the impact of training on clinical performance has varied. In the Camarata (Camarata, 1992; Camarata & Rassi, 1991) investigations, clinicians who scored videos of their own treatment sessions, improved the accuracy of targeted clinical behaviors whereas about half of the students in the Brasseur and Jimenez (1994) study but none of the clinicians in Francis' (1993) study increased their target behaviors. Some of the variables that may account for the differences in findings include:

- The length of time in which self-analyses were completed (whole term vs. part of the semester)
- The complexity of the analysis (two or three behaviors vs. an interaction analysis system)
- Feedback on or evaluation of the completed analysis
- Consequences for completing the assigned analysis and completing it on time

Camarata (1992) questioned whether the positive effects could be achieved if supervisees were to score a portion of the therapy session rather than the entire session. In a follow-up study of the same subjects (Brasseur & Jimemez, 1994), Brasseur and Jimenez (1996) concluded that some didactic training in the supervisory process might have been an important prerequisite to self-analysis. At minimum, supervisors probably need to share their philosophy of supervision, as well as their expectations and goals for the supervisory process with supervisees if supervisee attitudes and behaviors are to change. All of the bulleted variables could be systematically manipulated in future studies with supervisees who have different levels of experience, and who are at different stages of their careers (e.g., students, clinical fellows, speech-language pathologists in medical and school settings, etc.).

Another aspect of self-analysis that is important is that of commitment. Shapiro and Anderson (1989) found that clinicians demonstrated greater completion of commitments when written commitments were introduced early in the supervisory relationship and gradually faded. Written commitments proved more effective for beginning clinicians than for experienced clinicians. Experienced clinicians completed commitments when no written agreement was required and seemed to benefit from less structured, collegial interactions. Maloney (1994) investigated the influence of clinician journal writing on interpersonal communications skills and the affective nature of the relationship with clients. Lubinsky and Hildebrand (1996) examined the impact of journal writing in facilitating the attainment of personal goals in practicum. With these latter two studies, some of the same variables that were noted previously (target behaviors or skills, time, feedback, contingencies for completion) seemed to influence the results.

Gillam, Strike-Roussos, and Anderson (1990) demonstrated the functional relationship between joint analysis of session data and desired changes in clinicians' therapy behaviors. This experimental study introduced yet another variable to consider. Specifically, it may be important to ease clinicians into the process of self-analysis by jointly developing observation and data analysis strategies.

These studies do not represent an exhaustive review of relevant literature. Rather, they serve to highlight some of what we currently know from research and to spark some interest in conducting new investigations to demonstrate the effectiveness of analysis and self-analysis in particular.

Organizing the Data for Feedback

Once data have been collected by either supervisor or supervisee, they are then categorized. Interactions are analyzed to determine the amount of client learning that has occurred, clinical competencies apparent in the interactions, and so on. Client and clinician behaviors to be strengthened, extinguished, or modified are identified. Decisions are made about achievement of objectives.

Goldhammer et al. (1980) discussed at length the principles of organizing the data to determine patterns related to learning. Although they stressed the importance of being able to demonstrate consequences of behavior in the data and the ability to support the patterns on the basis of theory, they also said that patterns may be selected simply because one has hunches about them. The latter principle is discouraged because it is less persuasive, most likely to be wrong, and implies that "hunching one's way through supervisory practice" (p. 88) is acceptable.

Cogan (1973) suggested first analyzing the data on the behavior and learning of the student (client) and relating both to the objectives to determine if they have been met; then, analyzing the teacher's (clinician's) behaviors and forming hypotheses about the relationships between the behaviors and the learning. He also stressed the importance of dealing with interaction, not isolated parts. Some patterns will be more obvious than others, some will be more important than others, and some will reflect biases and inaccurate perceptions.

Cogan (1973) suggested that **critical incidents** should receive a high priority in the analysis because the one-time occurrence that has a profound impact on an individual's learning affect outcomes. Cogan's examples with regard to teaching involve aggressive teacher behaviors—behaviors related to discipline, and incidences that have positive consequences—where students gain insights that have lasting effects. Certain skills for managing clients affect the clinical interaction and may constitute a critical incident. On the positive side, the clinician's ability to capitalize on spontaneous learning—for example, the sudden insight of the client (an "aha moment"), or the unexpected accomplishment of a task—might be a critical incident, that once identified, the supervisor and supervisee may want to convert to a strategy.

The supervisor may very well have seen important patterns of behavior emerge during the observation and recorded them. If not, analysis is where the search begins. Data are perused, categories of behavior are quantified, and consequences of certain behaviors are identified (i.e., when the clinician did X, the client did Y). Some questions to be asked in analyzing data were listed previously (see Analysis by Supervisors section). Additional areas of interest in analysis might include: clarity of instructions and directions; task difficulty; pacing; clinician talk time; turn taking in group therapy; number, variety, creativity of activities; client response rate; client self-evaluations; and so on. It might be advisable to complete a functional behavior analysis (IDEA Partnership, n.d.). Gradually, the detective work will yield results and the data will fall into place. Out of this quantification and categorization both the supervisor and supervisee begin to draw some conclusions, make some inferences, and state some hypotheses to be tested. As treatment efficacy and clinical effectiveness studies reveal, there is no single variable, strategy, or technique or simple cause-effect solution that results in a perfect session. When session goals are or are not achieved, it is important to examine all the plausible reasons for success or failure.

Consider the following scenario. Session data reveal that 60% of the client's responses were incorrect. Incorrect responses increased as the session progressed. Two patterns are immediately obvious in the clinician's behavior: 1) he positively reinforced 35% of the incorrect responses; 2) direction giving and modeling for all productions (accurate and inaccurate) followed the same pattern throughout the session. Twenty percent of the time, the client had observable nonverbal reactions (facial grimaces, head shaking, or sighing) to his own incorrect productions. The clinician did not respond to these reactions but presented the task again in the same way. The nature of individual tasks and task difficulty obviously need to be analyzed. Consequences for correct responses and frequency with which they were applied are among the other variables that should be examined. Additional questions might emerge as the data are analyzed.

What follows such a session will depend on the dyad's place on the continuum. In the direct-active style at the Evaluation-Feedback Stage, feedback will be delivered by the supervisor in writing or during the conference and consist of value judgements and/or strategies the supervisee is directed to use in the next session.

In the Collaborative Style, there are a variety of ways to use the collected data. During the early part of the Transitional Stage, the supervisor will complete the analysis by categorizing and quantifying the behaviors, quantifying types of interactions, comparing clinician behaviors with client responses, summarizing client nonverbal reactions, and other methods. Data and the analysis are presented to the supervisee in the conference. As an alternative, the analysis might be done jointly to demonstrate the process. A bit further along the continuum, the supervisor will give the analyzed data, and later the raw data, to the clinician for study prior to the conference. At whatever point it seems appropriate, the clinician will begin tabulating data from audio or video recordings in preparation for the later stage of self-analysis.

In the beginning stages of analysis, the clinician may be assisted by using a technique that has a built-in method for analysis (e.g., KISS, Boone and Prescott, and Analysis of Behavior of Clinicians) or by certain questions that provide a focus and some structure. For example, "What evidence is there that your objectives were met or not met?" or "Can you see anything in your models and directions that are related to the client's responses?" Here is where supervisors might want to use the Supervision, Questioning, Feedback strategy for clinical teaching to guide questions that will facilitate analysis. For example, supervisees at the Evaluation-Feedback Stage and D1 level (unconsciously and consciously incompetent learner) will benefit from "what" questions that require recalling facts and basic knowledge. Supervisees at the Transitional Stage and D2 level (consciously competent learner) will receive "so what" questions to compel them to compare, analyze, synthesize, or apply knowledge. Or the supervisor may choose to have supervisees examine data with a wide-lens approach or in terms of long-range objectives.

Finally, as clinicians progress along the continuum, they assume more responsibility for data collection and self-analysis. Supervisors and supervisees analyze data separately. The analyses are brought to the conference where they become the basis for the conference agenda.

One may ask, "Why take the time to do all this when it is so much easier to tell them and get on to other matters?" First, self-analysis is essential to the skills listed at the beginning of this chapter. Second, learners must be actively involved in their own learning. Third, although teaching self-analysis skills may take more time than giving direct evaluations or feedback, over time there will be payoffs in terms of the supervisee's increasing independence, and ability to analyze and problem solve. Fourth, time should not be the prime consideration. It is assumed that if supervisors and supervisees are assigned to each other for a learning experience that some time is spent together. The question then becomes one of the quality of that time. Fifth, teaching these skills contributes to the accountability in supervision. Analyzed data can be compared across sessions and thus, clinician growth can be accurately documented, not "guestimated." More accurate hypotheses can be made about methodologies and their results. Sixth, a skill is being taught in the analysis stage which clinicians must have if they are to continue to grow and be self-sufficient, competent clinicians. Further, this skill is absolutely essential when clinicians become supervisors themselves. **And finally, the process of planning, observing, collecting and analyzing data are vital/fundamental to meaningful and productive reflective practice.**

DETERMINING THE CONTENT OF THE SUPERVISORY CONFERENCE

One purpose of analysis is to determine the content of the conference. Analysis that really reduces the data and places a priority on items to be discussed in the conference leads to an efficient, organized, and focused conference. It is the prelude to the conference. Here is another place where components overlap—analysis and planning flowing together.

The content of the conference will be discussed in the next chapter but the possibilities for topics are almost limitless. In addition to general topics, which may vary by situation, the infinite amount of behavior observed in most clinical sessions makes it reasonable to think that not everything observed or identified through analysis can be dealt with in the conference, although it often seems that participants in conferences try to do just that. The premise, here, is that conferences or other forms of feedback, must be planned. In the first edition of this textbook, Anderson (1988) stated that her observations of many hours of recordings of conferences made it obvious that conferences frequently are unplanned, unfocused, and disorganized and contain an unbelievable amount of trivia. Analysis does not assure the elimination of trivia—trivia are trivia, even when quantified. But analysis does make it easier to establish higher priorities for the discussion of some events or issues than others.

Three criteria for selecting items for the conference from all the patterns were provided by Goldhammer et al. (1980).

- *Saliency.* The frequency with which behaviors are found in the data, their significance, their relationship to theory, their relationship to other patterns or to commonalties among teachers (clinicians), and the relationship to what the supervisee sees as important or has requested to discuss.

- *Accessibility of patterns for treatment.* The patterns related to emotionally charged issues that may be too threatening for the supervisee.

- *Fewness.* Because time in conferences is limited and supervisees may only be able to assimilate a certain amount of input, patterns of behavior can be selected or rejected on the basis of certain criteria. These criteria include easy and clear identification of patterns in the data, the subsuming of some patterns under others, the similarity or difference to other patterns, the emotional content of the patterns, the amount of time needed to cover the patterns adequately, and the orderly transition from one issue to another. In other words, each pattern of behavior does not stand alone. It is related to others.

There are other important decisions to be made during the analysis that directly influence the content and organization of the conference. The foundation for an organized, problem-solving, meaningful conference is built during the analysis. Questions that must be asked are:

- Are there data on clinician strengths as well as weaknesses?
- Are there appropriate data to measure the accomplishment of objectives?
- Have clinicians participated in the analysis to an extent that will enable them to have meaningful input into structuring the conference?
- How much should they be expected to participate in the analysis?
- Are there enough data for an analysis? How much data are enough?

Although there is some indication that 3 to 5 minutes of observation and data collection are sufficient to represent the entire session (Boone & Prescott, 1972; Schubert & Laird, 1975), these findings came from the use of specific interaction analysis systems with limited numbers of behaviors. The same kind of information does not exist for other kinds of clinical analysis. The answer to this final question may depend on what clinical skills are being addressed.

> Is the information from the analysis to be considered as infallible? Will there be times when it is nonconclusive? Will there be crises times—or even noncrisis times—when the analyzed data will need to be discarded in favor of some more urgent issues? Is it possible to miss some important issues through the effort to be analytical? Supervisors need to be sensitive to the fact that overutilization of analyzed data can lead to a conference that is too structured.

There are many factors that need to be considered in planning the agenda for the conference. The use of the analyzed data is only one facet, but it is an important one in promoting a scientific approach to supervision and in helping supervisees to become aware of their own behavior and their own needs.

EVALUATION

What about evaluation? The reader is probably asking at this point. Is it eliminated entirely? Is it legitimate for supervisors to provide a direct evaluation? Certainly; in fact, it is the responsibility of supervisors to evaluate *at appropriate times*. It is unrealistic and unprofessional to assume that evaluation should never happen; it is not the intent of the writers to imply that. As stated previously, CAA (2017) standards mandate formative assessments. Thus, periodic evaluation must be built into each practicum experience. It is also a part of the clinical fellowship and likely a part employment in any setting. Additionally, studies about what supervisees want and expect indicate a desire for critique, identification of weaknesses, and guidance about specific techniques. Thus, expectations may not be met unless supervisees 1) receive some evaluation or 2) understand the reasons why the supervisor is encouraging self-evaluation and not providing it all themselves.

When the supervisor goes directly from the observation to evaluation it should be done rationally, however. Clinicians who are at the Evaluation-Feedback Stage and are unable to participate in joint- or self-analysis, can be assumed to need some direction which must come through evaluation and direct feedback. If certain behaviors have been identified as needing specific attention and it has been agreed that the supervisor will provide a rating of these occurrences of the behavior, this type of feedback is essential. Sometimes the use of direct evaluation is a more efficient procedure and certain features of the situation make it reasonable to employ direct evaluation: the seriousness of the impact of the behavior on the client may demand immediate evaluative feedback; the behavior may be too trivial or too obvious to justify any lengthy analysis procedure; the behavior may be one that is being dealt with on an ongoing basis and the clinician may need only a reminder; or the significance of the issue may be too complex for the clinician at the moment either intellectually or emotionally. Supervisors must use their best judgement here as to when to provide direct evaluation as related to teaching or when to involve the supervisee in self-analysis or self-evaluation. The important point of the decision should be, "What will the supervisee learn and how will she or he learn it best?"

The topic of feedback will be dealt with in greater depth in the next chapter on Integrating. The broader topic of formal, organizationally based evaluation is another issue. It will be included in Chapter 8. Formative evaluations should be scheduled periodically during a practicum and should include data collected and analyzed to substantiate ratings. Educational programs often conduct midterm and end of term evaluations using a single instrument designed to assess a supervisee's skills in evaluation, treatment and overall therapeutic management (e.g., Zylla-Jones, 2006).

SUMMARY

The analysis component of the supervisory process, like the observation component, is a point where the scientific approach is essential. It is a time when the supervisor and supervisee use the recorded data to hypothesize about what has happened and to plan subsequent events. Analysis is not synonymous with evaluation, but it is a necessary step that leads to objective, disciplined judgements by the supervisor and to independence through self-analysis and self-evaluation by the supervisee.

REFERENCES

Acheson, K., & Gall, M. (1980). *Techniques in the clinical supervision of teachers.* New York, NY: Longman, Inc.

American Speech-Language-Hearing Association. (1985). *Clinical supervision in speech-language pathology and audiology* [Position statement]. Retrieved from https://www.asha.org/policy/PS1985-00220/

American Speech-Language-Hearing Association. (2008). *Knowledge and skills needed by speech-language pathologists providing clinical supervision* [Knowledge and Skills]. Retrieved from https://www.asha.org/policy/KS2008-00294/

American Speech-Language-Hearing Association. (2016). *Code of ethics* [Ethics]. Retrieved from www.asha.org/policy/

Andersen, C. F. (1981). *The effect of supervisor bias on the evaluation of student clinicians in speech/language pathology and audiology* (Doctoral Dissertation). Retrieved from ProQuest Dissertations & Theses Global. (Accession No. 8112499) http://proxyiub.uits.iu.edu/login?url=https://search.proquest.com/docview/303153045?accountid=11620

Anderson, J. (1988). *The supervisory process in speech-language pathology and audiology.* Boston, MA: College-Hill.

Boone, D., & Prescott, T. (1972). Content and sequence analysis of speech and hearing therapy. *Asha, 14,* 58-62.

Boone, D., & Stech, E. (1970). *The development of clinical skills in speech pathology by audiotape and videotape self-confrontation* [Final report]. (Project No. 1381—Grant No. OEG-9-071318-2814). Washington, DC: U.S. Department of Health, Education, and Welfare.

Brasseur, J., & Jimenez, B. (1994). Supervisee self-analysis and changes in clinical behavior. In M. Bruce (Ed.), *Proceedings of the 1994 International & Interdisciplinary Conference on Clinical Supervision: Toward the 21st century* (pp. 111-125). Council of Supervisors in Speech-Language Pathology and Audiology, Cape Cod, MA.

Brasseur, J., & Jimenez, B. (1996). Novice supervisees' attitude changes after active participation in the supervisory process. In B. Wagner (Ed.), *Proceedings of the 1996 Conference on Clinical Supervision—Partnerships in supervision: Innovative and effective practices* (pp. 80-89). Council of Supervisors in Speech-Language Pathology and Audiology, Cincinnati, OH.

Brookshire, R. (1967). Speech pathology and the experimental analysis of behavior. *Journal of Speech and Hearing Disorders, 32,* 215-227.

Camarata, M. (1992). Facilitating self-analysis of videotaped treatment: A generalization effect. In S. Dowling (Ed.), *Proceedings of the 1992 National Conference on Supervision—Total quality supervision: Effecting optimal performance* (pp. 46-52). Council of Supervisors in Speech-Language Pathology and Audiology, Nashville, TN.

Camarata, M., & Rassi, J. (1991). *Facilitating self-analysis of videotaped treatment: Supervision efficacy factors.* Paper presented at the annual convention of the American Speech-Language-Hearing Association, Atlanta, GA.

Cogan, M. (1973). Clinical supervision. Boston, MA: Houghton Mifflin Co.

Council for Clinical Certification in Audiology and Speech-Language Pathology of the American Speech-Language-Hearing Association (2014). *2014 standards for the certificate of clinical competence in speech-language pathology.* Rev 2016. Retrieved from http://www.asha.org/Certification/2014-Apeech-Language-Pathology-Certification-Standards/

Council on Academic Accreditation in Audiology and Speech-Language Pathology (2017). *Standards for accreditation of graduate education programs in audiology and speech-language pathology.* Retrieved from http://caa.asha.org/reporting/standards/2017-standards/

Culatta, R., & Seltzer, H. (1976). Content and sequence analysis of the supervisory session. *Asha, 18,* 8-12.

Culatta, R., & Seltzer, H. (1977). Content and sequence analysis of the supervisory session: A report of clinical use. *Asha, 19,* 523-526.

Dowling, S. (2001). *Supervision: Strategies for successful outcomes and productivity.* Boston, MA: Allyn & Bacon.

Dowling, S., Sbaschnig, K., & Williams, C. (1991). *Supervisory training, objective setting and grade contingent performance.* Paper presented at the annual convention of the American Speech-Language-Hearing Association, Atlanta, GA.

Dwight, D. (2014). *Here's how to do therapy: Hands on core skills in speech-language pathology* (2nd ed.). San Diego, CA: Plural.

Francis, B. (1993). *Effects of speech-language pathology students' interaction analyses on clinical behaviors.* Unpublished master's thesis, California State University, Chico, Chico, CA.

Freeman, G. (1982). Consultation. In R. Van Hattum, *Speech-language programming in the schools.* Springfield, IL: Charles C. Thomas.

Gillam, R., Strike-Roussos, C., & Anderson, J. (1990). Facilitating changes in supervisees' clinical behaviors: An experimental investigation of supervisory effectiveness. *Journal of Speech and Hearing Disorders, 55,* 729-739.

Goldberg, S. (1997). *Clinical skills for speech-language pathologists.* Clifton Park, NJ: Cengage.

Goldhammer, R. (1969). *Clinical supervision.* New York, NY: Holt, Rinehart and Winston.

Goldhammer, R., Anderson, R., & Krajewski, R. (1980). *Clinical supervision* (2nd ed.). New York, NY: Holt, Rinehart and Winston.

Hegde, M. N., & Davis, D. (2010). *Clinical methods and practicum in speech-language pathology* (5th ed.). Clifton Park, NJ: Cengage.

IDEA Partnership. (n.d.) *Functional Behavior Assessment.* Retrieved from http://www.ideapartnership.org/documents/ASD-Collection/asd-dg_Brief_FBA.pdf

Ingram, K., Bunta, F., & Ingram, D. (2004). Digital data collection and analysis: Application for clinical practice. *Language, Speech and Hearing Services in Schools, 35,* 112-121. doi:10.1044/0161-1461

Lougeay-Mottiger, J., Harris, M., & Stillman, R. (1987). Use of a videotaped coding system to change clinician behavior. In S. Farmer (Ed.), *Proceedings of A National Conference on Supervision—Clinical supervision: A coming of age* (pp. 86-91). Council of University Supervisors of Practicum in Speech-Language Pathology and Audiology, Jekyll Island, GA.

Lubinsky, J., & Hildebrand, S. (1996). Journal keeping to help students attain personal goals in practicum. In B. Wagner (Ed.), *Proceedings of the 1996 Conference on Clinical Supervision—Partnerships in supervision: Innovative and Effective practices* (pp. 235-242). Council of Supervisors in Speech-Language Pathology and Audiology, Cincinnati, OH.

Maloney, D. (1994). Client-centered student journaling: A way of reflecting on clinical learning. In M. Bruce (Ed.), *Proceedings of the 1994 International & Interdisciplinary Conference on Clinical Supervision: Toward the 21st century* (pp. 191-195). Council of Supervisors in Speech-Language Pathology and Audiology, Cape Cod, MA.

Mawdsley, B. (1985). *Kansas inventory of self-supervision.* Paper presented at the annual convention of the American Speech-Language-Hearing Association, Washington, DC.

Mowrer, D. (1969). Evaluating speech therapy through precision recording. *Journal of Speech and Hearing Disorders, 34,* 239-245.

Olswang, L. (1990). Treatment efficacy research, a path to quality assurance. *Asha, 32*(1), 45-47.

Olswang, L., & Bain, B. (1994). Data collection: Monitoring children's treatment progress. *American Journal of Speech-Language Pathology, 3*(3), 55-66. doi:10.1044/1058-0360.0303.55

Orlikoff, R., Schiavetti, N., & Metz, D. (2015). *Evaluating research in communication disorders* (7th ed.). Upper Saddle River, NJ: Pearson.

Peaper, R., & Mercaitis, P. (1987). The nature of narrative written feedback provided to student clinicians: A descriptive study. In S. Farmer (Ed.), *Proceedings of A National Conference on Supervision—Clinical supervision: A coming of age.* Council of University Supervisors of Practicum in Speech-Language Pathology and Audiology, Jekyll Island, GA.

Roberts, J., & Smith, K. (1982). Supervisor-supervisee role differences and consistency of behavior in supervisory conferences. *Journal of Speech and Hearing Research, 25,* 428-434.

Roth, F., & Worthington, C. (2016). *Treatment resource manual for speech-language pathology* (5th ed.). Clifton Park, NJ: Cengage.

Schubert, G., & Gudmundson, P. (1976, November). *Effects of videotape feedback and interaction upon nonverbal behavior of student clinicians.* Paper presented at the annual convention of the American Speech-Language-Hearing Association, Houston, TX.

Schubert, G., & Laird, B. (1975). The length of time necessary to obtain a representative sample of clinician-client interaction. *Journal of National Student Speech and Hearing Association,* 26-32.

Schubert, G., Miner, A., & Till, J. (1973). *The analysis of behavior of clinicians (ABC) system.* Unpublished manuscript, University of North Dakota, Grand Forks, ND.

Schubert, G., & Nelson, J. (1976). *Verbal behaviors occurring in speech pathology supervisory conferences.* Paper presented at the annual convention of the American Speech-Language-Hearing Association, Houston, TX.

Shapiro, D., & Anderson, J. (1988). An analysis of commitments made by student clinicians in speech-language pathology and audiology. *Journal of Speech and Hearing Disorders, 53,* 202-210.

Shapiro, D., & Anderson, J. (1989). One measure of supervisory effectiveness in speech-language pathology and audiology. *Journal of Speech and Hearing Disorders, 54,* 549-557.

Silverman, F. (1998). *Research design in speech pathology and audiology.* Boston, MA: Allyn & Bacon.

Smith, K., & Anderson, J. (1982). Relationship of perceived effectiveness to content in supervisory conferences in speech-language pathology. *Journal of Speech and Hearing Research, 25,* 243-251.

Tufts, L. (1983). *A content analysis of supervisory conferences in communicative disorders and the relationship of the content analysis system to the clinical experience of supervisees* (Doctoral dissertation). Retrieved from ProQuest Dissertations and Theses Global. (Accession No. 8401588) http://proxyiub.uits.iu.edu/login?url=https://search.proquest.com/docview/303266850?accountid=11620

Ventry, I. M., & Schiavetti, N. (1980). *Evaluating research in speech pathology and audiology.* Reading, MA: Addison-Wesley.

Walz Garrett, J. (2013). Technology to support data collection and management in the public schools. *SIG 16 Perspectives on School-Based Issues, 14*(1), 10-14. doi:10.1044/sbi 14.1.10

Zylla-Jones, E. (2006). Using mid-semester student self-evaluations to improve clinical performance. *SIG 11 Perspectives on Administration and Supervision, 16*(2), 8-12. doi:10.1044/aas16.2.8

 This chapter is a revision of that appearing in the 2003 edition of this book.

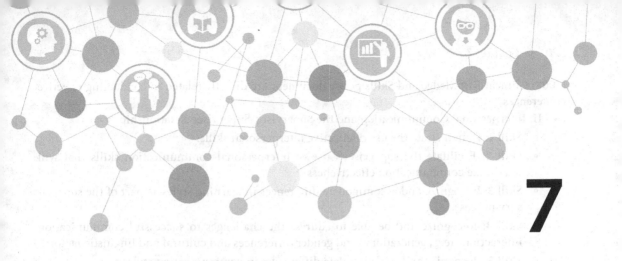

Integrating the Components

Judith A. Brasseur, PhD, CCC-SLP, F-ASHA and
Elizabeth S. McCrea, PhD, CCC-SLP, F-ASHA

At some point, everything that happens in the supervisory process—the preparation, the observation, the analysis—must be integrated through some form of communication between supervisor and supervisee. This typically occurs during a conference. Communication about the tasks and associated competencies for effective supervision (American Speech-Language-Hearing Association [ASHA], 1985) and the knowledge and skills needed to supervise (ASHA, 2008) usually occurs during the conference as well. Traditionally, the conference was viewed as a time when the supervisor provided feedback to the supervisee about the observation. This feedback was perceived to be something of a one-way street—from supervisor to supervisee. This is characteristic of the Direct-Active Style. For the Collaborative or Consultative Styles, Anderson (1988) stated that the broader term of *integrating* seems more appropriate than feedback in describing the interaction that takes place when supervisor and supervisee meet. Although feedback will be one aspect of the integration component, it is here where the components of understanding, planning, observing, and analyzing will merge. Since those components have been discussed previously, the content of this chapter will be related to the communication that takes place about them and their results and will suggest a richer synthesis of ideas than the old concept of supervisor-to-supervisee feedback. The integration component includes other activities such as planning, problem solving, analyzing, and many other topics necessary to maintain a productive relationship. The conference itself will not only include feedback about the clinical session but also discussion of procedural topics such as administrative issues or report writing, the supervisory process, professional issues, personal concerns, and general information relevant to the development of all participants. Task 8 (interacting with the supervisee in planning, executing, and analyzing supervisory conferences) and its nine competencies (ASHA, 1985) are focused on the conference. Core Area II and VI in ASHA's

McCrea, E. S., & Brasseur, J. A. *The Clinical Education and Supervisory Process in Speech-Language Pathology and Audiology* (pp 219-258). © 2020 Taylor & Francis Group.

(2008) Clinical Knowledge and Skills policy document are directly related to conducting effective conferences.

- II. Interpersonal Communication and the Supervisor-Supervisee Relationship
  - ○ Skill 1: Demonstrate the use of effective interpersonal skills.
  - ○ Skill 2: Facilitate the supervisee's use of interpersonal communication skills that will maximize communication effectiveness.
  - ○ Skill 3: Recognize and accommodate differences in learning styles as part of the supervisory process.
  - ○ Skill 4: Recognize and be able to address the challenges to successful communication interactions (e.g., generational and gender differences and cultural and linguistic factors).
  - ○ Skill 5: Recognize and accommodate differences in communication styles.
  - ○ Skill 6: Demonstrate behaviors that facilitate effective listening (e.g., silent listening, questioning, paraphrasing, empathizing, and supporting).
  - ○ Skill 7: Maintain a professional and supportive relationship that allows for both supervisee and supervisor growth.
  - ○ Skill 10: Use appropriate conflict resolution strategies.
- VI: Supervisory Conferences or Meetings of Clinical Teaching Teams
  - ○ Skill 1: Regularly schedule supervisory conferences and team meetings.
  - ○ Skill 2: Facilitate planning of supervisory conference agendas in collaboration with the supervisee.
  - ○ Skill 3: Select items for the conference based on saliency, accessibility of patterns for treatment, and the use of data that are appropriate for measuring the accomplishment of clinical and supervisory objectives.
  - ○ Skill 4: Use active listening as well as verbal and nonverbal response behaviors that facilitate the supervisee's active participation in the conference.
  - ○ Skill 5: Ability to use the type of questions that stimulate thinking and promote problem solving by the supervisee.
  - ○ Skill 6: Provide feedback that is descriptive and objective rather than evaluative.
  - ○ Skill 7: Use data collection to analyze the extent to which the content and dynamics of the conference are facilitating goal achievement, desired outcomes, and planned changes.

In examining other Core Areas and concomitant knowledge and skills (ASHA, 2008), it becomes apparent that many of the skills are an integral part of the self-exploring, critical thinking and problem solving necessary for growth. Consider, for example:

- III. Developing Critical Thinking and Problem-Solving Skills
  - ○ Skill 2: Assist the supervisee in objectively analyzing and interpreting the data obtained and in understanding how to use it for modification of intervention plans.
- IV. Developing Competence in Assessment
  - ○ Skill 1: Facilitate the supervisee's use of best practices in assessment, including the application of current research to the assessment process.
  - ○ Skill 4: Assist the supervisee in providing rationales for the selected procedures.
- V. Developing Competence in Intervention
  - ○ Skill 2: Facilitate the supervisee's consideration of evidence in selecting materials, procedures, and techniques, and in providing a rationale for their use.
  - ○ Skill 3: Assist the supervisee in selecting and using a variety of clinical materials and techniques appropriate to the clients served, and in providing a rationale for their use.

    ◦   Skill 5: Assist the supervisee in analyzing the data collected in order to reformulate goals, treatment plans, procedures, and techniques.

• VII. Evaluating the Growth of the Supervisee Both as a Clinician and as a Professional

    ◦   Knowledge 2: Understand the evaluation process as a *collaborative activity* [emphasis added] and facilitate the involvement of the supervisee in this process.

    ◦   Skill 2: Identify and develop and appropriately use evaluation tools that measure the clinical and professional growth of the supervisee.

    ◦   Skill 3: Analyze data collected prior to formulating conclusions and evaluating the supervisee's clinical skills.

SCHEDULED CONFERENCES

Core Area VI, Skill 1, focuses on regularly scheduling conferences. For some time, conferences have been the most commonly used structure for communicating feedback in professions where there is applied training—education, social work, counseling psychotherapy, health care and certainly speech-language pathology. Regularity is a critical factor. Geoffrey (1973) reported that 96% of the 111 facilities responding to her survey conducted regularly scheduled conferences. Of the 501 supervisors studied by Schubert and Aitchison (1975), 98% reported the use of post-therapy conferences. The importance of regular conferences continues to be emphasized (Brasseur, 1989; Christodoulou, 2016; Dowling, 2001; Mandel, 2015; McCrea, 1994; Mormer & Messick, 2016; O'Sullivan, Peaper-Fillyaw, Plante, & Gottwald, 2014; Strike, 1988) and is a basic expectation of supervisees (Dowling & Wittkopp, 1982; Larson, 1981; Tihen, 1983). Dowling (2001) emphasized the "catch me when you can" method is ineffective—it "will negatively affect the establishment of trust, the quality of the interpersonal relationship, and the effectiveness of the conference" (p. 128). Dowling suggested that weekly conferences be scheduled for students in training. Clinical fellows and professional staff may not need, nor may they want weekly conferences, but there needs to some regularity and a definite schedule (e.g., monthly) if the conferences are to be productive and facilitate professional growth.

COMMUNICATION IN THE CONFERENCE

The implementation of the continuum of supervision is dependent upon the communication skills of both supervisor and supervisee. The ability to be clear, specific, and concrete is essential to sharing feedback, perceptions, expectations, planning, discussion of data, and to determining the effectiveness of the supervisory interaction. Further, the supervisor's ability to encourage supervisee participation in self-exploration, critical thinking and problem solving during the conference is essential to movement along the continuum. Supervisors need to monitor their talk time to prevent dominating the conference. At times supervisees will need to plan some of their verbal behavior to achieve clear, concise discourse.

Clarity in Communication

Nothing is more powerful and frequently distressing to speakers than to see their verbal behaviors written in script. Even some of the most proficient language users are horrified by their excessive and irrelevant fillers (e.g., "OK," "you know," "um," "er," and "uh"), redundancies, fragmented sentences, and incorrect syntax or grammar. Consider the following excerpt from a supervisee in an actual conference:

Um, I think that—I guess that some or a lot of—well, you know—I think a lot of the words we've worked on—not, you know—I think it's near the, it's the same type of sound that we've been working on—you know—the voiceless—well, it's not a stop plosive, you know—um the other sounds we um—you know—worked on were stop plosives but the poorer articulation was—you know—would be /s/—you know—pretty much the same, I think....

This was in response to a supervisor question asking where they needed to go with the client. This type of utterance may be the result of several conditions—the supervisee's natural lack of facility with the language, anxiety, lack of preparation, poorly stated objectives, and other reasons.

Supervisors are not immune to such cluttered and imprecise verbalizations, as any number of conference transcripts reveal. Individually, they produce confusion and sometimes frustration for the listener. Multiplied for an entire conference or a whole semester, they are inefficient, time wasting, and nonproductive.

Listening to an audio recording or viewing a video recording of a conference early on in the supervisory relationship will likely reveal many types of behaviors that are obvious targets for objectives for supervisors and supervisees. The basis of such scattered, unclear communication may be in the planning and analysis components. If the agenda is planned carefully and the plan followed (Core Areas VI.2 and VI.3), there may be less rambling. If that planning is combined with skill in analysis, the data can be presented clearly and concisely.

One role of supervisors is to improve the communication behavior of their supervisees and themselves. Not only can improvement in verbal and nonverbal skills increase the efficiency and effectiveness of the conference, it should carry over to the clinical process. The supervisee who cannot clarify issues in the conference probably cannot give clear, precise directions to clients either, and may fill clinical sessions with unnecessary verbiage.

Strategies for this task must be carefully planned. Supervisees may perceive their verbal style as a personal characteristic that no one has a right to change. That may be true with regard to an individual's private life; when it becomes an issue in terms of professional interactions, it is another story. Anderson (1988) reported on a student in a supervision practicum who demonstrated a voice and manner of speaking that was coy, passive, flirtatious, and that conveyed an attitude of dependence and immaturity. In actuality, the student was a highly intelligent, mature, and capable professional. The behaviors were easily identified by Anderson and the student and objectives were set for modifying them. The student was highly motivated and made significant changes. In her final conference, she shared, "My friends tell me I don't sound like a little girl anymore."

Some of the techniques for collecting and analyzing data in the clinical process are applicable to the supervisory process. For example, one method for decreasing the verbosity of supervisor or supervisee is to complete verbatim transcripts of a portion of a conference recording. The individual who is redundant ad nauseum can then rewrite the transcribed text in a clear, concise style. This individual soon becomes conscious of the behavior in subsequent conversations and better able to change it.

From the counseling literature (Carkhuff & Truax, 1964), four facilitative dimensions in interpersonal interactions have been identified. McCrea (1980) adapted them for use in analyzing supervisors' behavior in speech-language pathology and audiology (Appendix 8-4). One of these dimensions is concreteness, and it is relevant to the issue of clarity discussed here. Concreteness means being specific, and the scale used for its measurement ranges from the lowest level (i.e, Level 1—supervisor statement which is extremely vague, causes confusion and greatly detracts from the flow of the discussion) to the highest l (e.g., Level 7—supervisor statements must be specific with an example and a rationale). Roberts and Smith (1982) indicated that supervisors do not give rationales and justification for their statements, and McCrea (1980) found that concreteness in supervisor behavior in the conferences she studied occurred below the minimally facilitative level of functioning needed for self-exploration. Because examples and rationales clarify topics being discussed, the findings of these studies suggest that supervisors need to examine their own conferences. Further, supervisors are expected to model professional conduct (Core Area XI) and what better way to induct supervisees into evidence-based practice than to provide rationales that are grounded in research.

SKILLS FOR FACILITATING
COMMUNICATION IN THE CONFERENCE

A multitude of books on counseling, the helping relationship, and interviewing contain descriptions of skills that facilitate communication (Brammer, 1985; Condon, 1977; Goldberg, 1997; Hackney & Nye, 1973; Knapp, 1972; Luterman, 1984; Molyneux & Lane, 1982; Shipley, 1997; Tannen, 1990, 1994). Such information may be familiar to many supervisors, having been part of their basic training as clinicians. Today, however, basic communication theory and methods for effective interpersonal communication may or may not be part of the curricular offerings in training programs. Thus, it may be necessary to provide some didactic training for supervisees or to upgrade skills through reading, self-study and continuing education.

Listening Skills

Core Areas II.6 and VI.4 focus on the skill of active and effective listening (ASHA, 2008). Effective listening is essential in counseling, therapy, and in conversations with friends. Kagan (1970) noted that people, in general, are not particularly good listeners. "We really don't listen to each other. I tell you about how much I hurt and you're just waiting for me to finish so you can tell me how much you hurt" (p. 95). Pickering and McCready (1990) stated that the skill of listening is related to intent—deciding if you really want to hear what someone has to say—if that person is valuable enough to listen to.

The literature on expectations reveals that supervisees want to be listened to, to have supervisors pay attention to them, and to take them seriously. In addition, if supervisors want supervisees to be active in conferences, they must not only listen but also must offer encouragers to talk. Encouragers are signals to continue talking and include behaviors such as saying, "fine," "I see," "good," "yes," "mmm," or "uh huh" (Shipley, 1997). Verbally and nonverbally attending to and acknowledging the supervisee and restating or paraphrasing the speaker's basis message are important basic skills (Pickering & McCready, 1990). Eye contact, positive head nods, appropriate facial expression, forward body leans, and at times touching are ways to convey that you are listening and function as minimal prompts to a speaker to continue. One of the categories in Blumberg's (1974, 1980) interaction analysis system is "accepts or uses teacher's ideas," and is defined as statements that clarify, build on, or develop ideas or suggestions by teachers. This is an activity extremely important to both the Collaborative and Consultative Styles. It should be apparent that listening is more than just hearing what the supervisee has said. It is responding to the input, rephrasing it to test understanding, clarifying it, restating it to better interpret intent, focusing the discussion, and checking the accuracy of listener perceptions. The flip side of active listening is apparent in a "yes, but..." response. It's difficult to think of anything that squelches communication quicker than a "yes, but..."

Barbara (1958) maintained that there are at least four essential factors in effective listening: concentration, active participation, comprehension, and objectivity. Concentration requires mental alertness and clearing the environment of distractions. Active participation requires openness, flexibility, and the use of some of the attending behaviors listed in the previous paragraph. Comprehension necessitates attending to the content, intent, and feelings being conveyed in a message. Objectivity requires that listeners not allow their personal feelings or attitudes to interfere with the message or their regard for the speaker.

Listening is not a one-way street in which supervisors must assume all responsibility. Supervisors can help supervisees become aware of their own listening patterns. A brief look at a video recording of a conference will reveal quickly what is happening between participants. If the supervisee is not using good listening skills in the conference, she or he may not be using them in the clinical session either. Establishing active listening skills as a supervisory objective and working on it as part of the supervisory process should facilitate generalization to the clinical process.

Rogers (1980), in a retrospective discussion of the development of his theories about dealing with people, related that in his early years as a therapist he discovered that simply listening to clients was important in being helpful. "So, when I was in doubt as to what I should do in some active way, I listened. It seemed surprising to me that such a passive kind of interaction could be so useful" (p. 137).

Questioning Skills

The ability to ask questions may be the most important skill in the supervisor's repertoire—questions that generate thinking by the supervisee, questions that do not already contain the answer desired by the supervisor, questions that have a purpose and are carefully thought out before they are uttered. In fact, it is possible that the type of questions asked by supervisors may, in many instances, be the determining factor in whether or not supervisees move along the continuum. Their impact may be either positive or negative.

Carin and Sund (1971), Cunningham (1971), and Davies (1981) suggested that learning in the classroom is determined largely through questioning techniques. Carin and Sund amplified this further when they said:

> Involved in any deep communication between persons is the ability to ask appropriate questions and to listen. This is the genius of communication. To listen and question at just the right place and degree delineates the truly brilliant instructor from the average. An insightful question appropriately delivered may stimulate the individual to reach a new level of mental mediation. We learn to think only by thinking. We become creative only by having opportunities to be creative. A properly phrased question often is the necessary "input" needed to ignite student's thinking and creative process (p. 2).

The use of questions in the classroom has received extensive coverage in education literature. Questioning is the most frequently used utterance of teachers, but questions are least commonly used to stimulate thinking. Rather, teachers use questions in giving directions, managing the classroom, initiating activities, and in other learning situations. Critical thinking, however, seems not to be stimulated by teachers through questioning (Cunningham, 1971). Is this true of supervisors?

Questioning has many purposes—to obtain feedback or responses, to get data, to encourage thinking, to promote problem solving, to evaluate the student's preparation or participation in planned activities, to determine strengths and weaknesses, to review or summarize, to help the student recall, understand, synthesize, or apply, and to focus (Carin & Sund, 1971; Cunningham, 1971; Davies, 1981; Whiteside, 1981). Pederson and Ivey (1993) maintain that "questions have a great deal to do with power" (p. 131). Questions can provide a means to control a conversation.

There is an assumption that high levels of questioning behavior raises the cognitive level of students, forcing them to reflect, refocus, clarify, expand, and be more creative in their thinking, although the research is somewhat contradictory. Nevertheless, many systems for classifying and studying questions have been proposed and they are worthy of attention in the self-study of verbal behaviors in the conference. Sanders (1966) used seven categories: memory, translation, interpretation, application, analysis, synthesis, and evaluation. Lowery (1970) suggested three categories: broad, narrow, and miscellaneous; with broad questions subcategorized into open-ended and valuing, narrow into direct information and focusing. Probably the most useful category system for questioning is presented by Cunningham (1971), who divided questions into narrow and broad categories, which he then broke down further. The narrow category includes cognitive memory questions (recall, identify and observe, yes or no, define, name, designate) and convergent questions (explain, state relationships, compare and contrast). The broad category includes divergent questions (predict, hypothesize, infer, reconstruct) and evaluative questions (judge, value, defend, justified choice). It is easy to see the increasing complexity of these classifications of questions. Recognition of the importance of these levels of questioning in encouraging thinking and problem solving by supervisees is an important part of any supervisor's approach to supervision.

Questioning in Speech-Language Pathology and Audiology

Interest in questioning by speech-language pathologists increased with the profession's involvement with the language-disordered child and the emphasis on the study of children's questions and answers (Ervin-Tripp, 1970; James & Seebach, 1982; Leach, 1972; Tyack & Ingram, 1977). Interest in discourse analysis focused attention on questions in relation to language development (Gallagher & Prutting, 1983). Although questioning has always been a tool of the clinician and, thus, a concern of supervisors, there was no indication of it having been a major topic of study as related to clinician behavior until recently. ASHA's (2008) Clinical Supervision Knowledge and Skills policy document stipulates that supervisors must be able "to use the type of questions that stimulate thinking and promote problem solving by the supervisee."

One structured method of clinical teaching, developed in athletic training, that has gained recent popularity in speech-language pathology and audiology is the supervision, questioning, and feedback (SQF) approach (Barnum, Guyer, Levy, & Graham, 2009). Described in the ASHA Practice Portal for Clinical Education and Supervision, in a workshop of the Council on Academic Programs in Communication Sciences and Disorders (Barnum & Guyer, 2015) and an ASHA convention preconference (Mormer & Messick, 2016), "strategic questioning" is used to stimulate thinking and promote clinical reasoning and problem solving. Strategic questioning, based on Bloom's revised taxonomy (Anderson & Krathwohl, 2001), involves planning the timing, sequencing, and linguistic content of questions to assist supervisees' abilities to process information at increasing levels of complexity. Six categories include: remember, understand, apply, analyze, evaluate and create; these tap different levels of cognition ranging from recall to deep critical thinking. A similar questioning method is evident in the implementation of Socratic questioning. Mormer and Messick (2016) adapted Oermann's (1997) Socratic approach in nursing education to assist clinical educators in formulating: clarification questions, questions to probe assumptions, questions to probe reasons, questions on differing perspectives, and questions on consequences. Research demonstrates that teachers overwhelmingly use low-level questions that do not stimulate critical thinking (Tofade, Elsner, & Haines, 2013), thus, highlighting the need to train supervisors to formulate effective questions and avoid using questions that create confusion, intimidate students and stifle higher level cognitive thinking.

Questioning in the Supervisory Conference

Questioning in the supervisory conference was an important issue to Blumberg and Cusick (1970) in the development of their interaction analysis system for studying the supervisory process, as evident by their inclusion for both participants of items related to requesting information, opinions, and suggestions. Their analysis of conferences revealed certain information related to questioning—supervisors did less asking for ideas and suggestions than telling, and less asking of opinions than giving of opinions. In fact, asking for suggestions was the least-used supervisory behavior, and supervisees never asked "Why?" when given advice. Thus, they said, teachers are not involved in problem solving about conditions they face in their classrooms. The interaction is not collaborative. Additionally, teachers reacted most negatively to supervisors asking for information, assuming that they were being "trapped." Blumberg and Cusick did not analyze the type of questions being asked but, if they had, they might have found a clue to the hostility engendered by such question asking.

Blumberg and Cusick (1970) also reported that conferences rated high direct-high indirect and those rated low direct-high indirect were perceived as more productive than the high direct-low indirect and the low direct-low indirect. Recall from Chapter 2 that high direct-high indirect includes telling, suggesting, giving information, criticizing, as well as reflecting and asking for information and suggestions. The low direct-high indirect contains less telling and more reflecting and asking. It is not known, of course, from Blumberg and Cusick's data if the conferences were more effective, only that teachers perceived them in that way. Thus, although there was a preference in terms of productivity or effectiveness for both kinds of behavior, there was a stronger emphasis on the asking and reflecting behaviors.

Smith and Anderson (1982b) also found questioning behaviors of supervisors and supervisees to be related to the perceived effectiveness components (direct and indirect supervisory behaviors) of the conference. Smith (1979), in another study, provided an extensive description of questions used in 45 supervisory conferences in speech-language pathology and audiology. Questions were usually cognitive and dealt with objectives or methods and materials. They asked primarily for factual information such as "What did Mary do when you asked her...." and "What are John's objectives?" (p. 11). Thus, they would fall in Cunningham's (1971) narrow category, and probably in the cognitive-memory subcategories. Smith found that supervisors asked 81% of the questions. The only difference in type of questions was that supervisees asked more opinion questions than supervisors. It did appear that supervisors varied their types of questions on the basis of such supervisee variables as experience and grade point average. Smith concluded that supervisors are dominating the questioning process and, by asking for the type of factual information indicated in her study, they are depriving supervisees of a vital opportunity for problem solving. She reflected: "If, as clinical supervisors, we intend to relinquish power and authority and utilize the clinical supervision model while training supervisees to problem solve, self-analyze, and self-direct their own behavior, we must critically analyze and change, if necessary, our use of questions during conference interactions" (p. 9).

Sbaschnig, Dowling, and Williams (1992) analyzed 45 conferences for 15 supervisor-supervisee pairs from two universities and found that supervisors talked more than six times as much as supervisees. Further, they asked twice as many questions as did supervisees. The supervisors had a direct, unchanging style. These results are consistent with those of K. Smith (1979) and K. S. Smith (1979).

The way in which questions are posed will determine not only the answer but also the type of thought that must go into the answer. This is readily apparent, in examining Cunningham's (1971) classification. For example:

Narrow or Cognitive Memory Questions
- *Recall*: How many responses did you elicit with X activity?
- *Identify-Observe*: What kinds of disfluencies are apparent when he talks with his dad?
- *Yes/No*: Did the stickers work as a reinforcer?
- *Define*: What do you mean when you say he is hyperactive?
- *Name*: What is the term for a slushy /s/ and other sibilants that is characterized by airflow over the sides of the tongue?
- *Designate*: Who shared video recordings in the last conference?

Narrow and Convergent Questions
- *Explain*: What happened when you used toys instead of pictures to elicit your targets?
- *State relationships*: What is the impact of doing therapy with Mrs. Jones at 10:00 a.m. vs. 4:00 p.m.?
- *Compare and contrast*: Which of the three strategies resulted in the most correct responses?

Broad and Divergent Questions
- *Predict*: What would happen if…?
- *Hypothesize*: How could you determine if X is really causing the change in his behavior?
- *Infer*: Given these varied research findings, what techniques seem to be the most plausible for your aphasia group?
- *Reconstruct*: Given these facts about adult learning styles, what things might you have done differently with the parent support group last Tuesday?

Broad and Evaluative Questions
- *Judge*: What theories and research suggest that full inclusion is the best service delivery mode for these students?
- Which strategies will likely effect the greatest amount of generalization?
- *Value*: Why might you be inclined to do that?
- *Defend*: Why do you think that is so?
- *Justified choice*: Despite the fact that all of the treatment goals have not been achieved, why do you think he is ready to be dismissed from therapy?

Using Cunningham's (1971) classification, Strike (1988) trained supervisors to use broad questions and subsequently examined the cognitive level of supervisor questions and supervisee responses. Her results suggested that without specific education, supervisors tend to use predominantly narrow questions, and that the frequency of higher level questions increases in conjunction with education. "More interestingly, the effectiveness of the higher-level questions in facilitating higher level thinking by supervisees also improves after supervisors participate in an educational program focused on question asking" (p. 17).

Some questions have an effect opposite of that intended. Consider, for example, the clinician who utters to her 4-year-old client, "Can you say____?" That question probably evokes other familiar yes-or-no questions that have been observed in treatment sessions where clinicians are attempting to encourage a client to talk. One of the first lessons the inexperienced clinician may learn is to avoid such questions; yet, it is easy to do, even with experience, unless there is constant monitoring and planning of new behaviors. The same can be said of supervisor utterances. Asking "Do you think it would be better if he wrote it out?" is deceptive. It may appear to request an opinion, but to the supervisee, is a directive and requires an automatic "yes" answer.

In addition to yes-or-no questions, Cunningham (1971) listed several other problem questions. The ambiguous question does not include enough criteria to enable the respondent to define a good answer. Asking "What about the session?" may appear to be a broad question to the supervisor, but the supervisee may feel that he or she must play a guessing game to find out what the supervisor wants to hear.

Another type of problematic question is the "spoon-feeding" question, sometimes called the leading or rhetorical, where the answer is embedded in the question. This type of question ranges from simple to complex. From transcripts of recordings of conferences, the following stand out as spoon-feeding: "That's more appropriate, isn't it?" and "That was mostly nonverbal wasn't it?"

Confusing questions, according to Cunningham (1971), include too many factors for the answerer to consider at one time. Consider this example from a recording of a conference: "What would you say—how high a success rate? Have you noticed, like, if he is succeeding at 60% or 70% of the time, is he usually okay vs. 20% of the time if he's getting one out of five right? Does that make a big change in behavior for you, in your situation or not? Or have you been able to determine any of that? What do you think?" The obvious answer is, "I think this is a very confusing question," but most supervisees would not have the courage to answer that way. This supervisee responded, "What do you mean? In the group?"

Shipley (1997) cautioned the use of "why" questions "because they put many respondents on the defensive" (p. 59). He suggested "could" questions are a better alternative. For example, "Could you explain that a little?" as opposed to "Why do you think that is a good thing to try?" Whiteside (1981) reported on "tugging questions" such as "Well, come one, you know that" or "What did you do? Come on now, you can tell me about that. What did you do?" These are perhaps more commonly used by clinicians in attempts to get a response from an unresponsive client. Molyneux and Lane (1982) included in their categories of interview questions, a similar type, which they labeled "bombardment"—one that contains three or more questions of any type. This appears to be what Tofade et al. (2013) labeled "shotgun" questions—questions containing several content areas with no particular link, and "funnel" questions which are multiple questions starting broadly and gradually leading to more focused inquiry. They note that these types usually cause confusion.

The kinds of questions posed not only influence the kinds of responses evoked, but also the kinds of thinking the respondent must use to answer the question. Furthermore, they can impact the relationship. Trust, respect, and a psychologically safe environment are necessary for taking risks and thinking creatively. In addition to providing a psychologically safe environment, Tofade et al. (2013) offered these addition practical considerations:

- *Phrasing and clarity*: Avoid compound questions, limit the number of action verbs in a question to one, and mix question types depending on instructional objectives.
- *Sequencing and balance*: Order questions and ask both convergent and divergent questions at varying knowledge and cognitive levels. Balance also relates to the frequency of question asking relative to time spent providing information, examples and engaging students in learning activities. Too many questions may leave learners feeling interrogated or threatened.

The Answers

The importance of listening has been stressed. Acceptance of answers to questions and the responses to them are important in the future participation and problem solving. Responses to incorrect or inaccurate answers require diplomacy, involving response, redirecting, helping the respondent move closer to a better answer, not blocking communication by responding negatively (Carin & Sund, 1971). In supervisory conferences, there are often answers that are neither right nor wrong and appropriate responses will encourage further discussion.

Responses are important but, frequently, silence is just as important. Silence may mean resistance or simply mean that the responder is engaged in exploring the issue (Brammer, 1985). Wait time—the lapse of time between question and response—influences the quality and quantity of learner responses. Wait time has been a popular area for study in education. Carin and Sund (1971) reported on a study that found that a teacher's wait time was one second. When the wait time was extended, it resulted in longer student responses, less "I don't know" answers and more whole sentences, increased speculative thinking, more questions from children, revised teacher expectations of children, and a wider variety of questions asked by the teacher. Depending on the type of question, educators should wait at least 20 seconds and up to 1 to 2 minutes for a complex question that requires higher cognitive effort (Tofade et al., 2013). Further, they should factor in think time—an imposed a period of uninterrupted silence to enable all students to process a question and formulate a response (Tofade et al., 2013). Supervisors need to learn to tolerate silence. Some people need more time to get their thoughts together than others, and the wait may result in a better answer.

INTERPERSONAL ASPECTS OF THE CONFERENCE

It was stated earlier that the interpersonal aspects of the supervisory process would not be treated extensively in this book—that addressing that topic requires a book of its own. There are volumes of material on interpersonal communication, helping relationships, and the helper skills needed to facilitate change in the helpee. Readers are implored to make themselves familiar with some of this literature. Among the many sources from the counseling and communication literature are Anderson and Guerrero (1998), Brammer (1985), Danish and Kagan (1971), Deetz and Stevenson (1986), Duck (1997), Faiver, Eisengart, and Colonna (2000), Feltham (2000), George and Cristiani (1981), Luft (1969), and Young (2001). Regardless of the coverage, it must be clear to readers that the approach presented here is based on assumption of attitudes of respect, empathic understanding, facilitative genuineness, concreteness of expression, unconditionality of regard, congruence, and self-exploration-all the interpersonal qualities proposed by Rogers (1957, 1961), Carkhuff (1969a, 1969b), Carkhuff and Berenson (1967), and the many others who followed them.

Although Pickering (1986) stated that the profession of speech-language pathology has not been exemplary in "probing aspects of interpersonal communications in its helping, clinical relationship" (p. 16), it is encouraging that there has been some focus in recent years on the interpersonal communication aspects of the supervisory process. The research of Pickering (1979, 1984) and McCrea (1980) were discussed earlier. In addition, Pickering has continued to explore this area (1987a, 1987b), as have many others, including Caracciolo, Rigrodsky, and Morrison (1978a, 1978b), Crago (1987), Hagler, Casey, and DesRochers (1989), Klevans, Volz, and Freidman (1981), Volz (1975), Volz, Klevans, Norten, and Putens (1978), McCready et al. (1996), and McCready, Shapiro, and Kennedy (1987). Ghitter (1987) explored the relationship between the interpersonal skills of supervisors and the impact on supervisees' clinical effectiveness in 88 dyads. Her results affirmed what has been demonstrated in Caracciolo et al. (1978a) and other studies in helping professions—when supervisees perceive high levels of unconditional positive regard, genuineness, empathic understanding, and concreteness, their clinical behaviors change in positive directions. Perceptions of those core behaviors facilitates high levels of clinical effectiveness.

The supervisory relationship may be one of the most intense interpersonal experiences in which a person can engage. The emotional dimensions of this vital relationship may influence both participants in ways that have not even begun to be identified. Mosher and Purpel (1972), in discussing the personal development of prospective teachers during student teaching, asserted that not only does learning to teach require the student to change what she or he does, it also requires "that he change what he is" (p. 115). They stressed the need to assist the student in his or her process of changing from a person to a professional person and offered suggestions for supervisors to deal with this critical period in a student's life. In examining actual behaviors, not merely perceptions, Pickering (1984) and McCrea (1980) found only minimal evidence of facilitative interpersonal interaction between supervisor and supervisee in speech-language pathology. Is this the state of the art today? Hagler et al. (1989) found that providing supervisors with data about their facilitative behaviors from analyses of conferences, along with some suggestions for change was not sufficient to induce a change in supervisors' behaviors.

Decades ago, Ward and Webster (1965a, 1965b) expressed their concern about personal needs of students in their growth and development as clinicians. Pickering (1977) stressed the importance for supervisors to have an understanding of four concepts of human relationships—authenticity, dialogue, risk taking, and conflict. In a later report of her research, Pickering (1984) contended that neither students nor supervisors appear to know "how to analyze the interpersonal dimensions of therapeutic relationships" (p. 194).

Much of the counseling literature reflects the need of counselors to help counselees express themselves about their feelings, their concerns, and their anxieties. Although supervisors are not counselors and a line must be drawn between the two roles, supervisors will find times when they need to reflect the supervisees' words and focus on their feelings. There are situations when dealing with feelings is essential.

Despite the data that suggest that supervisors have traditionally focused on teaching and instruction to the neglect of attending to supervisees interpersonal needs, there are signs that the profession is turning its attention to this area of study. If it is as important as it seems to be, then every supervisor in her or his role as facilitator of the supervisory process should become familiar with the literature and assist supervisees in learning about it. More than that, however, they need to study their own interpersonal interaction to determine its possible impact upon the supervisory process.

PLANNING FOR THE CONFERENCE

The first three skills in Core Area VI of ASHA's 2008 Knowledge and Skill policy document substantiate the importance of planning. These skills include conducting regular conferences/team meetings for which agendas are collaboratively planned and based on clinical and supervisory objectives. Planning the interaction between supervisor and supervisee is a primary aspect of the clinical supervision model. Cogan (1973) and Goldhammer, Anderson, and Krajewski (1980) discussed strategies for planning the conference and emphasized the importance of planning for maximizing the teaching-learning process in supervision. This planning comes out of the analysis of the clinical and/or supervisory processes, when decisions are made about what to do with the collected data and priorities are set for conference discussion. Goldhammer and colleagues discussed such issues as doing a full or partial analysis of the data; the order in which such issues will be presented; dealing with strengths or weaknesses; the balance between the past (analysis of previous data), the future (planning), and the present (discussion of the supervisory process); how to record what is happening in the conference; reviewing the contract, if there is one, for possible modification; and how and when to end the conference. They suggested that although there may be appropriate times for an open conference, it is easy to "squander an open conference on superficialities or on peripheral or irrelevant issues" (p. 136). The link between analyzed data and planning the conference has also been discussed in the previous chapter.

Although most studies of conferences have centered on what has already happened, Peaper (1984) conducted one of the first studies that focused on planning for the conference. Graduate students were divided into two groups. One group planned agendas for their conferences after listing potential topics for discussion under three categories-client-centered, clinician-centered, and supervisor-centered issues. Students in the other group did not participate in such a listing. Students in Peaper's study valued the conference, as opposed to the subjects of Culatta, Colucci, and Wiggins (1975), who did not feel a need for regularly scheduled conferences. The group that preplanned agendas for their conferences felt that they set the tone of the conference—not a surprising fact, but an important consideration for the supervisor who wish to have supervisees feel more "ownership" for the experience.

Experimental studies by McFarlane and Hagler (1992a, 1992b) and Jans, Hagler, and McFarlane (1994) have demonstrated the positive effects of supervisee-prepared agendas. These investigations substantiated that students were more actively involved in conferences for which they prepared agendas. Students initiated more and were less reflexive in conferences they planned. Sbaschnig et al. (1992) examined conference outcomes when supervisors planned agendas, when they were jointly planned and when supervisees planned them. Their dependent measures were talk time and question usage and the results revealed that supervisors talked more and dominated the conferences regardless of who planned the agenda. However, how the agendas were used in conferences was unknown. McFarlane and Hagler (1992a) suggested that supervisees may not accept ownership even when they planned the agenda. The ownership issue may be related to supervisee experience and should be investigated. Specifically, as students gain experience in their dual roles as clinicians and supervisees, they may be better able to assume responsibility for agenda planning and to be more active in conferences. Establishing goals for the supervisory process, to decrease supervisor control and increase supervisee participation, and monitoring progress in goal attainment also should be examined more closely. Obviously, goals should be directed toward the supervisee's movement along the continuum.

The agenda will identify conference content but how feedback will be provided also needs to be planned. Such planning should include decision making about purpose, type, content, amount, timing, and rationale, as well as evaluation of the appropriateness of the feedback. Feedback should usually result from the analysis of data collected during the observation. Kurpius and colleagues are among the many experts who have clarified the purposes and established criteria for giving helpful feedback (Kurpius, 1976; Kurpius, Baker, & Thomas, 1977; Kurpius & Christie, 1978).

When given to another person, feedback has three primary purposes (Kurpius, 1976):

1. To identify discrepancies between what the recipient assumes and what actually exists that is, the difference between perceptions and reality
2. To support or reinforce desired behaviors
3. To modify behavior so content and actions are congruent with the intended message or outcome

A supervisor should delineate these purposes for supervisees, and should also state the criteria for giving feedback. Criteria include (Kurpius & Christie, 1978):

- Be descriptive rather than evaluative.
- Be specific in describing behaviors.
- Consider the appropriateness (i.e., based on recipient rather than self needs).
- Determine usefulness of feedback—to be useful, the recipient must be able to act on it).
- Assess who desires the feedback—solicited is the most helpful.
- Attempt to determine receiver readiness—feedback must be well timed (i.e., timely feedback is provided close to the time when the event occurred and to a recipient who is psychologically ready to receive it).
- Seek clarification—check to see if the recipient understood, encourage questions, ask the recipient to restate in his or her own words, and so on.
- Check the accuracy of feedback prior to giving it. It should be objective—for example, derived from data collected during observation, based on standards (ASHA, American Psychological Association) or clearly identified competencies.

Further, it is important to control the amount of information the user receives, since too much will be overwhelming.

A slightly different perspective about the purposes of feedback is offered by Stone and Heen (2014). They identified the following three types, each with an explicit purpose. Appreciation is intended to motivate and acknowledge the actions of the learner. For example, providing positive reinforcement of specific observable behaviors. Coaching is designed to improve target skills—providing corrective measures to improve or refine a technique or clinical behavior. Evaluative feedback provides assessment based on a set of standards.

The previous discussion should make it clear that feedback is not solely evaluative, or just the end product of the supervisory process, or exclusively provided by the supervisor. It is, instead, an exchange of ideas that occurs throughout the entire interaction, emanating in a variety of ways from all the participants in all directions. It may come during or immediately after an observation, or it may be delayed. It may be verbal or written. Optimally, it is based on data collected during the observation but at times it may consist of judgmental or evaluative statements. Whatever its form, it serves both as closure to preceding events and transition to further planning. The conference is the typical vehicle for this interchange (Cogan, 1973). Supervisors and supervisees will be both recipients and providers of feedback for each other, their peers, and themselves. Dowling (2001) emphasized the importance of reciprocity and stated that "reciprocity is achieved by encouraging the supervisee to question, ask for clarification, compare analyses of data, and to provide feedback to the supervisor regarding the helpfulness of the information" (p. 85).

Readers are reminded that the integration component includes but is not restricted only to feedback. Given that feedback has not been thoroughly addressed in the previous chapters, some expanded discussion seems prudent.

FEEDBACK

Many of the expectations of supervisees about supervision are related to feedback behaviors of both supervisors and supervisees. In fact, feedback may constitute a major portion of what many supervisees think of as "supervision."

Studies on expectations reviewed in Chapter 3 revealed a variety of views about what supervisees and supervisors want and need with regard to feedback. Supervisees frequently expressed a desire for direct feedback about their work—a critique. This issue must be clarified in operationalizing the continuum. Supervisees must learn the appropriate balance between direct feedback from the supervisor and self-analysis. Unless this is clarified, it may be a source of frustration and dissatisfaction for the supervisee in conferences. Anderson (1988) offered an anecdote to illustrate. In the early days of the doctoral program in supervision at Indiana University, a PhD student and an insightful, advanced clinician were paired in supervision practicum and had established an excellent collaborative relationship. The supervisor trainee was observed to be supportive, encouraged problem solving, and stimulated creative thinking. The clinician was self-analytical, creative in planning, self-evaluative, and participated productively in conferences. A supervisory dyad created in heaven! Yet, about two thirds of the way into the semester, as the two walked down the hall after a conference, the student said, "Well, when are you going to start criticizing me?" The implications in terms of expectations, unexplored and unmet, need not be belabored. The experience, Anderson said, provided a valuable lesson for her, the trainee, and the clinician. Expectations must be identified, discussed and ways to meet the ones deemed as important and appropriate must be incorporated into the planning.

Providing Feedback

Feedback may be provided in a variety of situations using many different methods. Although the scheduled conference seems to be the most frequently used setting for the exchange of feedback, there are other procedures. These include: written feedback, spontaneous verbal interaction, and feedback during sessions. These procedures are primarily one-way delivery of feedback—supervisor to supervisee—and, thus, are almost always direct evaluations or suggestions.

Written Feedback

Many supervisors use checklists, rating scales, evaluation forms, or messages written during the observation period which are given to the supervisee after the clinical session (Geoffrey, 1973); but the type of feedback provided and received about the supervisory process has received minimal attention in the literature. The conference rating scale developed by Smith (1977; Smith & Anderson, 1982a), modified by Brasseur (1980) and contained in Appendix 3-7 has been used to examine direct and indirect supervisory styles (Brasseur & Anderson, 1983; McFarlane & Hagler, 1992, 1992b; Smith & Anderson, 1982a, 1982b). Supervisors and supervisees may use this scale to obtain feedback about conferences and to compare perceptions.

Kennedy (1981) studied the effects of two types of preconference written feedback—subjective statements and verbatim transcripts of events—on verbal behaviors of supervisors in conferences. Both supervisor and supervisees showed differences in conference behaviors, depending on which form of feedback had been provided. Weller's (1971) Multidimensional Observational System for the Analysis of Interactions in Clinical Supervision (MOSAICS) was the dependent measure and the verbatim condition yielded more supervisor explanation, opinion, and talk about supervision than the subjective condition. Supervisees in the subjective condition used more justification of opinions than those in the verbatim condition. Despite some limitations, this study addressed an important issue: Does type of feedback make a difference?

Peaper and Mercaitis (1987) and Rocchio and Iacarino (1990) studied written feedback and found it to be highly evaluative. Jans et al. (1994) examined the effects of supervisors' written session comments on their verbal feedback during conferences. They compared supervisors who provided written feedback to those who withheld it and found no differences in verbal conference content between the two groups. Supervisors in both conditions tended to provide facts, explanations and suggestions rather than evaluations and opinions. Both supervisors and supervisees engaged in limited evaluative discussion. Jans and colleagues suggested that supervisor experience and the tools used to analyze feedback and verbalizations might account for differences in the evaluative behavior of supervisors. Education and training would also likely be a factor—that is, training supervisors to refrain from immediate evaluation and training supervisees to analyze their own behaviors. Noting that students receive conflicting feedback from one supervisor to the next over the course of their graduate programs, Cascia (2013) measured interrater agreement of assessment and feedback among 15 speech-language pathology supervisors using two methods. The first method was to watch three video sessions and "take notes as they would when observing therapy in the clinic" and in the second they observed the same 10-minute videos but were given a 14-item structured form that focused on core clinical behaviors to collect data and evaluate skill. The supervisors affirmed if a target behavior was observed and wrote descriptions or rationales for each item. Results revealed that supervisors had higher agreement when given guidelines and a structured way to collect observational feedback. Cascia concluded that the results suggest the need for training and consistency with regard to feedback and evaluation.

Herd, Epperly, and Cox (2011) compared handwritten feedback to electronic feedback using iPads, noting the current generation of students' need for instant gratification, and constant and immediate access to information on their mobile devices. Preferences and perceptions of nine first-year graduate students were assessed in this study. Students preferred the electronic mode of communication with regard to timeliness and clarity but handwritten because they received a greater quantity and quality of feedback and reported difficulty reading small print on their mobile devices. It would be interesting to replicate and examine the content of the feedback and the impact on supervisee self-analysis across supervisees at different levels of development/different stages on the continuum. Specifically, it is likely that the immediate feedback provided was evaluative and it would be interesting to know if and how feedback changed over the course of a term, with supervisees who have some experience and clinical skills and so on.

Lorio, Delehanty, and Woods (2016) combined a treatment protocol to improve fidelity as suggested by Cascia (2013), graphs to display performance/progress, and text messaging to provide feedback to five first-year graduate students enrolled in a summer community practicum. Three feedback conditions were compared: a) e-mails sent after treatment sessions, b) text messaging during sessions, and c) no e-mails or texts. All conditions were supplemented by a graph depicting progress on the fidelity checklist sent in an e-mail after the session. Students reported all forms of feedback as helpful but preferred specific, immediate feedback. The fidelity checklist supported students' ability to implement specific therapy techniques and supervisors' ability to provide detailed feedback.

The content of the written message is of great importance in encouraging the collaborative approach to supervision. If the written message delivered to the supervisee after the observation is observational data collected by the supervisor, it should be useful to the supervisees in the analysis that precedes the conference. Certain types of questions from the supervisor may also enhance self-analysis by the supervisee. If the written feedback is a direct evaluation, however, the opportunity or motivation for supervisee self-analysis and self-evaluation may be lost and the tone of the conference preset. If the written message is used without further verbal interaction, it may be misunderstood. The intent of the message may be clearer and the opportunity for misunderstanding reduced if the purpose and content have been discussed during joint planning. As indicated in the literature, novice learners—those who are unconsciously or consciously incompetent—will need directing and coaching to acquire knowledge and skills and grow as a professional. Supervisors need to be cognizant of the need to shift timing, frequency and specificity of written feedback to facilitate supervisee movement on the continuum.

Report writing is one area in which written feedback is always provided to supervisees. Task 10 and its associated competencies (ASHA, 1985) focused on reporting and editing. It is not uncommon to hear supervisees say that a report was returned with so much red ink that it appeared to have "bled to death." On the other hand, supervisors report that helping supervisees develop good report writing skills is one of their toughest challenges but one that can yield significant benefits. If a student can write coherently about behavior, they most likely understand it and their work with their client.

In an investigation of feedback on written reports, Gunter (1985) examined the degree of consistency between supervisors' judgments of the most important constituents of a report and their evaluations of an actual report. The components considered of highest value were related to content, as opposed to style. Analysis of comments on an actual report, however, were inconsistent with this because they revealed more comments on style than on content. It is obviously easier to provide written feedback on style than content and Gunter pointed out the great need for a method to ensure that feedback on both are provided. She also reported that supervisors' comments on the report were not consistent, indicating that important components of feedback may be left out. She urged some means of consistency, such as a checklist for supervisors to use in reacting to reports.

Ruder et al. (1996) developed several evaluation forms, designed to improve the "consistency from one supervisor's expectations to the next" (p. 107). Among their forms is one used to evaluate the written work of student clinicians, specifically semester treatment plans and end of semester reports. Twenty-four items are scored on a 5-point rating scale (5 = very good, 4.5 = good, 4.0 = satisfactory, 3.5 = less than satisfactory, 3.0 = poor, below 2.5 = unsatisfactory). The items are related to content, style, and general professional behavior.

Sample *content* items include:
- Background information accurate and complete, only pertinent history included
- Diagnostic data displayed in a table or figure
- Tests results are accurately scored
- Protocols are completed and attached to report
- Goals and objectives are appropriate for age, disorder, and severity level
- Clinical impressions thoroughly integrate information from other sections

Sample *style* items include:
- Spelling and punctuation
- Morphology and syntax (grammar use)
- Report is free of unnecessary words, repetitions and meanderings
- Information reported in terms that are appropriate for the recipient

Sample *professional* items include:
- Met deadline for report
- Report is in correct format
- Exercised caution in making statements outside professions

Ruder et al. (1996) developed a computer-assisted program for supervision in their university clinic. The program created a spreadsheet for individual students and enabled individual supervisors to enter data and for all to share ratings. The spreadsheet analysis allowed for comparison of strengths and weaknesses of a particular clinician across and between supervisors. This type of approach and the written feedback inherent in it would make it easy to monitor an individual's acquisition of clinical competencies and thus be very helpful in providing the kind of formative assessments mandated by the 2017 ASHA Council on Academic Accreditation (CAA) Standards (Council on Academic Accreditation in Audiology and Speech-Language Pathology, 2017).

To provide more formative and consistent feedback to improve clinical documentation skills, Staltari, Baft-Neff, Marra, and Rentschler (2010) developed a clinical documentation rubric. The rubric identifies students' strengths and weaknesses in professional writing across three dimensions: content, organization and writing mechanics. Additionally, the rubric was used to develop a clinical documentation checklist, given to students at various stages throughout practicum to provide quantitative information about their writing skills. Qualitative information in the form of line-by-line edits and suggestions for document change were also provided. The two-pronged approach proved beneficial and the rubric and checklist are likely to be useful to other training programs. Smith and Hardy (2017) recommended that clinical educators use the track changes tool to provide edits and comments in documents, avoid rewriting, and guide with comments and examples.

Spontaneous or Unscheduled Verbal Interaction

Supervisors and supervisees have many opportunities for verbal interaction between the time of the observation and the conference. Regardless of setting, they meet in halls, the lunchroom, or the classroom; they may be working together on other tasks; or they may interact in a variety of other ways. The opportunities and temptations to discuss fragments of the observed clinical session in such interactions may be great.

One must ask what purpose is to be served by such spontaneous interactions. If a very specific goal has been set for the supervisor to rate certain interactions during the session, feedback may be given to the supervisee immediately. If immediate reinforcement is the goal, then this type of feedback is appropriate. Supervisors should resist the temptation to respond automatically with a stereotypical positive or negative statement without considering its purpose or effect. Further, a brief interchange may not do justice to the complexities of a clinical session. There likely has been no time for analysis by either party. A quickly delivered message may be misinterpreted. As with the written message, the probability is high that this type of interchange will take the form of an "instant evaluation" or directive for the future, which removes the need for self-analysis or self-evaluation by the supervisee. On the other hand, if a session has been a devastating failure, the supervisee may be greatly in need of an understanding word that will sustain him or her until the scheduled conference. Social rules usually encourage some kind of verbal exchange when two people meet—no one would wish to be met with a stony stare after a session. Whatever is said, the tone of the subsequent discussion may be influenced by the supervisor's words.

The remarks made by supervisors between observation and conference may be more important than they realize, especially in terms of the Collaborative Style. Such spontaneous remarks may take any of several forms, but certainly deserve some thought—and their goals and purpose should be an important part of planning the supervisory interaction. If the activities that make up the observation and analysis components as well as the type of feedback have been planned previously, there will be less uncertainty about what to expect in the conference and probably less need for spontaneous verbal interaction.

Direct Feedback During Clinical Sessions

This form of feedback includes such behaviors as communication through the "bug-in-the-ear" referred to in Chapter 5 (and in the following "Supervision by Earphone" section), slipping notes to the clinician that suggest changes in activities, interruption of the session to make suggestions or to demonstrate, using mobile devices and smart watches to send messages, and other forms of attracting the attention of the clinician in an attempt to alter the direction of the session.

Interruption of the Session

No data are available on the topic of interruption of the session by the supervisor. Countless discussions with supervisees indicate, however, that there are mixed reactions to this technique, depending on the supervisee's maturity, the supervisor's manner, the relationship between the two, the purpose and nature of the intervention, the amount of planning that preceded it, and the culture of the clinic or organization. Demonstrating for and participating with the supervisee is a distinct supervisory task, but jointly determining when it is appropriate is essential for a positive, supportive relationship.

Some clinicians report that they consider "swooping into the clinical session" without warning and taking over the work with the client to be the most reprehensible behavior supervisors can exhibit. There is a general feeling that, when supervisors enter unexpectedly and begin to interact directly with clients or to make suggestions in the presence of clients, it threatens the professional status of the clinician and damages credibility, and is demeaning. Other clinicians indicate that they welcome suggestions or demonstration. In fact, when present or former students are asked what was missing from their preparation, they often express a wish to have had more demonstrations from their supervisors. They do, however, consistently prefer to have some warning that it is going to happen or to have requested it.

In keeping with the theme of collaboration presented here, such unannounced or unplanned intervention would be especially inappropriate. Sensitivity to the supervisee's feelings and advanced planning would deter feelings of resentment and threat that might occur. The optimal way to deal with the issue of intervention and demonstration is to include it in planning activities, both long range and specific instances, so the supervisor's presence can be explained to the client. For example, the supervisee may indicate in the conference that she or he wishes a demonstration of a particular procedure. Or the supervisor may be concerned about the supervisee's evaluation and reinforcement of client responses and may wish to join the supervisee to assist in discriminating responses. If planned, the supervisee can easily explain the supervisor's forthcoming visit and be prepared for the interruption. Without further study, it seems safe to surmise that unplanned interruption may reinforce the supervisee's subordinate role and increase supervisee dependence.

Anderson (1988) stated that the only justification for unplanned interruptions would be if the client's welfare was in serious jeopardy. This is a particularly cogent issue in settings where clients are paying fees. The client's right to high quality service must be considered; at the same time, supervisors must be sure that their judgments about negative features of a session are accurate and not merely from their own "square boxes." In other words, the techniques may be different from those the supervisor would use. The issue at stake here is the learning that is taking place.

A special situation is probably presented in the case assessment sessions, especially if it is a one-visit evaluation where there will be no other opportunity to obtain reliable data. Incorrect test administration may warrant interruption. However, adequate planning and preparation may prevent such problems, or at least alleviate potential defensiveness.

When there is no observation room, a totally different situation is created. In some settings, supervisors may have to sit in the room where the session is being conducted. Intervention in such cases might be planned in such a way that the supervisee could request the supervisor to join in the session or to demonstrate a specific activity without infringing on the supervisee's relationship with a client. In some situations, supervisors and supervisees may work cooperatively as a team on a fairly regular basis, thus, giving the supervisor a natural opportunity to demonstrate. Sensitivity and planning are obviously important when supervisor and supervisee share the same space.

Rassi (1978) described a supervisory procedure in audiology assessment in which the supervisor demonstrates for the student, explains rationale between questions of the patient, and then has the student perform the tasks while the supervisor remains in the room. The supervisor then listens in an adjacent room and "if deemed necessary and/or appropriate, supervisor may intervene to assist student or give him suggestions" (p. 46). Rassi stressed the dangers of dependence on the supervisor and said, "Beware of transforming the student into a robot" (p. 47). Rassi (2001) discussed some fundamental differences in supervision of student or staff clinicians in audiology as compared to their counterparts in speech-language pathology, suggesting a more apprenticeship approach. The nature of clinical tasks involved in the practice of audiology, the number and variety of clients served, the physical environment dictated by the equipment used in clinical audiology, time constraints, and the probability that students may not be present for a particular client's return visit necessitates a more directive supervisory style (explaining, telling, modeling).

Live Supervision

The term live supervision, referred to briefly in the discussion of observation, has developed in the training of professionals in marriage and family counseling (Goodman, 1985) and has potential applicability for speech-language pathology and audiology.

In the live supervision approach, the supervisor assumes the role of co-therapist. Kaslow (1977) noted that there are many advantages to this model, where "the student can be exposed to intensive learning by direct observation and participation with the supervisor. Such experiences can be exhilarating and highly productive" (p. 224). This type of supervision also has its disadvantages, according to Kaslow—the possible assertiveness of the supervisor, the modeling that may take place, and the repression of the supervisee's spontaneity. It is hoped that, for supervisees, "the supervisor will help them maintain their individualities, find their own styles, trust their hunches, and gradually feel free to move in more rapidly, so that ultimately the teams will be well balanced" (p. 225).

Does this approach have application in our professions? Discussions with supervisors have revealed instances where a comparable approach is used, but Rassi's (1978, 1987, 2001; Rassi & McElroy, 1992) approach to audiology supervision is the only detailed account in the literature. Anderson (1988) reported that she frequently encountered this approach in off-campus settings. Certainly, it deserves investigation. Although at first glance, it may appear to be the antithesis of the model advocated in this text, this approach may be suited to interactions at either end of the continuum. At the very early stages, there may be a need for modeling, demonstrating, immediate intervention, or reinforcement of beginning clinicians—to help them develop some foundation skills. This methodology may also be viable with the marginal student. At the consultative end of the continuum, it may be the ideal way for peers to work together in solving certain problems. Gillam (1999) advocated an apprenticeship model in which faculty function as master clinicians and clinical researchers who teach students a research approach to the clinical process through demonstration, mediated learning experiences, and coaching. Determining when an apprenticeship model is most efficient and what effect it has on the potential development of Collaborative and Consultative Styles provide interesting matter for efficacy research.

Supervision by Earphone

A form of live supervision that has received some attention in the literature is that of the bug-in-the-ear technique. This method uses electronic equipment such as an FM transmitter and receiver, allowing the supervisor to communicate directly with the clinician in such a manner that the client is not privy to the conversation. Called the most intrusive device in use in supervision, both cognitively and emotionally, by Loewenstein and Reder (1982), it has been used for many years in social work and psychotherapy (Kadushin, 1976). Numerous recent examples are evident in teacher education in which "virtual coaching," using advanced online and mobile bug-in-the-ear technology, is implemented to assist pre-service and novice teachers in the moment to achieve planned student outcomes (Hollett, Brock, & Hinton, 2017; Rock, Zigmond, Gregg, & Gable, 2011).

The speech-language pathology literature contains a few references to the bug-in-the-ear procedure. Brooks and Hannah (1966) reported it as a supervisory tool but warned that the supervisor must avoid dominating the instruction and "causing the student to become a voice-operated automaton." They also indicated that it is sometimes difficult for the supervisor "to hold himself in check in this regard" (Brooks & Hannah, 1966, p. 386) and cited dependency of students as one of the dangers of such a system. A similar procedure was described by Starkweather (1974) for use in behavior modification training of clinicians, but he warned, "the whole procedure rests on the assumption that the supervisor's judgment is perfect, which is obviously unrealistic"

(p. 610) and followed that with the cogent statement that the same problem exists in traditional training, but that the degree of independence of the student in traditional training "may enable the excellent student to overcome some of the shortcomings of his mentor" (p. 610). Hagler and Holdgrafer (1987) and Wilson, Welch, and Welling (1996) suggested that the technique has the advantage of enabling supervisors to provide immediate feedback to clinicians in an unobtrusive manner. Hagler and Holdgrafer used it to attempt to modify the amount of clinician talk time as they obtained language samples. Results demonstrated that directives to "talk more/less" had the desired effect on the amount of talking done by student clinicians. In a comparable study, Hagler (1986) found that supervisors were able to reduce their verbal behavior during conferences as a result of verbal directives to "try to talk less" delivered at 2-minute intervals.

Citing the need for hands-on clinical teaching with novices and the advantages of real-time feedback, Scott, Becker, and Simpson (2017) used a "bug-in-the-eye" (BITi) technique. Using an Apple Watch, a supervisor provided feedback to two novice supervisees about implementation of stimulus-response-consequence (S–R–C) contingencies. A staggered AB sequence was implemented with an extended baseline (A) for one of the two subjects. In the treatment (B) phase, the novice received 5 to 10 specific scripted messages about S–R–C throughout a 50-minute session. Results demonstrated a significant correlation between BITi with a smartwatch and an increase in S–R–C contingencies being implemented for the two novices. Based on qualitative interviews and exit rating scales the students reported BITi feedback was noninvasive and minimally distracting.

Other Structures for Feedback

Microteaching and video confrontation methodologies, described in Chapter 5, involve the provision of feedback, often from peers and usually immediate. In some settings, case presentations and discussion provide opportunities for feedback, which are typically client centered. The case presentation, or staffing, rather than the conference, has been the classical means of supervising in psychiatric education. With this method, the trainee evaluates a case, presents it to the supervisor and peer group, or conducts an interview before a group. The trainee's performance is then discussed and critiqued by the supervisor and group (Kagan & Werner, 1977). This format has been used in speech-language pathology but has not been formally studied. Group conferences are a commonly used opportunity for sharing feedback and will be given more detailed attention later. Demonstration therapy provides another method for providing feedback. Wagner, McCrea, and Spigarelli (1992) studied advantages and disadvantages of using e-mail to conference. They noted that it is an effective means for providing feedback about specific issues such as scheduling, lesson planning, or sharing information from observations but suggested that it not be used as a replacement to traditional face-to-face conferences.

CONFERENCES

ASHA's (2008) Core Area VI.7 stipulates that supervisors must involve supervisees in the analysis of supervisory interactions to determine the extent to which the content and dynamics of the conference facilitate goal achievement, desired outcomes and planned changes. Core Area II.8 states that supervisors and supervisees should apply research to the supervisory process to develop relationships and analyze supervisor and supervisee behaviors. To realize these skills and to encourage and motivate supervisee development, it seems imperative that supervisors understand the nature of conferences and what has been learned through research.

Anderson's (1988) thinking and study about conferences was initially influenced by a large body of descriptive literature in education. Work by Cogan (1973), Blumberg and associates (Blumberg, 1974, 1980; Blumberg & Amidon, 1965; Blumberg & Cusick, 1970; Blumberg & Weber, 1968), Dussault (1970), Goldhammer et al. (1980; Goldhammer, 1969), Weller (1969), and others provided a foundation for most of the dissertation studies Anderson directed for more than a decade at Indiana University. Although addressed more extensively in the first edition of this text (Anderson, 1988), salient findings from some of the key studies have been discussed in earlier chapters. A brief summary of a few major findings from selected studies follows; it provides a framework for the conference studies in speech-language pathology.

Education

The pioneering work of Blumberg and his associates addressed the nature of the human relationships between supervisor and teacher, the place where Blumberg believed most of the problems in supervision arose (Blumberg, 1974; Blumberg & Amidon, 1965; Blumberg & Cusick, 1970; Blumberg & Weber, 1968). The main point of interaction in these relationships is the conference and therefore Blumberg turned his attention to analyzing conferences.

Blumberg and Cusick (1970) developed an interaction analysis system and used it to analyze 50 conferences. The results provided the first published view of what was actually occurring in conferences and the first use of the terms *direct* and *indirect* to describe supervisor behaviors. In their analysis, Blumberg and Cusick found that supervisors talked slightly less than teachers (45% for supervisors, 53% for teachers, and 2% silence). What was more interesting than the amount of time, however, was the type of verbal interaction. Supervisors were about 33% more direct than indirect (e.g., they were giving information, telling or suggesting to teachers what they should do, giving opinions, criticizing). They gave information five times more than they asked for it. Supervisor talk was heavily weighted toward telling, as compared to asking, in both problem solving and task-oriented discussions. They spent about seven times as much time telling supervisees what to do as they did in asking teachers for their ideas or suggestions. Supervisors asked opinions of teachers about one and one-half times more often than they gave opinions, and this was interpreted by teachers as an attempt to "box them into a corner" (Blumberg, 1974, p. 109). Teachers asked very few questions.

Further discussion of results included the interpretation that supervisors did not deal directly with teachers' negative feelings in a way that helped teachers. Interaction was mainly instruction from supervisors. Teachers did not perceive supervision as helpful—probably the reason they asked so few questions.

During the time supervisors engaged in accepting and clarifying teachers' ideas, 90% of the time was spent in giving short responses such as, "I see" and "uh huh." Very little time was spent in clarifying the supervisees' remarks. When teachers did exhibit negative social-emotional behaviors, the responses from the supervisor were not "therapeutic" but tended to be hostile and defensive. In trying to create a positive atmosphere, supervisors often used brief praising such as "good" or "I like that."

In another discussion of the 1970 study, Blumberg (1974, 1980) proposed that the behavior of supervisors was antithetical to the accumulated knowledge about helping relationships. The supervisors studied did not maintain a collaborative, problem-centered relationship with teachers. This is particularly significant since they were talking about employed professionals—not inexperienced students.

Although their analysis system focuses only on behavior, not content, Blumberg and Cusick (1970) discussed their impressions and stated that supervisors tended not to deal directly with teachers' complaints; that when supervisors gave advice and information, teachers did not question or ask for a rationale; and that the bulk of discussion revolved around "maintenance procedures" such as schedules, movement of children in the room, and so forth. Further, supervisors backed away from dealing with teachers' defensiveness and the researchers perceived the whole process as a rather stereotyped, role playing process. Very little behavior was related to action or problem solving, resulting in conferences in which the interaction was not related to critical problems in the classroom, nor was it collaborative.

Other studies of the content of conferences in education at that time reported similar data (Heidelbach, 1967; Lindsey, 1969; Link, 1970; Michalak, 1969; Pittinger, 1971). Weller (1969), whose interaction analysis system will be discussed in the next chapter, found in a study of conferences that over 93% of the conference was spent in analysis of instruction. Items related to this analysis were evenly divided between methods and materials (37.3%) and instruction and interactions (35.9%), while objectives and content received only 20% of the time. Over two thirds of the conference content was cognitive, rather than affective or social-disciplinary.

These early descriptive studies of teacher education conferences formed an important foundation for the study of conferences in our professions. Substantial evidence indicates that conferences in speech-language pathology and audiology are very similar to those described in education.

Speech-Language Pathology

Several descriptive studies of conferences are available in the speech-language pathology literature. It seems reasonable to assume that the process information derived from these investigations may be generalizable to audiology and speech-language pathology assessment conferences. Content will obviously differ.

Hatten's (1965) pioneer work reported descriptive data concerning the temporal, topical content, and social-emotional characteristics of 40 mid-semester supervisory conferences in a university clinic. Supervisors talked approximately 60% of the time. In the 35% of the time supervisees spoke, there responses were brief, most frequently "uh huh" or other kinds of agreement. Mean length of conference was approximately 16 minutes and the range of topics discussed was from 4 to 10, with a mean of 6.5. The number of topic changes within a conference, including returns to a previous topic, ranged from 5 to 49, with a mean of 24. Topics, in the order of the time spent on each, were: therapy techniques (41.97%), client's qualities (21.86%), therapist's qualities (13.87%), motivation (7.54%), clerical (4.21%), social (2.86%), parents (2.74%), interpersonal (2.58%) theory (1.7%), and equipment (0.64%). Thus, the first three topics accounted for almost 78% of the conference time. Only one category (client's qualities) was present in all conferences. Hatten suggested that percentages might change depending on the time in the semester the conference was held.

Underwood (1973 [Seeley, 1973]) used Blumberg and Cusick's (1970) interaction analysis system to investigate speech-language pathology conferences and reported results similar to those of Blumberg and Cusick. However, she found that speech-language pathology conferences with students were longer than those with teachers—a 24-minute average vs. 13 minutes in education. The least used supervisory behavior was "supervisor asks for suggestions," as in Blumberg and Cusick's study. The least used supervisee behavior was "negative social emotional behavior."

Another view of speech-language pathology conferences comes from a study of 10 supervisor-clinician pairs over a 12-week period (Culatta & Seltzer, 1976). As a group, the trend was for supervisees to provide raw data about the sessions; supervisors then used the data to suggest strategies for the next session. Sixty-one percent of all strategies came from supervisors, who asked about 70% of the questions (although the types were not indicated). There were no conferences in which clinicians made more statements than supervisors. Culatta and Seltzer (1976) noted the absence of evaluation statements by supervisors or self-evaluation by supervisees. Only 9% of all responses were evaluative; two-thirds provided by supervisors. In addition, even though supervisors thought they changed their behaviors during the 12-week term, there was virtually no change in the relative proportion of responses of supervisors and clinicians, talk time, and the categories of response. In a follow-up study (Culatta & Seltzer, 1977), the same proportions occurred across conferences and confirmed the fact that supervisors did not change, even on self-selected behaviors.

Similar data were provided by Schubert and Nelson (1976) who used Underwood's interaction analysis system (modified from Blumberg & Cusick, 1970) to analyze nine conferences. Behavior used most frequently was clinician positive social, including responses such as "mmhm" and "OK" (21.4%). Next most frequent was supervisors providing opinions and suggestions (20.6%), followed by providing factual behavior. Supervisor talk consistently accounted for a larger part of conferences (65%) than supervisee talk. No supervisor criticism or negative social behavior from clinicians was found.

Irwin (1975, 1976) studied conferences that were conducted after microtherapy sessions and also found that the direct style (instruction, modeling, negative reinforcement) was used significantly more than the indirect style (asking questions, positive reinforcement). Supervisees responded to supervisors, rather than initiating.

Similar behavior was cited by Roberts and Smith (1982), who described behavior of 15 supervisor-supervisee pairs in 45 conferences over a 6-week period from data obtained in Smith's (1977) extensive dissertation study. Using Weller's (1971) MOSAICS as the dependent measure, they found that supervisors assumed the initiatory role by structuring and soliciting responses and by contributing more pedagogical moves (uninterrupted verbal utterances). Supervisees assumed a predominantly reflexive role—participating less and when they did, they responded and reacted to supervisor moves. Supervisors set the content and interaction patterns and directed the dialogue, thereby affecting and controlling the conference. Supervisors talked less about previous behavior and more about what should be done in future sessions. As in the Culatta and Seltzer (1976) study, supervisees appeared to present data about the session; supervisors prescribed what supervisees should do and gave opinions and suggestions for future sessions. Supervisors provided more facts, experiences, and observations than evaluative statements, again in agreement with Culatta and Seltzer. Both supervisor and supervisee used simplistic rather than complex statements, meaning there was little explanation, justification, or rationalization of statements from either party. Behavior did not change over time.

Tufts (1983) developed a content analysis system to quantify the topical content of supervisory conferences and found results similar to the other studies. About half the time in conferences was spent on two categories—clinical procedures (e.g., techniques, materials, client management) and lesson analysis (e.g., discussion of what the client did). When the category client information (e.g., general comments about the client not related specifically to the observed lesson) was added, approximately 70% of the time was accounted for. Less emphasis was placed on client information and planning for future sessions. Tufts looked for differences in content based on supervisee experience and found no major differences between three experience levels, except in lesson planning. Supervisees with the most experience spent much more time planning and assumed more responsibility for planning than those with less experience.

Shapiro's (1984) study of commitments made in conferences revealed that 47% of the total commitments made were in the areas of planning, analysis, and evaluation of the clinical process, with particular focus on the client. Second most frequent commitments (39%) addressed implementation of treatment or assessment techniques for the client. Only 8% of commitments included planning, analysis, or evaluation of supervisee behavior. Findings reinforce that conferences focus on client and the clinical process.

Two studies focused entirely on the interpersonal aspects of the conference. McCrea (1980) adapted scales developed by Gazda (1974) for measuring the supervisor facilitative behaviors of Empathic understanding, respect, facilitative genuineness, and concreteness as well as the ability of the supervisee to self-explore, all concepts from Rogerian theory (Carkhuff, 1967, 1969a, 1969b; Carkhuff & Berensen, 1967; Carkhuff & Truax, 1964; Rogers, 1951, 1957, 1961, 1962). She analyzed 28 conferences. Respect, facilitative genuineness, and concreteness were demonstrated only at minimal levels and empathic understanding and supervisee self-exploration were not identified often enough to be included in statistical analyses. Two limitations of this study were that conference audio recordings were used, thereby eliminating the nonverbal behavior through which much affect is carried, and that behaviors were identified by trained raters and did not reflect perceptions of supervisees. Despite this, it appears very clear that the emphasis in these conferences, too, was not on clinician affect or behavior, but on such cognitive content as client problems, discussion of activities, planning strategies, and procedural matters.

Pickering (1979) used a descriptive, naturalistic approach to examine interpersonal communication in 40 samples each of therapy sessions and supervisory conferences. Although her qualitative methodology was different from other studies of conferences, her results were not. Supervisors' communication in conferences was predominantly instructional, giving suggestions, advice, opinions, directives, and questions. Supervisors seemed to have an individual style which they maintained. Emphasis was on resolving issues regarding clients not supervisees; content was cognitive and analytical. Supervisors shared few feelings; they were sympathetic and supportive and reinforcing when supervisees expressed feeling and concerns but did not aid supervisees in expanding those feelings or expressing their own. Supervisors frequently failed to attend to supervisees' expressions of feeling associated with therapy, often asking a cognitive question to turn conversation back to solution of client problems. The supervisors and supervisees rarely discussed the supervisory relationship or their feelings about each other. At the same time, supervisors were keeping journals in which they indicated the importance of the students' feelings in the therapeutic relationship with the client. Supervisees, too, focused on cognitive issues, shared feelings more frequently than supervisors, but they were frequently vague and reflected past feelings rather than current (probably because the discussion was the typical recounting of the clinical session).

Group Conferences

Although one-to-one conferences seem to be the traditional method in speech-language pathology and audiology, group or team conferences appear to be increasingly popular. Supervisors may be motivated to use groups because their workloads prevent individual scheduling, or they may have strong beliefs in the value of group interaction in the learning process.

Among the advantages of group supervision are: economy in terms of time and effort in dealing with common issues, sharing experiences and problem solving, emotional support, safety in numbers creates a comfortable learning environment, and peer influence (Kadushin, 1976). A supportive environment for change, and one in which supervisees do not feel their anxieties or problems are unique, should enhance professional self-esteem. In addition, supervisees are exposed to a wider variety of cases so the context for learning is expanded. Supervisees are able to learn directly and vicariously. Problem-solving skills should be enhanced as supervisees explore various solutions to dilemmas and learn that several approaches may be effectively implemented to solve a particular problem. Participation in a group can also enhance an individual's interpersonal communication abilities as they practice active listening, questioning, giving and receiving feedback, and learn how to manage resistance to change. Supervisees will be more active in the supervisory process because all members must assume equal responsibility for group functioning and share the responsibilities in accomplishing the tasks involved in supervision. This should foster supervisee independence and decrease dependence on the supervisor and facilitate the development of a personal, individual clinical style. Risks to effective and efficient group functioning involve issues of cohesiveness, trust, and insuring that all members share the work and have comparable responsibilities. Obvious disadvantages of group conferences are that some individual needs will not be met and that supervisees do not receive the amount of attention that occurs in one-to-one interactions.

Historically, Dowling (1979) was the main proponent of group methodology in our professions with her work and research on the *Teaching Clinic*. Developed for teacher training, the Teaching Clinic is a specifically structured peer-group from of supervision. As described by Dowling (2001) the Teaching Clinic consists of six sequential phases: 1) review of the previous teaching clinic, 2) planning, 3) observation, 4) data analysis and critique preparation, 5) problem solving and strategy development, and 6) clinic review. The group consists of a demonstration clinician who contributes a video recording of a clinical session, and a clinic leader who serves as facilitator. Other participants are a group monitor, who observes the process to see if roles are being fulfilled and ground rules followed, and peers of the demonstration clinician.

Basic operation of the Teaching Clinic is as follows:

1. The previous clinic is reviewed to maintain continuity. The demonstration clinician discusses the results of implementing the suggestions made in the previous clinic. Any problems from the previous clinic are discussed. Ground rules are reiterated.

2. During the planning session, the demonstration clinician presents his or her therapy objectives and plans, and requests certain data she or he would like to have collected. The leader then discusses data collection tasks to be carried out by peers.

3. The team members, including the demonstration clinician, view about 10 minutes of the video.

4. The demonstration clinician leaves the room to analyze data independently and the leader and peers analyze their data, problem solve, and determine how to provide feedback in the most supportive manner.

5. The demonstration clinician returns, presents his or her self-analysis, which is followed by group feedback, problem solving, and the generation of strategies for the next clinical session.

6. In the review, the monitor assesses the effectiveness of the group interactions.

A number of studies have been completed to analyze the efficiency and effectiveness of the Teaching Clinic. Dowling and Shank (1981) compared it to conventional supervision and found the two yielded similar outcomes. In a subsequent analysis (Dowling, 1983), using a more sensitive dependent measure (MOSAICS), there were some differences in that the teaching clinic contained more direct behaviors. Johnson and Fey (1983) compared individual conferences and the Teaching Clinic and found no differences with regard to student attitudes about therapy or perceived clinical effectiveness. In a 1987 investigation, Dowling found that teaching clinics were clearly viewed more positively than typical conferences and were perceived by the 46 graduate students in her study to be more indirect than typical conferences. McCrea (1994) described using an adaptation of the Teaching Clinic as part of the curriculum for a master's degree thesis option in supervision. This provided opportunities for students to apply what they learned in a three credit-hour course the previous semester to their own supervisory practice. McCrea reported that students increased their self-awareness and abilities to self-analyze the supervisory process as a result of their experience. Dowling, Glaser, Shapiro, Mawdsley, and Sbaschnig (1992) described some adaptations and unique uses of the Teaching Clinic. Descriptive data and anecdotal information supported the use of the Teaching Clinic as a primary or augmentative procedure. It was useful in a) increasing satisfaction with the supervisory process; b) identifying parameters of effective therapy; c) teaching self-analysis, problem solving, and strategy development skills; and d) analyzing and enhancing the quality of supervision. Given her expertise, years of studying this approach, and consulting with others who have experimented with the Teaching Clinic, Dowling (2001) recommended that it be used "as a supplement to traditional supervision rather than a substitute" (p. 321).

McFarlane and Hagler (1992a) compared the traditional approach to peer groups in which 47 undergraduates with less than 16 clock hours served as subjects. The hypothesis that student clinicians would initiate more in conferences with a peer than with a supervisor was not substantiated. Overall, peer supervisors initiated significantly less than supervisors in conferences. Supervisees remained passive regardless of the type of supervision they experienced. The results "suggested a need to rethink past explanations of supervisors' apparent inability to alter their largely direct-evaluative behavior" (p. 80). An important variable seems to be the level of supervisee experience; supervisees at the Evaluation-Feedback end of the continuum need a Direct-Active Style and are not yet ready to assume a leadership role in conferences.

Bowline, Bunce, Polmanteer, and Wegner (1996) described an innovative approach to clinical teaching developed at the University of Kansas out of frustration with the traditional method of supervision and the need to teach students to be effective team leaders and members. Clinical faculty manage a team in an area of individual expertise (e.g., Augmentative and Alternative Communication, adult neurogenics, child language, etc.). Students are assigned to a team and each graduate clinician provides between 5 and 10 hours of therapy per week. Teams meet weekly for a 2-hour period; students rotate the facilitator and recorder roles. Students set their own agenda and run the meetings; supervisors may add items to an agenda. In addition, undergraduates in a pre-practicum course rotate through three different teams in 4-week blocks of time. They write observation reports, note team's skills, and track the team process. The major benefits of this team approach are "that it is more efficient in terms of clinical operations and instruction, provides broader and more self-directed learning experiences for students, and better teaching by faculty" because they can focus on individual interests and experiences (Wegner, 1999, p. 104). A clinical teaching team model has also been employed at the University of North Carolina at Greensboro (McCready & Wegner, 2006; Reuler, Messick, Gavett, McCready & Raleigh, 2011). It serves as a supplement to traditional one-to-one supervision and is apropos to millennial students who have functioned in group activities from a very early age and appreciate collaborative team work (Reuler et al., 2011).

Supervisors who wish to use group conferences should be sensitive to the needs of supervisees. Many students prefer to have the opportunity for some individual contact with the supervisor along with group interaction. Certain aspects of the Collaborative Style lend themselves to a group methodology. For example, much of the introductory aspects of the first component, understanding, could be done in a group, not only to save time, but to allow supervisees to share insights and experiences. Teaching supervisees data collection and analysis techniques, as well as demonstrating certain clinical techniques are other tasks that could be easily managed in groups. For the Consultative Style, groups may be especially appropriate. Self-supervising clinicians have much to share with each other and such conferences could be an effective means of promoting professional growth, whatever the setting.

An important issue in implementing group supervision is how well prepared supervisors are in group dynamics and group processes. There is an analogy to be found in group therapy. Most supervisors have observed so-called group therapy, which was simply a few minutes of individual therapy for each client who happened to be sitting in the group, experiencing individual therapy with an audience. Among the reasons for this are that a group has been defined on the basis of scheduling convenience rather than on common goals or problems or the ability to work together, and their needs are so varied that even the most skillful group leader would have difficulty managing the group. Another reason is the lack of preparation, experience, or insight about group processes, which results in ineffective use of group time. Clinicians become supervisors and their lack of skill in group management generalizes to the supervisory process. Although group supervision is thought to be valuable, effectiveness is contingent on the skills of the leader. As many experts (Bowline et al., 1996; Dowling, 2001; Farmer, 1994) have noted and as any instructor who has tried to implement problem-based learning or other forms of group teaching can substantiate, supervisees need some orientation to group work. Complaints about group members who do not carry their weight or conflicts between individuals are not uncommon. Techniques to insure trust, openness, cohesiveness, and goal accomplishment have to be planned. Any supervisor who wishes to use a group approach would be wise to investigate the vast resources on group processes in the counseling (therapeutic groups), business (task groups) or communication literature. Understanding how to form groups (e.g., homogeneity, optimal size, etc.), identifying how groups and individuals within groups will be evaluated, clarifying group goals, developing mutual understanding each person's roles, clarifying members' right and responsibilities, and establishing ground rules (e.g., regarding confidentiality, attendance, honesty) are among the many concerns that need to be considered. Understanding group dynamics will not only be an asset in supervision, but also in all other professional domains in which we find ourselves to be part of a working group. This is particularly true in light of professional trends and initiatives toward interprofessional collaborative practice (ASHA, 2015; CAA, 2017, sec. 3.1.1A and B)

Varying Perceptions of Conferences

There is evidence that supervisees and supervisors perceive the activities within conferences differently. This fact, coupled with the data that indicate the supervisory process is not discussed, increases the opportunity for misunderstanding and frustration (Brasseur & Jimenez, 1996; Culatta et al., 1975; Dowling, 2001; McCrea, 1980; Pickering, 1984; Roberts & Smith, 1982; Shapiro, 1985; Shapiro, 1984; Tufts, 1983).

Culatta et al. (1975) found that supervisees and supervisors frequently reported "completely contradictory interpretations of the same event" (p. 152). The discrepancies relative to lesson planning were reported in the chapter on planning. Other areas where discrepancies existed are relevant. For example, supervisors said they believed it was important to have supervisees review client's case history and confer with the supervisor before client contact. Seventy percent of the supervisees, however, reported that supervisors did not attend these conferences, resulting in disappointment and confusion on the part of supervisees. Supervisors felt positively about viewing video recordings, supervisees did not. There were differing views about the value of various types of reports and of the supervisory conference. Most important, the areas of difference were never discussed during conferences. Similar results have been reported by others (Anderson & Milisen, 1965; Russell, 1976).

Such differences in perceptions are illustrated by the following situation. An off-campus supervisor says to the university supervisor, "I wish the student would use more of her own ideas and not just do what I do," while the supervisee says, "I feel that I have to do therapy the way she does it. That is what she wants." As in the study by Culatta et al. (1975), they seldom discuss these differences except with the university supervisor. In fact, this may become a major function of the university of the off-campus practicum—bridging the "communication gap."

In an extensive study of the conference, Smith (1977) and Smith and Anderson (1982b) found that supervisors, supervisees, and trained raters each perceived different effectiveness variables in conference content. Such differences of perception are not surprising. What is significant is the lack of discussion about the differences. It might be assumed that such differences between expectations and reality would be clarified at some time, as an integral part of understanding, but such does not seem to be the case. Relevant to this fact is the recommendation that supervisors and supervisees should keep their self-perceptions of the conference at a conscious level, investigating them at frequent intervals to determine if perceptions are similar. A lack of information regarding the convergence or divergence of perceptions of those involved in conference interactions, if allowed to exist over time, may greatly diminish the effectiveness of the conference (Smith & Anderson, 1982a, p. 258).

The mass of descriptive data on the conference and the consistency of the finding that *supervisor behavior does not change over time or according to the supervisee's experience* raises some interesting issues. There are, admittedly, weaknesses in some of the studies. Change has been measured over a relatively short period of time, possibly not sufficient to expect change. The questions asked, the settings in which research was conducted, instruments used to measure change, and the preciseness of methodology varies across studies. It must be assumed that the outcomes do not typify every conference, yet the striking similarities enhance collective credibility. The knowledge that supervisors' perceptions of their own behavior and its change are inaccurate does not give comfort to the supervisor who says, "But my conferences are not like that. I use different styles and behaviors to meet the needs of individuals." Although this may be true, no one can say it with certainty until they have engaged in some type of objective study of their conferences.

WHAT'S A SUPERVISOR TO DO?

What do all these studies and all this discussion tell the supervisor about the provision of feedback or conferences? Except for general knowledge about learning, motivation, communication, interpersonal interaction, leadership, and other relevant topics, there is not enough specific information to support the merits of any method of feedback or any particular type of conference. Anderson (1988) maintained that this allows freedom to speculate—professional growth, including specific behavior change in supervisees, will or will not take place mainly as a result of the interaction in the conference. It is the thesis of this book that the conference, while only one of several types of interaction between supervisor and supervisee, is probably the most important. This belief comes not only from the fact that it appears to be the most commonly used occasion for communication, but also because of the sheer dynamic of this interpersonal "happening"—this event that can be so important to its participants. Further, there is an assumption that it is through the intensive study of the conference that the positives and negatives of the supervisory process will begin to unravel.

What is known about the conference from research, is that it is consistent with the Direct-Active Style appropriate to the Evaluation-Feedback Stage, not with the Collaborative Style nor with the Consultative Style. If the continuum and the styles appropriate to its different point are accepted, conference behavior can be measured against that standard.

The Collaborative Style

Some of the characteristics of the Collaborative Style, appropriate to the Transitional Stage, are listed here. This is not an all-inclusive list, nor are items listed in order of importance. Any single conference must not necessarily include all the items. Content will be determined by individual needs, place on the continuum within the Transitional Stage, supervisory objectives, and other factors.

- The conference will include some evidence that it has been planned—there will be some type of agenda.
- There will be evidence that both short- and long-range goals have been set for all participants: client, clinician, supervisee, and supervisor.
- There will be evidence of data collection on both client and clinician by both supervisor and supervisee.
- The data will be presented in an organized manner which gives some evidence of planning data collection. For example, it will be obvious that data are related to goals. It will be obvious that planning took place to determine what data would be collected, how, by whom and how they will be presented.
- There will be emphasis on analysis of data related to the relationship between client and clinician behavior, not a single focus on the client. Inferences will be drawn about the relationship between client and clinician.
- Analysis will be related to goals and objectives.
- There will be data collection, analysis, and discussion of goals and objectives for supervisee and supervisor, that is, the supervisory process will be studied to determine if appropriate learning is taking place.
- There will be a combination of direct and indirect supervisor behaviors. The balance will be determined by continuum placement.
- Topics other than data from sessions will include procedural or administrative issues, academic topics, research relevant to practice, personal or affective concerns, professional issues, unexpected events and other pertinent issues.

- Although the emphasis will be on analysis, particularly self-analysis by the supervisee, leading to self-evaluation, there is time and place for varying degrees of evaluative feedback and information giving by the supervisor.

- The supervisor will assume responsibility for structuring joint problem solving through open, thought-provoking questions, appropriate responses to the supervisee, types of objectives set, and other techniques. In turn, the supervisee will accept responsibility for participating in problem solving.

- Part of the learning process will be the expansion of verbal statements by supervisor and supervisee—explanations, justifications, rationale for opinions and suggestions, questioning each other for such expansions if they do not occur. Research demonstrates that traditionally, utterances are simple and short, rather than the type that lead to in-depth discussion and information exchange. To optimize learning and generalization, more discussion of options, justifications, and explanations of suggestions by supervisors should be apparent in conference dialogue.

- The interpersonal interaction in the conference will be supportive and facilitative, with both participants being sensitive to the needs and feelings of the other.

- Supervisor and supervisee will review periodically their own objectives for the supervisory process, compare their perceptions of whether or not objectives are being met, and make appropriate adjustments.

The Consultative Style

The Consultative Style, appropriate to the Self-Supervision Stage, is not as clear-cut as the Direct-Active and Collaborative Styles. It may include behaviors from each of the other styles, but the supervisor and supervisee will maintain a different type of relationship. Referred to commonly in the literature in other helping professions, consultation is not so frequently discussed in speech-language pathology and audiology.

According to Hart (1982), consultation in counseling is "an informal educational experience usually used in place of supervision" (p. 12). Kurpius and Robinson (1978) called the consultant a "collaborator who forms egalitarian relationships with the consultee to bring about change. In this collegial relationship, there is a joint diagnosis with emphasis on consultees finding their own solution to their problems" (p. 232). The consultant serves as a catalyst for problem solving. Kurpius, Baker, and Thomas (1977) said that consultation is a frequently employed approach to supervision and it "implies shared problem definition, problem solving, and evaluation...there is a suggestion in the literature that consultation becomes a more dominant mode of supervision as the trainee becomes increasingly able and professional in his performance" (p. 288).

The Consultative Style of supervision is a style that results from the need to solve a problem. It has a voluntary, and possibly an intermittent or temporary aspect not found in the other styles. The supervisee identifies the need. The supervisor's role is not only to help the supervisee solve the immediate existing problem, but also to develop problem-solving abilities so that future problems may be anticipated and managed. A democratic, collegial relationship is essential to this style. Developing this type of relationship requires that the supervisor exhibit nonjudgmental and nonevaluative behaviors (Kurpius & Christie, 1978), in addition to behaviors that convey openness, supportiveness, interdependence, equal power, and professional respect. The supervisor is responsible for building the relationship and for using skills to facilitate the problem-solving process. Supervisees have the knowledge and expertise in their area of work, as well as the necessary abilities and resources to solve their problem although some of these may need to be developed. Supervisees are responsible for acknowledging ownership of the problem and for learning new skills and behaviors to solve their problem. The nature of the situation and the presenting problem may require the supervisor to perform different roles and use various skills and approaches during the process. The process of problem solving must always remain primary focus even though at times during the relationship there may be attention to content and the supervisor provides information, share knowledge, gives rationales or assumes other content-related roles. The emphasis on problem solving, fundamental to this style, will enable supervisees to function more effectively in the future.

A brief description of the components of the "clinical problem solving" process seems appropriate here. The supervisor facilitates this process, while the supervisee functions as the actual agent of change. First, the presenting problem needs to be clearly defined. Next, information must be gathered. This may involve doing library research, administering tests or other assessment protocols, interviewing, and so on. As data are being collected, they are analyzed, weighted, and used to generate multiple hypotheses about the precise nature of the problem. The problem is clarified and refined and translated into a goal statement. The next step involves formulating optimal interventions or solutions to solve the problem/achieve the goal. It is important to brainstorm a variety of alternatives (Kurpius & Robinson, 1978) and creativity is important. During brainstorming, criticism is withheld, free-wheeling is encouraged, quantity is desired, and combination and improvement of ideas are sought. The forces that support and impede change should be examined. An action plan is then devised, which will enable the hypotheses that were generated to be tested and evaluated. When the plan is implemented, both the process and the product should be evaluated. It is essential to include evidence-based practice into the action plan strategies and criteria for evaluating the effectiveness of the results. The process is a dynamic, cyclic, reiterative process in which observation, analysis, synthesis, deduction, induction, hypothesis generation, hypothesis testing, strategy design and implementation are interrelated (Barrows & Pickell, 1991)

This Consultative Style may seem minimally different from the Collaborative Style. Actually, the difference is a matter of degree. Consultation is an expansion of the Collaborative Style to meet the needs of supervisees who have truly reached the point where they are capable of self-supervision, are able to analyze their clinical work, and can identify their own needs. The time at which an individual reaches this stage varies. If reached during the educational program, the supervisor may become a monitor, may help supervisees expand their clinical activities and assume new challenges, or may assist them in spending more time in the analysis of the supervisory process. If reached during off-campus practice or the clinical fellowship, consultants may need to adjust their expectations and behaviors to truly operate as a consultant, that is, to assist supervisees in using their knowledge and skills to solve problems. In the service delivery setting, where supervisor and supervisee are both fully qualified professionals, the interactions will vary even more. Conference content will be determined not only by the nature of the problem to be solved but also by the frequency with which the supervisor is able to interact with the supervisee in the work setting. Despite professional standards, not every professional in the work force has the ability to be self-supervising in every situation. A person may reach the Self-Supervision Stage in one area of clinical expertise but not in others. Herein, lie the hazards in the use of the Consultative Style in any setting—the possible inaccurate perception of supervisees of their own ability, either positive or negative, or the inability of the supervisor to accurately determine the true nature of the supervisee's skills. This is why the suggestions in Chapter 4 for determining placement on the continuum are important.

You'll know you've achieved a Consultative Style when:

- You say "we" and mean it
- You feel you've learned from your supervisee and can tell him or her so
- You're not afraid to say, "You're right—I was wrong"
- The supervisee solves a problem with little or no input from you
- You accept the supervisee's input as important as your own
- You are able to work jointly on the supervisee's performance evaluations

Reflective Practice

Although not a new supervisory strategy, reflective practice has gained popularity in speech-language pathology and audiology in the last several years (Geller, 2014; Geller & Foley, 2009; Mormer & Messick, 2016; Tepper & Vaughn, 2017). It seems most applicable for the Transitional and Self-Supervision Stages of the continuum because it requires some knowledge, experience, and a level of clinical competence to be able to implement. The importance of self-reflection is evident in training program accreditation standards. The CAA 2017 Standards address self-reflection in Professional Practice Competencies for both audiology (3.1.1A) and speech-language pathology (3.1.1B). CAA Standard 3.1.1 states that to demonstrate accountability, students must be able to "use self-reflection to understand the effects of his or her actions and make changes accordingly." Competency in clinical reasoning mandates using "clinical judgement and self-reflection." As part of individual's professional duty, skill in self-assessment is necessary to improve one's effectiveness in the delivery of services.

What is apparent in reviewing the literature on reflective practice is that it means different things to different people, resulting in a high degree of methodological variation. Schon (1983) described the two primary components of reflective practice as the ability to reflect on performance in a prior experience (i.e., reflection-on-action) and the ability to make changes in behavior while engaged in the activity (reflection-in-action). Self-reflection obviously involves thinking about one's behaviors and feelings and to be aware of the impact they have on those served (e.g., student, client, patient). But merely articulating one's perceptions of what happened, one or two things that went well and a couple that didn't, speculating about why something was successful or not, how you felt while these things were happening and then jumping to solutions of what you might do differently next time isn't congruent with a scientific approach to supervision. If we are committed to the professional development of critical thinking evidence-based practitioners, we must view identifying our hunches as a first step.

As an initial step for learning to be reflective, journals or diaries offer a systematic method of capturing a personal way to explore attitudes, thoughts and feelings. Crago and Pickering (1987) and Pickering and McCready (1983) advocated journaling as an effective means to get in touch with one's feelings, examine interpersonal dynamics and the impact on relationships. Tice (2004) provides suggestions for those who are new the process of reflection. Pickering (1990) believed that if we value the human connection we need to study the interpersonal aspects of both the clinical and supervisory relationships. Mormer and Messick (2016) offered guidelines for journal writing that provides a structure particularly helpful to those new to this process. Journal entries provide qualitative data. The task then becomes to accrue quantitative data to validate what we think and how we feel—to determine how congruent our perceptions are with reality.

In describing their integrated reflective, developmental approach to supervision, Young, Lambie, Hutchinson, and Thurston-Dyer (2011) noted that "reflectivity" is the process of reconstructing therapeutic experiences by processing multiple perspectives, images, and actions to reframe a difficult event to help develop the ability to problem-solve future complex situations. In the supervisory process, it involves codeveloping and coinvestigating hypotheses. Supervisees learn the process of reflective practice as supervisors help them recognize signals that something is amiss and how to think about a problem. Goodyear (2014) suggests that techniques such as interpersonal process recall (Kagan, 1971) and Socratic questioning are appropriate instructional strategies to facilitate this learning. He notes that reflective practice requires routinely monitoring client progress which requires self-observation and analyses. Developing hypotheses and using a scientific approach to observation and analysis are precisely what are described in Chapters 5 and 6 and the process inherent in the cycle of supervision in Anderson's (1988) continuum model.

But, as Dreyfus (2004) suggested, skill development takes time. So, becoming an effective reflective practitioner is a developmental process. A supervisee has to be consciously competent to engage in meaningful reflective practice. Novice learners, those at the Evaluation-Feedback Stage of the continuum, can begin to learn with guidance from their supervisors but self-reflection is more appropriate for advanced supervisees who are observant, alert, and attentive (Goodyear, 2014). Reflective practice fits best at the Transitional and Self-Supervision Stages of the continuum—with Collaborative and Consultative Styles.

RESEARCH NEEDS

As a beginning in the process of validating the competencies for effective supervision, several studies have examined the impact of supervisee input into conference agendas (Jans et al., 1994; McFarlane & Hagler, 1992a, 1992b; Peaper, 1984; Sbaschnig, Dowling, & Williams, 1992) and a couple have investigated the effects of written and verbal commitments (Gillam, Strike, & Anderson, 1987; Shapiro, 1984). The effect of involving supervisees in preparing conference agendas on their active involvement in conferences is mixed. Written commitments appear to facilitate follow through with beginning clinicians while verbal commitments are sufficient in promoting action for more advanced clinicians. It is evident that more research is needed to identify the competencies that enhance the effectiveness of the supervisory process at various stages on the continuum.

Only the surface has been scratched in investigating the effect that communication skills have on supervisees' decision making, problem solving, and critical thinking abilities. For example, Strike (1988) demonstrated that supervisors can be trained to use convergent and broad questions and these higher level questions facilitate higher level thinking in supervisees. The limited sample size in her study makes replication essential. A number of other studies have examined supervisors' interpersonal skills. Caracciolo et al. (1978a, 1978b) and Ghitter (1987) have demonstrated that it is important for supervisees to perceive high levels of unconditional positive regard, genuineness, empathic understanding, and concreteness being offered by supervisors but McCrea (1980) and Pickering (1979) have shown that in actuality, these behaviors occur in conferences only minimally if at all. Hagler et al. (1989) found that providing data to supervisors about the amount of these behaviors in their conferences and written suggestions for change was not sufficient to induce change. They suggested that subsequent studies should attempt to train specific facilitative behaviors, including opportunities to role play or practice. Active listening, on the part of both supervisees and supervisors, is another communication behavior that needs to be examined. What is the extent of active listening in individual and group conferences—and what impact does it have on problem solving and decision making? Other behaviors, such as supervisor self-disclosure have been identified as important facilitators for supervisee change (Pickering & McCready, 1990) but their frequency of occurrence and influence on supervisee behaviors has not been investigated. There remain many important questions about the supervisory relationship and interpersonal skills that facilitate supervisee growth that need to be answered.

In looking at the composite characteristics of conventional speech-language pathology conferences, described in Chapter 2, we need to find out if things have changed in the last couple of decades. For example, past research indicated that very little explanation and justification, and few rationales are offered for ideas and strategies by either supervisors or supervisees (Hatten, 1965; Roberts & Smith, 1982; Smith and Anderson, 1982b). If evidence-based practice is to be the norm, as mandated by certification standards (CAA, 2017), rationales for practice should be abundant in conferences. Culatta and Seltzer (1976) noted the absence of supervisor evaluations and supervisee self-evaluations and this was evident in a number of other studies (Jans et al., 1994; Roberts & Smith, 1982; Schubert & Nelson, 1976; Tufts, 1983). Other studies have reported that written feedback from supervisors is highly evaluative (Peaper & Mercaitis, 1987; Rocchio & Iacarino, 1990). There is a compelling need to examine conference content in today's world.

Although Dowling (1981, 1983a, 1983b, 2001; Dowling et al., 2001) has conducted numerous studies on the Teaching Clinic, the advantages and disadvantages of other group models needs to be established through careful study. It seems that groups and teams are appropriate for specific kinds of tasks at the Evaluation-Feedback Stage (e.g., orienting supervisees to the supervisory process, teaching data collection strategies, etc.) and as supervisees progress through the Transitional Stage, peers may be able to assume more leadership in conferences. Training in the supervisory process and in group dynamics are apparent prerequisites to effective functioning in group conferences but this remains to be demonstrated. Because of the exposure to clients being served by peers, groups would also appear to be conducive to providing numerous opportunities to critically evaluate and incorporate research relevant to professional practice. Comparing and contrasting the information to support clinical decision making acquired in group vs. individual conferences would be interesting.

Readers will notice that the many references to support practices in Chapters 3 through 7 are dated. This highlights the compelling need to replicate older studies, try to regain the momentum and productivity that was apparent in the late 1970s and 1980s and to generate initiatives to advance the science and art of supervision. Lemoncello and Ness (2013) review the concepts of evidence-based practice, discuss the paucity of efficacy evidence and offer a complementary model of practice-based evidence that could easily be applied to design, implement, and evaluate supervisory practices.

SUMMARY

This last component, integrating, is also the beginning. It is the place where everything that has happened in the other components comes together and the future is determined. Understanding, planning, observing, and analyzing feed into this component.

Because the other components have been discussed individually, this chapter focuses on the communication that takes place between supervisor and supervisee. The conference is discussed at some length because this is the usual place where communication between supervisor and supervisee occurs.

This chapter includes extensive discussion about feedback, which is defined as interaction between all participants about all components of the process, not as jut the traditional reporting on observation. This component, then, becomes the culmination of all the effort and time that have gone into the supervisory process.

REFERENCES

American Speech-Language-Hearing Association (n.d.). *Practice portal for clinical education and supervision*. Retrieved from https://www.asha.org/Practice-Portal/Professional-Issues/Clinical-Education-and-Supervision/

American Speech-Language-Hearing Association. (1985). *Clinical supervision in speech-language pathology and audiology*. [Position statement]. Retrieved from https://www.asha.org/policy/PS1985-00220/

American Speech-Language-Hearing Association. (2008). *Knowledge and skills needed by speech-language pathologists providing clinical supervision* [Knowledge and skills]. Retrieved from https://www.asha.org/policy/KS2008-00294/

American Speech-Language-Hearing Association. (2015). *Strategic pathway to excellence—strategic objective 2*. Retrieved from https://www.asha.org/uploadedfiles/asha-strategic-pathway-to-excellence.pdf

Anderson, J. (1988). *The supervisory process in speech-language pathology and audiology*. Boston, MA: College-Hill.

Anderson, J., & Milisen, R. (1965). *Report on pilot project in student teaching in speech and hearing*. Bloomington, IN: Indiana University.

Anderson, L. & Krathwohl, D. (Eds.). (2001). *A taxonomy for learning, teaching and assessing: A revision of Bloom's taxonomy of educational objectives* (2nd ed). NY: Longman.

Anderson, P., & Guerrero, L. (1998). *Handbook of communication and emotion: Research, theory, applications, and contexts*. San Diego, CA: Academic Press.

Barbara, D. A. (1958). *The art of listening*. Springfield, IL: Charles C. Thomas.

Barnum, M., & Guyer, S. (2015). *The SQF mode of clinical supervision*. Workshop presented at the Council on Academic Programs in Communication Sciences and Disorders (CAPCSD) Newport Beach, CA.

Barnum, M., Guyer, S., Levy, L., & Graham, C. (2009). Supervision, questioning, feedback model of clinical teaching: A practical approach. In T. Wiedner (Ed.), *The athletic trainers' pocket guide to clinical teaching*. Thorofare, NJ: SLACK Incorporated.

Barrows, H., & Pickell, G. (1991). *Developing clinical problem-solving skills: A guide to more effective diagnosis and treatment*. New York, NY: W.W. Norton.

Blumberg, A. (1974). *Supervisors and teachers: A private cold war*. Berkeley, CA: McCutchan.

Blumberg, A. (1980). *Supervisors and teachers: A private cold war* (2nd ed.). Berkeley, CA: McCutchan.

Blumberg, A., & Amidon, E. (1965). Teacher perceptions of supervisor-teacher interaction. *Administrator's Notebook*, *14*, 1-4.

Blumberg, A., & Cusick, P. (1970). Supervisor-teacher interaction: An analysis of verbal behavior. *Education*, *91*, 126-134.

Blumberg, A., & Weber, W. (1968). Teacher morale as a function of perceived supervisor behavior style. *Journal of Educational Research*, *62*, 109-113.

Bowline, W., Bunce, B., Polmanteer, K., & Wegner, J. (1996). There's no "I" in team. In B. Wagner (Ed.), Proceedings of the 1996 Conference on Clinical Supervision—Partnerships in supervision: Innovative and effective practices (pp. 127-131). Council of Supervisors in Speech-Language Pathology and Audiology, Cincinnati, OH.

Brammer, L. (1985). *The helping relationship*. Englewood Cliffs, NJ: Prentice-Hall.

Brasseur, J. (1980). *The observed differences between direct, indirect, and direct/indirect videotaped supervisory conferences by speech-language pathology supervisors, graduate students, and undergraduate students* (Doctoral dissertation). Retrieved from ProQuest Dissertations & Theses Global. (Accession No. 8029212) http://proxyiub.uits.iu.edu/login?url=https://search.proquest.com/docview/303031314?accountid=11620

Brasseur, J. (1989). The supervisory process: A continuum perspective. *Language, Speech, and Hearing Services in Schools*, *20*, 274-295.

Brasseur, J., & Anderson, J. (1983). Observed differences between direct, indirect, and direct/indirect videotaped supervisory conferences. *Journal of Speech and Hearing Research*, *26*, 349-355.

Brasseur, J., & Jimenez, B. (1996). Novice supervisees' attitude changes after active participation in the supervisory process. In B. Wagner (Ed.), *Proceedings of the 1996 Conference on Clinical Supervision—Partnerships in supervision: Innovative and effective practices* (pp. 80-89). Council of Supervisors in Speech-Language Pathology and Audiology, Cincinnati, OH.

Brooks, R., & Hannah, E. (1966). A tool for clinical supervision. *Journal of Speech and Hearing Disorders*, *31*, 383-387.

Caracciolo, G., Rigrodsky, S., & Morrison, E. (1978a). Perceived interpersonal conditions and professional growth of master's level speech-language pathology students during the supervisory process. *Asha*, *20*, 467-477.

Caracciolo, G., Rigrodsky, S., & Morrison, E. (1978b). A Rogerian orientation to the speech-language pathology supervisory relationship. *Asha*, *20*, 286-290.

Carin, A., & Sund, R. (1971). *Developing questioning techniques*. Columbus, OH: Merrill.

Carkhuff, R. (1967). Toward a comprehensive model of facilitative processes. *Journal of Counseling Psychology*, *14*, 67-72.

Carkhuff, R. (1969a). *Helping and human relations: A primer for lay and professional helpers—I*. New York, NY: Holt, Rinehart and Winston.

Carkhuff, R. (1969b). *Helping and human relations—II*. New York, NY: Holt, Rinehart and Winston.

Carkhuff, R., & Berensen, B. (1967). *Beyond counseling and therapy*. New York, NY: Holt, Rinehart and Winston.

Carkhuff, R., & Truax, C. (1964). Concreteness: A neglected variable in research in psychotherapy. *Journal of Clinical Psychology*, *20*, 264-267.

Cascia, J. (2013). Analysis of clinical supervisor feedback in speech-language pathology. *Perspectives on Administration and Supervision*, *23*(2), 39-58. doi:10.1044/aaa23.2.39

Christodoulou, J. (2016). A review of the expectations of speech-language pathology externship student clinicians and their supervisors. *Perspectives in Administration and Supervision, Vol 1* (Part 2) 42-53. doi:10.1044/persp1.SIG11.42

Cogan, M. (1973). *Clinical supervision*. Boston, MA: Houghton Mifflin.

Condon, J. (1977). *Interpersonal communication*. New York, NY: Macmillan.

Council on Academic Accreditation in Audiology and Speech-Language Pathology. (2017). *Standards for accreditation of graduate education programs in audiology and speech-language pathology*. Retrieved from http://caa.asha.org/reporting/standards/2017-standards/

Crago, M. (1987). Supervision and self-exploration. In M. Crago & M. Pickering (Eds.), *Supervision in human communication disorders: Perspectives on a process*. San Diego, CA: Little Brown-College Hill Press.

Crago, M., & Pickering, M. (Eds.). (1987). *Supervision in human communication disorders: Perspectives on a process*. San Diego, CA: Little Brown-College Hill Press.

Culatta, R., Colucci, S., & Wiggins, E. (1975). Clinical supervisors and trainees: Two views of a process. *Asha*, *17*, 152-157.

Culatta, R., & Seltzer, H. (1976). Content and sequence analysis of the supervisory session. *Asha*, *18*, 8-12.

Culatta, R., & Seltzer, H. (1977). Content and sequence analysis of the supervisory session: A report of clinical use. *Asha*, *19*, 523-526.

Cunningham, R. (1971). Developing question-asking skills. In J. Weigand (Ed.), *Developing teacher competencies*. Englewood Cliffs, NJ: Prentice-Hall.

Danish, S. J., & Kagan, N. (1971). Measurement of affective sensitivity: Toward a valid measurement of interpersonal perception. *Journal of Counseling Psychology*, *18*, 51-54.

Davies, I. (1981). *Instructional techniques*. New York, NY: McGraw-Hill Co.

Deetz, S., & Stevenson, S. (1986). *Managing interpersonal communication*. New York, NY: Harper and Row.

Dowling, S. (1979). Developing student self-supervisory skills in clinical training. *Journal of National Student Speech and Hearing Association, 7*, 37-41.

Dowling, S. (1983). An analysis of conventional and teaching clinic supervision. *The Clinical Supervisor, 1*, 15-29.

Dowling, S. (2001). *Supervision: Strategies for successful outcomes and productivity*. Boston, MA: Allyn & Bacon.

Dowling, S., Glaser, A., Shapiro, D., Mawdsley, B., & Sbaschnig, K. (1992). Implementing the teaching clinic. In S. Dowling (Ed.), *Proceedings of the 1992 National Conference on Supervision—Total Quality supervision: Effecting optimal performance* (pp. 156-161). Council of Supervisors in Speech-Language Pathology and Audiology, Nashville, TN.

Dowling, S., & Shank, K. (1981). A comparison of the effects of two supervisory styles, conventional and teaching clinic, in the training of speech and language pathologists. *Journal of Communication Disorders, 14*, 51-58.

Dowling, S., & Wittkopp, M. (1982). Students' perceived supervisory needs. *Journal of Communication Disorders, 15*, 319-328.

Dreyfus, S. (2004). The five-stage model of adult skill acquisition. *Bulletin of Science, Technology, & Society, 24*(3) 177-181.

Duck, S. (Ed.). (1997). Handbook of personal relationships: Theory, research, and interventions (2nd ed.). New York, NY: John Wiley & Sons.

Dussault, G. (1970). *Theory of supervision in teacher education*. New York, NY: Teachers College, Columbia University.

Ervin-Tripp, S. (1970). Discourse agreement: How children answer questions. In J. Hayes (Ed.), *Cognitions and the development of language*. New York, NY: John Wiley and Sons.

Faiver, C., Eisengart, S., & Colonna, R. (2000). *The counselor intern's handbook* (2nd ed.). Belmont, CA: Brooks/Cole.

Farmer, S. (1994). Team supervision in communication disorders: A key to professional development. In M. Bruce (Ed.), *Proceedings of the 1994 International & Interdisciplinary Conference on Clinical Supervision: Toward the 21st century* (pp. 141-149). Council of Supervisors in Speech-Language Pathology and Audiology, Cape Cod, MA.

Feltham, C. (2000). *Handbook of counseling and psychotherapy*. Thousand Oaks, CA: Sage.

Gallagher, T., & Prutting, C. (1983). *Pragmatic assessment and intervention issues in language*. San Diego, CA: College Hill Press.

Gazda, G. (1974). *Human relations development—A manual for educators*. Boston, MA: Allyn and Bacon.

Geller, E. (2014). Broadening the "Ports of Entry" for speech-language pathologists: A reflective model of supervision. *SIG 11 Perspectives, 24*(2), 51-61. doi:10.1044/aas24.2.51

Geller, E., & Foley, G. (2009). Broadening the "ports of entry" for speech-language pathologists: A relational and reflective model for clinical supervision. *American Journal of Speech-Language Pathology, 18*(1), 22-41.

Geoffrey, V. (1973). *Report on supervisory practices in speech and hearing*. Unpublished report, Department of Hearing and Speech Sciences, University of Maryland, College Park, MD.

George, R., & Cristiani, T. (1981). *Theory, methods, and processes of counseling and psychotherapy*. Englewood Cliffs, NJ: Prentice-Hall.

Ghitter, R. (1987). Relationship of interpersonal and background variables to supervisee clinical effectiveness. In S. Farmer (Ed.), *Proceedings of A National Conference on Supervision—Clinical supervision: A coming of age* (pp. 49-56). Council of University Supervisors of Practicum in Speech-Language Pathology and Audiology, Jekyll Island, GA.

Gillam, R. (1999). ISSUE III: Models of clinical instruction. Adopting an integrated apprenticeship model in a university clinic. In P. Murphy (Ed.), *Council of Academic Programs in Communication Sciences and Disorders--Proceedings of the Annual Conference on Graduate Education* (pp. 97-99). Council of Academic Programs in Communication Sciences and Disorders, Minneapolis, MN.

Goldberg, S. (1997). *Clinical skills for speech-language pathologists*. San Diego, CA: Singular.

Goldhammer, R. (1969). *Clinical supervision*. New York, NY: Holt, Rinehart and Winston.

Goldhammer, R., Anderson, R., & Krajewski, R. (1980). *Clinical supervision* (2nd ed.). New York, NY: Holt, Rinehart and Winston.

Goodman, R. (1985). The live supervision model in clinical training. *The Clinical Supervisor, 3*, 43-59.

Goodyear, R. (2014). Supervision as pedagogy: Attending to its essential instructional and learning processes. *The Clinical Supervisor, 33*, 82-99. doi:10.1080/07325223.2014.918914

Gunter, C. (1985). Clinical reports in speech-language pathology: Nature of supervisory feedback. *Australian Journal of Human Communication Disorders, 13*, 37-51.

Hackney, H., & Nye, S. (1973). *Counseling strategies and objectives*. Englewood Cliffs, NJ: Prentice-Hall, Inc.

Hagler, P., Casey, P., & DesRochers, C. (1989). Effects of feedback on facilitative conditions offered by supervisors during conferencing. In D. Shapiro (Ed.), *Proceedings of the 1989 National Conference on Supervision: Supervision innovations* (pp. 155-158). Council of Supervisors in Speech-Language Pathology and Audiology, Sonoma, CA.

Hagler, P., & Holdgrafer, G. (1987). Effects of supervisory feedback on clinician and client discourse participation. In S. Farmer (Ed.), *Proceedings of A National Conference on Supervision—Clinical supervision: A coming of age* (pp. 106-111). Council of University Supervisors of Practicum in Speech-Language Pathology and Audiology, Jekyll Island, GA.

Hagler, P. H. (1986). *Effects of verbal directives, data, and contingent social praise on amount of supervisor talk during speech-language pathology supervision conferencing* (Doctoral dissertation). Retrieved from ProQuest Dissertations and Theses Global. (Accession No. 303410764) http://proxyiub.uits.iu.edu/login?url=https://search.proquest.com/docview/303410764?accountid=11620

Hart, G. (1982). *The process of clinical supervision*. Baltimore, MD: University Park Press.

Hatten, J. T. (1965). *A descriptive and analytical investigation of speech therapy supervisors-therapist conferences* (Doctoral dissertation). Retrieved from ProQuest Dissertations and Theses Global. (Accession No. 6513735) http://proxyiub.uits.iu.edu/login?url=https://search.proquest.com/docview/302175416?accountid=11620

Heidelbach, R. A. (1967). *The development of a tentative model for analyzing and describing the verbal behavior of cooperating teachers engaged in individualized teaching with student teachers* (Doctoral dissertation). Retrieved from ProQuest Dissertations & Theses Global. (Accession No. 302267757) http://proxyiub.uits.iu.edu/login?url=https://search.proquest.com/docview/302267757?accountid=11620

Herd, C., Epperly, R., & Cox, K. (2011). Clinical and technological innovations: Use of the Apple iPad in clinical supervision. *Perspectives on Administration and Supervision, 21*(3), 112-116. doi:10.1044/aas21.3.112

Hollett, N., Brock, S., & Hinton, V. (2017). Bug-in-the-ear technology to enhance preservice teacher training: Peer versus instructor feedback. *International Journal of Learning, Teaching and Educational Research, 16*(22), 1-10.

Irwin, R. (1975). Microcounseling interview skills of supervisors of speech clinicians. *Human Communication, 4*, 5-9.

Irwin, R. (1976). Verbal behavior of supervisors and speech clinicians during microcounseling. *Central States Speech Journal, 26*, 45-51.

James, S., & Seebach, M. (1982). The pragmatic function of children's questions. *Journal of Speech and Hearing Research, 25*, 2-11.

Jans, L., Hagler, P., & McFarlane, L. (1994). Effects of agenda use over time on participants' level of involvement in supervisory conferences. In M. Bruce (Ed.), *Proceedings of the 1994 International & Interdisciplinary Conference on Clinical Supervision: Toward the 21st century* (pp. 102-106). Council of Supervisors in Speech-Language Pathology and Audiology, Cape Cod, MA.

Johnson, C., & Fey, S. (1983). Comparative effects of teaching clinic versus traditional supervision methods. *SUPERvision, 7*, 2-4.

Kadushin, A. (1976). *Supervision in social work*. New York, NY: Columbia University Press.

Kagan, N. (1970). Human relationships in supervision. In J. Anderson (Ed.), *Conference on Supervision of Speech and Hearing Programs in the Schools*. Bloomington, IN: Indiana University.

Kagan, N., & Werner, A. (1977). Supervision in psychiatric education. In D. Kurpius, R. Baker, & I. Thomas (Eds.), *Supervision of applied training*. Westport, CT: Greenwood Press.

Kaslow, F. (1977). Training of marital and family therapists. In F. Kaslow & Associates (Ed.), *Supervision, consultation, and staff training in the helping professions*. San Francisco, CA: Jossey-Bass.

Kennedy, K. B. (1981). *The effect of two methods of supervisor preconference written feedback on the verbal behaviors of participants in individual speech pathology supervisory conferences* (Doctoral dissertation). Retrieved from ProQuest Dissertations and Theses Global. (Accession No. 8123492) http://proxyiub.uits.iu.edu/login?url=https://search.proquest.com/docview/303027541?accountid=11620

Klevans, D., Volz, H., & Friedman, R. (1981). A comparison of experimental and observational approaches for enhancing the interpersonal communication skills of speech-language pathology students. *Journal of Speech and Hearing Disorders, 46*, 208-213.

Knapp, M. (1972). *Nonverbal communication in human interaction*. New York, NY: Holt, Rinehart and Winston.

Kurpius, D. (1976). Implementing interpersonal communication in school environments. In J. Weigand (Ed.), *Implementing teacher competencies*. Englewood Cliffs, NJ: Prentice-Hall.

Kurpius, D., Baker, R., & Thomas, I. (Eds.). (1977). *Supervision of applied training*. Westport, CT: Greenwood Press.

Kurpius, D., & Christie, S. (1978). A systematic and collaborative approach to problem solving. In D. Kurpius (Ed.), *Learning: Making learning environments more effective*. Muncie, IN: Accelerated Development.

Kurpius, D., & Robinson, S. (1978). An overview of consultation. *Personnel and Guidance Journal, 3*, 231-233.

Larson, L. C. (1981). *Perceived supervisory needs and expectations of experienced vs. inexperienced student clinicians* (Doctoral dissertation). Retrieved from ProQuest Dissertations and Theses Global. (Accession No. 8211183) http://proxyiub.uits.iu.edu/login?url=https://search.proquest.com/docview/303157417?accountid=11620

Leach, E. (1972). Interrogation: A model and some implications. *Journal of Speech and Hearing Disorders, 37*, 33-46.

Lemoncello, R., & Ness, B. (2013). Evidence-based practice & practice-based evidence applied to adult, medical speech-language pathology. *Perspectives on Gerontology, 18*(1) 14-26. doi:10.1044/gero18.1.14

Lindsey, M. (1969). *Inquiry into teaching behavior of supervisors in teaching education laboratories*. New York, NY: Teachers College Press, Columbia University.

Link, C. H. (1970). *Teacher-supervisor conference interaction: A study of perceptions and their relation in selected variables* (Doctoral dissertation). Retrieved from ProQuest Dissertations and Theses Global. (Accession No. 7104376) http://proxyiub.uits.iu.edu/login?url=https://search.proquest.com/docview/302443067?accountid=11620

Loewenstein, S., & Reder, P. (1982). The consumers' response: Trainees' discussion of the experience of live supervision. In R. Whiffen & J. Byng-Hall (Eds.), *Family therapy supervision*. New York, NY: Grune and Stratton.

Lorio, C., Delehanty, A., & Woods, J. (2016). Digital platforms and supervisory feedback to graduate student clinicians. *Perspectives on Administration and Supervision, 1,* 18-34. doi:10.1044/persp1.SIG11.18

Lowery, L. (1970). *Learning about instruction: Questioning strategies: A personal workshop.* (ERIC Research Document # ED 113 297).

Luft, J. (1969). *Of human interaction.* Palo Alto, CA: National Press Books.

Luterman, D. (1984). *Counseling the communicatively disordered and their families.* Boston, MA: Little, Brown.

Mandel, S. (2015). Exploring the differences in expectations between supervisors and supervisees during the initial clinical experience. *Perspectives in Administration and Supervision, 25*(1), 4-15. doi:10.1044/aaa25.1.4

McCrea, E. (1994). Supervision as a Master's degree thesis option. In M. Bruce (Ed.), *Proceedings of the 1994 International & Interdisciplinary Conference on Clinical Supervision: Toward the 21st century* (pp. 221-229). Council of Supervisors in Speech-Language Pathology and Audiology, Cape Cod, MA.

McCrea, E. S. (1980). *Supervisee ability to self-explore and four facilitative dimensions of supervisor behavior in individual conferences in speech-language pathology* (Doctoral dissertation). Retrieved from ProQuest Dissertations and Theses Global. (Accession No. 8029239) http://proxyiub.uits.iu.edu/login?url=https://search.proquest.com/docview/303031 284?accountid=11620

McCready, V., Roberts, J., Bengala, D., Harris, H., Kingsley, G., & Krikorian, C. (1996). A comparison of conflict tactics in the supervisory process. *Journal of Speech and Hearing Research, 39,* 191-199.

McCready, V., Shapiro, D., & Kennedy, K. (1987). Identifying hidden dynamics in supervision: Four scenarios. In M. Crago & M. Pickering (Eds.), *Supervision in human communication disorders: Perspectives on a process.* San Diego, CA: College Hill Press.

McCready, V., & Wegner, J. (2006, April). *Team-based clinical education.* Presentation at Council of Academic Programs in Communication Sciences and Disorders (CAPCSD) annual conference. Destin, FL.

McFarlane, L., & Hagler, P. (1992a). An experimentally-based peer supervision component in a university clinic. In S. Dowling (Ed.), *Proceedings of the 1992 National Conference on Supervision—Total quality supervision: Effecting optimal performance* (pp. 78-84). Council of Supervisors in Speech-Language Pathology and Audiology, Nashville, TN.

McFarlane, L., & Hagler, P. (1992b). Effects of a supervisee-prepared agenda on conference interaction. In S. Dowling (Ed.), *Proceedings of the 1992 National Conference on Supervision—Total quality supervision: Effecting optimal performance* (pp. 85-91). Council of Supervisors in Speech-Language Pathology and Audiology, Nashville, TN.

Michalak, D. (1969). Supervisory conferences improve teaching. *Florida Educational Research and Development Council Research Bulletin, 5.*

Molyneaux, D., & Lane, V. (1982). *Effective interviewing: Techniques and analysis.* Boston, MA: Allyn and Bacon.

Mormer, E. & Messick, C. (2016, November 16). *Bringing the evidence to clinical education practices.* Pre-conference workshop presented at the American Speech-Language-Hearing Association Convention in Philadelphia, PA.

Mosher, R., & Purpel, D. (1972). *Supervision: The reluctant profession.* Boston, MA: Houghton Mifflin.

Oermann, M. (1997). Evaluation of critical thinking in clinical practice. *Nurse Educator, 22*(5), 25-28.

O'Sullivan, J., Peaper-Fillyaw, R., Plante, A., & Gottwald, S. (2014). On the road to self-supervision. *SIG 11 Perspectives, 24*(2), 44-50. doi:10.1044/aas24.2.44

Peaper, R. (1984). An analysis of student perceptions of the supervisory conference and student developed agendas for that conference. *The Clinical Supervisor, 2,* 55-64.

Peaper, R., & Mercaitis, P. (1987). The nature of narrative written feedback provided to student clinicians: A descriptive study. In S. Farmer (Ed.), *Clinical supervision: A coming of age.* Proceedings of a conference held at Jekyll Island, GA. Las Cruces, NM: New Mexico State University.

Pederson, P. B., & Ivey, A. (1993). *Culture-centered counseling and interviewing skills: A practical guide.* Westport, CT: Praeger.

Pickering, M. (1977). An examination of concepts operative in the supervisory process and relationship. *Asha, 19,* 607-610.

Pickering, M. (1979). *Interpersonal communication in speech-language pathology clinical practicum: A descriptive humanistic perspective* (Doctoral dissertation). Retrieved from ProQuest Dissertations and Theses Global. (Accession No. 7923892) http://proxyiub.uits.iu.edu/login?url=https://search.proquest.com/docview/303001992?accountid=11620

Pickering, M. (1984). Interpersonal communication in speech-language pathology supervisory conferences: A qualitative study. *Journal of Speech and Hearing Disorders, 49,* 189-195.

Pickering, M. (1986). *Communication. Explorations—A Journal of Research at the University of Maine.* Orono, ME: University of Maine.

Pickering, M. (1987a). Interpersonal communication and the supervisory process: A search for Ariadne's thread. In M. Crago and M. Pickering, (Eds.), *Supervision in human communication disorders: Perspectives on a process* (pp. 203-225). San Diego, CA: College-Hill Press.

Pickering, M. (1987b). Supervision: A person-focused process. In M. Crago & M. Pickering (Eds.), *Supervision in human communication disorders: Perspectives on a process.* San Diego, CA: College-Hill Press.

Pickering, M. (1990). The supervisory process: An experience of interpersonal relationships and personal growth. *National Student Speech-Language-Hearing Association Journal,* (17), 17-28.

Pickering, M., & McCready, V. (1983). Supervisory journals: An 'inside' look at supervision. *SUPER-vision, 7,* 5-7.

Pickering, M., & McCready, V. (1990). Interpersonal communication skills: A process in action. In *Clinical supervision across settings: communication and collaboration* (pp. 23-35). Rockville, MD: American Speech-Language-Hearing Association.

Pittinger, G.E. (1971). *An analysis of the patterns of verbal interaction and their relationship to self-reported satisfaction ratings and a measure of empathic accuracy in selecting secondary student teaching supervisory conferences* (Doctoral dissertation). Retrieved from ProQuest Dissertations and Theses Global. (Accession No. 7212847) http://proxyiub.uits.iu.edu/login?url=https://search.proquest.com/docview/302490167?accountid=11620

Rassi, J. (1978). *Supervision in audiology*. Baltimore, MD: University Park Press.

Rassi, J. (1987). The uniqueness of audiology supervision. In M. Crago & M. Pickering (Eds.), *Supervision in human communication disorders: Perspectives on a process* (pp. 31-54). San Diego, CA: Singular.

Rassi, J. (2001). A comparison of supervision practices in audiology and speech-language pathology. *California Speech-Language-Hearing Association (CSHA) Magazine, 30*(1), 12-13.

Rassi, J., & McElroy, M. (1992). Clinical teaching: Delineating competencies and planning strategies. In J. A. Rassi & M. D. McElroy (Eds.), *The education of audiologists and speech-language pathologists* (pp. 301-335). Timonium, MD: York Press.

Reuler, E., Messick, C., Gavett, E., McCready, V., & Raleigh, L. (2011, March). *Evidence-based practice for clinical education: What do we know and what can we do?* Proceedings of the Annual Conference of the Council of Academic Programs in Communication Sciences and Disorders, St. Petersburg, FL.

Roberts, J., & Smith, K. (1982). Supervisor-supervisee role differences and consistency of behavior in supervisory conferences. *Journal of Speech and Hearing Research, 25*, 428-434.

Rocchio, C., & Iacarino, J. (1990). *Written feedback provided to student clinicians*. Poster session presented at the annual convention of the American Speech-Language-Hearing Association, Seattle, WA.

Rock, M., Zigmond, N., Gregg, M., & Gable, R. (2011). The power of virtual coaching. *Educational Leadership, 69*(2), 42-48.

Rogers, C. (1951). *Client-centered therapy*. Boston, MA: Houghton-Mifflin Company.

Rogers, C. (1957). The necessary and sufficient conditions of therapeutic personality change. *Journal of Consulting Psychology, 21*, 95-103.

Rogers, C. (1961). *On becoming a person: A therapist's view of psychotherapy*. Boston, MA: Houghton Mifflin.

Rogers, C. (1962). The interpersonal relationship: The core of guidance. *Harvard Educational Review, 32*, 116-129.

Rogers, C. (1980). *A way of being*. Boston, MA: Houghton Mifflin.

Ruder, K., Simpson, K., Ruder, C., Smith, L., Trammel, R., & Landes, T. (1996). Laptop computer aids for supervision. In B. Wagner (Ed.), *Proceedings of the 1996 Conference on Clinical Supervision—Partnerships in supervision: Innovative and effective practices* (pp. 106-118). Council of Supervisors in Speech-Language Pathology and Audiology, Cincinnati, OH.

Russell, L. (1976). *Aspects of supervision*. Unpublished manuscript, Temple University, Philadelphia, PA.

Sanders, N. (1966). *Classroom questions: What kinds?* New York, NY: Harper and Row.

Sbaschnig, K., Dowling, S., & Williams, C. (1992). Agenda planning, talk time and question usage in the conference. In S. Dowling (Ed.), *Proceedings of the 1992 National Conference on Supervision—Total quality supervision: Effecting optimal performance* (pp. 92-96). Council of Supervisors in Speech-Language Pathology and Audiology, Nashville, TN.

Schon, D.A. (1983). *The reflective practitioner: How professionals think in action*. New York, NY: Basic Books.

Schubert, G., & Aitchison, C. (1975). A profile of clinical supervisors in college and university speech and hearing training programs. *Asha, 17*, 440-447.

Schubert, G., & Nelson, J. (1976). *Verbal behaviors occurring in speech pathology supervisory conferences*. Paper presented at the annual convention of the American Speech-Language-Hearing Association, Houston, TX.

Scott, C., Becker, T., & Simpson, K. (2017). Effect of real-time feedback using a smartwatch on clinical behavior of novice student clinicians. *Perspectives on Administration and Supervision, 2*, 79-90. doi:10.1044/persp2.SIG11.79

Seeley, J. U. (1973). *Interaction analysis between the supervisor and the speech and hearing clinician* (Doctoral dissertation). Retrieved from ProQuest Dissertations and Theses Global. (Accession No. 7329608) http://proxyiub.uits.iu.edu/login?url=https://search.proquest.com/docview/302664667?accountid=11620

Shapiro, D. (1985). *Clinical supervision: A process in progress*. National Student Speech-Language-Hearing Association Journal.

Shapiro, D. A. (1984). *An experimental and descriptive analysis of supervisees' commitments and follow-through behaviors as one measure of supervisory effectiveness in speech-language pathology and audiology* (Doctoral dissertation). Retrieved from ProQuest Dissertations and Theses Global. (Accession No. 8426682) http://proxyiub.uits.iu.edu/login?url=https://search.proquest.com/docview/303311796?accountid=11620

Shipley, K. (1997). *Interviewing and counseling in communicative disorders—Principles and procedures* (2nd ed.). Boston, MA: Allyn & Bacon.

Smith, K. (1979). *Supervisory conferences questions: Who asks them and who answers them*. Paper presented at the annual convention of the American Speech and Hearing Association, Atlanta, GA.

Smith, K., & Anderson, J. (1982a). Development and validation of an individual supervisory conference rating scale for use in speech-language pathology. *Journal of Speech and Hearing Research, 25*, 252-261.

Smith, K., & Anderson, J. (1982b). Relationship of perceived effectiveness to content in supervisory conferences in speech-language pathology. *Journal of Speech and Hearing Research, 25,* 243-251.

Smith, K. J. (1977). *Identification of perceived effectiveness components in the individual supervisory conference in speech pathology and an evaluation of the relationship between ratings and content in the conference* (Doctoral dissertation). Retrieved from ProQuest Dissertations and Theses Global. (Accession No. 7813175) http://proxyiub.uits.iu.edu/login?url=https://search.proquest.com/docview/302869635?accountid=11620

Smith, S., & Hardy, A. (2014). Use of iPad video-review feedback in the supervision of speech-language pathology student clinicians. *Perspectives on Administration and Supervision, 24*(2), 62-70. doi:10.1044/aas24.2.62

Smith, S. & Hardy, A. (2017). *Progressive clinical supervision practices for millennial clinicians.* Poster presentation at the American Speech-Language-Hearing Association Annual Convention, Los Angeles, CA.

Staltari, C., Baft-Neff, A., Marra, L., & Rentschler, G. (2010). Formative feedback for clinical documentation in a university speech-language pathology program. *Perspectives on Administration and Supervision, 20*(3), 117-123. doi:10.1044/aas20.3.117

Starkweather, C. W. (1974). Behavior modification in training speech clinicians: Procedures and implications. *Asha, 16,* 607-611.

Stone, D. & Heen, S. (2014). *Thanks for the feedback: The science and art of receiving feedback well.* New York, NY: Viking.

Strike, C. A. (1988). *Supervisors' implementation of trained information regarding broad questioning and discussion of supervision during their supervisory conferences in speech-language pathology* (Doctoral dissertation). Retrieved from ProQuest Dissertations and Theses Global. (Accession No. 8824185) http://proxyiub.uits.iu.edu/login?url=https://search.proquest.com/docview/303572273?accountid=11620

Tannen, D. (1990). *You just don't understand: Women and men in conversation.* New York, NY: William Morrow.

Tannen, D. (1994). *Talking from 9 to 5.* New York, NY: William Morrow.

Tepper, A., & Vaughn, A. (2017). *Reframing the big picture: Creating/sustaining a dynamic paradigm shift in clinical education via collaborative partnerships and transformative practices.* Presentation at annual American Speech-Language-Hearing Association national convention, Los Angeles, CA.

Tice, J. (2004). *Reflective teaching: Exploring our own classroom practice* [Teaching English/British Council/ BBC]. Retrieved from https://www.teachingenglish.org.uk/article/reflective-teaching-exploring-our-own-classroom-practice

Tihen, L. D. (1983). *Expectations of student speech/language clinicians during their clinical practicum* (Doctoral dissertation). Retrieved from ProQuest Dissertations and Theses Global. (Accession No. 8401620) http://proxyiub.uits.iu.edu/login?url=https://search.proquest.com/docview/303160597?accountid=11620

Tofade, T., Elsen, J., & Haines, S. (2013). Best practice strategies for effective use of questions as a teaching tool. *American Journal of Pharmaceutical Education, 77*(7), 155 doi:10.5688/ajpe777155.

Tufts, L. (1983). *A content analysis of supervisory conferences in communicative disorders and the relationship of the content analysis system to the clinical experience of supervisees* (Doctoral dissertation). Retrieved from ProQuest Dissertations and Theses Global. (Accession No. 8401588) http://proxyiub.uits.iu.edu/login?url=https://search.proquest.com/docview/303266850?accountid=11620

Tyack, D., & Ingram, D. (1977). Children's production and comprehension of questions. *Journal of Child Language, 4,* 211-224.

Underwood, J. (1973). *Interaction analysis between the supervisor and the speech and hearing clinician.* (Doctoral dissertation, University of Denver). Dissertation Abstracts International, 34, 2995B. (University Microfilms No.73-29,608)

Volz, H. B. (1975). *The effects on clinician performance, client progress, and client satisfaction of two programs to enhance the helping skills of undergraduate students in speech pathology* (Doctoral dissertation). Retrieved from ProQuest Dissertations and Theses Global. (Accession No. 7617239) http://proxyiub.uits.iu.edu/login?url=https://search.proquest.com/docview/302800387?accountid=11620

Volz, H., Klevans, D., Norton, S., & Putens, D. (1978). Interpersonal communication skills of speech-language pathology undergraduates: The effects of training. *Journal of Speech and Hearing Disorders, 43,* 524-541.

Wagner, B., McCrea, E., & Spigarelli, K. (1992). Supervisory conferences in speech-language pathology through computer electronic mail. In S. Dowling (Ed.), *Proceedings of the 1992 National Conference on Supervision—Total quality supervision: Effecting optimal performance* (pp. 97-105). Council of Supervisors in Speech-Language Pathology and Audiology, Nashville, TN.

Ward, L., & Webster, E. (1965a). The training of clinical personnel: I. Issues in conceptualization. *Asha, 7,* 38-41.

Ward, L., & Webster, E. (1965b). The training of clinical personnel: II. A concept of clinical preparation. *Asha, 7,* 103-106.

Wegner, J. (1999). K-TEAM: Empowering students. In P. Murphy (Ed.), *Proceedings of the Annual Conference on Graduate Education—New horizons* (pp. 100-106). Council of Academic Programs in Communication Sciences and Disorders, Minneapolis, MN.

Weller, R. (1971). *Verbal communication in instructional supervision.* New York, NY: Teachers College Press, Columbia University.

Weller, R. H. (1969). *An observational system for analyzing clinical supervision of teachers* (Doctoral dissertation). Retrieved from ProQuest Dissertations and Theses Global. (Accession No. 6918245) http://proxyiub.uits.iu.edu/login?url=https://search.proquest.com/docview/302414692?accountid=11620

Whiteside, J. (1981). *Analysis of question type in supervisory conferences and classroom in speech-language pathology.* Unpublished manuscript, Indiana University, Bloomington, IN.

Wilson, J., Welch, N., & Welling, R. (1996). Interactive supervision system: A tool for clinical teaching. In B. Wagner (Ed.), *Proceedings of the 1996 Conference on Supervision—Partnership in supervision: Innovative and effective practices* (pp. 196-198). Council of Supervisors in Speech-Language Pathology and Audiology, Cincinnati, OH.

Young, M. (2001). *Learning the art of helping: Building blocks and techniques* (2nd ed.). Upper Saddle River, NJ: Prentice-Hall.

Young, T., Lambie, G., Hutchinson, T. & Thurston-Dyer, J. (2011). The integration of reflectivity in developmental supervision: Implications for clinical supervisors. *The Clinical Supervisor, 30,* 1-18. doi: 10.1080/07325223.2011.532019

 This chapter is a revision of that appearing in the 2003 edition of this book.

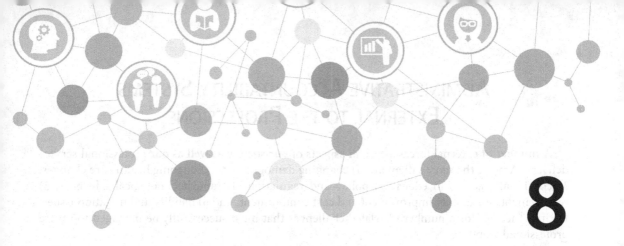

8

Accountability and Preparation of Clinical Educators and Supervisors

Elizabeth S. McCrea, PhD, CCC-SLP, F-ASHA and
Judith A. Brasseur, PhD, CCC-SLP, F-ASHA

The hallmark of any mature profession is the accountability it demonstrates for its processes and practices. There is ample evidence of this in what has become a rather vast literature for relatively young professions. There is further evidence in the continually increasing standards set by the Council for Accreditation of Academic Programs (CAA) and the Council for Clinical Certification (CFCC) to assure that patients and clients served by the professions receive the best possible services.

As the professions have continued their concern for clinical accountability, certain formalized systems have been developed through the CAA and CFCC and other agencies external to the professions that focus on administrative accountability and also influence supervisory practices. The thesis for this book is on supervisors as facilitators of objective supervisee self-analysis or on joint analysis as a teaching process that enables the participants to make changes in behavior to better meet objectives that have been set to support supervisee professional growth. It is argued that this learning process will result in greater generalization of knowledge and skill and greater self-awareness by supervisees and enable them to measure their own progress. As a result, they become accountable for their own continued growth as well as accountable for their work with their patients and clients. The role of the supervisor is pivotal in this teaching dynamic and, consequently, the preparation of supervisors to competently fulfill their role is important to the fidelity of the professions' training practices. Preparing to function as a supervisor is another aspect of supervisor accountability that is fundamental to the work that we do with our supervisees, and by extension, to the service that is provided to patients and clients.

McCrea, E. S., & Brasseur, J. A. *The Clinical Education and*
Supervisory Process in Speech-Language Pathology and Audiology (pp 259-310).
© 2020 Taylor & Francis Group.

Administrative Accountability Systems External to the Professions

A number of external forces affect all aspects of our society as well as our professional service delivery. Among the more salient are: 1) changing demographics, 2) ongoing health care changes, 3) continual changes in education policy and regulation, 4) rapid technological advances, 5) requirements for quality improvement and cost containment, and 6) liability and litigation issues. Each of these yields a number of related challenges that must successfully be managed to insure professional viability.

Demographics

Lubinski and Fratalli (2001) identified four factors with regard to the increasing and changing population. First is the growing number of persons with disabilities. Second is the number of clinically complex cases. In a report released to coincide with the anniversary of the American with Disabilities Act in 2012, the U.S. Census Bureau (2016b) indicated that there were 56.7 million Americans who reported that they had a disability and about one half of that number indicated that it was a severe condition. The prevalence of clients with comorbidities and multiple disabilities present assessment and intervention challenges.

Third is the aging of Americans. According to the Kaiser Family Foundation (n.d.), 28% of the population is 55 years old or older. Many of these individuals are beginning to retire and will have an impact on the demand for health care and related services. Conversely, the youngest members of the population who are between 0 and 18 years old comprise 24% of the population and will pose some challenges for the educational system. This Net Generation—those growing up with the Internet, computers and technology, and social media, and who expect rapid and continuous connectivity—will be a significant driver in the changes in education and ultimately the workforce.

Simultaneously, there has been an explosion the diversity of those living in the United States. The number of persons identifying as Black or African American according to the U.S. Census Bureau (2016b) is 13.4% of the population. According to the 2016 American Community Survey (U.S. Census Bureau, 2016a), those of Hispanic or Latino heritage composed 17.3% of the total population of the United States and those of Asian heritage composed 5.2%. While these are the primary minority populations at the current time, there are also individuals from Africa, the Caribbean, and the Pacific Islands who also contribute to the complexity of the population. This complexity challenges the social, health care, and educational systems that must try and meet their needs.

Health Care

The utilization of health insurance has become a challenge in light of the repeal of some aspects of the Affordable Care Act and the modification of it through changes in regulation. Complicating the insurance landscape even more is the fact that Medicare, Medicaid, and private insurers all have their own frameworks for what services they will support as well as the nature of supervision of students in the provision of those services to their insureds. Technological advances are influencing service delivery as well as the documentation of health care. The Health Insurance Portability and Protection Act governs the manner in which patient information can be shared and transmitted. The internet is increasing the level of sophistication of consumers about their health care as well as influencing their participation in it. The Human Genome Project and other genetic mapping research will continue to yield powerful opportunities for disease prevention as well as treatment. Payer sources are demanding greater cost effectiveness through coordinated care between collaborating specialties, which has implications for increased interprofessional practice .

Education

Federal legislation and regulation have influenced school practices for several decades. The Family Educational Rights and Privacy Act gives parents certain protections with regard to their children's educational record. General education and functional behavior assessments impact individualized education program content and implementation. Mirroring population trends, students are more culturally diverse and some do not speak English as their first language. Speech-language pathologists are increasingly combining classroom-based service delivery with more traditional pull-out service delivery and this requires collaboration and interprofessional practice with regular and special education colleagues. The Americans with Disabilities Act has provided access to augmentative communication (AAC) technology to support both the communication and education processes.

Technology

Technology plays a significant and vital role in service delivery. Procedures for swallowing assessment, vocal tract imaging, infant hearing screening, cochlear implant rehabilitation, and AAC are only a few of the technological advances that influence the practice of speech-language pathology and audiology. Treatment options have been extended and enhanced for both children and adults through the use of iPads and similar electronic platforms. In addition, information technology has had an impact both on consumers and service providers. Telehealth practices are increasingly more evident and are being regulated by both governmental and payer sources. Web-based teaching and distance learning are providing self-paced, self-directed learning opportunities for increasing numbers of students and practitioners alike.

Quality Improvement and Cost Containment

The Joint Commission, which accredits health care organizations, and the Joint Commission on Accreditation of Rehabilitation Facilities, which accredits rehabilitation facilities, both mandate quality improvement initiatives for their organizations. Quality improvement programs enable service providers to demonstrate treatment effectiveness and to contribute to the knowledge base about clinical outcomes. Universities, public schools, and health care settings all are demanding that workers do more with fewer resources. Cost containment can also mean fewer, less expensive, and more multiskilled personnel.

Liability and Litigation

In today's litigious society, it is inconceivable to practice without liability insurance. As the professions continue to engage in invasive and technologically complex procedures, risks increase. The ability to demonstrate competent evidence-based practice to document procedures and outcomes and to demonstrate accountability for our work is imperative. Importantly, professionals must keep abreast of current state and federal legislation and laws that govern our practice in their immediate work environment. The American Speech-Language-Hearing Association's (ASHA) governmental affairs website provides an excellent resource for this.

ADMINISTRATIVE ACCOUNTABILITY SYSTEMS INTERNAL TO THE PROFESSIONS

American Speech-Language-Hearing Association's Position Statement on Clinical Supervision

The professions, through the then legislative council, adopted the "Position Statement of Clinical Supervision in Speech-Language Pathology and Audiology" (ASHA, 1985). This statement identified clinical supervision as a distinct area of professional practice and specified 13 tasks and 81 supporting competencies fundamental to its competent execution. Subsequently, in 2008, the ASHA (2008a, 2008b) Ad Hoc Committee on Supervision reinforced the notion of supervision as a distinct area of practice and reorganized the original 13 knowledge areas into 11 core areas of knowledge along with their attendant skills. The knowledge and skills identified in these two documents need to be understood and implemented by those who function as supervisors of clinical activity.

Subsequently, the professions through the board of directors, adopted the reports of ASHA (2013) Ad Hoc Committee on Supervision (AHCS) and Ad Hoc Committee on Supervision Training (AHCST, 2016d), both of which also recognized that supervision is a distinct area of practice. In addition, the 2013 report also identified five distinct groups of people and settings that can present unique supervision challenges and recommended supervisors working in these settings and with these groups have specific training to ensure effective supervision. These groups include 1) individuals in academic training programs who supervise graduate students, 2) individuals in clinical or educational settings who provide externship or off-campus supervision to graduate students, 3) practitioners who supervise audiology or speech-language pathology assistants, 4) speech-language pathologists who supervise clinical fellows and audiologists who supervise audiology clinical doctoral students in the final externship, and 5) speech-language pathologists and audiologists who supervise credentialed colleagues who are changing their primary clinical focus or work setting (ASHA, 2013). The AHCST (ASHA, 2016a) identified supervision knowledge and skills goals specific to each of the five unique supervision groups and suggested a sequenced approach for supervisor training.

Council for Clinical Certification and the Council on Academic Accreditation

The Certificate of Clinical Competence (CCC) in either speech-language pathology or audiology is awarded to those applicants who have met the established standards developed by the CFCC. The standards identify the master's degree as the entry-level for professional practice in speech-language pathology and the Doctor of Audiology in audiology and stipulate the practicum requirements that must be incorporated into the course of study. These standards are reviewed and revised periodically to reflect the current Scope of Practice in Speech-Language Pathology and Audiology (ASHA, 2016e); in addition to recognition of practice in disorder areas, the current document recognizes supervision as a distinct area of practice. The Preferred Practice Patterns in Audiology and in Speech-Language Pathology (ASHA, 2006) contain a concrete statement by the professions about the minimum education and training standards requisite for the provision of competent services to communicatively disordered persons.

In addition to the standards for coursework and practica, the CFCC also stipulates the minimum standards for supervision of students during their practica experiences in speech-language pathology "must be provided by individuals who hold the ASHA CCC in the appropriate profession (V-E). The amount of direct supervision must be commensurate with the student's level of knowledge, skills, and experience, must not be less than 25% of the student's total contact with each client/patient, and take place periodically through the practicum and was sufficient to ensure the welfare of the client/patient" (CFCC, 2014). In audiology, applicants for the certificate must document a course of study and supervised clinical practicum sufficient in breadth and depth to achieve knowledge and skills identified in the (academic) standards and supervised by someone holding the CCC in audiology.

These requirements focus on the administrative aspects of the supervisory process and have been a part of the standards in one form or another since their inception. The CAA (2017) standards also imply clinical education processes that are consistent with the continuum model of supervision foundational to this book: The amount of supervision must be appropriate to the student's level of knowledge, experience, and competence (Stds. 3.7B and 3.8B in speech-language pathology and 3.6A, 3.7A, and 3.8A in audiology). Additionally, the standard requiring "demonstration of processes used in research and of the integration of research principles into evidence-based practice" (Std. 3.5B) is also consistent with this book's foundation in that evidence-based practice is dependent on the scientific method and necessitates the application of data and scientific evidence to clinical decision making.

The Code of Ethics

The Code of Ethics (ASHA, 2016c) recognizes that "the preservation of the highest standards of integrity and ethical principles is vital to the responsible discharge of obligations by audiologists, speech-language pathologists, and speech, language, and hearing scientists who serve as clinicians, educators, mentors, researchers, supervisors and administrators." Fully three of the four Principles of Ethics (and their implementing Rules of Ethics) speak to this obligation in regard to the supervisory process.

- Principle of Ethics I: Individuals shall honor their responsibility to hold paramount the welfare of persons they serve professionally or who are participants in research or scholarly activities, and they treat animals involved in research in a humane manner.
- Principle of Ethics II: Individuals shall honor their responsibility to achieve and maintain the highest level of professional competence and performance.
- Principle of Ethics IV: Individuals shall uphold the dignity and autonomy of professions, maintain harmonious interprofessional and intraprofessional relationships, and accept the profession's self-imposed standards.

Given the intent as well as the content of the previous two documents, it is clear that the Code of Ethics compels those engaged in the supervisory process to develop and maintain current skills both as a clinician and as a clinical educator/supervisor.

PREPARATION FOR THE SUPERVISORY PROCESS

The 1985 position statement (ASHA, 1985) and its counterpart in 2008 (ASHA, 2008a) both legitimized supervision as a distinct area of professional practice and expertise and stipulate that special preparation is needed to enable individuals to function competently as supervisors. Even before these documents, however, a number of early surveys in our disciplines revealed that supervisors felt the need for training in supervision (Anderson, 1972, 1973a; Schubert & Aitchison, 1975; Stace & Drexler, 1969). In a survey of the membership of Special Interest Group 11, Administration and Supervision in 2010, 67.6% of those responding (406/1,051) indicated that they felt formal training in supervision was very important (Victor, 2010). But, the notion "that anyone who has been supervised, can supervise" remained alive and well until 2013. This was a watershed year during which the 2013 Council of Academic Programs in Communication Sciences and Disorders

(CAPCSD) issued a white paper that called for training, and the ASHA (2013) Ad Hoc Committee on Supervision also called for training and preparation of supervisors. The 2016 AHCST continued to call for training and offered topics for supervision training in its final report (ASHA, 2016d and Appendix 8-1), which suggested supervisor training targets based on core knowledge and skills identified in the 2008 policy document.

Beginning in January 2020, the CFCC will implement a standard that will require that those who supervise students in practicum hold the CCC for at least 9 months and will document 2 hours of approved professional development in supervision before they may supervise a student (Flahive, 2018). To help supervisors meet this new and important standard, CAPCSD's Web-Based Professional Development Initiative, which contains learning modules in support of best practices in clinical education and supervision and is available for continuing education (CE) credit to member programs, is an important and powerful resource. Currently, two modules are available (Foundations of Clinical Education and Effective Student-Clinical Educator Relationships) with 2 to 4 additional modules scheduled to be developed in the near future. In addition, the ASHA Practice Portal (https://www.asha.org/Practice-Portal/Professional-Issues/) contains multiple resources in support of individual clinical educators and supervisors, including materials from the report of the Ad Hoc Committee on Supervision Training (ASHA, 2016a, 2016b, 2016d). However, given the welcome challenge of the CFFC's 2020 standard, other approaches to the preparation of supervisors are important to consider.

Training for Clinical Educators and Preceptors in Allied Disciplines

The 2013 CAPCSD white paper contained a brief survey of preparation initiatives fielded by other allied health disciplines. At that time, only two (physical therapy and occupational therapy) offered training; however, it was not required, even though the curriculum was formalized and structured, and it did not result in any kind of credential. Athletic training, on the other hand, did not require a specific curriculum but did require training that results in a credential. The remaining disciplines (nursing, psychiatry, social work and counseling, therapeutic recreation, speech-language pathology, audiology) were silent on training and, therefore, silent on curriculum.

Borders (2005) in a comprehensive 5-year review of published journal articles on counseling and counselor education recognized the absence of a consistent framework for preparation of the supervisors of counseling supervisees, but, through her review, identified several themes that could provide direction for such training:

- Continued evidence of and concern for a lack of clinical supervision for counseling practitioners, especially those in the schools—of particular concern the "extensive misunderstanding" of what clinical supervision is and the confusion of it as program management and administration, not clinical education
- Absolute critical role of the supervisory relationship and supervisor responsibility to create a safe, trusting, challenging, and open environment
- Greater attention to relationship dynamics, especially how to manage difficult relationship issues
- Need to discuss similarities and differences in multicultural supervision was identified
- Feedback as a challenge for supervisors who seemed reluctant to give negative feedback and preferred indirect over direct methods
- Management of ethical issues

Most importantly, this review found further support for the need for training of supervisors, including supervised practice.

Milne, Sheikh, Pattison, and Wilkinson (2011) conducted a systematic review of 11 controlled studies that assessed the implementation of evidenced-based practices in supervisor training in psychotherapy and counselling in the United Kingdom. The authors noted the salience of supervision as the cornerstone in training supervisors but, yet, no concerted effort to train them for that role. Further, although there were a number of supervision courses referenced in these studies, there was no apparent consensus about what constituted good training. This review also suggested that clear empirical support existed for supervisor training and that feedback, educational role play, and modeling (live or video demonstration) were provisionally supported training methods.

PREPARATION IN SPEECH-LANGUAGE PATHOLOGY AND AUDIOLOGY

Previously, impetus for preparation was primarily one of self-motivation; however, with the advent of the 2020 CFCC standard requiring documented professional development in supervision, it will be mandatory to acquire minimal training.

Content of Supervisory Preparation

Content will vary depending on the orientation of the program and the instructor's philosophy. This book presents Anderson's (1988) approach, which was based on the clinical supervision model of Cogan (1973; Goldhammer, 1969; Goldhammer, Anderson, & Krajewski, 1980) and influenced by situational leadership theory (Hersey & Blanchard, 1982). Anderson (1988) stated, "It has never been assumed that this is the only way to supervise" (p. 229) and she acknowledged the merit of other approaches. What is assumed to be absolutely essential is that those who supervise or those who teach others about the supervisory process have some model, some theoretical base, some solid foundation on which they can build their procedures, form hypotheses, and develop their plans. Without this foundation, supervision and instruction are likely to be fragmented, inconsistent, and lacking in direction and focus, with no rationale and justification.

There are certain types of information and certain skills related to the supervisory process that supervisors must acquire. The question about the content of such preparation is not what it should be, but what can be selected from the vast array of core knowledge and skills that are important to the supervisor within a variety of supervisory environments. Appendix A of the ASHA (2016a) Ad Hoc Committee on Supervision Training can be very helpful in this regard and provide a focus for training. Gazzola, DeStefano, Theriault, and Audet (2013) citing Falender et al. (2004), support the notion of a competency-based framework for supervisors as a precursor to developing training goals and outcomes specific to supervision competence.

MODELS OF PREPARATION IN THE SUPERVISORY PROCESS

There are many ways in which preparation in the supervisory process can be implemented. The approaches suggested here range from inclusion of information in early clinical management courses, to preparation at the doctoral level, to CE opportunities for practicing professionals. In each instance, there are different purposes and different strategies of implementation.

Inclusion in Clinical Management Courses

Training programs typically offer a course on clinical methods/clinical management procedures prior to or in conjunction with practica. It is highly recommended that basic information about the supervisory process be included in such a course. A basic introduction to the supervisory process at this point makes it easier for individual supervisor/supervisee dyads to begin a discussion of their own individual interaction. The purpose at this level is to assist supervisees in learning what to expect of supervision, their role and responsibilities, and how to maximize their clinical training.

McCrea (1985), in describing a component on supervision in an undergraduate clinical management class, listed the objectives as the following: 1) to encourage undergraduate students to view the clinical and supervisory processes as complementary and interactive; 2) to introduce undergraduate students to the participants and their primary roles and responsibilities within both processes; and 3) to introduce undergraduate students to problem-solving strategies to enhance both processes. McCrea then made the point that each part of the clinical process has its counterpart in the supervisory process and that they can be taught in such a way that the complementary and interactive natures of the two processes is emphasized. For example, assessment of and goal setting for the client have their counterparts in goal setting for the clinician's development, as do observation, data collection, and data analysis. Because time may be limited in such courses for inclusion of the topic, the instructor must be knowledgeable about the process and able to distill the information into meaningful concepts appropriate to the students' level. Such content should extend beyond the undergraduate level.

Even advanced graduate students will profit from opportunities to discuss their changing roles as supervisees. McCrea (1985) suggested such procedures as lectures, problem solving, and in-class discussion, as well as "hand on experiences...through the presentation of actual samples of supervisory problems, experiences with observation tools, and viewing and analysis of videotaped samples of supervisory conference behavior" (p. 3).

Some programs pair inexperienced clinicians with more advanced clinicians, easing inexperienced clinicians into the clinical process by having them first observe then gradually assume some responsibility for therapy interaction. This is an excellent opportunity for the supervisor to present some basis supervisory concepts to the advanced clinician and to provide them with opportunities to "test drive" the supervisory process with the assistance of the supervisor. They are able to learn something about the dynamics of the process at an early stage in their careers.

Basic Course in Supervision

Coursework in supervision is provided for master's degree or doctoral-level students in some colleges and universities. It is also often taken by professionals in the field who are supervising or preparing to do so. The wisdom of providing a course in supervision as part of the master's degree curriculum is borne from the fact that, historically, the major portion of the supervision of practica is performed by professionals who hold master's degrees, most of them without preparation or even much clinical experience (Anderson, 1972, 1973a, 1973b; Schubert & Aitchison, 1975; Stace & Drexler, 1969). Additionally, it is reasonable to assume that students and professionals who have the opportunity to take a course in supervision become better participants in the process. Knowledge of the process seems to give them more confidence about their own participation and an understanding of what they can expect to gain from the process.

The wisdom of such a course for doctoral-level students is similar. Most intend to obtain positions in academe where responsibilities are apt to include supervision of students, preparing them to become clinicians, or supervising in other settings. Further, if they have the CCC, they may be engaged in the supervision as doctoral students at the time they are taking the course. Such a course should include at least the following topics: relevant information on supervision from related disciplines; preparation for the role of supervisor; professional issues in supervision in speech-language pathology and audiology; the planning, and analysis role of the supervisor relative to both the clinical and supervisory processes; supervisory techniques; interpersonal aspects of the supervisory process; variations in supervision across sites; accountability and evaluation in the supervisory process; preparing supervisees for the process; and research in supervision. Assignments should include extensive readings from the speech-language pathology and audiology literature as well as from other disciplines; viewing of conferences; self-study of interactions within these conferences as a supervisor or supervisee; a research proposal or literature review on a specific topic in supervision or other assignments that meet individual needs and interests. The course content should be oriented so that it could be taken by both speech-language pathologist and audiologists.

Such courses and their content were discussed by Anderson, Rassi, Laccionle, Casey, Brasseur, McCrea, Ulrich, Ganz, and Hunt-Thompson in an ASHA Convention Short Course moderated by Smith (1985). Rassi described an introductory course for advanced students in the audiology graduate program who aspire to supervisory positions or have an interest in supervision in on-and off-campus experiences. Rassi noted that the course provided an opportunity for potential supervisors to study the process as they experienced it. Content included an examination of supervision research, methodology and theory in communication sciences and disorders, leadership and supervisory styles, data collection, conference analysis, interpersonal relationships, observation, attribution and judgment, and evaluation and self-evaluation. Activities included participation in laboratory experiences or practicum that was monitored by a regular staff supervisor, listening to conference interactions, keeping a journal, and role-playing of supervision interactions.

Coursework described by Casey (1985) had content and requirements similar to Rassi's (see Smith, 1985) but focused more on ASHA's core knowledge and skill areas. It included a practicum experience, conference analysis, and use of self-assessment instruments based on the ASHA knowledge and skill areas. Casey reported that the material in the course not only prepares individuals to supervise, but also enhances the student's performance as a supervisee. Dowling (1993, 1994) has repeatedly demonstrated the benefits that completing a course in supervision has for graduate students. Harris, Ludington, Roberts, Hooper, and Ringwalt (1992), in a training project conducted in North Carolina, noted that the graduate students who completed a course in supervision appeared to be more self-analytical and able to function within the framework of Anderson's (1988) model better that those who did not.

Practicum Experiences in Supervision

Each of the courses described has included a very important laboratory or practicum component. Just as clinicians need practice in developing clinical skills, supervisors also need opportunities to "field test" the skills they are learning about. Appendix A of the ASHA (2016) Ad Hoc Committee on Supervision Training report provides a basis for identifying such skills.

The practicum experience as part of a doctoral-level preparation program was described by Anderson (1981) as probably the most significant component of a training program. "This experience is a necessary step in gaining insight about the supervisory process, in the modification of the supervisory behavior of trainees, and in defining the questions that lead to research in the supervisory process" (p. 80). Interestingly enough, 37 years later, Borders (2005), in her 5-year review of clinical supervision training in counselor education, found empirical evidence that supervised supervision experiences are requisite to supervisor development and she recommended supervisor training programs include experiential components—ongoing practice with feedback—as well as didactic instruction.

Procedures for Anderson's doctoral level practicum (1981) in supervision was a function of need. Some doctoral students had experience in supervision and all had the CCC. They were assigned a certain number of master's-level student clinicians to supervise. The doctoral student planned, observed, analyzed the clinical work and held conferences with the students. Similarly, their work was planned, observed, analyzed, and discussed in conferences with the faculty directing the supervision practicum. Extensive use of audio and video recordings and interaction analysis systems provided the conference content.

Practicum or laboratory experience for the master's level students must be handled differently because they do not hold the CCC and, therefore, cannot be independently responsible for supervising student clinicians. They will need to be assigned to a clinical supervisor and involved in the supervisory process at whatever level is appropriate. At the beginning of the experience, the faculty supervisor, the student supervisor, and the student clinician to be supervised discussed the purpose of the experience, set objectives, and developed a plan for the semester. This plan included the student supervisor's role in observation, data collection, and analysis of clinical sessions. It also included procedures for observation, data collection, and analysis of conferences between the student supervisor, the student clinician, and the faculty supervisor. The plan specified procedures to be used: observation systems or other data collection methods, journal writing, observation of others, methods of analysis and reporting in the conference, and other suitable activities. The use of portfolios certainly provided a useful procedure for measuring growth. Conferences may be held between the two supervisory dyads (student clinician–student supervisor and faculty supervisor–student supervisor) or in a supervisory triad (faculty supervisor, student supervisor, and student clinician). In each case, the opportunity for self-analysis, discussion, and determination of progress toward set objectives was important. The use of contemporary electronic record keeping systems enhances the functionality of documentation procedures for both the clinical and supervisory processes and increases the efficiency of building and maintaining records for both.

Master's Level Preparation

McCrea (1994) developed a two-part master's degree option that included a three-credit hour seminar and a modified practicum experience. The seminar fully developed the dynamics of each component of Anderson's model. For example, strategies for implementing the integration phase in the context of supervisory conferences were discussed as were concept of immediacy, relational communication, conflict resolution and the importance of both verbal and nonverbal communication strategies. Students learn a variety of strategies to observe, analyze, and evaluate both the clinical and supervisory processes. The second component involved a modification of the Teaching Clinic (Dowling, 2001; Michalak, 1969) to allow students to apply what they learned in the seminar in the development of their own supervisory process skills. In using the Teaching Clinic for guided practice in supervision, each demonstration supervisee contributes a segment of a video-recorded supervisory conference and indicates what data he or she wanted to be collect to determine if objectives were met. The demonstration supervisee also indicated what data collection tools were to be used. The peer observers then viewed the recording, gathered and analyzed the data, problem solved the interaction, and decided how to provide feedback to the demonstration supervisee in the most complete and supportive manner. The demonstration supervisee remained in the room or not, at his or her discretion. Once the analysis phase was completed, the demonstration supervisee presented his or her own self-analysis followed by group feedback, problem solving, and generation of strategies for the next conference. This cycle repeated itself for as many student supervisees and weeks as there were available.

In a case study, Dowling and Biskynis (1993) examined the impact of a course in supervision and a subsequent practicum on the behavior of a graduate student. Pre- and post-measures of conferencing ability were obtained using a simulation experience to assess course outcomes. After studying Cogan's (1973) clinical supervision model and Anderson's (1988) continuum model of supervision and discussions with the instructor, the student established three goals and contracted to change these behaviors in her final conference at the end of the term. In the subsequent term, the student trainee enrolled in practicum. She was assigned to supervise a first semester clinician, teaming with the faculty supervisor who was certified. Over the course of the semester, the trainee assumed increasing responsibility for the student clinician although the instructor met regularly with the trainee and also observed supervisory conferences. They also completed joint analyses of conferences. Academic training resulted in changes in the trainee's talk time. Those behaviors for which grade contingencies were established consistently improved as well.

The practicum portion of each of these models highlight the importance of providing opportunities to apply concrete concepts learned in a course as well as the opportunity to practice these same skills. As stated previously, developing new behaviors requires practice, analysis of performance, and feedback. These approaches also provided workable models of how a practicum in supervision can be arranged for master's students in the absence of the CCC which is required for autonomous supervisory practice.

Preparation of Off-Campus Supervisors

Virtually every training program makes use of off-campus external placements to provide students with the variety of clinical populations and the intensity of practicum experience necessary to meet academic and certification standards. If preparation can make a difference in the effectiveness of on-campus supervisors, as is assumed, mechanisms for providing similar experiences should be available to off-campus sites as well. In 2020, with the requirement that all supervisors demonstrate 2 hours of CE in the supervisory process, what has been discretionary, will be mandatory. As noted earlier in this chapter, CAPCSD has developed a series of web-based, high-quality, dynamic e-learning courses to promote best practices in clinical supervision; these courses will be available at no cost to council member programs and their affiliated external supervisors and will carry CE units through ASHA and American Academy of Audiology. In addition, many programs provide educational offerings for off-campus supervisors in the form of regular credit courses or in-service offerings; however, with the availability of the CAPCSD modules for program-affiliated supervisors, these kinds of opportunities may not be as readily available nor as necessary on a program by program basis.

Even with this availability of systematic training, it is the university supervisor who will remain pivotal in helping off-campus supervisors apply that information in a productive way to the supervision of students. Brasseur (1985) developed a three-semester nine-credit hour program that included didactic, classroom-based content as well as a practicum in the supervisory process for off-campus supervisors who worked in public schools. The CAPCSD training modules obviate the need for traditional classroom instruction but the application of the instruction may need some support from the university supervisor. Brasseur's approach to a practicum seminar might be a case in point to support this process. It used a variety of formats: direct on-site observation of the site supervisor by the university supervisor, recorded interactions between the student and the site supervisor, and group discussions between the university supervisor and all of the site supervisors. Just as the site supervisor and student planned, so the work of the site supervisor was planned, observed, analyzed, and discussed with the faculty supervisor in periodic conferences. Once a month, all site supervisors met on campus to view and analyze video recordings, discuss problems, and plan objectives and strategies to enhance their supervisory competencies. In follow-up evaluations, the site supervisors indicated that the practicum was an essential component to their total preparation in the supervisory process.

Doctoral-Level Preparation

Beginning in 1972, a doctoral-level program, in which the main emphasis was preparation in the supervisory process, was funded by the U.S. Department of Education at Indiana University under the direction of Jean Anderson, (1981, 1985). The program was funded for 10 years and was, subsequently, continued by the university. McCrea secured additional funding from the Department of Education from 1990 to 1993. Since 1972, 19 dissertations and numerous theses on aspects of the supervisory process have been completed. The program was refined so that the following guidelines can be presented for others who are interested in developing a similar initiative:
- The objectives of a doctoral-level program should be a) to prepare personnel who can teach other supervisors and b) to prepare researchers in the supervisory process.

- The core content of the program should include at least the following: a) an introductory course that provides a framework and introduces the supervisory literature in speech-language pathology and audiology; b) an advanced seminar in which research in the supervisory process is studied extensively (this must include the 25 or more dissertations that have been identified in speech-language pathology supervision); c) practicum experiences directed toward ASHA core knowledge and skill (ASHA, 2008a, 2008b, 2013, 2016d); d) independent study as needed to fill the areas not covered in coursework and practica; e) research experiences; and f) dissertation.

- Programs for doctoral students should be individually planned, based on students' experience and needs. In addition to coursework, practicum, and research experience in supervision, each program should include a concentration in another area of speech-language pathology so that the student will be able to contribute to the total teaching mission of the university once they attain their degree. This is important, because the reality is that most university programs are not currently able to employ a faculty member to teach only supervision coursework. Although many programs desire someone who has preparation in supervision, their budgets require that they find prospective employees who can teach in more than one area.

- Programs should include a strong research emphasis—both academic and experiential—because of the significant need for research about the supervisory process. Research competencies to be achieved should be identified.

- Programs should meet all the basic requirements of the regular doctoral program in the university: research, dissertation and qualifying examinations.

- Whenever possible, courses from other departments of the university that are relevant to students' goals should be included in their program: business management, counseling, education, psychology, cognitive science, special education, instructional technology, and so on.

- Because most doctoral students are preparing themselves to teach in universities, they should have an opportunity for teaching experience. This experience should be supervised by faculty in the content area. Many campuses also offer noncredit programs that prepare individuals for their role as instructors and help them develop competencies for effective classroom teaching.

In addition, a minor concentration consisting of coursework and practicum should be available for doctoral students who prefer to concentrate in another area but wish to obtain some information about and experience in the supervisory process.

Continuing Education

Standards for renewal of the CCC in the professions mandate continued professional development for maintenance of the certificate. Every 3 years, certificate holders must accrue three CE units (30 hours) to renew their CCC and a portion of those hours might be acquired in supervision and clinical education. Additionally, almost all states require CE requirements for the renewal of licenses and/or public school credentials.

CE hours to be used to renew the CCC must be earned from an approved CE provider. Many states, universities, for-profit and not-for-profit providers and most importantly, ASHA are eligible providers. Within ASHA, Special Interest Groups (e.g., Special Interest Group 11, Administration and Supervision) offer CE sessions at ASHA and through their online journal, *Perspectives*. As 2020 approaches, it is likely that an increasing number of CE experiences will be available at both national and state conferences which will provide content in support of supervisors and the supervisory process. These opportunities will be especially important to supervisors of clinical fellows, speech-language pathology assistants, and others working in settings without a direct affiliation with a training program and access to the CAPCSD training modules.

IS EDUCATION IN SUPERVISION EFFECTIVE?

As preparation in the supervisory process continues to grow, the professions will need to ask themselves some searching questions. Any kind of educational program costs time and money and effort on the part of the teacher and the learner. The effectiveness of the teaching-learning process needs to be demonstrated. Further, the variety of possible approaches to preparation must be investigated. We need to know if preservice preparation is effective; in other words, if education at the graduate level carries over into the future when the supervisee becomes the supervisor. There is also a need to know if CE can be designed to meet the needs of adult professionals in a skill area such as supervision. Particularly important at the present time, because many of the offerings appear to be CE, are certain questions about their effectiveness:

- What is the effect of convention presentations with their wide variety from scientific reports, to didactic, tutorial sessions?
- What is the value of a 3- or 6-hour workshop that may include a period of group discussion or experimental activity in changing attitudes that help participants develop a philosophy about supervision or identify and modify their skills?
- What is learned by the professional who has supervised for years, whose habits are firmly established, and who is taking a course merely to meet certification or organizational requirements?
- Is the use of distance and web-based instruction and other new communication systems more effective than face-to-face instruction?

The work of Borders (2005) in counselling and Milne et al. (2011) in psychotherapy each found that training in supervision was important to supervisor development but it was unclear what aspects of training were the most salient. Gazzola et al. (2013, citing Lyon, Heppler, Leavitt, & Fisher, 2008) found that the total number of supervision activities (both didactic and practical), together with the total number of supervision hours were found to predict overall supervisory development and more hours of training seemed to predict better development. Edrich (2014) found that a basic 3-hour online training workshop could increase knowledge but did not change supervisor's expectations or attitudes.

Need for Research on the Preparation of Supervisors

With the adoption of the position statements (ASHA, 1985, 2008a) on supervision and subsequent reports of the Ad Hoc Committees on Supervision (ASHA, 2013, 2016d), the need to prepare supervisors for their roles was officially recognized. With that came the need for research, not only to validate the tasks and competencies/knowledge and skills contained in those documents, but also to determine how to effectively and efficiently prepare supervisors to evidence the tasks and execute the skills.

Dowling (1986) analyzed the task behavior of two supervisors enrolled in a doctoral program with emphasis on the clinical supervision approach (Cogan, 1973; Goldhammer, 1969). She found their behavior to be different than that of supervisors in other descriptive studies involving supervisory conferences (Culatta & Seltzer, 1976; Roberts & Smith, 1982; Smith, 1979). Conferences included more equality in the relationship; supervisors did not dominate and supervisees were not passive. Another difference was that conference behavior varied between supervisees; demonstrating that supervisors did modify their styles. Although experimental studies need to be designed to determine if differences can be attributed to academic and practicum work, descriptive studies such as this provide a foundation.

One study (Hagler, 1986) that used the "bug-in-the-ear" technique attempted to modify the amount of verbal behavior of supervisors during the conference by providing feedback through an earbud that delivered immediate feedback to subjects. The findings showed that supervisors were able to reduce their verbal feedback as a result of the verbal directive to "try to talk less" which was delivered through the earbud at 2-minute intervals. Data provided to the subjects about the amount of verbal praise and contingent social praise delivered in the same manner did not produce change. Generalization to other behaviors cannot be supported without further research, but, as the author stated, the study does constitute a "first step toward systematic modification of a supervisor's conferencing behavior, which someday may lead to strategies for teaching supervisory styles" (p. 67).

Hagler, Casey, and DesRochers (1989) examined the effects of feedback on facilitative conditions offered by supervisors during conferencing. They attempted to increase facilitative behaviors by providing supervisors with data about their use of concreteness, facilitative genuineness, respect, and empathic understanding and instruction for change. Analysis of two consecutive conferences, using McCrea's Adapted Scales, revealed no significant differences between experimental and control groups. They concluded that simple, written suggestions pertaining to each behavior has too little substance and impact to induce change. They suggested that subsequent studies train facilitative behaviors, including opportunities for role play and practice.

Using a multiple baseline across behaviors design, Strike (1988) examined the effects of training supervisors to ask a variety of questions and to talk about the supervisory process during conferences with supervisees. A three-phase program for each of the two behaviors was implemented, each phase involving a 1-hour training session. Phase I was designed to teach supervisors to distinguish between the clinical vs. the supervisory process and broad vs. narrow questions. In Phase II, subjects received verbal feedback about their use of a target behavior in actual conferences, and in Phase III, subjects engaged in self-analysis of a target behavior and was implemented only if a subject failed to reach criterion after training for the previous phase. The results revealed that the teaching methodology was effective in causing an increase in the amount of broad questions asked as well as discussion of the supervisory process during conferences for the seven subjects. Strike noted that without specific education about the use of questions, supervisors tended to use predominately narrow questions but that the frequency of higher-level questions increased with training. Importantly, she observed the effectiveness of the use of higher-level questions in facilitating higher-level thinking by supervisees. Data indicated supervisees demonstrated an increased capacity to compare/contrast, analyze, synthesize, evaluate information in response to supervisors' questions after supervisors participated in training focused on developing their higher-level question asking skills.

Dowling (1995) investigated if supervisor and supervisee questions and responses changed as a function of academic training. In a 9-hour module and a subsequent 15-week regular academic course, 29 graduate students, or "supervisees-in-training," participated in lecture, discussion, role play, and simulations. Simulated therapy and conferences were used to assess the trainees' skills in decreasing conference talk time, collecting at least three different pieces of data during their observations for use in conferences, and one goal of their own choosing. Supervisors' use of open and closed questions and supervisees' simple-elaborated responses were measured. Supervisory training resulted in a dramatic change in supervisors' use of open questions and supervisee elaborated responses.

Dowling (1992, 1993, 1994) and colleagues (Dowling, Sbaschnig, & Williams, 1991) examined the effects of graduate student supervisory training. At the beginning of a regular 3-hour academic course, the "supervisors in training" baseline conference behavior were measured, three professional development goals were set, and progress was measured at the end of the semester. Findings have consistently demonstrated the value of preprofessional training in supervision in changing target behaviors and philosophies.

Research of this nature must continue. Demonstrating that supervisors who have been trained are more effective than those who have not will confirm the need and provide the momentum to sustain the academic preparation and practicum for the fundamentally important role of the clinical educator and supervisor.

SUPERVISOR ACCOUNTABILITY
THROUGH SELF-ASSESSMENT AND STUDY

Accountability for Supervision Through Research

More than 30 years ago, Douglas (1983) stated that a "major consideration in clinical account-ability is the effectiveness and efficiency of treatment" (p. 116). This statement is just as true today as our Code of Ethics compels us to our clinical experience and expertise, client preferences, and best current evidence to provide quality services (ASHA, 2016c). Applying this principle to supervision would suggest that the effectiveness and efficiency of supervision should be the main considerations in accountability. Efficiency involves the skill with which supervisors use the pro-cedures and tasks of supervision. Effectiveness in supervision is based on whether or not what supervisors do makes a difference in the subsequent behavior of supervisees and ultimately in change in their clients.

One of the first in our professions to question efficacy of supervision was Nelson (1974), who presented a paper at an ASHA convention entitled, "Does Supervision Make a Difference?" Nelson assigned 24 inexperienced students to three different conditions—individual supervision, group supervision, and no supervision—and then rated supervisees on 24 competencies. Her data indi-cated that the individual and group subjects were rated higher than those who had no supervision. Thus, Nelson concluded that supervision does make a difference. Other early studies examined the effects of different methodologies of supervision (see Dowling, 1976; Engnoth, 1973; Goodwin, 1977; Hall, 1970; Nilsen, 1983), searching for answers about supervision efficacy and, despite meth-odological problems, these studies were instrumental in raising questions such as whether confer-ence length or individual vs. group conferences or immediate vs. delayed feedback impact certain clinician behaviors. Underwood (1973), on the basis of descriptive gathered with the Blumberg analysis system (1974) and ratings of perceptions of conference effectiveness, proposed guidelines for effective conferences. These include:

- There should be more clinician than supervisor talk.
- Silence should be followed by clinician talk.
- Supervisors should minimize asking for and giving information and spend more time asking for clinician opinions, ideas, and suggestions.

Smith (1977) studied both the content and perceived effectiveness of components of conferenc-es, using Weller's (1971) Multidimensional Observational System for the Analysis of Interactions in Clinical Supervision (MOSAICS) and the Individual Conference Rating Scale (Smith & Anderson, 1982) as dependent measures. Results revealed that both direct and indirect supervisor behaviors were perceived to be effective and that supervisors, supervisees, and trained raters perceived an effective conference differently. Both Underwood and Smith had findings similar to earlier studies of Blumberg and his colleagues, reported earlier in this text.

The basic questions that must be answered are:

- Does supervision make a difference?
- Is one methodology better than another?
- What variables in the conference make a difference in subsequent behaviors of supervisees?
- Which tasks and competencies/knowledge and skills (ASHA, 1985, 2008b) are important for facilitating supervisee growth at various points on the continuum?

A few studies have begun to address these issues. The effectiveness of commitments by super-visees to carry out specific activities in subsequent sessions was examined by Shapiro (1985). As reported earlier, a commitment is in essence, a form of a contract and beginning clinicians demonstrated better follow-through with written commitments while more advanced clinicians needed only verbal commitments to effect desired outcomes. Thus, commitments are an effective supervisory method.

Gillam, Strike and Anderson (1987), using a single-subject design, conducted a study to determine if supervisees would alter their clinical behaviors as a direct consequence of supervision conducted in accordance with the clinical supervision model (Cogan, 1973; Goldhammer, 1969). Three behaviors—informative feedback, number of explanations per activity, and clinician responses to off-task utterances—were targeted for change. Results indicated that supervisees changed the targeted clinical behaviors as a function of data-based discussions with their supervisors, jointly developed observation and data analysis strategies, and written conference agreements.

Schill and Glick (1994) evaluated the impact of portfolio review on students' ability to self-evaluate. Twelve randomly selected undergraduate clinicians were divided into two groups. Both constructed portfolios and one group had a midterm review with a partner and two supervisors. Results revealed that portfolio development was a viable method to use to assist clinicians in self-evaluation. Both groups demonstrated positive attitudes about the use of portfolios but the group who had a review were more positive than those who did not. These studies emphasize the need for increased research in the supervisory process. It is encouraging to note that many supervisors are teaming with colleagues who may be more knowledgeable than they in research techniques to conduct studies. Research is certainly a compelling way to demonstrate accountability. As Lemoncello and Ness (2013) suggested, conducting practice-based evidence investigations is a way to collect high-quality evidence that is developed in everyday practices. Using multiple baseline single-case experimental designs or controlled case studies can empower any supervisor to provide evidence to support practices.

Accountability Through Self-Assessment

It is equally as important for individual clinical educators to ensure the effectiveness of their practice as it is to document the effectiveness of training clinical educators and supervisors for the professions. Studying the supervisory process in one's own behavior is the first step to accountability in the clinical teaching aspect of the supervisory process. Studying the manner in which one might implement the dynamics of the supervisory process in one's own practice is also the platform upon which an individual supervisor can build his or her own program of lifelong learning. Certainly, the core knowledge and skills for clinical supervision (ASHA, 2008b) provide a framework for activity and behavior that is fundamental to the process; however, it is not only what one does but how it is done that is also important.

Self-study of the supervisory process will include some, if not all of the following steps:

- The task of learning about what actually occurs in the interaction may begin with unstructured, open-ended listening to an audio or video recording. Since most supervisors or supervisees have never done this, they may find themselves in the same place as beginning clinicians who are told to observe a recording without guidelines. What do they do? They probably see a constellation of behavior for which they have no labels or guidelines. Redundant behaviors, certain responses to the supervisee may stand out, or even missing behaviors might be apparent. It may be easy to see who dominated the discussion; what topics were discussed most frequently or at the greatest length; what kind of questions were asked. This first step should be unstructured, with viewers remaining open and nonjudgmental although it may be difficult to avoid the "instant evaluation."

- The next step is analogous to screening in the clinical process—subjective identification of certain behaviors, to which further, more specific attention will be given. For instance, the supervisee may be contributing to the conference in a manner that is inconsistent with their placement on the continuum. The supervisor may interrupt frequently. The supervisee may engage in lengthy monologues. The supervisor may ask too many questions or questions that do not promote supervisee analytic or reflective responses. From these behaviors, determination can be made of what aspects need further in-depth observation and analysis.

Another way to obtain preliminary information is to use an interaction analysis system (IAS) as a screening device. Certain systems are better for this purpose than others. As a result of their use, however, some patterns may emerge that might not be noticed through unstructured observation or that might be misperceived or misinterpreted during the subjective observation.

- Once behavior or patterns to be further studied have been identified, the interaction can be observed in greater depth. As with the clinical process, data collection techniques include individually devised tally systems, verbatim or selective verbatim recordings, anecdotal reports, checklists, or interactive analysis systems. The type of behavior, the availability of appropriate systems, the goal of the observation, and the complexity of the interaction will determine the methodology. Most importantly, the elements chosen for observation and data collection, should be reflective of the supervisory process goals identified in the planning phase.

- After data are collected, they will be analyzed. Behaviors will be categorized, counted, sequences identified, inferences proposed and hypotheses stated.

- Objectives will then be set for further study, for supervisor and supervisee behavior changes, and for subsequent data collection after changes have been attempted.

OBTAINING FEEDBACK ABOUT THE SUPERVISORY PROCESS

If the supervisory process is to be discussed and analyzed by supervisor and supervisee, information must be gathered to form the nucleus of this discussion. Attitudes, perceptions, actual behaviors, and needs are all important to this analysis and are most often the raw material and data for supervisory conference discussion.

In addition to the objective data obtained by the observation systems to be discussed next, there is a need to obtain subjective feedback about the supervisory conference. Rosenshine (1971) and Rosenshine and Furst (1973) have strongly urged the use of high-inference ratings (subjective ratings) along with low inference category counts which are more objective, as have Ingrisano and Boyle (1973) and Smith and Anderson (1982). How is this feedback obtained? Three methods are useful to varying degrees: 1) general discussion with the supervisee; 2) the use of rating scales or evaluation forms; and 3) the collection of objective behavioral data through the use of interaction analysis systems.

General Discussion

One drawback of attempting to obtain feedback directly from the supervisee is that it may be difficult, if not impossible, to obtain honest feedback, especially if it is negative. Supervisors do give grades to supervisees, or write recommendations and evaluations. There may be behaviors that are difficult to discuss with the supervisor. How do supervisees tell supervisors that they talk too much, that they don't give supervisees a chance to use their own ideas, that they always tell them about the negative aspects of their clinical work, not the positive—Or a host of other complaints one hears from supervisees—some justified, some not? Supervisors, too, may find it difficult to engage in this general discussion of supervisees' activities. They may not know how to structure such a conversation or they may find it difficult to accommodate supervisees in discussion of sensitive issues. Mormer and Messick (2016) shared three tools that can be helpful to supervisors in gaining some insight into their behavior, the way it is perceived, and therefore, its effect on the supervisee—which supervisors should take into account as they plan their work with their student: The Supervisory Relationship Questionnaire (Chapter 4; Appendix 4-5);

Providing Constructive Feedback—A Self-Checklist; and the Clinical Educator Self-Evaluation Form (Chapter 11; Appendix 11-4). Waller, Sanford, and Caswell (2018) described the utilization of the ASHA (2016b) AHCST final report as a strategy for identifying the strengths and needs of the clinical educators who participated in the study. Clinical educators self-rated supervisory knowledge and skills ASHA (2016b). Supervisor competencies were further explored through utilization of a reflective questionnaire, which was completed by the supervisees assigned to the participating supervisors. In the context of ICREATE, a social communication program for adolescents on the autism spectrum, supervisors and supervisees utilized the AHCST resources and found them useful in recognizing strengths and areas of need in aspects of learning environment, links to clinical decisions, level of independence, data collection, and clinical reflection. The gathering of feedback about areas of supervisory competency from supervisees was found to be a mutually informative process. Bidirectional feedback led to ongoing goals for supervisor development and future directions for ICREATE.

The success of analysis of the conference depends on each individual situation. The manner in which the supervisory process is presented at the beginning of the interaction will certainly influence ongoing conversations. Adequate information about the components of supervision and knowledge and skills will facilitate discussion. The interpersonal skills of the supervisor will make a difference in the supervisee's ability and willingness to be open and frank. The specificity of the objectives set for the supervisory process will also influence the productivity of the discussions; the more specific they are, the more likely they are to contribute to clarity of communication within the conference.

It is important to think of the discussion and feedback in the conference in its early stages as perception, which may or may not be accurate. The validity of it can be tested through the collection of data, but until that point, they must be dealt with as reality, as least for the perceiver.

Rating Scales

Rating scales or evaluation forms are high-inference tools that are a slightly more objective way of obtaining feedback about the supervisory interaction than open-ended discussion. Such forms may be developed and used by the training program/agency or supervisors may develop their own. In Chapter 3, the rating form developed by Powell (1987) and Brasseur and Anderson (1983) are a good basis for early discussion of the process and in setting objectives for supervisor and supervisee. They are also valuable guides to support ongoing discussion. The Supervisory Relationship Questionnaire (see Chapter 4) is also a productive tool to gather feedback about the supervisor-supervisee dynamic to facilitate understanding, communication, and planning.

Interaction Analysis Systems

Although there is a place for the high-inference methods just reviewed, they cannot be considered objective measures of what happened in the conference. The use of interaction analysis systems for observation and data collection of behaviors in the supervisory conference is perhaps more important in the supervisory conference than it is in the clinical session (Anderson, Brasseur, Roberts, & Smith, 1979). Although subjectivity is never completely eliminated, the use of such systems in conjunction with other methods is necessary for full study of the conference. From the collected data, inferences can be made and compared with the results of ratings. This is particularly important for the conference when there is little information about variables and their effectiveness.

Interaction analysis systems for the clinical process were discussed in the chapter on the Observation phase. Those systems were an outgrowth of similar systems for recording interaction in the classroom, based on the notion that a better understanding of classroom dynamics will help teachers do a better job. This concept has now been transferred to supervisory activity and clinical teaching. To review what was said about clinical interaction analysis systems, they are not evaluations. They are low-inference instruments for collecting data on behaviors within the context of the conference, which can then be examined, analyzed, and categorized so that inferences can be drawn about the interaction of the participants and its effects on their learning.

Systems from the education literature and from speech-language pathology for analyzing the supervisory process will be discussed here in relation to their objectives, content, usefulness, methodology, strengths and weaknesses, validity and reliability, and how closely they meet the criteria for interaction analysis systems proposed by Herbert and Attridge (1975).

Blumberg's System for Analyzing Supervisor-Teacher Interaction

Originally printed in *Mirrors on Behavior* (Simon & Boyer, 1970a, 1970b, 1974), Blumberg's system was developed to quantify supervisor-teacher interaction. It was used in Blumberg's (1974, 1980) studies of the supervisory conference. Based on analysis instruments for use in the classroom (Bales, 1951; Flanders, 1967, 1969), the basic assumption of the system is that learning in the conference and satisfaction with the supervisory process are directly related to the supervisees' level of independence and ability to participate in the conference. This system is designed to help supervisors develop some insight into their behavior and its effect on the course of their interaction with teachers. Underwood (1973) indicated that it is equally appropriate for speech-language pathology supervisors.

The system is time based; that is, behaviors are recorded every 3 seconds or when a change of behavior occurs within the 3-second interval. It is a single-scoring system, meaning that only one category number is applied to a verbal behavior.

The system incorporates 10 categories for supervisors, four for teachers (supervisees), and one that applies to both. Supervisor behaviors are: 1) support-inducing communication behavior; 2) praise; 3) accepts or uses teacher's ideas; 4) asks for information; 5) gives information; 6) asks for opinions; 7) asks for suggestions; 8) gives opinions; 9) gives suggestions; and 10) criticism. Supervisee behaviors are: 1) asks for information, opinion, or suggestions; 2) gives information, opinion, or suggestions; 3) positive social-emotional behavior, and 4) negative social-emotional behavior. The final category, silence or confusion, applied to both participants.

The Blumberg system is easily learned and used. The directions are clear and specific and include a description of each category and a form for collecting data from a recording. It also includes a unique method for transferring data to a matrix, which makes it possible to analyze data both quantitatively and qualitatively.

Blumberg (1980) did not present reliability or validity data, but addressed reliability of observation by providing what he called "ground rules," which are helpful in training reliability in recording. Brasseur (J. Brasseur, 1980; J. A. Brasseur, 1980), who used the system, stated:

> The amount of training needed to use the Blumberg system depends upon the user's objective-self-study or research. For personal self-study, categories are easy to learn and it is rather easy to establish consistency with one self in assigning behaviors to given categories. Learning to tally every three seconds on a time-based system is sometimes difficult but can be dealt with by using a recording containing a series of beeps at three second intervals or coding all behaviors during the learning process. For research purposes the time required for training would depend on the number of coders and the percentage of agreement to be obtained. (J. Brasseur, 1980, p. 72)

The system relates to cognitive behaviors. It is possible, however, to make assumptions about affective aspects from some of the categories and especially from the use of the matrix, which identifies what Blumberg called "building and maintaining interpersonal relationships."

The content of conference behaviors is not identified by the system; therefore, significance of behaviors cannot be fully interpreted. There are, however, many questions that can be answered that relate particularly to the questions of balance of direct-indirect (active/passive) behaviors. For example, how talk time is used—asking, telling, criticizing; what behavior follows what behavior; and identifying other categories that then allow for inference making, interpretation, and value judgment.

The system is not intended to be used as an evaluation. It is recommended for self-analysis, peer analysis, or research. It enables users to identify patterns of behavior and to devise ways to modify those that are not consistent with one's goals for the supervisory process.

Underwood System for Analyzing Supervisor-Clinician Behavior (Appendix 8-2)

After using Blumberg's system in her 1973 unpublished dissertation study, Underwood (1973, 1979; Seeley, 1973) modified the system. Her unpublished version includes the following categories for supervisor behavior: 1) supportive, 2) praise, 3) identifies problem, 4) uses clinician's ideas, 5) requests factual information, 6) provides factual information, 7) requests opinions and suggestions, 8) provides opinions/suggestions, and 9) criticism; for supervisees, behaviors include: 10) identifies problem, 11) requests factual information, 12) provides factual information, 13) requests opinions/ suggestions, 14) provides opinions/suggestions, 15) positive social behavior, and 16) negative social behavior. Underwood also includes Category 7 which is behavior indicating silence or confusion and can be identified for both supervisor and supervisee behavior. The system contains a fairly detailed description of each category and some ground rules for making certain decisions about categorizing verbalizations, a scoring sheet, and two analysis sheets to assist in interpretation.

Purposes, procedures, uses, and strengths and weaknesses are comparable to those of the Blumberg system. Underwood's items are, in several instances, more specific than Blumberg's and she does include more supervisee categories. Her items for both supervisors and supervisees combine opinion/suggestion, and it might be beneficial to separate them because only suggestions imply an evidence-based orientation while opinions infer a subjective, personal preference.

Like the Blumberg system, Underwood's system is relatively simple and easy to learn; it focused on behaviors and it enables users to make inferences about Direct-Indirect Styles. Although it is a cognitive system, it is again possible to make inferences and assumptions about affect from the data. Underwood did not attend to the sequences of behavior as Blumberg did; rather she stops with having users summarize data by computing percentages for individual categories.

The major weakness of the revised system by Underwood was that the lack of reliability and validity information renders its use for research questionable. It is, nonetheless, an interesting and useful tool for self-study.

Content and Sequence Analysis of the Supervisory Session (Appendix 8-3)

This system, developed by Culatta and Seltzer (1977) was the first published system for study-ing the supervisory process in speech-language pathology and has been used in several studies. The authors identified the importance of isolating the interaction variables in the supervisory conference and grouping them into manageable categories. To do this, they modified the Boone and Prescott (1972) Content and Sequence Analysis System for recording clinician-client behavior. The theoretical base for both systems is behavior theory (Roberts, 1980).

The Content and Sequence Analysis System provided for recording behavior on one dimension only and in the cognitive domain only. It is a frequency-based system, recoding all verbal behaviors as they occur. The authors provided directions, defined categories, and gave an example of each. Despite the title, users can record only the type of behavior, not the content of the interaction. Categories are divided equally and include for supervisors: 1) good evaluation, 2) bad evaluation,

3) strategy, 4) observation, 5) question, 6) information, and 7) irrelevant. Categories for supervisees include 1) good self-evaluation, 2) bad self-evaluation, 3) question, 4) strategy, 5) observation, 6) information, and 7) irrelevant. Just as the in the Boone and Prescott (1972) system, a chart is provided for marking the behaviors and then, adding connecting marks to produce a line graph.

In addition, although this is a frequency-based system, Culatta and Seltzer (1977) presented a unique methodology for changing from a time-free analysis, which may produce misleading information, to a graph that also charts the number of seconds spent in each behavior. They presented an example of the way in which the two methodologies may provide entirely different pictures of what actually happened. For example, the time-free analysis may show a relatively equal interchange between supervisor and supervisee while the addition of the time component may reveal that the supervisor used long verbal statements while the supervisee responded with "uh huh."

The system's main strengths were its practicality, simplicity, and clarity. It can be learned easily and a large amount of valuable data can be collected rather quickly. It is particularly useful as an early introduction to isolating behavior in the conference. It can serve as a screening instrument to identify behaviors that may be studied in greater detail (Roberts, 1980). The data collected can be used to answer many questions: Most frequent categories used? Ratios of behaviors? Balance of input (using the time-based methodology)? Sequence of behavior?

The system has several weaknesses, despite its usefulness. Its theoretical bias may not be congruent with all approaches in supervision. Therefore, it may not measure all appropriate behaviors (Roberts, 1980). Categories are broad and unidimensional. Categories do not describe all components of the conference or represent all possible interactions. Some are not mutually exclusive. The authors give no ground rules for coding, so there is no structured way to resolve confusion between categories. They also do not include a method for analysis of data, as in Blumberg's and Underwood's systems. Because of its questionable reliability and validity, Dowling, Sbaschnig, and Williams (1982) concluded it has serious limitations as a research tool.

McCrea's Adapted Scales (Appendix 8-4)

None of the previous systems provide for recording data in the affective or interpersonal domain. The McCrea Adapted Scales for the Assessment of Interpersonal Functioning in Speech-Language Pathology Supervisory Conferences addresses this complex issue (McCrea, 1980).

Developed from the work of Carkhuff (1969a, 1969b) and Gazda (1974), these scales are based on the work of Carl Rogers (1957) and test his theories, which stated that if certain core facilitative conditions are present within a clinical relationship and are perceived by the client, the client will experience positive change. The original concepts were developed for use in mental health, but workers in other helping professions have assumed that these constructs are applicable not only in psychotherapy, but to other interpersonal situations such as parent-child, student-teacher, and supervisor-supervisee interactions (McCrea, 1980).

The McCrea Adapted Scales provides data about the presence or absence of four interpersonal categories of supervisor behavior: empathic understanding, respect, facilitative genuineness, and concreteness, and one category of supervisee behavior—self-exploration, which is assumed to be analogous to self-supervision.

The system is frequency based as well as rating based—that is, the presence or absence of the behaviors is noted, and then the behavior is rated according to its degree of facilitation on a scale of 1 to 7, with the higher ratings being facilitating and the lower ratings, non-facilitating.

The categories are clearly described, as are each of the seven points on each rating scale. Very specific ground rules and procedures are given for the use of each scale. Score sheets and an analysis sheet are included. The system is easily used and is not difficult to learn. McCrea (1980) estimated 5 to 7 hours of training results in reliable use for self-study, however, more training might be needed to reach agreement/reliability for research purposes.

Although the reliability study for these scales appeared to indicate that it can be used to observe and analyze interpersonal processes in supervision in speech-language pathology, reliability was only demonstrated for respect, facilitative genuineness, and concreteness. Because of the infrequent occurrence of empathic understanding and self-exploration, reliability for the entire instrument could not be established. McCrea (1980) indicated, however, the likelihood that reliability could be achieved if those behaviors were present in greater numbers.

The system can be used for self-study or research to obtain baseline levels of interpersonal functioning and to measure attempts to modify behavior in the interpersonal processes within supervision.

Weaknesses of the system are in the ambiguity and subjectivity of the scales on which the system was based (Carkhuff, 1969a, 1969b; Gazda, 1974). Because of the system's base in Rogerian theory, the only supervisee behavior identified is self-exploration, defined as the ability to talk objectively about personal behavior and its consequences (e.g., self-reflection). This is an important behavior in the facilitation of the continuum described here because self-supervision is perceived as a natural consequence of the ability to self-explore (McCrea, 1980).

Another weakness in the system is that it does not identify or categorize nonverbal behavior. A major portion of affect is carried nonverbally; therefore, data obtained from this scale can be assumed to be incomplete.

Despite these weaknesses, the system has strengths. It is the first system in speech-language pathology supervision to record and analyze interpersonal behavior. It has a strong theoretical base in the works of Rogers, Carkhuff, and Gazda (McCrea, 1980).

Smith's Adapted MOSAICS Scale (Appendix 8-5)

Smith (1977) adapted and validated the MOSAICS for use in speech-language pathology. The system provides an analysis of both content and process of the interaction in individual or group conferences.

The system is multidimensional, each unit of discourse (pedagogical move) being scored in six different dimensions. For example, each move is scored as follows: 1) according to the person doing the speaking—supervisor, supervise, or observer; 2) according to type-structuring, soliciting, responding, reacting, or summarizing, and 3) according to topic, which, in turn, is broken down into instructional and related. Although the system appears to be somewhat formidable, Weller (1971) provided extensive procedures and definitions for its use. Smith (1977), in her adaptation, rewrote certain definitions to fit speech-language pathology, clarified some of the rules for scoring and developed a score sheet for recording behaviors.

Extensive suggestions were given by Weller (1971) about the interpretation of the data that can be gathered with this system. The most useful are the analysis of the teaching cycles or the sequence of the pedagogical moves and the critical ratios produced by manipulating certain data. The analysis procedures counteract what is probably the main weakness of the system which is the massive amount of data obtained. Another weakness of the system is its complexity which makes it appear difficult to learn, and for research purposes, to obtain agreement between coders.

The strengths of the system are so great, however, that the weaknesses are almost inconsequential in consideration of its strengths. Of all the system presented here, it comes closest to meeting the standards set by Herbert and Attridge (1975). It is the only one which addresses content, and its multidimensional nature provides in-depth information. Categories are clearly described, exhaustive, and, for the most part, mutually exclusive. Directions for use and analysis are clear. No transcript is needed for coding because coding can be done directly from a recorded audio-recorded replay. Weller's suggestions for data reduction through critical ratio calculations and teaching cycle analysis make it possible to manipulate the data for in-depth interpretations.

MOSAICS can be used for self-analysis, peer analysis, and for individual or group interactions. Its greatest advantage, however, is its appropriateness for research. No other system described here approaches it in terms of its use as a research tool or in it multidimensional nature. It provides a highly reliable and valid dependent measure for descriptive and experimental design.

Use of Interaction Analysis Systems

There has been some uncertainty about the sampling process for studying clinical interactions using interaction analysis systems. The question applies to the supervisory conference as well. Some attempts have been made to determine whether or not sampling a segment of a conference is adequate to represent the entire conference.

Casey (1980) researched the validity of analyzing only a portion of a conference with McCrea's Adapted Scales. She asked what portions of the conference, if any, can be considered representative of the entire conference. Findings were that "scores derived for respect, facilitative genuineness, and concreteness (the only categories that occurred frequently enough to be analyzed by McCrea [1980]) during the 1) the beginning 5-minute segment, 2) the ending 5-minute, 3) a random 5-minute segment from the middle of the conference, and 4) two random 2.5-minute segments from the middle of the segment were representative of scores derived from coding the entire conference with McCrea's Adapted Scales" (Casey, 1980, p. 65). No such conclusions can be drawn for empathetic understanding or self-exploration because of their infrequent occurrence.

Casey (1980) further stated that it is possible to generalize the results of her investigation to all systems used for supervisory conference analysis. This statement is based only on the fact that all these systems are frequency based, not on the fact that they are all equally adequate instruments for analyzing conferences. Generalization cannot be made to clinician-client interaction from Casey's study. Further, Casey cautioned that the time segments would not be valid for categories of behavior which have minimal frequency of occurrence during the segment. Minimal frequency is defined as between 20% and 25% percent of behaviors in the segment.

Hagler and Fahey (1987) investigated the use of short segment samples of supervisory conferences with the MOSAICS system (Weller, 1971) and found 5-minute segments samples to be generally valid representations of events of the entire conference. All of these studies evidence some problems that result in a reluctance to wholeheartedly recommend small-segment sampling for study. Certainly, it would further the study of the process if one could assume the representative nature of a small time sample; however, questions must be asked about the purpose of the study and the content and variability within the conference before depending upon small samples.

For those who profess an interest in learning about themselves as supervisors, there is no better way at the present time than the methods suggested here even though they may seem daunting, if not impossible. Observing, confronting, engaging one's own behavior is often not easy but it is one of the most powerful and effective ways to become aware of and reflective about its consequences. For, those who wish to learn more about their practice as a supervisor, they are encouraged to start slowly, to use the simpler systems first to gain some insights, and then to devise a plan for their ongoing study.

REFERENCES

American Speech-Language-Hearing Association. (n.d.). *Practice Portal.* https://www.asha.org/Practice-Portal/Professional-Issues.

American Speech-Language-Hearing Association. (1985). *Clinical supervision in speech-language pathology and audiology.* [Position statement]. Retrieved from https://www.asha.org/policy/PS1985-00220/

American Speech-Language-Hearing Association. (2006). *The preferred practice patterns in audiology and in speech language pathology.* [Policy statement]. Retrieved from https://www.asha.org/policy/PP2006-00274

American Speech-Language-Hearing Association. (2008a). *Knowledge and skills needed by speech-language-pathologists providing clinical supervision.* [Position statement]. Retrieved from https://www.asha.org/policy/PS2008-00295

American Speech-Language-Hearing Association. (2008b). *Knowledge and skills needed by speech-language pathologists providing clinical supervision.* [Knowledge and skills]. Retrieved from https://www.asha.org/policy/KS2008-00294

American Speech-Language-Hearing Association. (2013, December). *Knowledge, skills and training considerations for individuals serving as supervisors.* [Final report of the Ad Hoc Committee on Supervision]. Retrieved from https://www.asha.org/uploadedFiles/Supervisors-Knowledge-Skills-Report.pdf

American Speech-Language-Hearing Association. (2016a). *Appendix A of final report of the Ad Hoc Committee on Supervision Training.* Retrieved from https://www.asha.org/uploaded Files/Topics-for-Supervision-Training.pdf

American Speech-Language-Hearing Association. (2016b). *Appendix E of final report of the Ad Hoc Committee on Supervision Training.* Retrieved from http://www.asha.org/uploaded Files/Self-Assessment-of-Competencies-in-Supervision.pdf

American Speech-Language-Hearing Association. (2016c). *Code of ethics* [Ethics]. Retrieved from www.asha.org/policy

American Speech-Language-Hearing Association. (2016d). *Final report of the Ad Hoc Committee on Supervision Training.* Retrieved from http://www.asha.org/uploaded Files/A-Plan-for-Developing-Resources-and-Training-Opportunities-in-Clinical-Supervison.pdf

American Speech-Language-Hearing-Association. (2016e). *Scope of practice.* Retrieved from https://www.asha.org/uploaded Files/SP2016-0343.pdf

Anderson, J. (1972). Status of supervision in speech, hearing and language programs in the schools. *Language, Speech and Hearing Services in Schools, 3,* 12-23.

Anderson, J. (1973a). Status of college and university programs of practicum in the schools. *Asha, 15,* 60-68.

Anderson, J. (1973b). Supervision: The neglected component of the profession. In L. Turton (Ed.), *Proceedings of a Workshop on Supervision in Speech Pathology.* University of Michigan, Ann Arbor, MI.

Anderson, J. (1981). Training of supervisors in speech-language pathology and audiology. *Asha, 23,* 77-82.

Anderson, J. (1985). Doctoral level emphasis. In K. Smith (Moderator), *Preparation and training models for the supervisory process* [Short course]. Presented at the annual convention of the American Speech-Language-Hearing Association, Washington, DC.

Anderson, J. (1988). *The supervisory process in speech-language pathology and audiology.* Boston, MA: College-Hill.

Anderson, J., Brasseur, J., Casey, P., Roberts, J., & Smith, K. (1979, November). *Studying the supervisory process* [Short course]. Presented at the annual convention of the American Speech and Hearing Association, Atlanta, GA.

Bales, R. (1951). *Interaction process analysis.* Reading, MA: Addison-Wesley.

Blumberg, A. (1974). *Supervisors and teachers: A private cold war.* Berkeley, CA: McCutchan.

Blumberg, A. (1980). *Supervisors and teachers: A private cold war* (2nd ed.). Berkeley, CA: McCutchan.

Boone, D., & Prescott, T. (1972). Content and sequence analysis of speech and hearing therapy. *Asha, 14,* 58-62.

Borders, L. D. (2005). Snapshot of clinical supervision in counseling and counselor education: A five year review. *The Clinical Supervisor, 24*(1-2), 69-113. doi:10.1300/J001v24n01_05

Brasseur, J. (1980). System for analyzing supervisor-teacher interaction—Arthur Blumberg. In J. Anderson (Ed.), *Proceedings—Conference on Training in the Supervisory Process in Speech-Language Pathology and Audiology* (pp. 71-73). Indiana University, Bloomington, IN.

Brasseur, J., & Anderson, J. (1983). Observed differences between direct, indirect, and direct/indirect videotaped supervisory conferences. *Journal of Speech and Hearing Research, 26,* 349-355.

Brasseur, J. A. (1980). *The observed differences between direct, indirect, and direct/indirect videotaped supervisory conferences by speech-language pathology supervisors, graduate students, and undergraduate students* (Doctoral dissertation). Retrieved from ProQuest Dissertations & Theses Global. (Accession No. 8029212) http://proxyiub.uits.iu.edu/login?url=https://search.proquest.com/docview/303031314?accountid=11620

Carkhuff, R. (1969a). *Helping and human relations: A primer for lay and professional helpers—I.* New York, NY: Holt, Rinehart and Winston.

Carkhuff, R. (1969b). *Helping and human relations—II.* New York, NY: Holt, Rinehart and Winston.

Casey, P. (1985). *Course and practicum in supervision at graduate level. In K. Smith (Moderator), Preparation and training models for the supervisory process* [Short course]. Presented at the annual convention of the American Speech-Language-Hearing Association, Washington, DC.

Casey, P. L. (1980). *The validity of using small segments for analyzing supervisory conferences with McCrea's Adapted System* (Doctoral dissertation). Retrieved from ProQuest Dissertations & Theses Global. (Accession No. 8024566) http://proxyiub.uits.iu.edu/login?url=https://search.proquest.com/docview/302969751?accountid=11620

Cogan, M. (1973). *Clinical supervision.* Boston, MA: Houghton Mifflin.

Council for Academic Accreditation of Graduate Programs in Audiology and Speech-Language Pathology. (2017). *Standards for accreditation of graduate programs in audiology and speech-language pathology.* Retrieved from https://www.asha.org/wp-content/uploads/Acred-Standards-for-Grad-Programs.pdf

Council for Clinical Certification in Audiology and Speech-Language Pathology of the American Speech-Language-Hearing Association. (2014). *2014 standards for the certificate of clinical competence in speech-language pathology* (Rev. 2016). Retrieved from http://www.asha.org/Certification/2014-Speech-Language-Pathology-Certification-Standards/

Council of Academic Programs in Communication Sciences and Disorders. (2013). *Preparation of speech-language-pathology clinical educators* [White Paper]. Retrieved on June 16, 2018, from http://www.capcsd.org

Culatta, R., & Seltzer, H. (1976). Content and sequence analysis of the supervisory session. *Asha, 18,* 8-12.

Culatta, R., & Seltzer, H. (1977). Content and sequence analysis of the supervisory session: A report of clinical use. *Asha, 19,* 523-526.

Douglas, R. (1983). Defining and describing clinical accountability. *Seminars in Speech and Language, 4,* 107-119.

Dowling, S. (1986). Supervisory training: Impetus for clinical supervision. *The Clinical Supervisor, 4,* 27-35.

Dowling, S. (1992). *Implementing the supervisory process: Theory and practice.* Englewood Cliffs, NJ: Prentice Hall.

Dowling, S. (1993). Supervisory training, objective setting, and grade contingent performance. *Language, Speech, and Hearing Services in Schools, 24,* 92-99.

Dowling, S. (1994). Supervisory training effects of grade contingent/non-contingent objective setting. In M. Bruce (Ed.), *Proceedings of the 1994 International and Interdisciplinary Conference on Clinical Supervision: Toward the 21st century* (pp. 180-183). Council of Supervisors in Speech-Language Pathology and Audiology, Cape Cod, MA.

Dowling, S. (1995). Conference question usage: Impact of supervisory training. *The Supervisors' Forum, 2,* 11-14.

Dowling, S. (2001). *Supervision: Strategies for successful outcomes and productivity.* Boston, MA: Allyn & Bacon.

Dowling, S., & Biskyni, R. (1993). Effects of supervisory training and practicum: A case study. *The Supervisor's Forum, 1,* 9-12.

Dowling, S., Sbaschnig, K., & Williams, C. (1982). Culatta & Seltzer: Content and analysis of the supervisory session: Question of reliability and validity. *Journal of Communication Disorders, 15,* 353-362.

Dowling, S., Sbaschnig, K., & Williams, C. (1991). *Supervisory training, objective setting and grade contingent performance.* Paper presented at the annual convention of the American Speech-Language-Hearing Association, Atlanta, GA.

Dowling, S. S. (1976). *A comparison to determine the effects of two supervisory styles, conventional and teaching clinics, in the training of speech pathologists* (Doctoral dissertation). Retrieved from ProQuest Dissertations & Theses Global. (Accession No. 7701883) http://proxyiub.uits.iu.edu/login?url=https://search.proquest.com/docview/302804338?accountid=11620

Edrich, M. (2014). *Effects of online training on off-campus clinical supervisors' knowledge, attitudes and expectations regarding the supervisory process.* Unpublished doctoral dissertation. Nova Southeastern University, Ft. Lauderdale, FL.

Engnoth, G. L. (1973). *A comparison of three approaches to supervision of speech clinicians in training* (Doctoral dissertation). Retrieved from ProQuest Dissertations and Theses Global. (Accession No. 7412552) http://proxyiub.uits.iu.edu/login?url=https://search.proquest.com/docview/302670407?accountid=11620

Falender, C. A., Cornish, J. A., Goodyear, R., Hatcher, R., Koslow, N. J., & Leventhal, G. (2004). Defining competencies in psychotherapy supervision. A consensus statement. *Journal of Clinical Psychology, 60*(7), 771-785. doi:10.1002/jclp.20013

Flahive, L. (2018, April). *CFCC update. Presentation at the CAPCSD Conference.* Retrieved from https://www.asha.org/uploadedFiles/CFCC-2018-Update.pdf

Flanders, N. (1967). Teacher influence in the classroom. In E. Amidon & J. Hough (Eds.), *Interaction analysis: Theory, research, and application.* Reading, MA: Addison-Wesley.

Flanders, N. (1969). *Classroom interaction patterns, pupil attitudes, and achievement in the second, fourth and sixth grades* (Cooperative Research Project No. 5-1055 [OE 4-10-243]). Ann Arbor, MI: The University of Michigan.

Gazda, G. (1974). *Human relations development—A manual for educators.* Boston, MA: Allyn and Bacon.

Gazzola, N., DeStefano, J., Theriault, A., & Audet, C. (2013). Learning to be supervisors: Investigation of difficulties experienced by supervisors in training. *The Clinical Supervisor, 32,* 15-39. doi:10.1080/0735223.2013.778678

Gillam, R., Strike, C., & Anderson, J. (1987). *Facilitating change in clinical behaviors: An investigation of supervisory effectiveness.* Unpublished manuscript, Indiana University, Bloomington, IN.

Goldhammer, R. (1969). *Clinical supervision.* New York, NY: Holt, Rinehart and Winston.

Goldhammer, R., Anderson, R., & Krajewski, R. (1980). *Clinical supervision* (2nd ed.). New York, NY: Holt, Rinehart and Winston.

Goodwin, W. (1977). *The frequency of occurrence of specified therapy behaviors of student speech clinicians following three conditions of supervisory conferences* (Doctoral dissertation). Retrieved from ProQuest Dissertations and Theses Global. (Accession No. 7701892) http://proxyiub.uits.iu.edu/login?url=https://search.proquest.com/docview/302822373?accountid=11620

Hagler, P., Casey, P., & DesRochers, C. (1989). Effects of feedback on facilitative conditions offered by supervisors during conferencing. In D. Shapiro (Ed.), *Proceedings of the 1989 National Conference on Supervision: Supervision innovations* (pp. 155-158). Council of Supervisors in Speech-Language Pathology and Audiology, Sonoma, CA.

Hagler, P., & Fahey, R. (1987). *The validity of using short segments for analyzing supervisory conferences in speech pathology.* Human Communication Canada.

Hagler, P. H. (1986). *Effects of verbal directives, data, and contingent social praise on amount of supervisor talk during speech-language pathology supervision conferencing* (Doctoral dissertation). Retrieved from ProQuest Dissertations and Theses Global. (Accession No. 303410764) http://proxyiub.uits.iu.edu/login?url=https://search.proquest.com/docview/303410764?accountid=11620

Hall, A. S. (1970). *The effectiveness of videotape recordings as an adjunct to supervision of clinical practicum by speech pathologists* (Doctoral dissertation). Retrieved from ProQuest Dissertations and Theses Global. (Accession No. 7118014) http://proxyiub.uits.iu.edu/login?url=https://search.proquest.com/docview/302574772?accountid=11620

Harris, H., Ludington, J., Roberts, J., Hooper, C., & Ringwalt, S. (1992). A documentation of the effectiveness of instruction in the supervisory process. In S. Dowling (Ed.), *Proceedings of the 1992 National Conference on Supervision—Total quality supervision: Effecting optimal performance* (pp. 57-61). Council of Supervisors in Speech-Language Pathology and Audiology, Nashville, TN.

Herbert, J., & Attridge, C. (1975). A guide for developers and users of observation systems and manuals. *American Educational Research Journal, 12*, 1-20.

Hersey, P., & Blanchard, K. (1982). *Management of organizational behavior* (4th ed.). Englewood Cliffs, NJ: Prentice-Hall.

Ingrisano, D., & Boyle, K. (1973). *A study of effectiveness and efficiency variables in a supervisory interaction.* Unpublished manuscript, University of Wisconsin, Madison, WI.

Kaiser Family Foundation. (n.d.). https://www.kff.org

Lemoncello. R., & Ness, B. (2013). Evidence-based practice and practice-based evidence applied to adult medical speech-language pathology. *SIG 18 Perspectives on Gerontology, 18*(1), 14-26. doi:10.1044/gero18.1.14

Lubinski, R., & Frattali, C. (2001). *Professional issues in speech-language pathology and audiology* (2nd ed.). San Diego, CA: Singular Thompson Learning.

Lyon, R.C., Heppler, A., Leavitt, L., & Fisher, L. (2008). Supervisory training experiences and overall supervisory development in predoctoral interns. *The Clinical Supervisor, 27*(2), 268-284. doi:10.1080/073252208024490877.

McCrea, E. (1985). Supervision component in undergraduate clinical management class. In K. Smith (Moderator), *Preparation and training models for the supervisory process* [Short course]. Presented at the annual convention of the American Speech-Language-Hearing Association, Washington, DC.

McCrea, E. (1994). Supervision as a Master's degree thesis option. In M. Bruce (Ed.), *Proceedings of the 1994 International & Interdisciplinary Conference on Clinical Supervision: Toward the 21st century* (pp. 221-229). Council of Supervisors in Speech-Language Pathology and Audiology, Cape Cod, MA.

McCrea, E. S. (1980). *Supervisee ability to self-explore and four facilitative dimensions of supervisor behavior in individual conferences in speech-language pathology* (Doctoral dissertation). Retrieved from ProQuest Dissertations and Theses Global. (Accession No. 8029239) http://proxyiub.uits.iu.edu/login?url=https://search.proquest.com/docview/303031 284?accountid=11620

Michalak, D. (1969). Supervisory conferences improve teaching. *Florida Educational Research and Development Council Research Bulletin, 5.*

Milne, D. L., Sheikh, A. I., Pattison, S., & Wilkinson, A. (2011). Evidenced-based training for clinical supervisors: A systematic review of 11 controlled studies. *The Clinical Supervisor, 30*, 53-71. doi:10.1080/07325223.2011.5649555

Mormer, A., & Messick, C. (2016, November 16). *Bringing evidence to clinical education practices.* Preconference workshop presented at the American Speech-Language-Hearing Convention in Philadelphia, PA.

Nelson, G. (1974). *Does supervision make a difference?* Paper presented at the annual convention of the American Speech and Hearing Association, Las Vegas, NV.

Nilsen, J. F. (1983). *Supervisor's use of direct/indirect verbal conference style and alteration of clinical behavior* (Doctoral dissertation). Retrieved from ProQuest Dissertations and Theses Global. (Accession No. 8309991) http://proxyiub.uits.iu.edu/login?url=https://search.proquest.com/docview/303165270?accountid=11620

Powell, T. (1987). A rating scale for measurement of attitudes toward clinical supervision. *SUPERvision, 11*, 31-34.

Roberts, J. (1980). Content and sequence analysis system. In J. Anderson, *Proceedings—Conference on Training in the Supervisory Process in Speech-Language Pathology and Audiology.* Indiana University, Bloomington, IN.

Roberts, J., & Smith, K. (1982). Supervisor-supervisee role differences and consistency of behavior in supervisory conferences. *Journal of Speech and Hearing Research, 25*, 428-434.

Rogers, C. (1957). The necessary and sufficient conditions of therapeutic personality change. *Journal of Consulting Psychology, 21*, 95-103.

Rosenshine, B. (1971). Research on teacher performance criteria. In B. Smith (Ed.), *Research in teacher education.* Englewood Cliffs, NJ: Prentice-Hall.

Rosenshine, B., & Furst, N. (1973). The use of direct observation to study teaching. In R. Travers (Ed.), *Second handbook of research on teaching.* Chicago, IL: Rand McNally.

Schill, M., & Glick, A. (1994). Use of a portfolio review process to enhance self-evaluation by student clinicians. In M. Bruce (Ed.), *Proceedings of the 1994 International and Interdisciplinary Conference on Clinical Supervision: Toward the 21st century* (pp. 207-212). Council of Supervisors in Speech-Language Pathology and Audiology, Cape Cod, MA.

Schubert, G., & Aitchison, C. (1975). A profile of clinical supervisors in college and university speech and hearing training programs. *Asha, 17*, 440-447.

Seeley, J. (1973). *Interaction analysis between the supervisor and the speech and hearing clinician.* (Doctoral dissertation). Retrieved from ProQuest Dissertations and Thesis Global. (Accession No. 7329608). http://proxyiub.uits.iu.edu/login?url=https://search.proquest.com/docview/302664667? accountid=11620. See Underwood (1973).

Shapiro, D. (1985). Clinical supervision: A process in progress. *National Student Speech-Language-Hearing Association Journal.*

Simon, A., & Boyer, E. (Eds.). (1970a). *Mirrors for behavior: An anthology of classroom observation instruments* (Vol. A). Philadelphia, PA: Research for Better Schools.

Simon, A., & Boyer, E. (Eds.). (1970b). *Mirrors for behavior: An anthology of classroom observation instruments* (Vol. B). Philadelphia, PA: Research for Better Schools.

Simon, A., & Boyer, E. G. (1974). *Mirrors for behavior III: An anthology of observation instruments.* Wyncote, PA: Communication Materials Center, in cooperation with Humanizing Learning Program Research for Better Schools.

Smith, K. (1979). *Supervisory conferences questions: Who asks them and who answers them.* Paper presented at the annual convention of the American Speech and Hearing Association, Atlanta, GA.

Smith, K. (Moderator). (1985). *Preparation and training models for the supervisory process.* Short course presented at the annual convention of the American Speech-Language-Hearing Association, Washington, DC.

Smith, K., & Anderson, J. (1982). Development and validation of an individual supervisory conference rating scale for use in speech-language pathology. *Journal of Speech and Hearing Research, 25,* 252-261.

Smith, K. J. (1977). *Identification of perceived effectiveness components in the individual supervisory conference in speech pathology and an evaluation of the relationship between ratings and content in the conference* (Doctoral dissertation). Retrieved from ProQuest Dissertations and Theses Global. (Accession No. 7813175) http://proxyiub.uits.iu.edu/login?url=https://search.proquest.com/docview/302869635?accountid=11620

Stace, A., & Drexler, A. (1969). Special training for supervisors of student clinicians: What private speech and hearing centers do and think about training their supervisors. *Asha, 11,* 317-320.

Strike, C. A. (1988). *Supervisors' implementation of trained information regarding broad questioning and discussion of supervision during their supervisory conferences in speech-language pathology* (Doctoral dissertation). Retrieved from ProQuest Dissertations and Theses Global. Ihttp://proxyiub.uits.iu.edu/login?url=https://search.proquest.com/docview/303572273?accountid=11620

Underwood, J. (1973). Interaction analysis between the supervisor and the speech and hearing clinician (Doctoral dissertation, University of Denver). *Dissertation Abstracts International, 34,* 2995B. (University Microfilms No. 73-29, 608).

Underwood, J. (1979). *Underwood category system.* Unpublished manuscript, University of Northern Colorado, Greeley, CO.

U.S. Census Bureau. (2016a). *American community survey.* Retrieved from https://www.census.gov./programs-surveys/acs/.

U.S. Census Bureau. (2016b). *Quick facts.* Retrieved from https://census.gov/quickfacts/fact table/US/PST045217

Victor, S. (2010). Coordinator's column. *Perspectives in Administration and Supervision. 20*(3), 83-84. doi:10.1044/aas20.3.83

Waller, J., Sanford, M., & Caswell, T. (2018, May). Building competencies in clinical supervision: Outcome of integrating self-assessment resources from the American Speech-Language-Hearing Association Ad Hoc Committee on Supervision Training. *SIG 11 Perspectives on Administration and Supervision,* 4-20. doi:10.1044.persp.3.SIG11.4

Weller, R. (1971). *Verbal communication in instructional supervision.* New York, NY: Teachers College Press, Columbia University.

i This chapter is a revision of that appearing in the 2003 edition of this book.

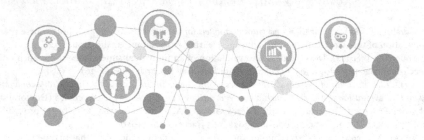

APPENDIX 8-1
TOPICS FOR SUPERVISOR TRAINING

Notes

1. The knowledge and skills listed in this document as well as the supervision goals for the five constituent groups are adapted from the Final Report of the 2013 Ad Hoc Committee on Supervision, titled *Knowledge, Skills and Training Consideration for Individuals Serving as Supervisors*.

2. The topic area for each group's specific set of knowledge and skills was determined by the 2016 Ad Hoc Committee on Supervision Training.

3. It is recognized that specific knowledge and skills might pertain to other constituent groups—that is, just because an item is identified only for clinical educators of graduate students does not mean that it cannot apply to supervisors in other groups.

Supervision Goals for Five Constituent Groups

Topic Areas / Knowledge and Skills	Clinical Educators of Graduate Students	Preceptors of Audiology Externs	Mentors of Clinical Fellows	Supervisors of Support Personnel	Supervisors of Those in Transition
	Develop clinical and professional knowledge and skills for entry-level practice	*Facilitate transition from supervised/mentored student to independent practitioner*	*Facilitate transition from supervised student to mentored professional to certified independent practitioner*	*Facilitate the acquisition of skills needed for the provision of efficient and effective services within the scope of practice under the supervision of a credentialed provider*	*Facilitate the acquisition of knowledge and skills needed for those professionals transitioning to a new area of practice or those reentering the profession*
I. Supervisory process and clinical education **Supervisor will:**					
a) Possess knowledge of collaborative models of supervision	•	•	•	•	•
b) Possess knowledge of adult learning styles	•	•	•	•	•
c) Possess knowledge of teaching techniques (e.g., reflective practice, questioning techniques)	•	•	•	•	•
d) Define supervisor and supervisee roles and responsibilities appropriate to the setting	•	•	•	•	•

	Graduate Students	Audiology Externs	Clinical Fellows	Support Personnel	Those in Transition
e) Adhere to research/evidence-based practice, convey that information/analysis to supervisee and encourage supervisee to seek applicable research and outcomes data and to use methods for measuring treatment outcomes	•	•	•	•	•
f) Connect academic knowledge and clinical procedures	•				
g) Explore existing knowledge and skills, including transferable skills	•				•
h) Sequence knowledge and skills development	•				
i) Facilitate the supervisee's ability to respond to various clinical settings and expectations of SORs	•				
j) Provide appropriate balance of direct observation and other monitoring activities consistent with the Clinical Fellow's skills and goals while maintaining compliance with ASHA Clinical Fellowship guidelines			•		
k) Provide opportunities to achieve independence in the workplace			•		
l) Develop a multifaceted experience for the student within the scope of the profession		•			
m) Allow the student to develop increasing independence in the externship		•			
II. Relationship development and communication skills Supervisor will:					
a) Develop a supportive and trusting relationship with supervisee	•	•	•	•	•
b) Create an environment that fosters learning and exploration of personal strengths and needs of supervisee	•	•	•	•	•
c) Transfer decision-making and social power to supervisee, as appropriate	•	•	•	•	•
d) Educate supervisee about the supervisory process		•	•	•	•

	Graduate Students	Audiology Externs	Clinical Fellows	Support Personnel	Those in Transition
e) Define expectations, goal setting, and requirements of the relationship	•	•	•	•	•
f) Define and demonstrate expectations for interpersonal communication and other modes of communication	•	•	•	•	•
g) Define and demonstrate evidence of cultural competence and appropriate responses to different communication styles	•	•	•	•	•
h) Demonstrate recognition of and access to appropriate accommodations for supervisees with disabilities	•	•	•	•	•
i) Engage in difficult conversations, when appropriate, regarding supervisee performance	•	•	•	•	•
j) Demonstrate use of technology, when appropriate, for remote supervision	•	•	•	•	•
k) Collaborate with other supervisors where and when applicable	•	•	•	•	
l) Build and foster professional identity and engagement	•	•	•		
m) Promote self-reflection to learn new skills and hone existing skills					•
n) Establish and maintain professional boundaries and appropriate relationships		•	•		
o) Facilitate efficiency, team building, and interprofessional relationships				•	
p) Empower support personnel to (a) work at their top potential and (b) continue to develop relevant skills				•	
q) Model and develop appropriate relationships with support personnel and within the organizational structure				•	

	Graduate Students	Audiology Externs	Clinical Fellows	Support Personnel	Those in Transition
III. Establishment/implementation of goals **Supervisor will:**					
a) Develop goals/objectives with the supervisee that allow for growth in critical thinking and problem solving	•				•
b) Set personal goals to enhance supervisory skills	•	•	•	•	•
c) Observe sessions and collect and interpret data with supervisee	•	•	•	•	•
d) Give the supervisee objective feedback to motivate and improve performance	•	•	•	•	•
e) Understand the levels and use of questions to facilitate learning	•	•	•	•	•
f) Adjust supervisory style based on level and needs of supervisee	•	•	•	•	•
g) Review relevant paperwork and documentation	•	•	•	•	•
h) Establish goals for the Clinical Fellow experience through a collaborative process of development/assessment			•		
IV. Analysis and evaluation **Supervisor will:**					
a) Examine collected data and observation notes to identify patterns of behavior and targets for improvement	•	•	•	•	•
b) Assist supervisee in conducting self-reflections until independence is achieved	•	•	•	•	•
c) Assess supervisee performance	•	•	•	•	•
d) Determine if progress is being made toward supervisee's goals	•	•	•	•	•
e) Modify or add to goals, if needed	•		•	•	•
f) Analyze existing skills of the support person				•	

	Graduate Students	Audiology Externs	Clinical Fellows	Support Personnel	Those in Transition
g) Provide ongoing assessment and objective (data-based) feedback, including the use of any reporting tools		•	•		•
h) Conduct ongoing and measurable competency assessment				•	
i) Evaluate support personnel through performance-based measures rather than developmental assessment				•	
j) Assign responsibilities to support personnel based on skills assessment				•	
V. Clinical and performance decisions Supervisor will:					
a) Model/guide supervisee to respond to ethical dilemmas	•	•	•	•	•
b) Model/guide supervisee to apply regulatory guidance in service delivery	•	•	•	•	•
c) Model/guide supervisee to access payment/reimbursement for services	•	•	•	•	•
d) Guide supervisee in use of reflective practice techniques to modify performance	•	•	•	•	•
e) Provide guidance regarding both effective and ineffective performance	•	•	•	•	•
f) Determine if progress is being made toward goals	•	•	•	•	•
g) Identify Issues of concern about supervisee performance	•	•	•	•	•
h) Create and implement plans for improvement	•	•	•	•	•
i) Assess response to plans and determine next steps	•	•	•	•	•
j) Identify the need for continuing education and training and develop a plan for achieving necessary skills/knowledge				•	•

	Graduate Students	Audiology Externs	Clinical Fellows	Support Personnel	Those in Transition
k) Adapt to changes in the service delivery environment				●	
l) Understand the relationship defined by the agreement between the university and clinic site, and adhere to the requirements and serve as an effective liaison	●	●			
m) Accept and adhere to ASHA roles and responsibilities for mentoring Clinical Fellows			●		
n) Assist in the development of workplace navigation skills, including becoming part of the team and adhering to the policies and procedures of the facility		●	●		●
o) Facilitate the supervisee's utilization of information to support clinical decision making and problem solving	●	●	●		
p) Guide the supervisee in reflective practice to encourage flexibility, growth, and independence		●	●		
q) Delegate responsibilities effectively				●	
r) Focus on client-centered care				●	
s) Hold appropriate credentialing for the professional and supervisory roles				●	
t) Know and ensure compliance with state, federal, regulatory, and ASHA guidelines for duties and responsibilities; reimbursement; and legal and ethical repercussions in relation to the scope of practice of the supervisor				●	
u) Understand and communicate, to others in the setting, respective roles and responsibilities, including appropriate ASHA guidelines and state regulations					
v) Guide the supervisee in developing advocacy skills for clients, himself/herself, and the profession		●	●	●	
w) Match/develop skills with job assignments				●	

APPENDIX 8-2
UNDERWOOD CATEGORY SYSTEM FOR ANALYZING SUPERVISOR-CLINICIAN BEHAVIOR

Supervisor Behavior

1. Supportive
2. Praise
3. Identifies problem
4. Uses clinician's idea
5. Requests factual information
6. Provides factual information
7. Requests opinions/suggestions
8. Provides opinions/suggestions
9. Criticism

Clinician Behavior

10. Identifies problem
11. Requests factual information
12. Provides factual information
13. Requests opinions/suggestions
14. Provides opinions/suggestions
15. Positive social behavior
16. Negative social behavior

Other Behavior

17. Silence or confusion

Category Definitions

Supervisor Behavior

1. **Category 1—Supportive:** Supervisor talk which enhances the supervisor-clinician relationship. This category does not include praise. Supervisor behaviors which encourage the clinician to continue talking (e.g., "Mmhmm") are categorized "supportive". In instances where supervisor supportive behavior is followed immediately by another supervisor behavior, the supportive behavior is not scored. (e.g., "Mmhmm, that was a good idea." This sequence is scored 2; not 1, 2.)

2. **Category 2—Provides opinion:** Supervisor behavior which connotes positive value judgment is categorized . This may relate to the clinician's behaviors or thoughts. Supervisor praise of client or other person's behavior (e.g., "Her /r/ sounds good." Or "He (parent) is really helping her at home.") is categorized, *Provides Opinion not Praise.*

3. **Category 3—Identifies problem:** Supervisor statements which help pinpoint a problem requiring some kind of solution. The word "problem" need not be in the statement.

4. **Category 4—Uses clinician's idea:** Supervisor repeats, clarifies, extends or develops clinician's thoughts. Also supervisor asks clinician to modify or develop her or his own ideas (e.g., "How could you carry that idea further?") Often praise precedes this category.

5. **Category 5—Requests factual information:** Supervisor attempts to gain information. This category is factually oriented and not concerned with opinions. A response is scored Category 5 if the information being requested is about something that has already happened and there is only one right answer. The question, "How did you (clinician) respond to her (client)?" is categorized as, since what has already occurred is fact and cannot be changed. The question, "How would you respond to that behavior next time?" is categorized as .

6. **Category 6—Provides factual information:** Supervisor behavior much like Category 5, only the supervisor is giving instead of asking for information. Any lecture-type behavior is included here.

7. **Category 7—Requests opinions/suggestions:** Supervisor attempts to learn clinician's feelings, thoughts, or ideas. This category includes supervisor behavior which asks the clinician to analyze, evaluate, or think about alternative procedures.

8. **Category 8—Provides opinions/suggestions:** Supervisor behavior much like Category 7 only the supervisor is giving instead of asking for analysis, evaluation or alternative procedures. Included are supervisor's feelings, thoughts, ideas.

9. **Category 9—Criticism:** Supervisor behavior which connotes negative value judgment is categorized "criticism". This may relate to the clinician's behaviors or thoughts. Supervisor criticism of any person other than the clinician is categorized "provides opinions/suggestions," not "criticism". The supervisor's tone of voice and body language must be considered in determining whether or not a response fits into Category 9. An evaluative statement with a "but" in it often fits in this category.

Clinician Behavior

10. **Category 10—Identifies problem:** Clinician behavior which helps pinpoint or shows recognition of a problem requiring some kind of solution. The word "problem" need not be in the statement.

11. **Category 11—Requests factual information:** Clinician attempts to gain information. This category is factually oriented and not concerned with therapy techniques. The question, "Is it OK to have therapy outside?" is categorized . "What would you have done in that situation." Is scored .

12. **Category 12—Provides factual information:** Clinician behavior much like Category 11, only the clinician is giving instead of asking for information.

13. **Category 13—Requests opinions/suggestions:** Clinician attempts to learn supervisor's feelings, thoughts, or ideas. This category includes clinician behavior which asks the supervisor to analyze or evaluate therapy techniques.

14. **Category 14—Provides opinions/suggestions:** Clinician behavior much like Category 13 only the clinician is giving instead of asking for analysis, evaluation or alternative procedures. Included here are clinician's feelings, thoughts, ideas.

15. **Category 15—Positive social behavior:** Clinician behavior which is the counterpart to Category 1. Statements which convey agreement by choice are categorized here, but those that indicate compliance related to supervisor's authority are Negative Social Behavior. In instance where clinician positive social behavior is followed immediately by another clinician behavior, that positive social behavior is not scored (e.g. "Mmhmm, I don't think that would work with this client.") This sequence is scored 14, not 15, 14. Positive social behavior is typically one word or a short phrase or sentence.

16. **Category 16—Negative social behavior:** Clinician behavior which tends to produce tension, convey defensiveness, or is disruptive. Compliance related to supervisor's authority and rationalizations are included here. Negative social behavior is typically one word or a short phrase or sentence.

Other Behavior

17. **Category 17—Silence or confusion:** This category is used when there is silence or both supervisor and clinician are talking at the same time, so that it becomes impossible to categorize behavior specifically. An exception would be when there is silence that seems to produce defensiveness (either Category 9 or 16). Any pause of four seconds or longer is scored as silence.

General Note About Scoring Procedures

If there is a topic change within any category, that category is scored again. This could occur any number of times.

In order to facilitate high reliability in scoring, Blumberg's guidelines presented below were followed:

- View each act as a response to the last act of the other person or as an anticipation of the next act of the other. The point is that we are dealing with sequentially related behavior and not that which occurs in isolation. Operationally, this means that interaction is recorded from the point of view of the recipient of the behavior, not the giver. This is because we are interested in recording the behavior, not the intentions of the person behaving.
- Difficulty is apt to arise in differentiating behavior in the following categories: 1 and 2; 5 and 7; 6, 8, and 9; 15 and 16 and so on. In these cases the ground rule is, after replaying the sequence to understand the context, choose the lower numbered category of those that are in question.
- The use of "ohh-h" or "hmm" by itself is taken to be encouragement and is in Category 1. When "uh huh" is followed by a rephrasing or use of the teacher's idea it is in Category 4.
- Start and end the tallying with a "15"—silence. It is assumed that the conference begins and ends in silence.

Underwood Analysis Sheet

Supervisor-Clinician Conference Analysis

Date: _____

Supervisor: _____

Clinician: _____

Supervisor Category Counts		**Clinician Category Counts**	
Category	*# of Events*	*Category*	*# of Events*
2	_____	10	_____
3	_____	11	_____
4	_____	12	_____
5	_____	13	_____
6	_____	14	_____
7	_____	16	_____
8	_____		_____
9	_____		_____

Supervisor Significant Total (SST) _____ $= \dfrac{SST}{ST} =$ ___%   Clinician Significant Total (CST) _____ $= \dfrac{CST}{ST} =$ ___%

Significant Total (ST = Supervisor Significant Total + Clinician Significant Total) = _____

Category	# of Events
17	_____
1	_____
15	_____

Grand Total (GT = Total Events in Session) = _____

Summary Data

Supervisor Talk : Clinician Talk $\dfrac{SST}{ST} : \dfrac{CST}{ST} =$ _____% : _____%

Supervisor Supportive Behavior $\dfrac{\text{Category 1}}{GT} =$ _____ $=$ _____%

Supervisor Praise $\dfrac{\text{Category 2}}{ST} =$ _____ $=$ _____%

Supervisor Use of Clinician's Ideas $\dfrac{\text{Category 4}}{ST} =$ _____ $=$ _____%

Supervisor Use of Criticism $\dfrac{\text{Category 9}}{ST} =$ _____ $=$ _____%

Supervisor Request for Factual Information $\dfrac{\text{Category 5}}{ST} =$ _____ $=$ _____%

Supervisor Request for Opinions or Suggestions $\dfrac{\text{Category 7}}{ST} =$ _____ $=$ _____%

Factual Information Exchange $\dfrac{\text{Categories } 5 + 6 + 11 + 12}{ST} =$ _____ $=$ _____%

Problem Solving Behavior $\dfrac{\text{Categories } 3 + 4 + 7 + 8 + 10 + 13 + 14}{ST} =$ _____ $=$ _____%

*Direct Supervisory Behaviors $\dfrac{\text{Categories } 6 + 8 + 9}{\text{Total Supervisor Behaviors}} =$ _____ $=$ _____%

*Indirect Supervisory Behaviors $\dfrac{\text{Categories } 1 + 2 + 4 + 5 + 7}{\text{Total Supervisor Behaviors}} =$ _____ $=$ _____%

(*Additions made to original system by authors)

Reprinted from from Seeley, J. (1973). Interaction analysis between the supervisor and the speech and hearing clinician. Doctoral dissertation). Retrieved from ProQuest Dissertations and Thesis Global. (Accession No. 7329608). http://proxyiub.uits.iu.edu/login?url=https://search.proquest.com/docview/302664667? accountid=11620.

APPENDIX 8-3
CONTENT AND SEQUENCE ANALYSIS OF
SUPERVISORY SESSION

Categories

SUPERVISOR		
Category	*Title*	*Definition*
1	**Good Evaluation**	Supervisor evaluates observed behavior or verbal report of trainee and gives verbal or nonverbal approval.
	Example	Supervisor: You did a good job in reinforcing the correct production of the X sound.
2	**Bad Evaluation**	Supervisor evaluates observed behavior or verbal report of trainee and gives verbal or nonverbal disapproval.
	Example	Supervisor: You made a mistake by not reinforcing correct productions of the X sound.
3	**Question**	Any interrogative statement made by the supervisor relevant to the client being discussed.
	Example	Supervisor: Why did you choose candy as a reinforcer?
4	**Strategy**	Any statement by the supervisor given to the clinician for future therapeutic intervention.
	Example	Supervisor: I think you will probably keep his attention longer if you give him a piece of candy for a correct response.
5	**Observation/ Information**	Provision by the supervisor of any relevant comment pertinent to the therapeutic interaction that is not evaluating, questioning, or providing strategy.
	Example	Supervisor: It appeared that when you sat on the floor the child gave you more correct responses.
6	**Irrelevant**	Any statement or question made by the supervisor which has no direct relationship to the supervisory process.
	Example	Supervisor: Pittsburgh sure is a beautiful city in the fall.
CLINICIAN		
Category	*Title*	*Definition*
7	**Good Self-Evaluation**	Clinician provides a positive statement about his own behavior or strategy.
	Example	Clinician: Sitting on the floor was a really good idea with this child.
8	**Bad Self-Evaluation**	Clinician provides a negative statement about his own behavior or strategy.
	Example	Clinician: Boy, it was dumb to sit on the floor with this child.

9	**Question**	Any interrogative statement made by the clinician relevant to the client being discussed.
	Example	Clinician: Do you think I should sit on the floor with this child?
10	**Strategy**	Any statement or suggestion made by the clinician for future therapeutic intervention or justification of past therapeutic intervention.
	Example	Clinician: I think in the next session he would pay more attention if I positioned him so that we maintained better eye contact.
11	**Observation/ Information**	Any statement made by the clinician relevant to the therapeutic interaction that is not evaluating, questioning or suggesting strategy.
	Example	Clinician: I notice that when he looks at me he can follow directions better.
12	**Irrelevant**	Any statement or question made by the clinician which has no direct relationship to the supervisory process.
	Example	Clinician: It sure looks like the Steelers are going to win the Super Bowl.

Reprinted with permission from Culatta, R., & Seltzer, H. (1976). Content and sequence analysis of the supervisory session. *Asha, 18,* 8-12.

Procedures and Ground Rules for Using the Culatta and Seltzer System

Procedures

1. Audio or video record the conference.
2. Select a random 5-minute segment to analyze.
3. Time the statements of both speakers and any silent periods.
4. Categorize each statement and place a mark in the appropriate place in the scoring grid code every time there is a change in behavior.
5. Connect the marks in each square to get a picture of the types of utterance and sequence of behaviors.

Ground Rules

1. Determine from the context if verbal lubricants (e.g., "um hmm," "OK," etc.) should be ignored or categorized as a good evaluation.
2. Consider any period of silence lasting 5 seconds or longer as a silent period.

Coding for Culatta and Seltzer System

Name: _____   Date: _____   Time: _____

Supervisor: _____   Trainee: _____   Silence _____

Totals: _____

1. Good eval																												
2. Bad eval																												
3. Question																												
4. Strategy																												
5. Obs./info																												
6. Irrelevant trainee																												
7. Good self-eval																												
8. Bad self-eval																												
9. Question																												
10. Strategy																												
11. Obs/info																												
12. Irrelevant																												

Data Analysis Form

SUPERVISOR CATEGORY	FREQUENCY (TOTAL NUMBER OF BEHAVIORS IN EACH CATEGORY)	PERCENTAGE OF TOTAL
1. Good evaluation		
2. Bad evaluation		
3. Question		
4. Strategy		
5. Observation/information		
6. Irrelevant		
Total participation time:		

CLINICIAN CATEGORY	FREQUENCY	PERCENTAGE
7. Good Self-Evaluation		
8. Bad Self-Evaluation		
9. Question		
10. Strategy		
11. Observation/Information		
12. Irrelevant		
Total Participation Time:		

Reprinted with permission from Culatta, R., & Seltzer, H. (1976). Content and sequence analysis of the supervisory conference. *Asha, 18*, 8-12.

APPENDIX 8-4
McCREA'S ADAPTED SCALES FOR ASSESSMENT OF INTERPERSONAL FUNCTIONING IN SUPERVISORY CONFERENCES

Five categories of interpersonal functioning are scored according to the following rules:

Procedures

1. Generally you will begin by making two passes through the segment of audio recording that you want to analyze. The first time you will record the speaker and the first few words of his/her utterance. This information is the unit of coding. The second time you will:
   - Decide the category/categories for the utterance.
   - Rate each category.

   You may make several passes through the data if necessary.

2. A set of formal scoring procedures is unavailable. Scorers may use their own methods for recording.

Ground Rules

1. The utterance is the unit of observation. An utterance changes when the speaker changes or the topic of conversation changes.

2. Generally, the pattern of transcription will follow the CHANGE IN SPEAKER. However, there are some exceptions to this rule:
   - Background "umhmms," "OKs," etc. will not be transcribed.
   - "Umhmm," "OK," "right" that stand out as separate because of a break in the primary speaker's speech will not be transcribed if they appear to be a social lubricant, a filler, acceptance that the message is being received. They will be transcribed when they appear to be meant as positive reinforcement or agreement; this will, in part, be determined by context and/or nonverbal cues.
   - In extended utterances, segments will change when they do not relate to or focus upon the previous segment.
   - When within-speaker off-topic interjections occur: transcribe the original statement, transcribe the off-topic interjection, do not transcribe the concluding statement but bracket it with the preceding two statements.
   - In instances of parallel talk, transcribe each speaker's utterances separately. Do not try to keep track of the multiple overlaps in the transcript.
   - When utterances are completely unintelligible, transcribe with a ____ as unintelligible.
   - When utterances are partially unintelligible, transcribe the audible portion and utilize a ____ for the part that is not understood. This will allow coding and rating of the audible portion.

3. Rate each utterance. A Level 5 represents a neutral statement, 6 and 7 add to the statement and below 5 subtracts from the statement.

1	2	3	4	/	5	/	6	7
	subtracts				neutral		adds	

4. The following are general clues to aid category selection:

- ○ Empathic understanding is scored only when the supervisor deals with the supervisee's feelings.
- ○ With the exception of tag questions, all supervisor questions are scored at some level of respect. Negative and positive reinforcement of the supervisee is scored as respect.
- ○ Facilitative genuineness is scored when the supervisor is relating his/her opinion.
- ○ All supervisor statements are scored under concrete.

5. Score the supervisor utterances in as many categories that apply.
6. Supervisee self-exploration is scored only when the supervisee is discussing his/her own behavior or feelings. If a supervisee has no self-exploration, score the utterance as NA (i.e., not appropriate).
7. In rating behavior categories, utilize Time Rule, i.e., in extended utterances when several rating of a behavior seem to occur, only apply the rating associated with longest segment of the utterance.

Supervisor Categories

CONCRETENESS
Concreteness means being specific. It is often complementary to empathy because one needs to be specific to show understanding.
Scale for Measuring Concreteness During a Supervision Conference

1	Supervisor statement, which is extremely vague, causes confusion and greatly detracts from the flow of discussion.
2	Vague statements by the supervisor, which have no focus on the topic being discussed.
3	Supervisor statements, which are vague but have focus related to the immediate past utterance.
4	Supervisor statements that have a previous focus and include some specific terms along with some vague terms. A new supervisor statement, which is general with some focus.
5	Supervisor uses no vague terms. No use of indefinite pronouns in place of nouns. Statements are specific.
6	Supervisor statements will be specific (like Level 5) but will include example or reasons.
7	Supervisor statements must be specific with an example and rationale.

FACILITATIVE GENUINENESS

Facilitative genuineness is expressing one's self naturally and openly. It is revealing one's own feelings and thoughts rather than acting strictly in terms of one's role as supervisor. To be genuine is to be honest, real, or authentic. In the early stages, a relationship only requires an absence of phoniness. The supervisor is silent or refrains from communicating his judgments. Facilitative genuineness is being open when it is helpful to the supervisee. However, higher levels of genuineness may require the supervisor to give negative feedback to the supervisee. When negative feedback is necessary, the supervisor tries to take out the hurt.

Scale for Measuring Facilitative Genuineness During a Supervision Conference

1	Supervisor's opinions are stated in a sarcastic or insulting manner.
2	An apparent discrepancy between the supervisor's intent and what he/she says.
3	Supervisor may teach about a disorder, technique, supervisory process, etc. Supervisor reinforces client behavior and/or the therapy activity.
4	Supervisor as teacher but he/she includes some of his/her feelings.
5	Supervisor requests feedback from the supervisee or gives a suggestion directed toward the supervisee. Veiled negative evaluation.
6	Supervisor gives opinion that disagrees with supervisee's. Supervisor gives positive and negative evaluation. If negative evaluation is hurtful score Level 5. Veiled positive evaluation.
7	Supervisor takes a risk and evaluates with justification.

RESPECT

Respect involves accepting the Supervisee as a separate person with potentialities, apart from any evaluation of his behavior or thoughts; a Supervisor may evaluate behavior or thoughts and still rate high respect if it is quite clear that his valuing of the supervisee is unconditional. The supervisor must believe in the supervisee's ability to deal with a problem constructively when given proper guidance. For example, the supervisor does not give the supervisee advice off the top of his head. By avoiding this and encouraging the supervisee to offer his own ideas, the supervisor conveys to the supervisee that he believes the supervisee has the ability to find his own solutions. Respect is rarely found alone in communication. It is frequently paired with responses in other dimensions.

Scale for Measuring Respect During a Supervision Conference

1	Supervisor relates a clear lack of respect for the supervisee in a sarcastic manner.
2	Supervisor may deliberately put the supervisee off by changing the topic of discussion or by communicating a statement with no focus to the previous one made by the supervisee.
3	Supervisor may ask the supervisee for clarification of an activity on a client. Also coded at this level are information and self-answered questions. Questions which seek rote or mechanical answers. Statements of the type "yes, but...." are Level 3.
4	Supervisor may ask for clarification of the supervisee's behaviors or feelings. Questions which guide the clinician to a specific answer.
5	Supervisor provides clarification of supervisee's previous utterance. Supervisor mirrors supervisee's thought, ideas, etc. Supervisor asks open-ended questions which ask the supervisee for analysis or opinion regarding therapy. Supervisor makes a suggestion.

| 6 | Supervisor clarifies the supervisee's utterance and goes further to interpret the supervisee's evaluation. Supervisor gives positive opinion about supervisee's behavior. |
| 7 | Supervisor positively evaluates the supervisee and goes further to take a risk for the supervisee related to the positive evaluation. |

EMPATHIC UNDERSTANDING

Basically this behavior communicates understanding. It involves more than the ability of the supervisor to sense the supervisee's private world; it involves both the supervisor's sensitivity to current feelings. The Supervisor does not need to feel the same emotions but he must demonstrate an appreciation for and sensitive awareness to those feelings.

Scale for Measuring Empathic Understanding During a Supervision Conference

1	Supervisor denies the feelings reflected by the supervisee. Denial may be accompanied by a hurtful or sarcastic manner.
2	Supervisor ignores feelings reflected by the supervisee.
3	Supervisor communicates only partial awareness of the supervisee's feelings.
4	Supervisor recognizes the supervisee's feelings without accepting or refuting them.
5	Supervisor recognizes and accepts the supervisee's feelings. Exact repetition or reflection of supervisee's feelings.
6	Supervisor recognizes and elaborates upon the supervisee's feelings. This may include providing a label for the supervisee's feelings when the clinician him/herself may not have labeled his/her feelings.
7	Supervisor recognizes, labels, elaborates upon, and accepts supervisee's feelings.

Supervisee Category

SELF-EXPLORATION

The ability to objectively talk about one's own behavior and its consequences.

Scale for Measuring Self-Exploration During a Supervision Conference

1	Supervisee is dishonest about his/her feelings or behaviors.
2	Supervisee holds back or refuses to self-explore when the opportunity is presented.
3	Supervisee gives a limited direct response to the supervisor's question about his/her feelings.
4	Supervisee may report that his/her behavior had a certain effect on the client or the therapy activity (e.g., cause and effect relationships).
5	Supervisee analyzes the consequences of his/her behavior with no reporting.
6	Supervisee analyzes his/her behavior and relates his/her feelings about the behavior.
7	Supervisee analyzes his/her feelings or elaborates on his/her feelings about his/her behavior.

Reprinted with permission from McCrea, E. S. (1980). Supervisee ability to self-explore and four facilitative dimensions of supervisor behavior in individual conferences in speech-language pathology (Doctoral dissertation). Retrieved from ProQuest Dissertations and Theses Global. (Accession No. 8029239) http://proxyiub.uits.iu.edu/login?url=https://search.proquest.com/docview/303031284?accountid=11620.

APPENDIX 8-5
MULTIDIMENSIONAL OBSERVATION SYSTEM FOR ANALYSIS OF INTERACTION IN CLINICAL SUPERVISION (MOSAICS)

Categories

Speaker

S: Supervisor—The individual who has major responsibility for the conference.

C: Clinician—The individual who participates with the supervisor in the conference.

Pedagogical Moves

STR: *Structuring*: Structuring moves set the context for subsequent behavior by 1) launching or halting/excluding interactions between participants, focusing attention on a problem; or 2) indicating the nature of the interaction in terms of time agent, activity, topic, and cognitive process, regulations, reasons, and instructional aids. Structuring moves from an implicit directive by launching discussion in specified directions and focusing on topics and procedures. Structuring may occur either by announcing or stating propositions for subsequent discussion. In general, structuring serves to move the discussion forward.

SOL: *Soliciting*: Soliciting moves intended to elicit 1) an active verbal response on the part of persons addressed; 2) a cognitive response (e.g., encouraging persons to attend to something); 3) a physical response. Soliciting moves may be questions, commands, or requests. Rhetorical questions are not counted as solicitations.

RES: *Responding*: Responding moves bear a reciprocal relation to soliciting moves and occur only in relation to them. Their function is to fulfill the expectation of the solicitation. Responses may be in the form of answers, statement of not knowing, etc. In general every solicitation must be intended to elicit a response, and every response must be directly elicited by a solicitation.

REA: *Reacting*: Reacting moves are occasioned by prior structuring, soliciting, responding, or reacting moves but are not directly elicited by them. Pedagogically, these moves serve to modify (clarifying, synthesizing, or expanding) and/or to rate (positively or negatively) what has been said in the moves that occasioned them. Reacting moves may evaluate, discuss, rephrase, expand, state implications, interpret, or draw conclusions from a previous move.

RSM: *Summary Reaction*: A summary reaction is occasioned by more than one previous move and serves the function of a genuine summary or review.

Substantive Areas (Content Analyses)

A. Instructional

1. Generality

S: *Specific*. Pedagogical moves that focus on the objectives, methods, or instructional interactions for the particular client(s) on which the supervision is based. These may be related to the client(s) in the past, present, or future.

G: *General*. Pedagogical moves that focus on generalized objectives, methods, or instructional interactions. These may include generalizations, past experiences, or applications of theory from speech pathology and audiology or related fields (e.g. child development, linguistics, psychology).

2. Focus

O: *Objective and Content.* Expected therapy outcomes and the content or subject matter related to these outcomes.

M: *Methods and Materials.* Materials of therapy and strategic operations designed to achieve objectives.

X: *Execution and Instructional Interactions.* Interactions between clinician, client(s), and content therapy, either as the execution of a particular therapy plan or unexpected interactions and critical incidents.

3. Domain

C: *Cognitive.* Pertaining to cognition, knowledge, understanding, and learning. The cognitive domain is here restricted to cognitive interactions between client(s) and therapy.

A: *Affective.* Pertaining to interest, involvement, and motivation. Affective interaction between client(s) and therapy.

D: *Social and Disciplinary.* Pertaining to discipline, control and social interactions. Interactions between clinician and client(s) or client(s) and client(s).

B. Related Areas (Discussion that does not focus on the analysis of instruction)

SBJ: *Subject.* Discussion of content and subject matter where the intent is to have the clinician understand the topic of discussion.

SPR: *Supervision.* Discussion of topics related to supervision, the supervisory process, and training of clinicians.

GRL: *General Topics Related to Speech Pathology and Audiology.* Discussion of topics such as school, other professionals, parent interactions, and referrals, which are only indirectly related to therapy interactions.

GNR *General Topics Not Related to Speech Pathology and Audiology.* Discussion of topics unrelated to speech pathology and audiology such as the weather or sports.

Substantive-Logical Meanings (Logical Analysis)

A. Process Relating to the Proposed Use of Language

DEF: *Defining.* A statement of what a word means, how it is used, or a verbal equivalent. Definitions may be in the form of the characteristics designated by a term or specific instances of the class designated by a term.

INT: *Interpreting.* Rephrasing the meaning of a statement; a verbal equivalent which makes the meaning of a statement clear. Interpreting bears the same relationship to statements that defining does to terms.

B. Diagnostic Processes

FAC: *Fact Stating.* Giving an account, description, or report of an event or state of affairs which is verifiable in terms of experience or observational tests. Included are statements of what is, what was, or what will be, as well as generalizations and universal statements.

XPL: *Explaining.* Explanations or reasons which relate one object, event, action, or state of affairs to another object, event, action, or state of affairs, or which show relationship between an event or state of affairs and a principle or generalization. Included are conditional inferences, explicit instances of compare and contrast; and cause and effect relationships.

EVL: *Evaluation.* Statements about the fairness, worth, importance, value, or quality of something.

JUS: *Justification.* Justification or vindication of an evaluation. Reasons for holding an evaluation; support or criticism for explicit or implicit opinions and evaluations.

C. Prescriptive Processes

SUG: *Suggestions.* Suggestions, alternatives, and possible actions and goals which might be used or could have been used in therapy.

SGX: *Explanations of Suggestions.* Reasons for offering a suggestion; relationships between suggestions and other objects, events, actions, states of affairs, principles, or generalizations.

OPN: *Opinions.* Directives or opinions of what should be done or ought to have been done in a given situation. A definite evaluative overtone is presumed.

OPJ: *Justifications for Opinions.* Justification or vindication of an opinion; reasons for opposing an opinion; support or criticisms for opinions.

Summary of MOSAICS Scoring

Speaker

S: Supervisor
C: Clinician

Pedagogical Moves

STR: Structuring, launching or halting move that directs the flow of discussion.
SOL: Soliciting, asking for a physical or verbal response.
RES: Responding, answering or fulfilling the expectation of a solicitation.
REA: Reacting, amplifying, qualifying, or making an unsolicited reaction.
RSM: Summary reaction to more than one move or genuine summary or review.

Substantive Areas (Content Analysis)

A. Instructional

1. Generality
   S: Specific, pertinent to the specific client(s) being discussed.
   G: General, pertinent to generalized objectives, methods, theory or related fields.
2. Focus
   O: Objectives and content to be taught.
   M: Methods and materials, strategic and planned aspects of implementing objectives.
   X: Execution, critical incidents, tactical and unexpected interactions.
3. Domain
   C: Cognitive, pertaining to knowledge, learning, information, understanding.
   A: Affective, pertaining to effective interactions—interests, motivation, attending.
   D: Disciplinary and social interactions.

B. Related Areas

SBJ: Content and subject matter to be learned by the clinician.
SPR: Supervision and clinician-training.
GRL: General topics related to speech pathology and audiology.
GNR General topics NOT related to speech pathology and audiology.

Substantive-Logical Meanings (Logical Analysis)

A. Processes Relating to the Proposed Use of Language

DEF: Defining, definitions and verbal equivalents.
INT: Interpretations and rephrasing.

B. Diagnostic Processes

FAC: Fact stating, accounts, descriptions, or reports.
XPL: Explanations, reasons, or relationships.
EVL: Evaluations.
JUS: Justifications, reasons for evaluations.

C. Prescriptive Processes

SUG: Suggestions, alternatives, and possible actions.

SGX: Explanations, reasons, and relationships for suggestions.

OPN: Opinions, directives of what should or ought to be done.

OPJ: Justifications for opinions, reasons, support and criticisms.

Rules for Scoring MOSAICS

General Rules

1. Listen to recording and score: speaker and pedagogical move.
2. Rewind recording, listen and score: instructional or related substantive areas.
3. Rewind recording, listen and score: substantive-logical meanings.

Specific Rules

General Coding Instructions

A. Code from the viewpoint of an observer, with pedagogical meaning inferred from the speakers' verbal behaviors.

B. Grammatical form may give a clue, but it is not decisive in coding. For example, SOL maybe found in declarative, interrogative, or imperative form. Likewise, RES may be in the form of a question, indicating a tentative answer on the part of the speaker.

C. Coding is done in the general context of the discussion. When two people are speaking at once, or when a person makes an interruption which is not acted upon (the interrupted party continues speaking on the original topic), the interruption is not counted and coding continues in the basic context.

D. When one individual is making an extended pedagogical move which is periodically encouraged by grunts and statements such as "uh huh" and "go on," without actually changing discourse or pausing for longer than 2 seconds, their interruptions are not counted as separate pedagogical moves.

Pedagogical Moves

A. STR moves from an implicit directive by launching discussion in specific directions and focusing on topics or procedures. The function of STR is either launching or halting-excluding, generally by the method of announcing or stating propositions. When a choice may be made between STR and REA, code STR for statements which move the discourse forward or bring it back on the track after a digression. For example, a new SUG or OPN is almost invariably found in a structuring move.

B. In general, internal or parenthetical shifts of topic or emphasis are not separately coded unless they constitute a relatively permanent change in the discourse. The discourse in the overall context.

C. Checking Statements (e.g., "Follow me?") are not coded as SOL within the context of another move unless some cue indicating a desired RES is present.

D. Implicit in any SOL is the concept of knowing or not knowing. Therefore, code RES for any of the range of possible responses, including invalid ones and those indicating knowing or not knowing alone (e.g., "I don't know").

E. A SOL which calls for a face is coded FAC, but if the RES gives both a fact and explanation, the response is coded RES/XPL. In the same way, complex responses to solicitations of EVL, SUG, and OPN are coded as JUS, SGX, and OPJ.

F. A speaker cannot respond to his or her own solicitation. An immediate self-answer to a question indicates that it was a rhetorical question, which is not coded SOL in the first place. If a speaker answers his or her own question after an intervening incorrect answer, the correction is coded as a reaction to the incorrect answer. If the speaker answers his or her own question after a pause, the answer is coded as JUS, SGX, and OPJ.

G. When a reaction to a previous move is followed by genuine summary reaction (RSM), both moves are scored for the same speaker.

H. RSM frequently occurs when a unit of discussion is concluded by a speaker, who then turns to a new topic. The coder must determine when RMS ends and STR begins.

I. A reaction to a solicitation occurs only when the reaction is about the solicitation and not a response to the SOL.

J. A reaction may follow the absence of other reactions to a move such as STR. For example, a speaker may make a proposal and then react to the absence of any positive reactions from the other participants.

Substantive Areas

A. Coding of Substantive Areas is in terms of the main context of discussion. However, in non-directive discussions shifts of substantive area are common. In order to code these shifts, which are an important aspect of supervision, the following rules are observed:

B. Code Instruction Areas in preference to Related Areas if a conflict arises. For example, if it is difficult to determine whether discussion of subject content (e.g., language) is in the context of objectives for the clients (SOC) or in the context of the understanding of the content by the clinician (SBJ), code SOC in preference to SBJ.

C. Code Instructional Domain (Cognitive, Affective, or Disciplinary-social) first. This is the most general of the content dimensions, it tends to persist longest in the discourse, and it is the most difficult to code out of context. If a conflict arises in coding, code Cognitive in preference to Affective and Affective in preference to Disciplinary-social.

D. Code Instructional Focus (Objective and content, Methods and materials, eXecution) second. Significant shifts in these areas occur more frequently than changes in Instructional Domain. If a conflict arises in coding, code Objectives in preference to Methods and Methods in preference to eXecution.

E. Code Instructional Generality (Specific or General) last. Moves commonly shift from Specific to General and back again. For a single move, code the area which occupies the most time or emphasis in the move, and code each move separately. If a conflict arises, code Specific in preference to General.

F. Indicate the Substantive Area of each move even if is not explicitly referred to.

Substantive-Logical Meanings

A. Only when DEF or INT are the main focus of the discourse are they coded as such. They are not coded when they are in the immediate context of other Substantive-Logical Meanings.

B. In a sequence of complex moves (XPL, SGX, OPJ, or JUS), individual simple moves (FAC, SUG, OPN, or EVL) are coded in the context of the complex moves. For example, in a series of explanations, a move stating a fact will generally be coded as XPL since one can consider the fact is intimately related to the interrelationships among the other explanations. However, when FAC represents a definite shift to a new topic or when it is in response to SOL/FAC, it is coded as FAC.

C. Complex moves (XPL, SGX, OPJ, and JUS) always involve relationships between their simple analogues (FAC, SUG, OPN, and EVL) and other factors, such as generalizations, other simple moves, etc. In the analysis of therapy particularly for objectives and methods, it is often difficult to determine when relationships are actually involved and when the move represents merely an extended description. As a general rule, these substantive-logical meanings are coded as complex whenever relationships are made to clients or specific therapy situations. In most other situations these moves are extended descriptions and codes as simple moves.

D. When more than one Substantive-Logical process occurs within a single pedagogical move and the overall context or emphasis is unclear, code according to the following order of priority; OPJ, JUS, SGX, XPL, OPN, EVL, SUG, FAC, INT, DEF. In effect, this means that complex is coded in preference to simple, prescriptive in preference to diagnostic.

Scoring Sheet for Adapted MOSAICS

NAME: _____   DATE: _____   TIME: _____

SPEAKER	MOVE	SUBSTANTIVE	SUBSTANTIVE-LOGICAL	NOTES
S, C	STR SOL RES REA RSM	S, G O, M, X C, A, D SBJ, SPR, GRL, GNL	OPJ, JUS, SGX, XPL, OPN, EVL, SUG, FAC, INT, DEF	

Reprinted with permission from Smith, K. J. (1977). Identification of perceived effectiveness components in the individual supervisory conference in speech pathology and an evaluation of the relationship between ratings and content in the conference (Doctoral dissertation). Retrieved from ProQuest Dissertations and Theses Global. (Accession No. 7813175) http://proxyiub.uits.iu.edu/login?url=https://search.proquest.com/docview/302869635?accountid=11620.

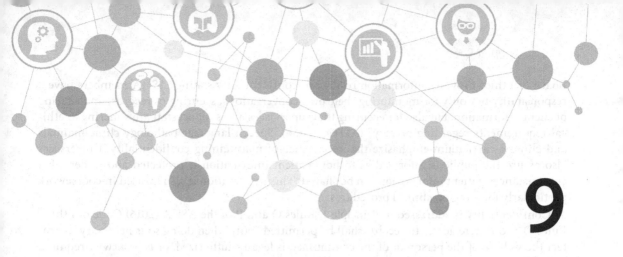

9

Ethical Practice in Clinical Education and Supervision

Wren Newman, SLPD, CCC-SLP, F-ASHA

PROFESSIONAL ASSOCIATIONS AND CODES OF ETHICS

The American Speech-Language Hearing Association (ASHA) and the American Academy of Audiology (AAA) each provide a code of ethics to support professionals in ethical decision making. The ASHA (2016) Code of Ethics includes Principles and Rules, several of which pertain directly to supervision. The Code of Ethics of AAA (2018) also includes rules pertinent to supervision. Professionals in audiology and speech-language pathology should reference these documents as well as state licensure guidelines pertinent to ethical behavior and supervision.

CONFIDENTIALITY AND THE SUPERVISEE, PATIENT, AND FAMILY

The supervisor supports the supervisee (including graduate student clinicians, clinical fellows, and speech-language pathology assistants) in understanding ethical behavior as it pertains to the patients we serve. Supervisees must demonstrate the ability to keep patient information confidential including patient history, patient progress, and records maintained in patient files. The concept of confidentiality applies to all settings, including but not limited to private practice, health care, and the educational setting. Training programs provide students detailed instruction in the area of confidentiality as it relates to patient information. Universities provide students with specific protocols to assure patient information is secured and shared appropriately. The ASHA (2013)

McCrea, E. S., & Brasseur, J. A. *The Clinical Education and Supervisory Process in Speech-Language Pathology and Audiology* (pp 311-319).
© 2020 Taylor & Francis Group.

Board of Ethics provides information relative to confidentiality stating "ASHA members have a responsibility not only for monitoring their own conversations, securing of records, and sharing of client information, but also for ensuring that supervisees and support staff are adhering to ethical requirements regarding privacy" (ASHA, n.d.-a). Speech-language pathology clinic manuals and clinical curriculum emphasize the importance of maintaining confidentiality. Universities also assure the public is informed as to how patient information is protected and under what circumstances patient information can be shared. This information is also infused in coursework particularly focusing on clinical procedures.

Confidentiality is addressed in Principle 1, Rules O and P of the ASHA (2016) Code of Ethics. Rules O and P state access to records shall be permitted "only when doing so is necessary to protect the welfare of the person or of the community, is legally authorized, or is otherwise required by law." Supervisees should understand confidentiality pertains to patient information (patient records) and to patient progress (O'Neil-Pirozzi, 2001). Course assignments are generally infused throughout the curriculum to assure students demonstrate knowledge in the area of patient confidentiality prior to beginning clinical experiences. Any regulations relating to confidentiality in off-site clinical placements should be part of the supervisee's orientation to the new setting. Procedures may vary from location to location. Accordingly, an off-site supervisor should not assume the supervisee is aware of the practices used in another setting and specific site procedures should be reviewed with all supervisees at the beginning of the off-site experience.

Some off-site placements will require students to participate in specific trainings relative to patient confidentiality. In school settings, a supervisee is permitted to access and review student records under the Family Educational Rights and Privacy Act of 1974 (U.S. Department of Education, n.d.). Families assume an unstated trust with the professionals with whom they work that information shared will remain between the clinician, the supervisee, others designated by the family, the family, and the patient.

In health care settings, a supervisee is permitted to have access to patient information under the Health Insurance Portability and Accountability Act of 1996, or HIPPA (U.S. Department of Health & Human Services, 2006). The definition of "health care operations" in the privacy rule provides for "conducting training programs in which students, trainees, or practitioners in areas of health care learn under supervision to practice or improve their skills as health care providers... [with facilities that] can shape their policies and procedures for minimum necessary uses and disclosures to permit medical trainees access to patients' medical information, including entire medical records."

The following scenarios provide examples of situations involving a supervisee and a confidentiality issue. In these types of ethical situations, it is always important to understand there is more than one way to approach the situation, and to view each situation as a teachable moment.

Scenario 1: A parent (Mrs. Smith) is sitting in the waiting room of a private practice while her daughter is in therapy. Mrs. Smith notices one of her neighbors leaving the center with her little boy. As the supervisee and Mrs. Smith walk to the treatment room to talk about her daughter's session, Mrs. Smith says she has "heard" the neighbor's little boy has autism and what a sad thing that must be. Mrs. Smith asks, "How is the little boy doing?" How does the graduate student address this scenario?

Scenario 2: A father of a child who is receiving treatment in a school setting asks the supervisee for a summary of the child's progress to date and he requests a copy of the child's records. The parents of the child are divorced and the supervisee indicates he will need to review the request with his supervisor before providing any documentation. The father persists saying, "I don't see why I cannot access my child's records now." How does the graduate student address this scenario?

Scenario 3: A hospitalized patient is receiving dysphagia treatment following a significant stroke and the family asks to speak to the speech-language pathologist and the graduate student outside of the hospital room. The patient signals he wants the discussion to take place in his room.

These three scenarios represent only a few of the possible ethical dilemmas pertinent to patient/client confidentiality a supervisor and supervisee may be faced with. To avoid problems with patient/client confidentiality, supervisors should discuss possible scenarios and solutions with the supervisee at the start of the clinical experience. It is important to assure the supervisee that discussion of these situations is a great first step. Supervisees should understand these situations present periodically and discussion should focus on assuring patients and families are protected appropriately.

In Scenario 1, it is important the supervisee continue to walk with the parent to the treatment room without discussion of the question presented by the parent. Whether the supervisor is in the treatment room or not, the supervisee should simply state she is not able to discuss anything about any other patients seen at the site. The supervisee should then move forward in the discussion of the parent's child's session and then, the supervisee should review the ethical situation with the supervisor. If the supervisee has made an error and addressed the question of the parent, it is also important for the supervisee to tell the supervisor what has happened. The supervisor can then address and document the situation if the supervisee has not managed the situation appropriately. This scenario touches on a very important concept relative to the supervisory process. Supervisees must feel comfortable in sharing concerns and possible errors in judgment. If the supervisor berates the supervisee, the supervisee will likely be hesitant to share judgment errors in the future. This situation should be addressed through discussion and explanation with a strategy for future situations which may present with similar circumstances.

In Scenario 2, the supervisee is in an awkward situation where there may be a court restriction as to whom may have access to the child's file. The supervisee should indicate he will check with his or her supervisor and someone will contact the parent later in the day. It is better to address a situation like this with a conservative approach than to provide information which may or may not be available to the parent. Should the supervisee have provided the records as requested by the father, the supervisor will need to be involved in notifying the appropriate individuals of the possible breach and address the situation accordingly. Certainly, this scenario would have a better outcome if the supervisee is provided with knowledge of procedures and policies relative to patient information prior to the presentation of a situation like this.

In Scenario 3, the supervisor and the graduate student should respect the patient's request to remain in the room. The family may or may not present all of the questions they wished to address however, leaving the patient to have a private discussion about the patient's current status with the family is not sensitive to the patient's request. This would likely be perceived by the patient as disrespectful and could be problematic legally.

In general, ethical situations can be seen from more than one perspective. In terms of a supervisory responsibility, it is not necessarily to show a supervisee the "right" answer to address the situation but rather, to help the supervisee look at a situation from more than one perspective. Taking the time to think about a situation from more than one viewpoint typically allows for the examination of multiple aspects of an ethical dilemma. Reviewing and discussing the dilemma from the family's perspective as well as the patient's perspective should assist in moving toward the best outcome.

As practitioners and as supervisors, we often discuss situations that present in our practice with colleagues to seek their opinion as we form our decision. This is an important skill to share with our supervisees.

ETHICAL CONSIDERATIONS

The discussion of confidentiality also applies to the supervisor and the supervisee. Whether the supervisee is performing well or is having difficulty in particular areas, the information should be between the supervisor and the supervisee. Confidentiality as it pertains to the supervisory relationship should be an area of awareness for supervisors and supervisees. Many times feedback to supervisees is presented in a walk down a school hallway or a hospital corridor. What may be easy for the supervisor to share with the supervisee, may be difficult for the supervisee to hear and certainly to process particularly in a public area.

The supervisor should work to provide an environment where the supervisee feels supported to learn and where clinical and professional growth is the focus. It is safe to say most supervisees are intimidated and unsure of their abilities when beginning a clinical assignment. Supervisees often feel their knowledge base is limited particularly as it pertains to clinical decision making and generalization of learning from classroom to clinic.

An example of a situation where supervisee confidentiality is jeopardized is as follows. Two graduate students are in the hallway of the university clinic. The students' supervisor walks up to the students and says "Allison, nice session. Mary, we have some things to talk about. I will be available later this afternoon." As this situation presents, both Allison and Mary have had their confidentiality compromised. It is possible Allison may be uncomfortable with her success being announced in the hallway. Some supervisees are embarrassed by recognition especially if they are aware other students are having difficulty. Mary is likely uncomfortable with the information that she and her supervisor have "some things to talk about." An alternative solution might have been for the supervisor to say, "Busy day today for you both, I'm sure. Allison, I think we have a meeting at 2:00 and then, Mary, I think I see you at 2:30. Look forward to seeing you both." In the recommended version of the conversation, there is no implied positive or negative evaluation of either supervisee and there is no reason for either supervisee to feel uncomfortable.

Supervisee confidentiality issues also present in off-site settings. Consider a supervisee who has difficulty with time management. This is a negative behavior no matter what the circumstances are. Late arrivals to a clinical assignment are not acceptable and typically result in a poorly organized session. Late arrivals can then impact the patients scheduled for the remainder of the day. Consider the scenario of a supervisee who is chronically 5 to 10 minutes late at least two times per week at a placement where productivity is monitored closely. When the supervisee enters the patient's room on a particular day, the supervisor says to the supervisee, "Nice of you to join us today. Mr. Jones was waiting for you but I thought I would go ahead and start. I wasn't sure when you would arrive." The issue of arriving on time for a scheduled appointment is a very important one. But this type of discussion should be presented away from the actual event. The supervisee may focus on the "jab" the supervisor provided rather than the fact he has a time management problem. If that is the case, the supervisee may divert his thinking about his own behavior and focus his thoughts on the behavior of the supervisor. It may be more meaningful to suggest to the supervisee that as the session has already begun, the supervisor will finish the session and the supervisee will be able to work with the patient tomorrow. It is important for the supervisee to understand the need to begin and end a session on time. Embarrassing a supervisee in front of a patient, will likely result in a negative impact on the supervisee with possible damage to the communication between the supervisor and the supervisee. The goal is to have the supervisee modify the behavior and enable timely arrival at the clinical placement. The goal is not to have the supervisee's focus on how "mean" the supervisor was and miss the concept of what the supervisee needs to change in her behavior. In this situation, the supervisee should be asked to develop strategies she can implement to address late arrivals. Discussion should center on the idea that arriving late can result in disorganization in providing treatment. Brainstorming together may result in the supervisee and supervisor establishing some ways to improve time management collaboratively, without embarrassing the supervisee in front of the patient. If the behavior is not successfully addressed by the supervisee, additional meetings will be needed with more stringent consequences. Significantly, these meetings should be conducted in private and documented so both the supervisor and supervisee have notes on the plan to address the concern as well as an understanding of the timeline to do so.

Consider a situation where supervisors from a variety of different disciplines including physical therapy, occupational therapy, and speech-language pathology are conversing in a meeting room where discussion comes up about their clinical students. As supervisees from the various disciplines mentioned walk down the hallway, they overhear a conversation pertaining to the student clinicians. The comments are both positive and negative relating to students' personalities, personal appearance, and students' performance in the setting. The idea of clinical supervisors in discussion about students' performance, appearance, or personality is not a good practice. The idea the supervisees can overhear the discussion is of even greater concern. This can result in supervisees hearing information about their performance or, the performance of others. Certainly, conversation about any supervisee's performance should remain between the supervisor and the supervisee. The consequence of this situation could be a reduction in trust in the supervisory process by the supervisees, and it may suggest a model of what a supervisor's role should not be to a supervisee. It is important to remember that we are not only assisting a supervisee in developing clinical skills, we are also providing a model of the role and behavior of a supervisor.

Finally, consider one more scenario in this area. A clinical fellow has a visit from his clinical fellowship mentor and the meeting is concluding. The clinical fellow is exiting the office, the door of the office is open, and the supervisor says, "I have never have had a male clinician as a clinical fellow before. I guess I should not be surprised, but you are doing very well."

In this last scenario, the clinical fellow's confidentiality is compromised and, the supervisee may either accept the information he has overheard without concern or, may be upset by the manner in which the information has been presented. The clinical fellow may feel he is receiving a compliment of some sort but he also may feel the supervisor does not have a particularly positive picture of male clinicians. Statements like these can also give the supervisee the idea that these types of comments are acceptable. The model from the supervisor should be one where comments about supervisees are not made publicly but rather are provided in a private conversation. Certainly, comments about ethnicity, gender, race, religion, and sexuality, should not be made unless it is pertinent to the clinical situation (e.g., a young boy might work more effectively with a male clinician than a female clinician). Again, supervisors have the responsibility to model the behaviors you would like your supervisees to emulate from your supervisory style.

Vicarious Liability

Vicarious liability means a supervisor is ultimately responsible for the client. There are several rules within the ASHA (2016) Code of Ethics that help to define the responsibility of the supervisor in the process. The Code of Ethics, Principle 1, rule D states "individuals shall not misrepresent the credentials of aides, assistants, technicians, support personnel, students, research interns, Clinical Fellows, or any others under their supervision, and they shall inform those they serve professionally of the name, role, and professional credentials of persons providing services." Supervisees may only perform procedures for which they have been appropriately trained and must be supervised accordingly. The responsibility for the patient remains with the certified and/or licensed professional. When the supervisor explains the education and training of the supervisee, the patient and family should understand the roles and responsibilities of each individual participating in the therapeutic process. Although supervisory requirements do not mandate 100% supervision (unless client needs mandate such), the supervisor is the individual who is ultimately responsible for the needs of the patient relative to communication and safety.

In a scenario where a supervisee is working with a patient and something happens (e.g., a patient falls off the chair, a child swallows a puzzle piece, a patient passes out), the individual who is ultimately responsible for the patient is the licensed provider of service. ASHA (2014) certification requirements indicate that the amount of direct supervision "must be commensurate with the student's knowledge, skills, and experience, must not be less than 25% of the student's total contact with each client/patient, and must take place periodically throughout the practicum. Supervision must be sufficient to ensure the welfare of the client/patient." It is generally not considered an ethical problem if a minor accident occurs during a session. It is the follow-up communication with the family that is key.

Respondeat superior is the legal terminology associated with vicarious liability. The supervisor oversees the care of the patient and is responsible for the actions of the supervisee with the patient even if the supervisor is not with the supervisee at the time a problem presents. The supervisor is also responsible for problems not shared by the supervisee. An example of this scenario is as follows: The supervisee is working with a child who is in kindergarten. During the session, the child slips off her chair and bumps her forehead on the table. She indicates she is fine, she rubs her forehead a few times and the session continues. When the mother picks the child up from school at the end of the day, she notices an "egg" on the child's forehead and phones the school to ask what happened. Eventually, the phone call is transferred to the speech-language pathology supervisor who was not in the session nor was she made aware of the child's accident. The supervisor, however, is responsible for not knowing about the event. In this scenario, the situation is likely not a serious one but should be a learning experience for the supervisee and the supervisor. Although the child was not injured, a phone call should have been made to the parent or a note should have been sent home with the child explaining what happened with a phone number for the mother to call if she has questions. A dialogue between the supervisor and the supervisee relative to these types of scenarios is beneficial at the beginning of the clinical experience. The supervisee should be aware of the importance of sharing anything that may present when the supervisor is not in attendance. Providing examples may help the supervisee understand why ongoing communication is important and may help to avoid a scenario like the one presented.

A supervisor may be held liable under the doctrine of respondeat superior, meaning the supervisor may be held accountable for problems caused by the supervisee. "This liability attaches whether or not the supervisor breached a duty. Supervisors may be held liable under this doctrine as either the 'master,' or as an employer (Saccuzzo, 1997, p. 123). Also, ASHA's (2016) Code of Ethics, Principle 1, rule E states tasks related to the provision of clinical services can be assigned to assistants, support personnel, or others "only if those persons are adequately prepared and are appropriately supervised." The responsibility for the welfare of individuals being served remains with the certified professional.

Situations relative to respondeat superior can present with more serious consequences. Consider the following: A patient who has suffered a significant stroke is left with severe oral communication problems. He is participating in a group setting and he writes a note indicating he does not want to live anymore. The note is handed to the graduate student clinician and the student brings the note to the supervisor immediately following the conclusion of the group. The supervisor is able to reach the wife, who contacts a psychologist who has worked with the patient in the past. In this scenario, the supervisee as well as the supervisor managed the situation appropriately and a possible serious situation was avoided. Had the supervisee thought the patient was having "a bad day," the outcome might have been very different. Should the patient have harmed himself, even if the supervisor was not aware of the situation, the supervisor is responsible for the care of the patient as well as the actions of the supervisee. Accordingly, communication must be ongoing, timely, and comprehensive. Again, the importance of ongoing and open communication between the supervisor and supervisee is of critical significance. The supervisor's communication with the supervisee at the onset of the experience should include examples of these possible circumstances.

Although supervisees may be providing assessment and treatment, patients and families have the right to expect the same level of service as would be provided by a certified or licensed professional.

DUAL RELATIONSHIP

This topic pertains to situations where the supervisor and the supervisee have more than the relationship of supervisor and supervisee. A dual relationship presents when the supervisor has an existing relationship with the supervisee or when a second relationship develops during the supervisory experience other than the existing supervisory relationship. An example would be Joan, a speech-language pathology assistant who works in a private practice and has done so for several years. Joan has been supervised by the practice owner as required by the state. She is now in the process of completing a master's degree in speech-language pathology and the practice owner is providing the supervision of the required clinical hours for graduation from the master's program and, ultimately, for certification and licensure requirements. The owner of the practice knows the speech-language pathology assistant very well and feels confident Joan is proficient in her work with children in the practice. Accordingly, the owner of the practice does not provide supervision at the level required and Joan is treating the clients with whom she worked as a speech-language pathology assistant but is not receiving the appropriate percentage of supervision as a graduate student. Joan is hesitant to discuss with the practice owner what she understands to be the differences between a speech-language pathology assistant and a speech-language pathologist in terms of supervision. The owner of the practice has been very supportive of her and Joan does not want to hurt her supervisor in any way. In this scenario, the dual relationship is negatively impacting Joan's ability to learn how to treat different types of cases, have regular ongoing supervisory meetings, and move along the supervisory continuum. The issue presents because of the existing relationship with the practice owner.

Having two different relationships with a supervisee can most definitely impact the supervisory relationship and can be a key factor in the success or failure of the experience. According to Kilminster and Jolly (2000), "the supervision relationship is probably the single most important factor for the effectiveness of supervision" (p. 827). The relationship between the supervisor and supervisee is already a fragile one. The power differential between the supervisee and the supervisor is substantial. The supervisee is in a position of reduced power in the relationship and generally does not want to disappoint, antagonize, or irritate the supervisor. The supervisor-supervisee relationship is such that the supervisee may not feel comfortable in expressing concerns about the process. When a second relationship exists between the supervisor and the supervisee, the impact can be substantial.

Another example of where the dual relationship presents and results in a challenging scenario is one where the supervisor asks the supervisee to do something not related to the supervisory relationship. If the supervisor is going on a vacation, and she requests the supervisee to stay at her house in her absence, the supervisee may not want to accept the request but may feel uncomfortable saying no to the supervisor. This example shows the effect of the power differential which can result in a situation where the supervisee may not feel she has a choice. These situations can of course become more complex if a problem presents when the supervisee has agreed to assist the supervisor. Should something go wrong while the supervisee is staying at the house (e.g., the bathroom floods, the dog is sick, etc.), the supervisee may feel the supervisor will think of her differently. The supervisee will likely worry as to how the situation will reflect on the supervisor's evaluation of the supervisee in the clinical setting. Sometimes the supervisor is thinking the supervisee will benefit from some extra income and likely most of these scenarios work out well. However, if the scenario results in a problem, the supervisor needs to understand the complexity of the outcome. Will the supervisor hold the supervisee responsible for the incident related to a nonsupervisory situation? Even if the supervisor does not hold the supervisee responsible, will the supervisee think the supervisor is holding him or her responsible?

There are other problematic dual relationship situations which can present in a supervision situation. If the supervisee is a friend of the supervisor, supervision can be problematic in at least two ways. The supervisee may resent the constructive suggestions the supervisor provides. It can be difficult to receive constructive feedback from someone you know well. On the other hand, the supervisor may not choose to provide feedback to a supervisee where there is an existing relationship. The supervisor may not want to damage a friendship and accordingly, may only provide positive feedback.

Consider the situation where the supervisee is asked by the supervisor to work on a submission of a poster session for the state association annual conference. The supervisee may move forward with this request because the supervisor has asked her to do so. This is an appropriate challenge for a student or a clinical fellow. The supervisee may not want to complete the submission, however, based on the supervisor's evaluative role, the supervisee will likely move forward with the request. The direction from the supervisor should result in a positive experience even if the supervisee's submission is not accepted. The supervisor has provided the supervisee with a first step in moving forward as a professional.

In contrast, consider a situation where there is an existing relationship and the supervisor asks the supervisee to work on a poster for the state association annual conference. The supervisee may feel comfortable saying, "I'm just not able to right now. I know you are always thinking about good things for me to do, but I'm really swamped now so it won't work. I'll hope to do something like that at another time." The supervisee may not have a clear picture of the role of the supervisor in this situation and may not understand the power differential. Another example of a situation that could present with a dual relationship is one where the supervisor may be more demanding of a supervisee she knows personally as she wants to be sure no one thinks she is giving preferential treatment to the family friend.

Overall, it is best for the supervisor and supervisee to have only one relationship. The supervisor-supervisee relationship is a fragile one simply by the nature of the evaluative component and the power differential. Maintaining a professional relationship reflecting mutual respect and value of the learning experience will likely result in the best outcome.

POWER DIFFERENTIAL AND THE ETHICS OF THE SUPERVISORY RELATIONSHIP

Principle 4, rule G of the ASHA (2016) Code of Ethics states "individuals shall not engage in any form of harassment, power abuse, or sexual harassment." According to Kilminster and Jolly (2000) "the supervision relationship is probably the single most important factor for the effectiveness of supervision." The relationship between the supervisor and supervisee is a fragile one. The power differential between the two individuals is substantial. Discussions of supervisory experiences often result in a speech-language pathologist or audiologist reporting a bullying relationship during some point in their training. The supervisee may share a perception nothing they did was ever right. Often, the supervisee will express a feeling of fear and an inability to perform. Sometimes the supervisee will share a sense of having no power in the situation and no ability to address the problem. From the supervisee's perspective, the treatment by the supervisor results in a feeling of not being able to do anything right. This situation is a very difficult one. The supervisor has the responsibility to treat the supervisee with respect. Feedback to the student should have a balance of skills the student is performing well as well as things to continue to work to improve. The lists of positive behaviors and skills to develop should be approximately the same in length. There are some students who do not perform well in a clinical setting even after successful performance in classes across the curriculum. In the situation where a student feels nothing they do is right, the ability to address the problem is intensified.

Supervisees should have a feeling of support. An atmosphere where the supervisee is disrespected or treated in a negative way will probably not result in a successful outcome. The supervision of a marginal student is challenging however, the supervisor needs to treat the individual with respect and provide an atmosphere where the student is supported. The supervisor who provides only negative comments will likely not move the student in a positive direction and can result in a student who is nearly paralyzed in their ability to perform.

Barnett, Erickson Cornish, Goodyear, and Lichtenberg, (2007) discuss the idea that supervisees need the freedom to experiment or try a new approach without fear. This is important. If supervisees are always concerned about evaluation, making the supervisor happy, and/or the fear of making mistakes, then they are less likely to share questions they have. This, in turn, may indicate a lack of knowledge or preparation to the supervisor. It is unethical to treat a supervisee in a manner that is disrespectful or cruel. The supervisee is already nervous, concerned about doing well, and in a position of reduced power. The supervisor's effort in establishing a positive relationship by balancing feedback that provides information on things the supervisee is doing well along with areas to be improved, should establish a foundation for a relationship of trust, open discussion, and positive interaction. Kilminster and Jolly (2000) identified that supervisees value being liked, appreciate a supervisor who is genuine, and respect a supervisor who is empathetic when difficult situations present. The supervisor should provide the supervisee a safe environment in which supervisees can openly address their work.

REFERENCES

American Academy of Audiology. (2018). *Code of ethics*. Retrieved from: https://www.audiology.org/sites/default/files/about/membership/documents/Code%20of%20Ethics%20with%20procedures-REV%202018_0216.pdf.

American Speech-Language-Hearing Association. (n.d.-a). *Frequently asked questions about student supervision*. Available from https://www.asha.org/slp/supervisionFAQs/#hipaa.

American Speech-Language-Hearing Association (2013). *Issues in ethics: Confidentiality*. Retrieved from: https://www.asha.org/Practice/ethics/Confidentiality/

American Speech-Language-Hearing Association. (2014). *2014 standards and implementation procedures for the certificate of clinical competence in speech-language pathology* (2014, revised March, 2016). Retrieved from https://www.asha.org/Certification/2014-Speech-Language-Pathology-Certification-Standards/

American Speech-Language-Hearing Association. (2016). *Code of ethics* [Ethics]. Available from https://www.asha.org/Code-of-Ethics/

Barnett, J. E., Erickson Cornish, J. A., Goodyear, R., & Lichtenberg, J. W. (2007). Commentaries on the ethical and effective practice of clinical supervision. *Professional Psychology: Research and Practice, 38*(3) 268-275.

Kilminster, S. M., & Jolly, B. C. (2000). Effective supervision in clinical practice settings: A literature review. *Medical Education, 34*, 827-840.

O'Neil-Pirozzi, T. M. (2001). Please respect patient confidentiality. *Contemporary Issues in Communication Science and Disorders, 28*, 48-51.

Saccuzzo, D. P. (1997). Liability for failure to supervise adequately mental health assistants, unlicensed practitioners and students. *California Western Law Review, 34*(1), 10.

U.S. Department of Education. (n.d.) *Protecting student privacy*. Retrieved from https://studentprivacy.ed.gov/node/548/

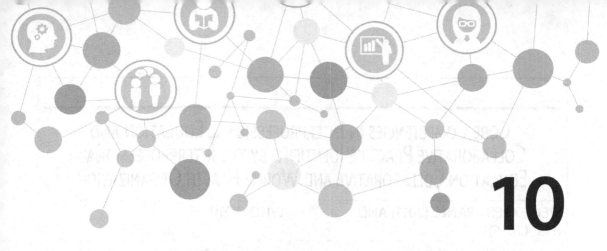

10

Simulations and Interprofessional Education and Practice in Communication Sciences and Disorders

A. Lynn Williams, PhD, CCC-SLP, F-ASHA, F-NAP and
Mindi Anderson, PhD, APRN, CPNP-PC, CNE, CHSE-A, ANEF, FAAN

Overview of Interprofessional Education and Interprofessional Practice in Health Care and Education

Per the World Health Organization (WHO) (2010) and other sources, interprofessional education (IPE) is a pedagogy where at least two professions of students are deliberately put together with defined educational outcomes (Buring et al., 2009; Interprofessional Education Collaborative [IPEC], 2016; IPEC Expert Panel, 2011; Thistlethwaite, 2015; WHO, 2010). One of the main purposes of IPE is for the students involved to experience functioning as a collaborative team within the health care or school environment for the betterment of patients or clients (Buring et al., 2009). Students should learn with other professions, exchanging thoughts and ideas, rather than education occurring in discipline-specific silos (IPEC, 2016; WHO, 2010).

The original IPEC report in 2011 included six different professions, including medicine, nursing, and others (IPEC, 2016). IPEC then expanded its membership beyond the original six national education associations of health to add additional members, including the American Speech-Language-Hearing Association (ASHA). IPEC specified a set of core competencies that have been widely adopted; it includes the necessary knowledge and skills to practice as an interprofessional (ASHA, 2016). These competencies are listed in Table 10-1.

McCrea, E. S., & Brasseur, J. A. *The Clinical Education and Supervisory Process in Speech–Language Pathology and Audiology* (pp 321-334).
© 2020 Taylor & Francis Group.

TABLE 10-1
CORE COMPETENCIES IN INTERPROFESSIONAL EDUCATION AND COLLABORATIVE PRACTICE IDENTIFIED BY THE INTERPROFESSIONAL EDUCATION COLLABORATIVE AND WORLD HEALTH ORGANIZATION

IPEC EXPERT PANEL (2011) AND IPEC (2016)	WHO (2010)
• Values and ethics for IPP • Roles and responsibilities • Teams and teamwork • Interprofessional communication	• Ethical practice • Roles and responsibilities • Teamwork • Communication • Relationship with the patient • Learning and reflection

Adapted from Interprofessional Education Collaborative. (2016). *Core competencies for interprofessional collaborative practice: 2016 update.* Washington, DC: Interprofessional Education Collaborative; Interprofessional Education Collaborative Expert Panel. (2011). *Core competencies for interprofessional collaborative practice: Report of an expert panel.* Washington, DC: Interprofessional Education Collaborative; and reprinted with permission from World Health Organization, *Framework for Action on Interprofessional Education & Collaborative Practice,* Copyright (2010). Retrieved from https://www.who.int/hrh/resources/framework_action/en/. Accessed May 31, 2019.

These competencies require academic programs to move beyond their own discipline-specific silos in order to engage students across professions to interact and learn with each other (Wilhaus et al., n.d.). A fundamental element of that learning for students involves working together effectively as a clinical team (Wilhaus et al., n.d.).

Changes in health care provided the drive for IPE, largely because new models of health care delivery required a team-based and collaborative approach (Institute of Medicine, 2001; WHO, 2010). However, IPE and interprofessional practice (IPP) also occur in academic settings in which the collective knowledge and skills of school professionals are utilized to create educational plans in which shared knowledge guides the development and implementation of integrated goals that are not fragmented across disciplines (ASHA, 2016). Similar to the desired patient-centered outcomes in health care, collaborative practice in school settings improves the educational, emotional, and social health of children, which incorporates the standards for educational best practices.

A number of professions have endorsed the concept of IPE, with changes in accreditation standards as a motivating drive for academic programs to incorporate aspects of IPE and IPP into their academic and clinical curricula (Buring et al., 2009). A short time ago, the Council on Academic Accreditation in Audiology and Speech-Language Pathology (CAA; 2017) revised accreditation standards to incorporate IPE and practice. Specifically, professional practice competencies (3.1.1A for audiology; 3.1.1B for speech-language pathology) include understanding "how to work on interprofessional teams to maintain a climate of mutual respect and shared values;" good communication skills among team members; knowing roles (including own and others); and understanding different roles in order to effectively operate as a team for optimal patient care (CAA, 2017, pp. 9, 19).

	TABLE 10-2	
	TYPES OF SIMULATION	
SIMULATION	**DESCRIPTION**	**EXAMPLES**
Standardized patients	Coaching an individual to simulate a patient realistically; can be standardized.	Traumatic brain injury, cerebrovascular accident
Mannequins	High- to low-fidelity life-size simulator that looks like a human; can be programmed by computers to demonstrate different functions.	Tracheostomy (Ward et al., 2014), audiological testing (Baby Isao, manufactured by Intelligent Hearing Systems; Alanazi et al., 2017)
Computer-based simulations	Interactive computer simulations of different clinical cases.	SimuCase (www.simucase.com) AudSim (audstudent.com)
Immersive virtual reality	Three-dimensional computer-based simulation, which feels like the student is immersed in the situation.	Avatars in *Second Life*

Reprinted and adapted with permission from American Speech-Language-Hearing Association, from *A national survey of simulation use in university programs in Communications Sciences and Disorders*, Dudding, C. C., & Nottingham, E. E., 27(1), 2018; permission conveyed through Copyright Clearance Center, Inc. and adapted from Lopreiato, J. O. (Ed.), Downing, D., Gammon, W., Lioce, L., Sittner, B., Slot, V., Spain, A. E. (Associate Eds.) and the Terminology & Concepts Working Group. (2016). *Healthcare Simulation Dictionary*. Rockville, MD: Agency for Healthcare Research and Quality; October 2016. AHRQ Publication No. 16(17)-0043.

INCORPORATING INTERPROFESSIONAL EDUCATION AND INTERPROFESSIONAL PRACTICE INTO CLINICAL EDUCATION

Although there are different educational models for incorporating IPE into the curriculum, several organizations, including the Society for Simulation in Healthcare (SSH) and the National League for Nursing (NLN), distinguished the intersection between IPE and simulation (referred to as Sim-IPE) as an opportunity to blend these two areas in clinical education (O'Rourke, Horsley, Doolen, Mariani, & Periseault, 2018; Tullmann, Shilling, Goeke, Wright & Littlewood, 2012). SSH is a society made up of multidisciplinary members throughout the world, including medicine, nursing, and others (Wilhaus et al., n.d.).

The International Nursing Association for Clinical Simulation and Learning (INACSL) in the INACSL Standards of Best Practice: Simulation[SM] Simulation Glossary (INACSL Standards Committee, 2016b) defines simulation as "an educational strategy in which a particular set of conditions are created or replicated to resemble authentic situations that are possible in real life" (p. S44). As discussed by Gaba (2004), different simulation modalities can be used (INACSL Standards Committee, 2016b).

The activity (or simulation) itself can be called a simulation-based experience (INACSL Standards Committee, 2016b). Other terms seen in the literature include simulated learning environment (Dzulkarnain, Wan Mhd Pandi, Rahmat, & Zakaria, 2015; MacBean, Theodoros, Davidson, & Hill, 2013), simulated and simulation learning experience (SLE; van Vuuren, 2016; Ryan et al., 2017), or clinical simulation (CS; ASHA, n.d.), can be defined as "an activity designed to mimic real functions or behaviors for education and training purposes" (Alanazi et al., 2017, p. 12).

There are different ways that simulation can be incorporated. Table 10-2 lists the most common SLEs along with examples from speech-language pathology and audiology.

Many of these SLEs have been incorporated within speech-language pathology and audiology clinical education programs. Several authors have written about SLE activities for those in the speech-language pathology and audiology professions. These include Theodoros, Davidson, Hill, and MacBean (2010), as cited in MacBean et al. (2013), and Wilson et al. (2011). These sources specify types of simulations, including standardized patients (SPs) and mannequin-based simulations (MacBean et al., 2010; Theodoros et al., 2010).

Incorporating simulation within an interprofessional context involves a number of shared elements, including responsibility, accountability, and others (Bridges, Davidson, Odegard, Maki, & Tomkowiak, 2011). A significant component of Sim-IPE is assisting students to understand not only others' roles and responsibilities, but their own as well (Bridges et al., 2011).

Benefits and Challenges of Sim-IPE

While Sim-IPE provides a platform to incorporate IPE within clinical experiences, it is important to understand both the benefits and challenges (INACSL Standards Committee, 2016c). Theodoros et al. (2010), as cited in MacBean et al. (2013), and Wilson et al. (2011) expand on benefits and challenges, specifically for those in speech-language pathology and audiology. One of the benefits is that multiple skills can be targeted; this may include communication and history-taking (MacBean et al., 2013; Theodoros et al., 2010). Research of SPs being engaged (McNaughton & Anderson, 2017) by speech-language pathology students has shown that SP performance is reproducible and accurate (Hill, Davidson, & Theodoros, 2013). Authors have described that SPs help increase student confidence and learning (Bressmann & Eriks-Brophy, 2012). Early literature has also shown that SLEs are effective for audiology student learning (Dzulkarnain et al., 2015).

A number of challenges have been identified for implementation of simulation, which may incorporate Sim-IPE, into academic and clinical programs. According to MacBean et al. (2013) and Theodoros et al. (2010), these include:

- Simulation space
- Finding and training SPs
- Case creation
- Financial commitment
- Time

SLEs and Sim-IPE are fairly new in the speech-language pathology and audiology curriculum (Dudding & Nottingham, 2018; Dzulkarnain et al., 2015; MacBean et al., 2013; Ward et al., 2014). Therefore, few publications exist (Dzulkarnain et al., 2015; MacBean et al., 2013) to support its use for these professions.

TABLE 10-3

RESOURCES FOR INTERPROFESSIONAL EDUCATION AND SIMULATED LEARNING ENVIRONMENT/EXPERIENCE

REFERENCE	SAMPLE IPE RESOURCES
ASHA https://www.asha.org/practice/interprofessional-education-practice/	• Repository of resources, publications, and presentations on IPE and IPP relative to audiology and speech-language pathology • Links to websites with resources
CAPCSD (n.d.) http://www.capcsd.org/academicclinical-resources/interprofessional-education-2/ipe-resources/	• Links to websites with resources • Link to guide: *Best practices in healthcare simulations in communication sciences and disorders* (CAPCSD, 2018)
National Center for Interprofessional Practice and Education (n.d.) https://nexusipe.org/	• Forums related to IPE • IPE conference information and research • Tools to evaluate IPE
Speakman, Tagliareni, Sherburne, & Sicks (2016) http://www.nln.org/newsroom/news-releases/news-release/2016/01/29/ipe-toolkit-and-vision-statement	• Checklist for IPE readiness • Exemplars for the different best practice models for IPE
University of Washington Center for Health Sciences Interprofessional Education Research and Practice (n.d.-b) https://collaborate.uw.edu/ipe-teaching-resources/	• Curriculum for educators, including a toolkit • Sample IPE activities and cases • Templates for cases and simulations • Tools for evaluating IPE and to debrief

INFORMATION FOR FACULTY TO BE INTERPROFESSIONAL EDUCATORS

There are multiple resources available for Sim-IPE. One example is the NLN toolkit (Speakman, Tagliareni, Sherburne, & Sicks, 2016) that may be helpful for any discipline considering IPE. The University of Washington Center for Health Sciences Interprofessional Education Research and Practice (n.d.-a, n.d.-b) provides resources for IPE activities, toolkits, and training opportunities for clinical faculty interested in developing Sim-IPE, along with other resources listed in Table 10-3. The Council of Academic Programs in Communication Sciences and Disorders (CAPCSD; 2018) created a task force to determine current best practices in simulations in communication sciences and disorders. The final guide noted that an important first step in getting started with Sim-IPE is to identify the desired student learning outcomes that are specific to each profession and to promote communication, professionalism, and teamwork among the professions (CAPCSD, 2018).

Jeffries, Dreifuerst, Kardong-Edgren, and Hayden (2015) illustrated a simulation framework within nursing and described faculty development that is needed in order to implement simulation. Five components included within the framework, now the NLN Jeffries Simulation Theory (Jeffries, Rodgers, & Adamson, 2015), are the facilitator (supervisor or possibly preceptor), participant (student or learner), educational practices, characteristics of simulation design, and anticipated learner outcomes. Within the simulation design, debriefing is a primary feature (Jeffries et al., 2015); an important aspect where learners engage in reflection about a simulated experience (Dreifuerst, 2010; NLN Board of Governors, 2015a). Debriefing transpires as the facilitator and students recall, reflect on, and analyze what happened in the simulation and the thought processes behind actions (Dreifuerst, 2010). It is needed to develop student clinical reasoning skills, enhance learning (Dreifuerst, 2010), and develop practitioners who can reflect (NLN Board of Governors, 2015a). It has been posited as needed not only after simulation, but within the classroom and clinical experience as well (NLN Board of Governors, 2015a).

The skills, therefore, of the debriefer are essential. Good debriefing, however, does not just happen. It requires training and development (NLN Board of Governors, 2015a). According to the INACSL Standards of Best Practice: Simulation[SM] Debriefing (INACSL Standards Committee, 2016a), the debriefing also needs to be structured.

There are multiple debriefing models or frameworks available to structure a debrief. In the Debriefing for Meaningful Learning (DML; Dreifuerst, 2010, 2015) model, the clinical educator uses the Socratic method to guide practitioners through a structured activity that involves reflection in, on, and through action. The goal is for students to learn how to be reflective and to develop clinical reasoning skills (Dreifuerst, 2010, 2015; Jeffries, Dreifuerst, et al., 2015). Promoting Excellence and Reflective Learning in Simulation (PEARLS; Eppich & Cheng, 2015) is another debriefing framework used in simulation-based education. It provides a structured framework to facilitate clinical decision making, teamwork, collaboration among professionals, as well as, enhance technical skills. It incorporates three education strategies in the debriefing: self-assessment of the learner, facilitated discussion, and feedback (Eppich & Cheng, 2015). These are but two examples of models or frameworks.

Evaluation of the debriefer is important as well. As stated in INACSL Standards of Best Practice: Simulation[SM] Debriefing (INACSL Standards Committee, 2016a), a debriefer's competence should be validated "through the ongoing use of an established instrument" (p. S22). Two commonly used debriefing evaluation tools are the Debriefing Assessment for Simulation in Healthcare (DASH; Simon, Raemer, & Rudolph, 2009) used by trained individuals to evaluate debriefing skills; and the Debriefing Experience Scale (DES; Reed, 2012) utilized by the learners to evaluate their debriefing experience.

Clinical educators must be prepared to develop and use Sim-IPE. Jeffries et al. (2015) described training that included three workshops of 2- to 3-days each created to teach faculty the following skills: how to conduct a simulation, debriefing, and how to utilize evaluation tools.

SIMULATION AND AMERICAN SPEECH-LANGUAGE-HEARING ASSOCIATION REQUIREMENTS

ASHA (n.d.) has provided guidelines and frequently asked questions about CS and what does and does not constitute clinical hours specifically for speech-language pathology and audiology professionals.

The 2014 Standards for the Certificate of Clinical Competence in Speech-Language Pathology (CFCC) were recently revised in 2016 by the Council for Clinical Certification in Audiology and

Speech-Language Pathology (CFCC, 2013); CS (or Alternative Clinical Education [ACE]) was added to Standard V-B. Specifically, programs who hold CAA accreditation are now allowed to use

> CS for as much as 75 hours (direct clinical contact). This modification of standards specified that CS experiences should allow students to a) interpret, integrate, and synthesize core concepts and knowledge; b) demonstrate appropriate professional and clinical skills; and c) incorporate critical thinking and decision-making skills while engaged in identification, evaluation, diagnosis, planning, implementation, and/or intervention. (ASHA, n.d., Standards reprinted with permission from ASHA.)

The minimum supervision requirement is still mandated within CS or SLE ("25% of a student's total contact with each client or patient") (ASHA, n.d.). The revised standard acknowledges that supervision takes different forms and can be synchronous or asynchronous but should include a debriefing component to ensure meaningful learning. When asynchronous, CS must "meet the 25% supervision requirement in asynchronous learning situations. In synchronous learning, observation" occurs while the student completes a task with an SP or within a SLE (ASHA, n.d.).

The revised CFCC standard also addresses the way clock hours are determined (CFCC, 2013). Some companies who publish computer-based simulations specify the average time the experience is projected to take. However, academic programs can either use the average time that a cohort of students takes to complete a simulation or determine a set time that is applied consistently across all student cohorts (CFCC, 2013).

Finally, the standard specifies that clinical hours can only be counted once although students have the option of repetitive practice within a SLE (CFCC, 2013). It is suggested that these guidelines be checked frequently for changes.

ASSESSMENT OF INTERPROFESSIONAL EDUCATION AND INTERPROFESSIONAL PRACTICE COMPONENTS AND STUDENT CLINICAL OUTCOMES

A number of tools has been created to evaluate various components of IPE and IPP. These include assessment of teamwork and professionalism, attitudes toward IPE and IPP, debriefing, and clinical skills. This section focuses on assessment of clinical skills, but Table 10-4 summarizes some of the assessment tools in each area.

Two frequently used measures for assessment of students' learning and clinical skills are the Objective Structured Clinical Examination (OSCE; Harden, 1988; Harden, Stevenson, Downie, & Wilson, 1975; Zraick, 2012) and the Assessment of Foundation Clinical Skills (AFCS; Hill, Davidson, McAllister, Wright, & Theodoros, 2014). The OSCE is often used with SPs (Zraick, 2012), and the AFCS is utilized with SLEs (Hill et al., 2014). Each of these assessment tools is briefly described below.

Originally created to evaluate medical students (Harden, Stevenson, Downie, & Wilson, 1975), OSCEs are widely utilized for formative and summative evaluation (Lopreiato et al., 2016) across a number of health fields, including allied health disciplines (Zayyan, 2011). They involve the development of a series of brief simulated clinical encounters (Harden, 1988; Lopreiato et al., 2016), often with an SP, that require students to perform specific tasks (e.g., history taking, test administration, interpersonal and professional communication skills) within a highly structured encounter that is timed (Zraick, 2012; Zraick, Allen, & Johnson, 2003). OSCEs require prior preparation, such as development of a case and training of SPs (Zraick, 2012; Zraick et al., 2003). They can be administered at different points across a semester or program of study. Currently, literature regarding OSCEs with speech-language pathologists is limited (Zraick, 2012). In one study, SPs were used with speech-language pathology students to address and then assess communication

TABLE 10-4

SUMMARY OF INTERPROFESSIONAL EDUCATION/INTERPROFESSIONAL PRACTICE ASSESSMENT TOOLS OF TEAMWORK/INTERPROFESSIONALISM, ATTITUDES, DEBRIEFING, AND CLINICAL SKILLS

ASSESSMENT AREA	ASSESSMENT TOOLS	DESCRIPTION
Teamwork and interprofessionalism	Interprofessional Professionalism Assessment (IPA; Interprofessional Professionalism Collaborative: http://www.interprofessionalprofessionalism.org/; Frost et al., 2018; Holtman, Frost, Hammer, McGuinn, & Nunez, 2011)	Twenty-six behavioral-item assessment tool used by preceptors and supervisors to rate how well a student or trainee demonstrates professionalism across six categories (altruism and caring, excellence, ethics, respect, communication, accountability) when interacting with other professionals
	Clinical Teamwork Scale (CTS; Guise et al., 2008)	Fifteen-item brief tool to evaluate teamwork as a unit; objective measure for short simulations or during care; includes five categories of teamwork, such as communication
	Mayo High Performance Teamwork Scale (MHPTS; Malec et al., 2007)	Sixteen-item assessment of teams, which measures key resource management skills in training settings
	Communication and Teamwork Skills Assessment (CATS; Frankel, Gardner, Maynard, & Kelly, 2007)	Twenty-one items assessment of teams in the categories of coordination, situational awareness, cooperation, and communication
	Team Strategies and Tools to Enhance Performance and Patient Safety (TeamSTEPPS; http://teamstepps.ahrq.gov)	Includes 25 items in the categories of team structure, e.g., leadership, situation monitoring, mutual support, and communication
	Interprofessional Socialization and Valuing Scale (ISVS; Zook, Hulton, Dudding, Stewart, & Graham, 2018)	Twenty-one-item self-report used to assess the impact of IPE programming across three subscales related to working with others (e.g., value and comfort)

continued

TABLE 10-4 (CONTINUED)

SUMMARY OF INTERPROFESSIONAL EDUCATION/INTERPROFESSIONAL PRACTICE ASSESSMENT TOOLS OF TEAMWORK/INTERPROFESSIONALISM, ATTITUDES, DEBRIEFING, AND CLINICAL SKILLS

ASSESSMENT AREA	ASSESSMENT TOOLS	DESCRIPTION
Attitudes (some as mentioned in Woermann, Weltsch, Kunz, Stricker, & Guttormsen, 2016)	Readiness of Health Care Students for Interprofessional Learning (RIPLS; Parsell & Bligh, 1999)	Self-report scales to assess attitudes toward IPE and care
	Interdisciplinary Education Perception Scale (IEPS; Luecht, Madsen, Taugher, & Petterson, 1990)	
	Attitudes Towards Health Care Teams Scale (as cited in Curran, Heath, Kearney, & Button, 2010)	
	University of the West England Interprofessional Questionnaire (Pollard, Meirs, & Gilschrist, 2005)	
Debriefing	Debriefing Assessment for Simulation in Healthcare (DASH; Simon, Raemer, & Rudolph, 2009; https://harvardmedsim.org/debriefing-assessment-for-simulation-in-healthcare-dash/)	Collection of tools used to develop and assess a debriefer's skills
	Debriefing Experience Scale (DES; Reed, 2012)	Rating scale of 20 items with 4 subscales; subjective tool utilized by learners to assess the debriefing
Clinical skills	Objective Structured Clinical Examination (OSCE; Harden, 1988; Lopreiato et al., 2016)	Timed assessment of students within a highly structured simulated encounter, often with SPs
	Assessment of Foundation Clinical Skills (AFCS: Hill, Davidson, McAllister, Wright, & Theodoros, 2014)	Assessment tool used within a SLE that incorporates 7 of the 11 clinical competency units assessed by the COMPASS

skills with aphasia patients (Zraick et al., 2003). Overall, skills were improved with a combination of didactic information and SP experiences, particularly after additional lecture. Students felt the SP and OSCE experiences were appropriate (Zraick et al., 2003).

The AFCS was designed specifically for evaluation of foundational clinical skills within a simulated clinical placement for speech-language pathology students (Hill et al., 2014). This tool, designed by Australian authors, is linked to the Australian clinical evaluation tool, COMPASS (Competency Assessment in Speech Pathology). The AFCS incorporates seven of the 11 clinical competency units that are assessed by COMPASS with consideration of the different learning objectives, as well as, clinical activities that can occur with this type of placement. The seven units include four professional competencies as well as three occupational competencies. The visual analogue scale (VAS) of the COMPASS is also included to evaluate students' competency. The VAS includes four categories that range from pre-Novice at one end, to Novice and Intermediate (middle), to Entry level at the other end. Behavioral descriptors are specified for each category based on the following three elements from McAllister, Lincoln, Ferguson and McAllister (2011): "transforming knowledge into practice, dealing with complexity, and level of independence" (Hill et al., 2014, p. 12). Preliminary results of a study by Hill et al. (2014) support the AFCS as a valid tool for simulated clinical placement to assess foundational clinical skills.

Next Steps

To meet the changes in educational and health care reforms, clinical programs for speech-language pathologists and audiologists need to embrace new pedagogies to prepare our students to be "practice ready" to work collaboratively with others outside our professions. In order to successfully plan and implement IPE, faculty may need to:
- Learn how to teach differently (NLN Board of Governors, 2015b)
- Attend continuing education and other development opportunities incorporating interprofessional collaboration and IPE content (Buring et al., 2009; NLN Board of Governors, 2015b)

Additionally, faculty should:
- Create an IPE committee comprised of all the health professions involved (Thistlethwaite, 2015)
- Determine shared content among the professions (Thistlethwaite, 2015)
- Read and incorporate the IPEC core competencies, which should be used a backbone (NLN Board of Governors, 2015b)
- Assimilate critical elements of IPE (Buring et al., 2009)
- Choose the right teaching method (Thistlethwaite, 2015)
- Ensure IPE is threaded throughout the curriculum (Buring et al., 2009; NLN Board of Governors, 2015b; Thistlethwaite, 2015)

If planning to utilize Sim-IPE, faculty needs to:
- Be formally trained in simulation pedagogy (Kardong-Edgren, 2015), including how to design, plan, manage, and debrief simulations, e.g., use simulation effectively (Texas Board of Nursing, 2015)
- Attend continuing education on simulation (Kardong-Edgren, 2015)
- Read and incorporate the INACSL Standards of Best Practice: Simulation[SM] (INACSL, n.d.) including the INACSL Standards of Best Practice: Simulation[SM] Simulation-Enhanced

Education (Sim-IPE; INACSL Standards Committee, 2016c) and the standards of practice related to SPs, e.g., the Association of Standardized Patient Educators (ASPE) Standards of Best Practice (SOBP; Lewis et al., 2017), as appropriate.

Opportunities exist for speech-language pathology and audiology professions to use and validate simulation pedagogy (MacBean et al., 2013; Ward et al., 2014). The optimal use of SPs for communication sciences and disorders has many areas that need to be researched (Zraick, 2014). Many questions still exist that need to be researched. For example:

- Are skills learned in simulation retained (Ward et al., 2014)?

- Is simulation (such as the engagement of SPs; McNaughton & Anderson, 2017) useful for enhancing speech-language pathology student knowledge and other outcomes (Hill, Davidson, & Theodoros, 2010)?

- Are outcomes of students in simulation similar to workforce placements (MacBean et al., 2013)?

- Are skills learned within simulation able to be translated to the clinical setting (MacBean et al., 2013)?

More studies are also needed to look at the reproducibility of standarized patient performance in different types of scenarios (Hill et al., 2013). OSCE studies incorporating SPs, particularly related to speech-language pathologists and audiologists are needed (Zraick, 2012).

In conclusion, faculty are encouraged to build on the work of colleagues in other health and education professions and to contribute to the evidence base within the speech-language pathology and audiology professions.

REFERENCES

Alanazi, A. A., Nicholson, N., Atcherson, S. R., Franklin, C. A., Nagaraj, N. K., Anders, M., & Smith-Olinde, L. (2017). Audiology students' perception of hybrid simulation experiences: Qualitative evaluation of debriefing sessions. *Journal of Early Hearing Detection and Intervention, 2*(1), 12-28. doi:10.15142/T32K8V

American Speech-Language-Hearing Association. (n.d.). *Certification standards for speech-language pathology frequently asked questions: Clinical simulation 2014 SLP Certification Standards.* Retrieved from https://www.asha.org/Certification/Certification-Standards-for-SLP--Clinical-Simulation/

American Speech-Language-Hearing Association. (2016, August). *Interprofessional education and interprofessional practice in communication sciences and disorders: An introduction and case-based examples of implementation in education and health care settings.* Retrieved from https://www.asha.org/uploadedFiles/IPE-IPP-Reader-eBook.pdf

Association of Standardized Patient Educators. (n.d.). Retrieved from http://www.aspeducators.org/

Bressmann, T., & Eriks-Brophy, A. (2012). Use of simulated patients for a student learning experience on managing difficult patient behavior in speech-language pathology contexts. *International Journal of Speech-Language Pathology, 14*(2), 165-173. doi:10.3109/17549507.2011.638727

Bridges, D. R., Davidson, R. A., Odegard, P. S., Maki, I. V., & Tomkowiak, J. (2011). Interprofessional collaboration: Three best practice models of interprofessional education. *Medical Education Online, 16*(10). doi:10.3402/meo.v16i0.6035

Buring, S. M., Bhushan, A., Broeseker, A., Conway, S., Duncan-Hewitt, W., Hansen, L., & Westberg, S. (2009). Interprofessional education: Definitions, student competencies, and guidelines for implementation. *American Journal of Pharmaceutical Education, 73*(4), 59. doi:10.5688/aj730459

Council on Academic Accreditation in Audiology and Speech-Language Pathology. (2017). *Standards for accreditation of graduate education programs in audiology and speech-language pathology.* Retrieved from https://caa.asha.org/wp-content/uploads/Accreditation-Standards-for-Graduate-Programs.pdf

Council of Academic Programs in Communication Sciences and Disorders. (n.d.). *IPE resources.* Retrieved from http://www.capcsd.org/academicclinical-resources/interprofessional-education-2/ipe-resources/

Council of Academic Programs in Communication Sciences and Disorders. (2018, May 21). *Best practices in healthcare simulations in communication sciences and disorders.* Retrieved from http://www.capcsd.org/wp-content/uploads/2018/05/Simulation-Guide-Published-May-18-2018.pdf

Council for Clinical Certification in Audiology and Speech-Language Pathology of the American Speech-Language-Hearing Association. (2013). *2014 Standards for the Certificate of Clinical Competence in Speech-Language Pathology.* Retrieved June 11, 2018, from http://www.asha.org/Certification/2014-Speech-Language-Pathology-Certification-Standards/

Curran, V. R., Heath, O., Kearney, A., & Button, P. (2010). Evaluation of an interprofessional collaboration workshop for post-graduate residents, nursing and allied health professionals. *Journal of Interprofessional Care, 24*(3), 315-318. https://doi.org/10.3109/13561820903163827

Dreifuerst, K. T. (2010). *Debriefing for meaningful learning: Fostering development of clinical reasoning through simulation.* (Order No. 3617512, Indiana University). Retrieved from ProQuest Dissertations and Theses, 212. http://search.proquest.com/docview/1527174151?accountid.7398

Dreifuerst, K. T. (2015). Getting started with debriefing for meaningful learning. *Clinical Simulation in Nursing, 11*(5), 268-275. http://dx.doi.org/10.1016/j.ecns.2015.01.005

Dudding, C. C., & Nottingham, E. E. (2018). A national survey of simulation use in university programs in Communication Sciences and Disorders. *American Journal of Speech-Language Pathology, 27*(1), 71-81. https://doi.org/10.1044/2017_AJSLP-17-0015

Dzulkarnain, A. A., Wan Mhd Pandi, W. M., Rahmat, S., & Zakaria, N. (2015). Simulated learning environment (SLE) in audiology education: A systematic review. *International Journal of Audiology, 54*(12), 881-888. doi:10.3109/14992027.2015.1055840

Eppich, W., & Cheng, A. (2015). Promoting excellence and reflective learning in simulation (PEARLS): Development and rationale for a blended approach to health care simulation debriefing. *Simulation in Healthcare, 10*(2), 106-115. doi:10.1097/SIH.0000000000000072

Frankel, A., Gardner, R., Maynard, L., & Kelly, A. (2007). Using the Communication and Teamwork Skills (CATS) assessment to measure health care team performance. *Joint Commission Journal on Quality & Patient Safety, 33*(9), 549-558. doi:10.1016/S1553-7250(07)33059-6

Frost, J. S., Hammer, D. P., Nunez, L. M., Adams, J. L., Chesluk, B., Grus, C., . . . Bentley, J. P. (2019). The intersection of professionalism and interprofessional care: Development and initial testing of the interprofessional professionalism assessment (IPA). *Journal of Interprofessional Care,* 1-14. https://doi.org/10.1080/13561820.2018.1515733

Gaba, D. M. (2004). The future vision of simulation in healthcare. *Quality and Safety in Healthcare, 13*(Suppl. 1), i2-i10. http://dx.doi.org/10.1136/qshc.2004.009878

Guise, J. M., Deering, S. H., Kanki, B. G., Osterweil, P., Li, J., Mori, M., & Lowe, N. K. (2008). Validation of a tool to measure and promote clinical teamwork. *Simulation in Healthcare, 3*(4), 217-223. doi: 10.1097/SIH.0b013e31816fdd0a

Harden, R. M. (1988). What is an OSCE? *Medical Teacher, 10*(1), 19-22.

Harden, R. M., Stevenson, M., Downie, W. W., & Wilson, G. M. (1975). Assessment of clinical competence using objective structured examination. *British Medical Journal, 1*, 447-451. https://doi.org/10.1136/bmj.1.5955.447

Hill, A. E., Davidson, B. J., McAllister, S., Wright, J., & Theodoros, D. G. (2014). Assessment of student competency in a simulated speech-language pathology clinical placement. *International Journal of Speech-Language Pathology, 16*(5), 464-475. doi:10.3109/17549507.2013.809603

Hill, A. E., Davidson, B. J., & Theodoros, D. G. (2010). A review of standardized patients in clinical education: Implications for speech-language pathology programs. *International Journal of Speech-Language Pathology, 12*(3), 259-270. doi:10.3109/17549500903082445

Hill, A. E., Davidson, B. J., & Theodoros, D. G. (2013). The performance of standardized patients in portraying clinical scenarios in speech-language therapy. *International Journal of Language & Communication Disorders, 48*(6), 613-624. doi:10.1111/1460-6984.12034

Holtman, M. C., Frost, J. S., Hammer, D. P., McGuinn, K., & Nunez, L. M. (2011). Interprofessional professionalism: Linking professionalism and interprofessional care. *Journal of Interprofessional Care, 25*(5), 383-385. doi:10.3109/13561820.2011.588350

INACSL Standards Committee. (2016a, December). INACSL standards of best practice: Simulation[SM] Debriefing. *Clinical Simulation in Nursing, 12*(S), S21-S25. https://www.inacsl.org/inacsl-standards-of-best-practice-simulation/

INACSL Standards Committee. (2016b, December). INACSL standards of best practice: Simulation[SM] Simulation glossary. *Clinical Simulation in Nursing, 12*(S), S39-S47. https://doi.org/10.1016/j.ecns.2016.09.012

INACSL Standards Committee. (2016c, December). INACSL standards of best practice: Simulation[SM] Simulation-enhanced interprofessional education (sim-IPE). *Clinical Simulation in Nursing, 12*(S), S34-S38. http://dx.doi.org/10.1016/j.ecns.2016.09.011

Institute of Medicine. (2001). *Crossing the quality chasm: A new health system for the 21st century.* Washington, DC: National Academies Press.

International Nursing Association for Clinical Simulation and Learning. (n.d.). *INACSL Standards of best practice: Simulation[SM].* Retrieved from https://www.inacsl.org/i4a/pages/index.cfm?pageid=3407

Interprofessional Education Collaborative. (2016). *Core competencies for interprofessional collaborative practice: 2016 update.* Washington, DC: Interprofessional Education Collaborative.

Interprofessional Education Collaborative Expert Panel. (2011). *Core competencies for interprofessional collaborative practice: Report of an expert panel.* Washington, DC: Interprofessional Education Collaborative.

Jeffries, P. R., Dreifuerst, K. T., Kardong-Edgren, S., & Hayden, J. (2015). Faculty development when initiating simulation programs: Lessons learned from the National Simulation Study. *Journal of Nursing Regulation, 5*(4), 17-23. https://doi.org/10.1016/S2155-8256(15)30037-5

Jeffries, P. R., Rodgers, B., & Adamson, K. (2015). NLN Jeffries Simulation Theory: Brief narrative description. *Nursing Education Perspectives, 36*(5), 292-293.

Kardong-Edgren, S. (2015). Initial thoughts after the NCSBN National Simulation Study. *Clinical Simulation in Nursing*, 11(4), 201-202. http://dx.doi.org/10.1016/j.ecns.2015.02.005

Lewis, K. L., Bohnert, C. A., Gammon, W. L., Hölzer, H., Lyman, L. . . . Gliva-McConvey, G. (2017). The Association of Standardized Patient Educators (ASPE) standards of best practice (SOBP). *Advances in Simulation*, 2(10). http://doi.org/10.1186/s41077-017-0043-4

Lopreiato, J. O. (Ed.), Downing, D., Gammon, W., Lioce, L., Sittner, B., Slot, V., Spain, A. E. (Associate Eds.), and the Terminology & Concepts Working Group. (2016). *Healthcare Simulation Dictionary*. Rockville, MD: Agency for Healthcare Research and Quality; October 2016. AHRQ Publication No. 16(17)-0043.

Luecht, R. M., Madsen, M. K., Taugher, M. P., & Petterson, B. J. (1990). Assessing professional perceptions: Design and validation of an Interdisciplinary Education Perception Scale. *Journal of Allied Health*, 19(2), 181-191.

MacBean, N., Theodoros, D., Davidson, B., & Hill, A. E. (2013). Simulated learning environments in speech-language pathology: An Australian response. *International Journal of Speech-Language Pathology*, 15(3), 345-357. https://doi.org/10.3109/17549507.2013.779024

Malec, J. F., Torsher, L. C., Dunn, W. F., Wiegmann, D. A., Arnold, J. J., Brown, D. A., & Phatak, V. (2007). The Mayo High Performance Teamwork Scale: Reliability and validity for evaluating key crew resource management skills. *Simulation in Healthcare*, 2(1), 4-10. doi:10.1097/SIH.0b013e31802b68ee

McAllister, S., Lincoln, M., Ferguson, A., & McAllister, L. (2011). A systematic program of research regarding the assessment of speech-language pathology competencies. *International Journal of Speech-Language Pathology*, 13(6), 469-479. doi:10.3109/17549507.2011.580782

McNaughton, N., & Anderson, M. (2017). Standardized patients: It's all in the words. *Clinical Simulation in Nursing*, 13(7), 293-294. http://doi.org/10.1016/j.ecns.2017.05.014

National Center for Interprofessional Practice and Education. (n.d.). Retrieved from https://nexusipe.org/

National League for Nursing Board of Governors. (2015a, June). *Debriefing across the curriculum: A living document from the National League for Nursing in collaboration with the International Nursing Association for Clinical Simulation and Learning*. Retrieved from http://www.nln.org/newsroom/nln-position-documents/nln-living-documents

National League for Nursing Board of Governors. (2015b, December). *Interprofessional collaboration in education and practice: A living document from the National League for Nursing*. Retrieved from http://www.nln.org/newsroom/nln-position-documents/nln-living-documents

O'Rourke, J., Horsley, T. L., Doolen, J., Mariani, B., & Periseault, C. (2018). Integrative review of interprofessional simulation in nursing practice. *Journal of Continuing Education in Nursing*, 49(2), 91-96. doi:10.3928/00220124-20180116-09

Parsell, G., & Bligh, J. (1999). The development of a questionnaire to assess the readiness of health care students for interprofessional learning (RIPLS). *Medical Education*, 33(2), 95-100. doi:10.1046/j.1365-2923.1999.00298.x

Pollard, K., Miers, M.E., & Gilchrist, M. (2005). Second year scepticism: Pre-qualifying health and social care students' midpoint self-assessment, attitudes and perceptions concerning interprofessional learning and working. *Journal of Interprofessional Care*, 19(3), 251-268. https://doi.org/10.1080/13561820400024225

Reed, S. J. (2012). Debriefing Experience Scale: Development of a tool to evaluate the student learning experience in debriefing. *Clinical Simulation in Nursing*, 8(6), e211-e217. https://doi.org/10.1016/j.ecns.2011.11.002

Ryan, C., Roy, S., O'Neill, B., Simes, T., Lapkin, S., & Riva, E. (2017). Designing simulation learning experiences to reduce technological burden on nursing academics: A discussion paper. *Australian Journal of Advanced Nursing*, 35(2), 6-11. http://www.ajan.com.au/

Simon, R., Raemer, D.B., & Rudolph, J.W. (2009). *Debriefing Assessment for Simulation in Healthcare*. Cambridge, MA: Center for Medical Simulation.

Speakman, E., Tagliareni, E., Sherburne, A., & Sicks, S. (2016). *Guide to effective interprofessional education experiences in nursing education*. Retrieved from http://www.nln.org/newsroom/news-releases/news-release/2016/01/29/ipe-toolkit-and-vision-statement

Texas Board of Nursing. (2015). *Texas Board of Nursing: 3.8.6.a. Education guideline: Simulation in pre-licensure nursing education*. Retrieved from https://www.bon.texas.gov/

Theodoros, D., Davidson, B., Hill, A., & MacBean, N. (2010). *Integration of simulated learning environments into speech pathology clinical education curricula: A national approach*. Health Workforce Australia. Retrieved from https://www.academia.edu/6618513/Integration_of_simulated_learning_environments_into_speech_pathology_clinical_education_curricula_A_national_approach

Thistlethwaite, J. E. (2015). Interprofessional education and the basic sciences: Rationale and outcomes. *Anatomical Sciences Education*, 8(4), 299-304. doi:10.1002/ase.1521

Tullmann, D., Shilling, A. M., Goeke, L., Wright, E. B., & Littlewood, K. E. (2014). Recreating simulation scenarios for interprofessional education: An example of educational interprofessional practice. *Journal of Interprofessional Care*, 27(5), 426-428. https://doi.org/10.3109/13561820.2013.790880

University of Washington Center for Health Sciences Interprofessional Education Research and Practice. (n.d.-a). *About us*. Retrieved from https://collaborate.uw.edu/

University of Washington Center for Health Sciences Interprofessional Education Research and Practice. (n.d.-b). *Resources and training*. Retrieved from https://collaborate.uw.edu/ipe-teaching-resources/

van Vuuren, S. (2016). Reflections on simulated learning experiences of occupational therapy students in a clinical skills unit at an institution of higher learning. *South African Journal of Occupational Therapy, 46*(3), 80-84. http://dx.doi.org/10.17159/2310-3833/2016/v46n3/a13

Ward, E. C., Baker, S. C., Wall, L. R., Duggan, B. L. J., Hancock, K. L., Bassett, L. V., & Hyde, T. J. (2014). Can human mannequin-based simulation provide a feasible and clinically acceptable method for training tracheostomy management skills for speech-language pathologists? *American Journal of Speech-Language Pathology, 23*(3), 421-436. doi:10.1044/2014_AJSLP-13-0050

Wilhaus, J., Palaganas, J., Manos, J., Anderson, J., Cooper, A., Jeffries, P., ... Mancini, M. E. (n.d.). *Interprofessional education and healthcare simulation symposium.* Retrieved from http://www.nln.org/docs/default-source/professional-development-programs/white-paper-symposium-ipe-in-healthcare-simulation-2013-(pdf).pdf?sfvrsn=0

Wilson, W., Goulios, H., Kapadia, S., Patuzzi, R., Kei, J., Vikovic, J., . . . Marshall, A. (2011). *A national approach for the integration of simulated learning environments into audiology education: Final report. Health Workforce Australia.* Retrieved from http://www.voced.edu.au/content/ngv:67212

Woermann, U., Weltsch, L., Kunz, A., Stricker, D., & Guttormsen, S. (2016). Attitude towards and readiness for interprofessional education in medical and nursing students of Bern. *GMS Journal for Medical Education, 33*(5), 1-20. Retrieved from https://dx.doi.org/10.3205%2Fzma001072

World Health Organization. (2010). *Framework for action on interprofessional education & collaborative practice.* Retrieved from https://www.who.int/hrh/resources/framework_action/en/

Zayyan, M. (2011). Objective Structured Clinical Examination: The assessment of choice. *OMAN Medical Journal, 26*(4), 219-222. doi:10.5001/omj.2011.55

Zook, S. S., Hulton, L. J., Dudding, C. C., Stewart, A. L., & Graham, A. C. (2018). Scaffolding interprofessional education: Unfolding case studies, virtual world simulations, and patient-centered care. *Nurse Educator, 43*(2), 87-91. doi:10.1097/NNE.0000000000000430

Zraick, R. I. (2012). Review of the use of standardized patients in speech-language pathology clinical education. *International Journal of Therapy & Rehabilitation, 19*(2), 112-118. https://doi.org/10.12968/ijtr.2012.19.2.112

Zraick, R. I. (2014, March). *The use of standardized patients in Communication Sciences and Disorders.* Retrieved from https://academy.pubs.asha.org/2014/04/the-use-of-standardized-patients-in-communication-sciences-and-disorders/

Zraick, R. I., Allen, R. M., & Johnson, S. B. (2003). The use of standardized patients to teach and test interpersonal and communication skills with students in speech-language pathology. *Advances in Health Sciences Education Theory and Practice, 8*(3), 237-248. doi:10.1023/A:1026015430376

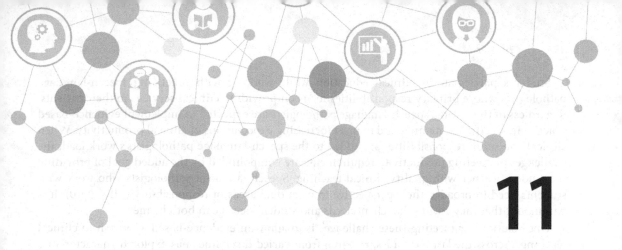

11

Clinical Education and Supervision of Graduate Students

Cheryl Messick, PhD, CCC-SLP, F-ASHA

Clinical education is a key component of graduate education in speech-language pathology, audiology, education, and other health-related fields (e.g., nursing, physical therapy, counseling). For many students, practicum experiences provide important confirmation that they have chosen the "right" profession (Cole & Wessel, 2008). When engaged in clinical education, students have the "opportunity to apply their academic knowledge to a clinical setting and develop understanding about the work they will be doing after graduation" (Sheepway, Lincoln, & McAllister, 2014, p. 199). Practicum experiences provide an important context for seeing and learning how to implement evidence-based practice (Christodoulou, 2016). Additionally, students see how theory is interpreted while they develop clinical competencies through interactions with patients in varied settings (Radtke, 2008). It is also through practicum experiences that students obtain an understanding of professionalism, develop professional oral and written communication skills, and learn case management skills.

Speech-language pathology graduate students are currently required to obtain at least 375 hours of "patient contact time" under the supervision of a certified speech-language pathologist (Council on Academic Accreditation in Audiology and Speech-Language Pathology, 2014). Consider that graduate students may be in the academic classroom a total of 12 to 15 hours per week in a typical graduate program. In contrast, during a clinical externship, students may attend practicum up to 5 days per week and be engaged in clinical education activities for 24 to 40 hours per week. From the perspective of time alone, clinical education experiences comprise a major portion of learning in speech-language pathology graduate education. More importantly, clinical education provides students the opportunity to apply content from coursework to clinical practice in a context that includes modeling, feedback and support from the clinical instructor (Burns, Beauchesne, Ryan-Krause, & Sawin, 2006).

McCrea, E. S., & Brasseur, J. A. *The Clinical Education and Supervisory Process in Speech-Language Pathology and Audiology* (pp 335-360).
© 2020 Taylor & Francis Group.

Students participate in clinical education while working with practicing speech-language pathologists whose primary responsibilities focus on providing clinical services to their patients. Regardless of the setting, speech-language pathologists are expected to implement evidence-based practice in an efficient manner and to meet increasing expectations of clinical productivity. When clinical education responsibilities are added to the speech-language pathologists's work load, the challenges of meeting productivity requirements are compounded by the added goal of providing the student learner with quality clinical teaching. Speech-language pathologists who work with students need to broaden their perspective to meet dual areas of responsibility (Ellis, 2010). It is paramount that they ensure that client needs and student needs can both be met.

One solution for meeting these challenges is to apply an evidence-based approach to clinical teaching. Across the last 2 decades, research from varied disciplines has explored characteristics associated with positive clinical learning experiences which can be applied to clinical education and supervision of speech-language pathology students. Through examination of the literature, key components can be identified which facilitate the development of effective clinical learning experiences. Additionally, through implementation of an evidence-based approach to clinical education supervisors (SORs) can enhance the quality and efficiency of clinical teaching.

Earlier chapters in this textbook address varied components of the supervisory process providing guidelines for structuring clinical education experiences from the viewpoint of SORs. In this chapter, the focus will be on applying multidisciplinary research in three specific areas which have been tied to creating successful clinical learning experiences in graduate clinical education:

1. Characteristics of SORs and supervisees (SEEs) associated with positive learning experiences

2. Developing positive relationships

3. Creating a supportive learning environment

The goal is to identify characteristics and strategies that can be implemented to set the stage for positive learning experiences in off-campus clinical education with speech-language pathology students.

Setting the Stage for Optimal Teaching and Learning

Characteristics of Supervisors and Supervisees Associated With Positive Learning Experiences

A wide range of studies have focused on describing the characteristics and attributes associated with optimal learning experiences. Many of these studies have approached the issue by gathering data on student perceptions and judgements of *effective* vs. *ineffective* instructor behaviors (Byrd, Hood, & Youtsey, 1997; Cole & Wessel, 2008; Laurent & Weidner, 2001; Löfmark & Wikblad, 2009; Öhrling & Hallberg, 2000; Taylor, White, Kaplan & O'Rourke, 2012). Other studies have approached the issue by eliciting descriptions of current SORs compared to ideal or preferred SORs (Papastavrou, Lambrinou, Tsangari, Saarikoski, & Leino-Kilpi, 2010; Papathanasiou, Tsaras & Sarafis, 2014; Saarikoski & Leino-Kilpi, 2002; Wagner & Hess, 1997). A third approach comes from literature reviews across studies aimed at defining key characteristics of SORS that have been associated with positive clinical education experiences (Christodoulou, 2016; Davis & Nakamura, 2010; Kilminster & Jolly, 2000; Levy et al., 2009; Radtke, 2008; Recker-Hughes, Wetherbee, Buccieri, Fitzpatric-Timmerberg & Stolfi, 2014; Weidner, 2009).

Across studies, a constellation of attributes associated with effective vs. ineffective instructors emerges. Broadly speaking, positive learning experiences are associated with clinical educators whose interpersonal style is perceived as being *empathetic, warm, flexible, dependable, approachable,* and *respectful* towards students (Burns et al., 2006; Cole & Wessel, 2008; Davis & Nakamura, 2010; Kilminster & Jolly, 2000; Laurent & Weidner, 2001; Levy et al., 2009; Wagner & Hess, 1997). On the flip side, characteristics such as being *rigid* and *judgmental, lacking respect,* and *having low empathy* have been associated with negative experiences.

Numerous studies report that an instructor's interest and attitude towards working with students influences perception of the clinical learning experience. SORs described as *enthusiastic, dynamic,* and *energetic* convey a positive attitude towards being a clinical educator (Burns et al., 2006; Carr, Spencer, Paulsen, & Chiu, 2016; Kilminster & Jolly, 2002; Laurent & Weidner, 2001; Levy et al., 2009; Taylor et al., 2012). Students value working with SORs who appear to enjoy teaching, and who do not view it as an extra burden (Cooper, Courtney-Pratt & Fitzgerald, 2015). Other attributes associated with positive learning center on student perception of the SORs clinical competence as indicated by the following desirable traits: *competent, knowledgeable, confident,* and *professional* (Levy et al., 2009; Taylor et al., 2012; Weidner, 2009). In a survey completed by 23 speech-language pathology student clinicians, attributes ranked highly included being supportive, realistic, as well as organized (Taylor et al., 2012). Behaviors identified as demonstrating professionalism in a study of physical therapy students included having a positive attitude, using evidence-based practice, showing respect for patients and students, and pursuing continuing education (Cole & Wessel, 2008). When considered holistically, students report that they learn best when working with clinical educators who are excited and positive about providing services to their patients and teaching students; that is, students value working with a professional perceived to be a positive role model (Carr et al., 2016; Cole & Wessel, 2008).

There is some evidence that characteristics viewed as important by SEEs may differ from the perceptions of SORs. Byrd et al. (1997) created a survey where 15 factors were ranked in terms of their relative importance in creating a positive clinical learning experience. The subjects in the study included both nursing instructors and nursing students. Factors identified as most important by instructors were ranked as least important by students and vice versa. For example, SORs ranked the ability to give and receive constructive criticism and clinical competence as the most important, while SEEs ranked those aspects as least important. In contrast students ranked knowledge of the preceptoring process, compatibility, and attitude towards teaching as most important, with SORs ranking those items as least important. The findings of this study support the value of discussions between clinical educators and students addressing aspects of importance to each.

There are only a few studies which have explored the attributes that instructors consider desirable in student clinicians (Burns, et.al., 2006; Carr et al., 2016; Chipchase et al., 2012; Hauer et al., 2015). One study included occupational therapy, physical therapy, and speech-language pathology clinical educator participants and found that a student's interest and willingness to engage in learning and the demonstration of professionalism were considered more desirable traits than arriving with an adequate knowledge base or clinical skills (Chipchase et al., 2012). Interest in learning was manifested by behaviors such as a willingness to try new techniques, to take on new and requested tasks, and to display responsibility for own learning. Positive signs of professionalism were conveyed through behaviors such as arriving on time, dressing appropriately for the setting, completing follow-up tasks from the previous day, and arriving prepared (e.g., bringing needed resources, completing readings). Carr et al. (2016) asked preceptors to rank 13 desirable traits in students with the highest ratings going to initiative and communication skills. Students who communicate their learning needs to the instructor, come prepared each day, and show an eagerness to learn are valued by clinical instructors. May, Morgan, Lemke, Karst and Stone (1995) identified 10 generic student abilities that are essential for successful clinical practice in physical therapy (described in Chapter 4). Their list focused on behaviors that were not discipline specific skills, but which contribute to success in clinical learning, and included behaviors and attributes such as commitment to learning, effective use of time and resources, responsibility, and use of constructive feedback. It is notable that the list of desired student attributes across studies includes behaviors that all students can achieve regardless of whether they are at a beginning or advanced level in their graduate program.

Creating a Positive Relationship

The relationship between a clinical educator and a student clinician has been identified as perhaps the most important variable affecting the quality of the clinical experience (Kilminster & Jolly, 2000; Levy et al., 2009; Papastravrou et al., 2010; Wagner & Hess, 1997). When the relationship between the SOR and the SEE is positive, students report a high level of satisfaction with the experience (Carlson, Wann-Hansson, & Pilhammer, 2009; Papastavrou et al., 2010). In contrast, difficulties in the relationship impact motivation and participation, and create stress and anxiety in SEEs which negatively impacts learning (Chesser-Smyth, 2005; Levett-Jones, Lathlean, Higgens, & McMillan, 2009). When the student-instructor relationship is positive, students are able to focus on the needs of the patients and clinical learning (Levett-Jones et.al, 2009).

While the impact of a positive relationship between the SOR and the SEE cannot be underestimated, it is important for clinical educators to realize that this relationship is not one of equality, particularly from the perspective of the student. Wagner and Hess (1997) described the social power issues inherent in the SOR–SEE relationship where the clinical educator is clearly in the power seat in terms of evaluating and grading the SEE's performance. SORs come to the table with clinical experience and expertise and students hope to gain knowledge and skills while under their supervision. Additionally, SEEs are well aware of the power related to professional influence held by the SOR, including the potential to provide letters of reference, facilitate professional networking, and open doors for later employment.

With the power base being in the hands of the SOR, it is their responsibility to initiate steps to build a positive relationship (Wagner & Hess, 1997). The development of a positive relationship begins with a foundation of mutual respect between the SOR and the SEE, where each partner values what the other brings to the experience. To start this process, it is important to structure opportunity for the SOR and SEE to learn about one another. Initial interactions often occur through email exchanges prior to the start of the placement and then continue in the first face-to-face meetings. These initial conversations start the process of developing a trusting relationship which is "prerequisite for quality preceptoring" (Carlson et al., 2009 p. 524). It can be helpful for the SOR to share background on their career and past clinical teaching experiences along with information about the caseload and the types of experiences the student may have during the term. Asking SEEs to describe their experiences to date including graduate coursework completed, previous clinical experiences, as well as relevant life experiences, starts the process of developing a relationship. Additionally, asking SEEs to outline their current strengths and areas they hope to develop during the upcoming placement can provide useful background to the SOR. When clinical educators invest a 30-minute segment up-front to become acquainted with the student, it provides SEEs and SORs an opportunity to listen and learn about one another. This simple step begins a foundation for creating a positive relationship.

One key component that contributes to relationship building is the creation of open pathways of communication. From the outset, it is important to encourage the SEE to share their ideas and thoughts; this can be facilitated by asking the SEE for input frequently and listening carefully when they respond. In a survey study by Taylor et al. (2012), the most important supervisory behavior implemented in face-to-face discussions was creating opportunity for the student to express their ideas and opinions. In today's fast-paced clinical environment, SORs need to consciously structure opportunities for student talk time and limit the duration of their own conversational turns. When discussions take the form of a dialogue with two-way communication, opportunities for active participation are reinforced. Encouraging students to ask questions any time and request help when needed facilitates the development of a supported learning environment (Levett-Jones et al., 2009; Öhrling & Hallberg, 2000). Teaching can be geared to the student's individual needs more readily when SEEs are comfortable voicing their ideas and concerns (Davis & Nakamura, 2010; Kilminster & Jolly, 2000; Laurent & Weidner, 2001; Levy et al., 2009; Öhrling & Hallberg, 2000; Recker-Hughes et al., 2014).

Student confidence levels increase when they are in an environment that encourages them to share ideas, ask questions, and discuss their learning needs openly (Levett-Jones et al., 2009). In a qualitative study of nursing students in their final clinical experience, students described how effective clinical educators create a "safe space for learning" (Öhrling & Hallberg, 2000, p. 30). Symbolically speaking, this referred to an environment where SEEs were comfortable voicing their fears and concerns, which often related to particular patient care tasks or situations. SORs then helped students recall background information and develop a plan of action which often included structured practice of the target skill. These steps helped the student develop competence in a new area which was possible because of mutual trust and open lines of communication.

Creating a Supportive Learning Environment

The research suggests that clinical instructors can set the stage for a positive experience by creating a clearly structured format for the initial weeks of the experience. Three components of structuring supportive learning will be explored: 1) having a culture that values teaching and learning; 2) providing orientation to the staff and facility; and 3) structuring clinical learning through setting expectations and implementing teaching strategies. By considering these areas, the clinical instructor can take steps to "create a safe space for learning" (Öhrling & Hallberg, 2000, p. 26) which sets the stage for a positive clinical experience.

A culture that values learning and teaching. There are numerous studies across clinical disciplines that have indicated that clinical education is enhanced in an environment that values teaching and learning activities (Burns et al., 2006; Cole & Wessel, 2008; Levett-Jones et al., 2009; Öhrling & Hallberg, 2000; Saarikoski & Leino-Kilpi, 2002). This begins with the culture conveyed (either directly or indirectly) at the department level. In a department where teaching and life-long learning are valued, there is an expectation that staff will be actively engaged in providing clinical education (Cooper et al., 2015; Recker-Hughes et al, 2014). A number of studies have reported that the perceived quality of the clinical learning environment is impacted by the overriding atmosphere of the department (Levett-Jones et al., 2009; Papastavrout et al., 2010; Saarikoski & Leino-Kilpi, 2002). Student perceptions of a department's receptivity are formed by their interactions with department staff beginning on the first day of a placement (Chesser-Smyth, 2005; Levett-Jones et al., 2009). When students feel welcomed to a site, not just by their assigned SOR but by the staff at large, they feel comfortable coming to the placement and they begin to participate in discussions early on in the clinical experience.

Orientation to the staff and facility. Activities which convey a culture that values teaching and learning, begin with an organized approach to onboarding a student. As noted by Kleffner (2010) an orientation process helps to create a positive learning experience and to define expectations of SEEs and SORs. While larger agencies often require students to complete a formal orientation to the facility, the focus here will be on components of orientation at the department level.

The following steps in the orientation process seem like common sense, but may not be implemented consistently or in an organized manner with students. Similar to the steps described for building a relationship, research suggests that these steps can help a student become comfortable at the facility and engaged in clinical learning (Cole & Wessel, 2008; Foley, 2007; Öhrling & Hallberg, 2000; Recker-Hughes et al., 2014). As part of the orientation process, the student should be introduced to all members of the team, with a brief description of each staff members' role in the department and how the student will interface with them (Recker-Hughes et al., 2014; Saarikkoski & Leino-Kilpi, 2002). On the flip side, introductions of the student to staff should minimally include the following: 1) designation of the university attended by the student (if multiple institutions send students to the facility), 2) delineation of the time period of the clinical placement, and 3) identification of team members the student will be directly working with. As Öhrling and Hallberg (2000) noted, these steps provide the student with a "symbolic key, giving them access to the place for learning" (p. 30). Formal introductions legitimize the student's presence at the facility and confirm the department's commitment to educate the student clinician (Cooper et al., 2015). Studies exploring factors that impact clinical learning have found that steps such as these facilitate student comfort at the facility and increase the likelihood of active participation in discussions, factors which are associated with positive learning experiences (Cole & Wessel, 2008; Löfmark & Wikblad, 2009; Papathanasiou et al., 2014; Papastavrou et al., 2010; Saarikoski & Leino-Kilpi, 2002).

In terms of navigating the physical space, it is important for the student to become familiar with the work areas where the speech-language pathology staff provide services as well as relevant locations throughout the agency (e.g. co-treatment areas, patient reception, cafeteria, elevators, stairwells). Another piece of the orientation process addresses logistical factors such as storage of personal items (e.g., lunch, purse, coat), expected arrival and departure times of a typical day and preferred methods for contacting the SOR if there is an emergency.

Similar to employees beginning a new position, students who participate in organized orientations adapt more quickly to the expectations defined and develop a concept that they are a member of the team (Cooper et al., 2015; Foley, 2007; Saarikoski & Leino-Kilpi, 2002). The notion of team membership contributes to the socialization process of a student and is tied to perceptions of a positive learning experience (Burns et al., 2006; Löfmark & Wikblad, 2001; Recker-Hughes et al., 2014).

Structuring clinical learning—Setting expectations. Setting expectations at the start of a clinical experience is an important component of creating a positive learning environment (Brown et al., 2011; Cole & Wessel, 2008; Lindahl, Dagborn, & Nilsson, 2009; McCrea & Brasseur, 2003; Mormer, Palmer, Messick, & Jorgensen, 2013). As noted by Mormer et al. (2013), "discussing expectations establishes a framework of learning, which allows students to feel comfortable in the clinical environment" (p. 397). When expectations are discussed openly and defined clearly it increases the likelihood of student satisfaction with the experience (Mormer et al., 2013). Student expectations and satisfaction in turn contribute to the development of a positive relationship between the SOR and SEE (Tihen, 1983; as discussed in Chapter 3). It is through the processes of discussing goals, needs, and expectations that open communication patterns develop and facilitate a cooperative relationship (McCrea & Brasseur, 2003). Appendix 11-1 includes an example of a Practicum Expectations Worksheet created to provide clinical educators and students with a structured outline of key areas to discuss during the initial weeks of a placement. This form was created to address expectations in terms of communication, logistics and clinical learning and was adapted from Mormer et al. (2013) and Rye (2008). Through the use of a structured form, expectations are considered and clearly defined.

Students often arrive to a clinical placement with some preconceived notions about the learning experience. Based on discussions with the university clinical coordinator and classmates who previously were at the site, the student may be aware that a placement serves pediatric and/or adult populations, takes place in a particular setting type (e.g., acute care, outpatient rehab, school-based settings) and will primarily consist of diagnostic or treatment services. By structuring a conversation where the SEE describes the types of experiences and clinical skills they hope to have, and the SOR confirms or clarifies the details of the clinical experiences typically available, realistic expectations can be framed.

Questions focusing on clinical learning provide an opportunity to discuss student learning and teaching preferences. Initiating the discussion by asking the student to describe how they best learn in new settings can help the clinical instructor consider ways to incorporate those preferences. Beginning level students may not have clinical learning preferences, but experienced students are able to discuss factors relevant to learning and teaching strategies including modalities for processing new information effectively, preferred timing and methods for receiving feedback, and consideration of the types of support they would like from the SOR during the initial weeks of the experience. Setting up a structure for how the student will be transitioned into clinical services in the early weeks is ideally based on SOR preferences and patient needs, balanced by the SEEs experience and comfort level. Defining the student's roles and responsibilities in seeing patients through a timeline (e.g., weeks 1 to 2; weeks 3 to 5; weeks 6 to 10) can help set clear expectations which can be modified if needed (Lindahl et al., 2009; Mormer et al., 2013). Appendix 11-2 includes an example of structuring expectations regarding student participation and responsibilities sequenced across a term for a school externship experience.

As noted in Chapter 3, studies in speech-language pathology and audiology have found differences in expectations based on a student's level of experience. As student experience increases, clinical skills and confidence levels grow, which influences the type of support viewed as helpful. Broadly speaking, beginning level students value high levels of support, direction, and oversight by the SOR. A number of studies have examined the expectations of beginning level students and found common themes such as wanting SORs to do co-planning of lesson plans and telling the student specific diagnostic and treatment methods to use. Novice clinicians expect to receive feedback and have scheduled conference times when support and guidance can be provided (Dowling & Wittkopp, 1982; Fitzgerald, 2009; Mandel, 2015; Taylor et al., 2012). More advanced students expect to have opportunities to transition from being a "student" to becoming a practicing clinician and hope to develop collegial relationships with their SOR and other members of the clinical team. They value opportunities to develop and propose treatment and diagnostic plans with the clinical educator giving input as needed. Conference meetings are valued most when they can be initiated by advanced students as needed (Christodoulouo, 2016; Dowling & Wittkopp, 1982; Fitzgerald, 2009; Mandel, 2015; Russell, 1976; Tihen, 1983; as discussed by McCrea & Brasseur, 2003, and in Chapter 3). Students across all levels value receiving guidance on appropriate treatment methods to meet the individual needs of their clients and appreciate the opportunity to be creative (Fitzgerald, 2009). They expect to receive feedback on what they are doing well and what they need to improve. Students across levels expect direct oversight by the licensed speech-language pathologists (Christodoulou, 2016; Dowling & Wittkopp, 1982; Fitzgerald, 2009) and should be assured that the SOR, who is the licensed professional, will be present and available at all times ensuring that quality services are provided to the patient while supporting and guiding clinical learning.

In many clinical settings, students initially observe the SOR providing services which gives the student an opportunity to learn preferred practice patterns of the clinician and the site. Qualitative studies have suggested that while observation experiences are valuable, advanced level students perceive that learning primarily occurs when actively engaged in service delivery with patients (Cole & Wessel, 2008; Cooper et al., 2015; Kilminster & Jolly, 2000; Levett-Jones et al., 2009). By asking advanced level students to describe their current clinical competencies and discuss situations where they have a high degree of comfort, the SOR and SEE can create a plan for moving the student more quickly into patient contact time with some types of cases while structuring observation time in situations where the SEE has less experience, knowledge, and confidence.

While the focus here is on the importance of defining expectations at the start of the term, in reality the process needs to be ongoing across the semester. As student clinical competencies increase their expectations in terms of support and guidance by the SOR changes. "Therefore there is a need for continuing exploration of perceived role as well as expectations and needs... on an ongoing basis" (McCrea & Brasseur, 2003, p. 53). While beginning level clinicians prefer a directive style of clinical teaching, across time preferences shift to non-directive approaches that incorporate higher-level questioning and reflective practice. It is notable that research has found that SOR's often continue to rely on lower-level questions and directive input despite student preferences for a non-directive style (McCrea & Brasseur, 2003). This tendency speaks to the need for clinical educators to make a concerted effort to solicit and listen to student input and consciously modify their approach to clinical teaching in line with changing student preferences. It is suggested that in a 12- to 15-week externship experience that the student and clinical educator structure check-in points approximately every 4 weeks to confirm/modify student expectations and learning needs. Students should be encouraged as well to initiate discussion with the SOR at any time so that adjustments can be made on a continuous basis.

Structuring clinical learning—Modifying supervision style in relation to the student needs. In considering how to approach clinical teaching with graduate students, the concept of individualized instruction emerges across studies. As described by Davis and Nakamura (2010) in relation to working with medical residents, the process involves consideration of the student's knowledge, experience, preferred modality or style, and personal goals to customize teaching. Carlson et al. (2009) describe a cyclical process where the SOR considers the level of teaching and support, implements teaching strategies, evaluates and reflects on the student's needs, and then adjusts the level of teaching and support after obtaining input from the SEE. This process of planning, implementing, evaluating, and modifying is not unlike the decision-making steps used by speech-language pathologists when assessing or treating communication disorders with patients. Carlson and colleagues describe steps in structuring student experiences moving from high levels of support towards independent interactions. The initial experiences are structured so that the student works with the patient after receiving direct instruction with the clinical educator next to the student throughout the tasks. As the second step, Carlson et al. suggest that the SOR's position during the patient interaction is within peripheral vision, but at a distance allowing the student the opportunity to complete the task seemingly independently but with the instructor remaining in the area. Finally, the last step allows the student to work with a client and then report back to the SOR to discuss their findings.

The format for modifying supervision style suggested by Carlson et al. (2009) is based on the idea that across time in a clinical placement the student's knowledge and skills increase allowing the SOR to take steps to expand their level of independence. Barnum, Guyer, Levy, and Graham (2009) developed the Supervision Questioning Feedback (SQF) model from their work with athletic training students, which proposes that a student's supervisory needs will vary in relation to the student, the situation and the task at hand. Rather than assuming that advanced students require less support and input, the SQF model is based on the notion that a student's understanding and competence level will vary depending on contextual factors including, for example, previous knowledge and experience with similar cases, and current clinical skill level. An experienced student may be comfortable working independently with clients who are similar to previous patients they have seen. In contrast, when seeing a patient with a complex or unusual profile, or when functioning in a situation requiring time-sensitive decision making, that same student may want and need direct instruction and constant input from the clinical instructor. In the SQF model the clinical instructor modifies their supervision strategies and style as well as their questioning techniques based on the student's need in the moment. The end goal is to provide adequate support and input while guiding the student towards independence as possible based on the situation. Appendix 11-3 provides an outline of the SQF model which includes delineation of characteristics of three developmental levels of student clinician learners (D1, D2, D3) and three styles of supervision modified in relation to the clinical situation (S1, S2, S3).

Structuring clinical learning—Teaching strategies. In reviewing studies on clinical teaching strategies and techniques, research from varied disciplines reveals a common set of techniques used by clinical educators that students associate with positive learning experiences (Beckman & Lee, 2009; Burns et al., 2006; Cole & Wessel, 2008; Davis & Nakamura, 2010; Carlson et al., 2009; Kilminster & Jolly, 2000; Levett-Jones et al., 2009; Öhrling & Hallberg, 2000). The following strategies described were selected because they were identified in at least four different studies and are applicable to speech-language pathology clinical teaching:

1. *Modeling* (Burns et al., 2006; Carlson et al., 2009; Cole & Wessel, 2008; Kleffner, 2010; Öhrling & Hallberg, 2000): Modeling or demonstrating a skill while working with a patient provides students with an opportunity to see the technique in practice. Modeling is most effective when

it includes a discussion of the strategy, the rationale for its use, and consideration of alternative approaches (Kleffner, 2010). In ideal situations, the SEE is given an opportunity to perform the task immediately after observing the demonstration.

2. *Thinking Aloud* (Burns et al., 2006; Cole & Wessel, 2008; Kleffner, 2010; Martin, Copley & Tyack, 2014; Öhrling & Hallberg, 2000): This technique, also referred to as the *Talk & Drive* approach (Burns et al., 2006) begins with the clinical educator providing an on-line commentary while working with a patient describing what they are doing, why they are doing it, and pointing out relevant features contributing to the decision making. This technique serves to provide ongoing instruction for the student, and provides a model of openly describing ones clinical observations and rationale for steps taken. When the student's participation in client interactions increase they in turn are encouraged to engage in the same dialogue describing what they are doing, noticing and giving rationale for their decision.

3. *Asking Questions* (Barnum et al., 2009; Beckman & Lee, 2009; Burns et al., 2006; Cole & Wessel, 2008; Levett-Jones et al., 2009; Öhrling & Hallberg, 2000; Spencer, 2003): Questioning techniques are considered an important method for promoting the development of critical thinking skills by students. Using strategic questioning, the SOR will begin with lower-level questions and then progress to higher-level items. Barnum et al. (2009) have created an elegant and simple set of three questioning forms designed to gauge student understanding and promote critical thinking skills which are summarized in Appendix 11-3 (Barnum et al., 2009): 1) "What?" questions focus on lower-level thinking and are aimed at determining a student's knowledge and understanding of issues; 2) "So what?" questions are considered at the mid-level of cognitive processing and push a student to apply knowledge to new situations and to compare and contrast issues; and 3) "Now what?" questions extend student thinking by evaluating information, making projections, and defending decisions. In addition to SORs using varied levels of questioning, SEEs should be encouraged to ask questions to gather needed information (Öhrling & Hallberg, 2000). This provides an opportunity to obtain a sense of a student's level of understanding by the level of questions they ask and from their answers to questions posed.

4. *Providing Feedback* (Barnum et al., 2009; Beckman & Lee, 2009; Burns et al., 2006; Cole & Wessel, 2008; Kilminster & Jolly, 2000): In study after study, students note that feedback received from SORs promotes learning. When feedback is used effectively in clinical teaching it provides students with an understanding of what they are doing well and what should be changed. Research on feedback in clinical teaching has found that instructors report that they provide students with feedback more often than they actually do, and students perceive that they receive feedback less often than indicated by data (Bienstock et al., 2007). Perceptions on both sides are somewhat skewed. One simple suggestion offered by Bienstock et al. (2007) is for feedback events to be clearly and overtly labeled (e.g., "I'd like to share some feedback; It's time for feedback"). Additionally, as noted by McCrea and Brasseur (2003), feedback should be based on data collected during observations providing quantitative measures of behaviors rather than subjective impressions.

Feedback is used for varied purposes including to confirm, validate or reinforce behaviors, to differentiate a desired behavior/outcome from an actual behavior, to provide coaching or guidance on how to modify a behavior, and to evaluate performance (Barnum et al., 2009; McCrea & Brasseur, 2003; Stone & Heen, 2014). In Chapter 7, McCrea and Brasseur describe suggestions by Kurpius and Christie (1976) for increasing student understanding of feedback by clarifying the purpose of the feedback and delineating criteria for conveying clear feedback. Feedback should be specific and descriptive. Additionally, it should be useful and relevant as perceived by the receiver. The impact of feedback on changing behavior is highly dependent on whether the recipient is open to the feedback and values it. Smither, London, and Reilly (2005) completed a meta-analysis of factors impacting the effect of feedback on employee performance. They found that feedback resulted in change when the SEEs had an open attitude towards receiving the feedback, believed that change was possible, and perceived the feedback as useful. Supervisor variables that impacted the likelihood of change by the SEE included conveying the information in a professional and respectful manner, and focusing on aspects that were important and critical to the SEE's job responsibilities.

Students benefit from balanced feedback that clearly describes strengths as well as areas to improve (Nottingham & Henning, 2014). As discussed in Chapter 7, it is critical for clinical educators to balance the use of direct feedback while also creating opportunities for students to self-evaluate. When feedback focuses on goals that the student clinician and clinical educator created together to promote the student's development in key areas, it is more likely to be valued and addressed (McCrea & Brasseur, 2003). For further details on other variables related to providing feedback effectively (e.g., clinical writing; spontaneous vs. unscheduled verbal interactions; and feedback interrupting a session), see the feedback sections in Chapter 7.

One of the challenges in providing feedback in externship settings arises from the pace of the clinical caseloads in many settings. One technique widely used and explored in medical and clinical settings is the *one-minute preceptor* technique (Henning, 2009; Salerno et al., 2002). This method, which admittedly takes more than one minute to complete, provides a structured and efficient method for providing feedback immediately after a patient session while also eliciting student thoughts in the process. The steps of the process include the following:

1. Get a commitment or assertion from the learner. (*So what do you think is going on with this patient?*)
2. Probe for rationale and supportive findings. (*Tell me how you got to this conclusion.*)
3. Reinforce the points made by the student that are on target/correct and give positive feedback. (*I was thinking along similar lines, but hadn't considered the other factors you noticed.*)
4. Provide constructive guidance about errors and omissions. (*One counter sign to the proposal is X, which is tied to the patient's difficulty in completing that task.*)
5. Provide a wrap up—emphasize a general principle or define a "take home" point. (*It's always important to consider....*)

With advanced planning and thought around key concepts which are typically covered with student clinicians, a clinical educator can create a list of target areas which might be appropriate to address using the one-minute preceptor structure. By writing out sample scenarios using the 1-minute preceptor format, the speech-language pathologist will become familiar with the structure of the prompts and be able to implement the strategy spontaneously and effectively when working with students. As SORs approach the task of providing supervision and clinical education with graduate students advanced planning that includes consideration of a student's individual needs can help create optimal learning experiences. Similar to a lesson plan used to guide a classroom teacher, a clinical instruction plan that incorporates the use of modeling, questioning techniques, and feedback strategies can set the clinician up to consciously and conscientiously provide clinical teaching.

Summary

The purpose of this chapter is to provide a summary of research on clinical teaching strategies that have been identified as promoting positive and effective learning experiences for students and which could be implemented in off-campus practicum settings. By incorporating evidence-based strategies to approach clinical teaching in a systematic way, speech-language pathologists can create a structure aimed at optimizing student learning in externship settings while providing quality clinical services with their patients. Below is a summary of aspects to consider and to incorporate in clinical teaching:

1. Desirable clinical educator characteristics include being flexible, empathetic, warm, dependable, and approachable.

2. Students value working with SORs who they perceive as competent, knowledgeable, and professional.

3. When the relationship between the SOR and the SEE is positive, students report high levels of satisfaction in the experience. Relationship building begins by taking time to learn about one another.

4. Learning is enhanced when students are encouraged to ask questions, share ideas, and request help whenever it is needed. Checking with SEEs frequently to determine if they have questions and to solicit their input helps to establish open communication lines.

5. On the first day of the placement, introduce the student to members of the staff and take time to provide a tour of the department and the facility.

6. Explore expectations by asking the student to define their goals for the placement and describe the types of clinical experiences they hope to experience. Gather information on the student's learning and teaching preferences. Work together to develop a plan that defines the SEE roles and responsibilities across the first weeks and describes how the SOR will provide support. Revisit the issue of needs and expectations periodically and modify the teaching plan based on student input. You might consider asking your student to develop an expectations guide for your facility.

7. Implement teaching strategies such as modeling/demonstration, the talk aloud technique, and use of questioning techniques to confirm student knowledge and promote critical thinking skills.

8. Provide feedback on a regular basis that is specific and addresses student strengths and areas to improve. Incorporate self-evaluation as part of the feedback cycle. In turn, ask the student to give you feedback on clinical teaching and identify aspects to modify to facilitate better learning.

Appendix 11-4 includes a Clinical Instructor Self Evaluation form, designed so that clinical educators can examine their use of strategies to optimize clinical education. By using the evidence to consider your own strengths and weaknesses to structure clinical education, the likelihood that the experience will be positive for both the SOR and the SEE will be enhanced.

REFERENCES

Barnum, M., & Guyer, M. S. (2015). *The SQF model of clinical supervision.* Invited presentation at the 2015 CAPCSD Conference. Newport Beach, California.

Barnum, M., Guyer, S., Levy, L., & Graham, C. (2009). Supervision, questioning, feedback model of clinical teaching: A practical approach. In T. Wiedner (Ed.), *The athletic trainers' pocket guide to clinical teaching* (p. 85-91). Thorofare, NJ: SLACK.

Beckman, T. J., & Lee, M. C. (2009). Proposal for a collaborative approach to clinical teaching. *Mayo Clinic Proceedings,* 84(4), 339-344.

Bienstock, J. L., Katz, N. T., Cox, S. M., Hueppchen, N., Erickson, S., & Puscheck, E. E. (2007). *To the point: medical education reviews-providing feedback.* American Journal of Obstetrics & Gynecology, 196(6), 508-513.

Brown, T., Williams, B., McKenna, L., Palermo, C., McCall, L., Roller, L.,…Aldabah, L. (2011). Practice education learning environments: The mismatch between perceived and preferred expectations of undergraduate health science students. *Nurse Education Today, 31,* e22-e328.

Burns, C., Beauchesne, M., Ryan-Krause, P., & Sawin, K. (2006). Mastering the preceptor role: Challenges of Clinical Teaching. *Journal of Pediatric Health Care, 20*(3), 172-187.

Byrd, C. Y., Hood, L., & Youtsey, N. (1997). Student and preceptor perceptions of factors in a successful learning partnership. *Journal of Professional Nursing, 13,* 344-351

Carlson, E., Wann-Hansson, C., & Pilhammar, E. (2009). Teaching during clinical practice: Strategies and techniques used by preceptors in nursing education. *Nurse Education Today, 29,* 522-526.

Carr, D. W., Spencer, T., Paulsen, J., & Chiu, J. (2016). Characteristics of athletic training students that preceptors find desirable. *Athletic Training Education Journal, 11*(1), 27-31.

Chesser-Smythe, P. A. (2005). The lived experiences of general student nurses on their first clinical placement: A phenomenological study. *Nurse Education in Practice, 5*, 320-327.

Chipchase, L. S., Buttrum, P. J., Dunwoodie, R., Hill, A. E. Mandrusiak, A., & Moran, M. (2012). Characteristics of student preparedness for clinical learning: clinical educator perspectives using the Delphi approach. *BMC Medical Education, 12*(112). Retrieved from http://www.biomedcentral.com/1472-6920/12/112

Christodoulou, J. N. W. (2016). A review of the expectations of speech-language pathology externship student clinicians and their supervisors. *Perspectives on Administration & Supervision,* 1(Part 2), 42-53.

Cole, B., & Wessel, J. (2008). How clinical instructors can enhance the learning experience of physical therapy students in an introductory clinical placement. *Advances in Health Sciences Education, 13,* 163-179.

Cooper, J., Courtney-Pratt, H., & Fitzgerald, M. (2015). Key influences identified by first year undergraduate nursing students as impacting on the quality of clinical placement: A qualitative study. *Nurse Education Today, 35,* 1004-1008.

Council for Clinical Certification in Audiology and Speech-Language Pathology of the American Speech-Language-Hearing Association. (2016). *2014 Standards and Implementation Procedures for the certification of clinical competence in speech-language pathology.* Retrieved from https://www.asha.org/Certification/2014-Speech-Language-Pathology-Certification-Standards/

Council on Academic Accreditation in Audiology and Speech-Language Pathology (2014). Standards for accreditation of graduate education programs in audiology and speech language pathology (2008, revised 2014). Retrieved from http://caa.asha.org/wpcontent/uploads/Accreditation-Standards-for-Graduate-Programs.pdf

Davis, O. C., & Nakamura, J. (2010). A proposed model for an optimal mentoring environment for medical residents: A literature review. *Academic Medicine, 85,* 1060-1066.

Dowling, S., & Wittkopp, J. (1982). Students' perceived supervisory needs. *Journal of Communication Disorders, 15,* 319-328

Ellis, M. V. (2010). Bridging the science and practice of clinical supervision: Some discoveries, some misconceptions. *The Clinical Supervisor, 29,* 95-116.

Fitzgerald, M. D. T. (Oct 2009). Reflections on student perceptions of supervisory needs in clinical education. *Perspectives on Administration and Supervision, 19,* 96-106.

Foley, K. (2007). *Occupational therapy professional students: level II fieldwork experience - is it broken?* PhD dissertation, Indiana University. Retrieved from ProQuest Dissertations Publishing. (Accession No. 3283103)

Hauer, K. E., Oza, S. K., Kogan, J. R., Stankiewicz, C. A., Stenfors-Hayes, T., ten Cate, O....O'Sullivan, P. S. (2015). How clinical supervisors develop trust in their trainees: a qualitative study. *Medical Education, 49,* 783-795.

Henning, J. M. (2009). The one-minute preceptor: A time efficient clinical teaching model. In T. Wiedner (Ed.), *The athletic trainers' pocket guide to clinical teaching* (p. 100-104). Thorofare, NJ: SLACK.

Kilminster, S. M., & Jolly, B. C. (2000). Effective supervision in clinical practice settings: A literature review. *Medical Education, 34,* 827-840

Kleffner, J. H. (2010). *Becoming an effective preceptor.* University of Houston College of Pharmacy, Texas Southern University College of Pharmacy and Health Sciences, Texas Tech Health Science Center School of Pharmacy, The University of Texas at Austin College of Pharmacy.

Kurpius, D., & Christie, G. S. (1978). A systematic and collaborative approach to problem solving. In D. Kurpius (Ed.), *Learning: Making learning environments more effective* (pp. 13-16). Muncie, IN: Accelerated Development.

Laurent, T., & Weidner, T. G. (2001). Clinical instructors' and student athletic trainers' perceptions of helpful clinical instructor characteristics. *Journal of Athletic Training, 36*(1), 58-61.

Levett-Jones, T., Lathlean, J., Higgens, I., & McMillan, M. (2009). Staff-student relationships and their impact on nursing students' belongingness and learning. *Journal of Advanced Nursing, 65*(2), 316-324. doi:10.1111/j.1365-2648.2008.04865.x

Levy, L. S., Sexton, P., Willeford, K. S., Barnum, M .G., Guyer, M. S., Gardner, G., & Fincher, A. L. (2009). Clinical instructor characteristics, behaviors and skills in allied health care settings: A literature review. *Athletic Training Education Journal, 4*(1), 8-13.

Lindahl, B., Dagborn, K., & Nilsson, M. (2009). A student-centered clinical education unit: Description of a reflective learning model. *Nurse Education in Practice, 9,* 5-12.

Löfmark, A., & Wikblad, K. (2009). Facilitating and obstructing factors for development of learning in clinical practice: a student perspective. *Journal of Advanced Nursing, 34*(1), 43-50.

Mandel, S. (2015). Exploring the differences in expectations between supervisors and supervisees during the initial clinical experience. *Perspectives on Administration and Supervision, 25,* 4-30.

Martin, P., Copley, J., Tyack, Z. (2014). Twelve tips for effective clinical supervision based on a narrative literature review and expert opinion. *Medical Teacher, 36,* 201-207.

May, W. W., Morgan, B. J., Lemke, J. C., Karst, G. M., & Stone, H. L. (1995). Model for ability-based assessment in physical therapy education. *Journal of Physical Therapy Education, 9*(1), 3-6.

McCrea, E. S., & Brasseur, J. A. (2003). *The supervisory process in speech-language pathology and audiology.* Boston, MA: Pearson.

Messick, C., & Mormer, E. (May 2012). *Bringing evidence to clinical teaching.* Invited presentation Communication Sciences & Disorders Department of the University of Utah, Salt Lake City, UT

Mormer, E., Palmer, C., Messick, C., & Jorgensen, L. (2013). An evidence-based guide to clinical instruction in audiology. *Journal of the American Academy of Audiology, 24*(5), 393-406

Nottingham, S., & Henning, J. (2014). Feedback in clinical education, Part II: Approved clinical instructor and student perceptions of and influences on feedback. *Journal of Athletic Training, 49*(1), 58-67.

Öhrling, K., & Hallberg, I. R. (2000). Student nurses' lived experience of preceptorship. Part 2–The preceptor-preceptee relationship. *International Journal of Nursing Studies, 37*, 25-36.

Palomo, M. (2004). *Development and validation of a questionnaire measure of the supervisory relationship.* Unpublished doctoral clinical thesis, Oxford University, Oxford, England.

Palomo, M., Beinart, H., Cooper, J.J. (June 2010). Development and validation of the Supervisory Relationship Questionnaire (SRQ) in UK trainee clinical psychologists. *British Journal of Clinical Psychology, 45*(Pt. 2), 131-149.

Papastavrou, E., Lambrinou, E., Tsangari, H., Saarikoski, M., & Leino-Kilpi, H. (2010). Student nurses experience of learning in the clinical environment. *Nurse Education in Practice, 10*, 176-182.

Papathanasiou, I. V., Tsaras, K., & Sarafis, P. (2014). Views and perceptions of nursing students on their clinical learning environment: teaching and learning. *Nurse Education Today, 34*, 57-60.

Radtke, S. (2008). A conceptual framework for clinical education in athletic training. *Athletic Training Education Journal, 2*, 36-42.

Recker-Hughes, C., Wetherbee, E., Buccieri, K. M., Fitzpatric-Timmerberg, J., & Stolfi, A. M. (2014). Essential characteristics of quality clinical education experiences: standards to facilitate student learning. *Journal of Physical Therapy Education, 28*, 48-55.

Russell, L. (1976). *Aspects of supervision.* Unpublished manuscript, Temple University, Philadelphia, PA.

Rye, K. J. (2008). Perceived benefits of the use of learning contracts to guide clinical education in respiratory care students. *Respiratory Care, 53*(11), 1475-1481.

Saarikoski, M., & Leino-Kilpi H. (2002). The clinical learning environment and supervision by staff nurses: developing the instrument. *International Journal of Nursing Studies, 39*, 259-267.

Salerno, S. M., O'Malley, P. G., Pangaro, L. N., wheeler, G. A., Moores, L. K., & Jackson, J. L. (2002). Faculty development seminars based on the one-minute preceptor improve feedback in the ambulatory setting. *Journal of General Internal Medicine, 17*, 779-787.

Sheepway, L., Lincoln, M., & McAllister, S. (2014). Impact of placement type on the development of clinical competency in speech-language pathology students. *International Journal of Language and Communication Disorders, 49*(2), 189-203.

Smither, J. W., London, M., & Reilly, R. R. (2005). Does performance improve following multisource feedback? A theoretical model, meta-analysis, and review of empirical findings. *Personnel Psychology, 58*, 33-66.

Spencer, J. (2003). Learning and teaching in the clinical environment. *BMJ 326*, 590-594.

Stone, D., & Heen, S. (2014). *Thanks for the feedback: The science and art of receiving feedback well.* New York, NY: Viking.

Taylor, K., White, E., Kaplan, R., & O'Rourke, C. M. (2012). The supervisory process in speech-language pathology: Graduate students' perspective. *Perspectives on Administration and Supervision, 22*(2), 47-54.

Tihen, L. D. (1983). *Expectations of student speech/language clinicians during their clinical practicum* (Doctoral dissertation). Retrieved from ProQuest Dissertations and Theses Global. (Accession No. 8401620)

Wagner, B. T., & Hess, C. W. (1997). Supervisees' perceptions of supervisors' social power in speech-language pathology. *American Journal of Speech-Language Pathology, 6*, 90-95.

Weidner, T. G. (2009). The effective approved clinical instructor. In T. Weidner (Ed.), *The Athletic Trainers' Pocket Guide to Clinical Teaching* (p. 85-91). Thorofare, NJ: SLACK.

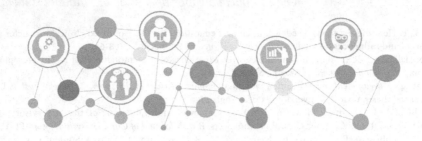

APPENDIX 11-1
PRACTICUM EXPECTATION WORKSHEET

This form is printed with permission from the Communication Science & Disorders Department of the University of Pittsburgh.

COMMUNICATION		
Names	1. Clinical instructor(s)	
Record methods of reaching clinical instructor and contact info (phone, email)	1. Emergency cancellation procedure (e.g., clinician illness; death in family)	
	2. Contact info at work	
	3. Contact at home (preferred or not?)	
What happens if...	1. I am ill	
	2. Clinical instructor is ill/absent from work	
	3. Inclement weather	
	4. Professional absence (e.g., attend conference)	
Preferred form of address for the supervisor and self	1. Clinical instructor	
	2. Clinical instructor in front of patient	
	3. Self (to patients)	
Background knowledge	1. **Student**—coursework; past experiences; strengths; goals (share clinical portfolio; send student vita)	
	2. **Clinical Instructor**—clinical experiences; areas of expertise; supervisory experiences	

LOGISTICS		
Preplacement requirements (e.g., orientation; badge; computer access)	1. What needs to be done; where/how and with whom	
Schedule	1. Specific days/times of clinic placement	
	2. Expected arrival and departure time (in relation to anticipated client services)	
Attire	1. Appropriate/Suggested	
	2. Inappropriate	
Materials	1. Materials/supplies student should bring; storage of personal items (e.g., purse)	
	2. Materials/supplies available for student to use (what and where kept)	
	3. Guidelines on use of computer and phone while on site	
Meals	1. Availability of food on site and storage of food; locations for eating; eat with other clinical educator, and other staff?	
Restrooms	1. Locations	
Introduction to other key staff	1. Other audiology and speech-language pathology staff on site	
	2. Support staff (names; roles)	
Patient scheduling	1. Where to get schedule	
	2. What happens if client cancels?	
	3. How to know appt type?	
	4. What to do when running behind?	
CLINICAL LEARNING		
Schedule and typical types of speech- language pathology services	1. Instructor's responsibilities and typical schedule with clinical services provided (that student will be involved)	

Role in seeing patients and clients	1. Weeks 1 to 2	
	2. Weeks 3 to 5	
	3. Weeks 6 to 10	
	4. Weeks 11 to 15	
Initial skills and goals on which to focus		
Feedback	**Clinical instructor to student**	
	1. Provide feedback on learning goals	
	2. Feedback during sessions	
	3. Feedback after sessions	
	4. Scheduled discussions (end of day; end of week?)	
	Student to clinical instructor	
	1. Preferred mode of receiving feedback	
	2. Preferred timing of feedback	
	3. Plan for student to provide feedback on supervisory techniques that are helpful/not helpful	

Adapted from Mormer, E., Palmer, C., Messick, C., & Jorgensen, L. (2013). An evidence-based guide to clinical instruction in audiology. *Journal of the American Academy of Audiology, 24*(5), 393-406 and Rye, K. J. (2008). Perceived benefits of the use of learning contracts to guide clinical education in respiratory care students. *Respiratory Care, 53*(11), 1475-1481.

APPENDIX 11-2
EXPECTATIONS FOR STUDENT CLINICIAN PARTICIPATION AND RESPONSIBILITIES SEQUENCED ACROSS A SEMESTER FOR SCHOOL EXTERNSHIP

This document is included with permission from the Communication Science and Disorders Department of the University of Pittsburgh. The structured set of expectations are designed to serve as a guideline for a 15-week experience that can be adapted and modified as appropriate.

PRIOR TO START OF TERM	1. School practicum assignment sent to student clinician and clinical educator confirming placement 2. Student contacts clinical educator to confirm placement and set up day/time for orientation meeting/discussion 3. Student clinician reads Communication Science and Disorders Department School Practicum Handbook and familiarizes themselves with the School Practicum Blackboard site resources 4. Orientation meeting/discussion held prior to start of term when possible (using *Practicum Expectations Worksheet*) 5. Clinical educator reviews American Speech-Language-Hearing Association Guidelines on Clinical Supervision
WEEKS 1 TO 2	1. Orientation meeting/discussion using *Practicum Expectations Worksheet* (if not held before start of the term) 2. Observe clinical educator provide services and complete responsibilities 3. Become acquainted with the site(s), and clinical educator's resources (including therapy and testing materials) 4. Review files and individualized education programs (IEPs) of pupils on caseload and become familiar with record keeping methods used by speech-language pathologists 5. Meet the principal, administrative staff, teachers, and support staff at the site 6. Complete orientation activities for site or district 7. Participate in structured activities as assigned by the clinical educator (e.g., help create schedule; collect data while clinical educator implements session; gather/organize materials for planned lessons with clinical educator; plan several lessons) 8. Observe students on caseload in at least one classroom 9. Confer with clinical educator daily and make plan for upcoming day 10. Interact with the pupils (as appropriate) 11. Master Clinician should have reviewed *School Practicum Handbook* 12. Discuss the scheduling process with clinical educator

WEEKS 3 TO 4	1. Continue observations of clinical educator as assigned 2. Plan sessions for 15% to 30% of the caseload and implement lessons with clinical educator assistance; assist with remaining caseload as planned with clinical educator 3. Work with clinical educator to collect session data and complete documentation for specific cases 4. Identify at least one case for student to participate with the clinical educator in the process of developing/updating an IEP and attending team meetings during term 5. Complete written self-evaluation of performance and share reflections with clinical educator 6. Discuss methods of reinforcing/motivating children to achieve maximal performance with clinical instructor 7. Assist with daily events (e.g., screenings; development of materials; monitoring of progress on IEP objectives) 8. Complete observations of children from caseload in varied school settings (e.g., classroom; lunch room; recess) and review their speech-language pathology and educational records 9. Collect children and bring them to and from their sessions as needed 10. Confer with clinical educator and develop specific student clinician training objectives for the next 2 weeks (use *School Practicum Formative Assessment Form*). Discuss modifications in expectations as needed.
WEEKS 5 TO 6	1. Plan sessions for 25% to 60% of the caseload, implement lessons, and record data 2. Participate in daily routines with clinical instructor 3. Develop new system of data collection for at least one case or group of children 4. Discuss use of the Pennsylvania Educational Standards in the speech-language pathology caseload with the clinical instructor 5. Confer with clinical instructor and develop specific student training objectives for the next 4 weeks

WEEKS 7 TO 8	1. Plan sessions for 60% to 80% of the caseload, implement lessons, record data, and document performance.
	2. Confer with clinical instructor on such topics as:
	   a. Collaborative service delivery with other school staff
	   b. Methods for maximizing carryover of objectives to other environments
	   c. Developing relationships with family members
	3. Identify several children for reassessment measures to be completed during the practicum experience
	4. Develop plan for completing measures and sharing results with family members and school staff
	5. Initiate suggestions for modifications in treatment programs for cases as needed and discuss ideas with clinical instructor
	6. Prepare for and complete midterm evaluation. Student should make sure clinical instructor has access to communication and speech disorders department forms via clinical education web system; meet with clinical educator for midterm evaluation meeting; complete self-evaluation form and bring hard copy to meeting
	7. Assess new children referred to speech-language services

WEEKS 9 TO 10	1. Plan sessions for 85% to 100% of the caseload, implement lessons, record data, and document performance
	2. Review progress of target cases on IEP goals and develop plan for moving children toward appropriate levels; confer with clinical educator on plans
	3. Complete assessment plan for targeted children and write IEPs and evaluation reports; attend IEP meeting
	4. Attend team meetings and participate as possible
	5. Confer with clinical instructor regarding
	   a. Professional development through continuing education
	   b. American Speech-Language-Hearing Association Code of Ethics and PA Code of Professional Practice and Conduct for Educators
	6. Clinical educator and student work together to develop a plan for the next 4 weeks including identification of specific training skills and competencies and responsibilities

WEEKS 11 TO 14	1. Plan sessions for 100% of the caseload, implement lessons, record data, and document performance 2. Complete all daily duties independently 3. Confer with professional staff as needed regarding caseload 4. Confer daily with clinical educator highlighting achievements and needs in terms of caseload 5. Schedule end of term conference with clinical educator
WEEK 15	1. Make up any sessions that were missed during the term 2. Complete end of term conference (bring completed self-evaluation form)

APPENDIX 11-3
SUMMARY OF THE SUPERVISION QUESTIONING FEEDBACK SUPERVISION MODEL

DEVELOPMENTALLY BASED LEARNER CHARACTERISTICS	SITUATIONAL SUPERVISION BEHAVIORS	STRATEGIC QUESTIONING LEVELS
D1. Unconsciously incompetent and consciously incompetent learner. Novice learner. Often highly enthusiastic and overly confident. Student does not yet know what they don't know.	**S1. Directing and motivating.** Provide direct instructions and coaching. Remains close to the student and client, and steps in to implement tasks correctly when needed. Checks the student's understanding of the situation. Facilitates the student to be able to complete tasks appropriately providing ongoing reinforcement and feedback. Clinical educator reviews basic concepts and provides opportunity to practice basic skills.	**Q1. WHAT questions.** Focus on determining what student knows and remembers. Goals are to differentiate the student's knowledge level. Questions push student to recall facts and identify key concepts to determine student's understanding of the situation.
D2. Consciously competent learner. The student is aware of the vast amount of information that they don't know and the skills they have not yet developed. Confidence level is often below that of the D1 learner. Is not able to do tasks at the level required on their own.	**S2. Coaching and motivating.** Provides prompts, cues, and feedback as needed. Creates space for student to work with the patient (e.g., stands behind). Reinforces student and encourages them so they can do the task well. Gives sincere feedback on what is done well, and lets them know they can ask for assistance or information when they need it. Goal is to move from lower-level cognitive processes to higher-level skills.	**Q2. SO WHAT questions.** Focus on getting the student to apply or to analyze. Pushes student to take known content and apply it to appropriate clinical situations.

| D3. Consciously competent learner. Student is able to bring in knowledge and implement skills with proficiency. Is aware of the need for assistance and asks for help. | S3. Supporting and motivating. Pushes student to develop plan and consider alternative approaches. Remains within "line of sight" but at a distance, giving the student permission to work with the patient fairly independently. Encourages student and reinforces appropriate plans and decisions. Acknowledges their ability to do the task. Goal is for student to use critical thinking skills and develop sound clinical reasoning abilities. | Q3. NOW WHAT questions. Push student to evaluate information, to develop plans, and to defend their decisions. |

Adapted from Barnum, M., & Guyer, M. S. (2015). *The SQF model of clinical supervision.* Invited presentation at the 2015 CAPCSD Conference. Newport Beach, California and Barnum, M., Guyer, S., Levy, L., & Graham, C. (2009). Supervision, questioning, feedback model of clinical teaching: A practical approach. In T. Wiedner (Ed.), *The athletic trainers' pocket guide to clinical teaching* (p. 85-91). Thorofare, NJ: SLACK.

Appendix 11-4
Clinical Educator Self-Evaluation Form

Use the following statements to rate yourself in terms of the consistency of implementing the following clinical instruction strategies when teaching student clinicians.

A. OPEN ENVIRONMENT As a clinical educator, I…	1. Never	2. Rarely	3. Sometimes	4. Usually	5. Always
A1. Let students know that I value their views and ideas					
A2. Work with my students as an equal partner in the clinical teaching process					
A3. Use a collaborative approach in clinical teaching					
A4. Create a safe supportive learning environment					
A5. Use a non-judgemental approach in clinical teaching					
A6. Treat my students with respect					
A7. Create an open-minded atmosphere					
A8. Encourage the students to be open with me					
A9. Promote clinical teaching as an exchange of ideas between the student and me					
A10. Provide feedback in a comfortable/safe manner					
A11. Treat the student as an adult learner					
A12. My students discuss their concerns with me					

B. UNDERLYING ORGANIZATION When teaching student clinicians…	1. Never	2. Rarely	3. Sometimes	4. Usually	5. Always
B1. At the start of the placement, time is spent defining clinical expectations for the term					
B2. At the start of the placement, the student is oriented to the facility (e.g., introduced to professional and support staff; location of restrooms; parking)					
B3. At the start of the placement, time is spent learning about the student (e.g., previous clinical experiences; relevant life experiences; strengths)					
B4. At the start of the placement, time is spent sharing information about myself (e.g., my career path; clinical interests/expertise)					
B5. Conference sessions are scheduled on a regular basis					
B6. My student and I both draw up agenda items for our conference discussions					
B7. Student goals are written down					
B8. Student goals are verbally defined					
B9. Conference discussions include addressing student learning goals					
B10. Student goals are modified and updated across the term					
B11. Conference discussions are kept free of interruptions					

C. COMMITMENT When working with students, I show that…	1. Never	2. Rarely	3. Sometimes	4. Usually	5. Always
C1. I am interested in being their clinical educator					
C2. I am interested in them as people					
C3. I like providing clinical instruction to students					
C4. I am approachable to my students					
C5. I want to be available to them					
C6. I pay attention and respond to their spoken feelings and anxieties					
C7. I convey interest in their development as a professional					

D. REFLECTIVE EDUCATION When teaching students, I…	1. Never	2. Rarely	3. Sometimes	4. Usually	5. Always
D1. Draw from a number of theoretical models					
D2. Give my students opportunity to learn about a range of models					
D3. Link theory and clinical practice through discussions					
D4. Encourage students to reflect on their skill development					
D5. Pay close attention to the processes of clinical teaching					
D6. Promote student learning by experimenting with different teaching strategies					
D7. Consciously use different questioning techniques to promote critical thinking					
D8. Consider the level of questions posed by student to better determine their understanding of clinical issues					
D9. Encourage students to reflect on their knowledge before answering a question					
D10. Encourage students to reflect on their knowledge before answering a question					
D11. Utilize journal reflections as a way to promote reflective thinking					

E. ROLE MODEL When teaching students, I…	1. Never	2. Rarely	3. Sometimes	4. Usually	5. Always
E1. Convey my knowledge to my students					
E2. Demonstrate clinical skills for my students					
E3. Share my professional goals with my students					
E4. Discuss my continuing education activities with my students					
E5. Help my students to understand the organizational structure of my agency					
E6. Convey enthusiasm in discussing our patients/clients with my students					
E7. Treat my colleagues with respect					
E8. Acknowledge the power differential between my student and myself					

F. FEEDBACK When teaching students, I…	1. Never	2. Rarely	3. Sometimes	4. Usually	5. Always
F1. Pay attention to the student's individual level of competence as I give feedback					
F2. Ask the student to tell me their preferences in regards to how/when feedback should be provided					
F3. Provide a balance of feedback (areas of strength and areas to develop further)					
F4. Give positive feedback on student performance (strengths)					
F5. Give negative feedback on student performance (areas to improve/develop further)					
F6. Include feedback on student performance that is constructive					
F7. Describe specific behaviors when giving feedback					
F8. Focus feedback on the student's learning goals					
F9. Provide timely feedback (close to the time the behaviors occurred)					
F10. Give feedback verbally					

F11. Give written feedback					
F12. Have the student self-evaluate before I share my feedback					
F13. Clearly delineate that feedback is going to be provided (e.g., "it's feedback time")					
F14. Give the student room to learn through making mistakes					
F15. Discuss professional issues that are impacting student performance					
F16. Help identify student's individual learning needs					
F17. Consider the impact of the student's previous skills & experience on their individual learning needs					
F18. Provide regular/ongoing feedback on student performance					
F19. Modify the teaching strategies as student skills and confidence grow					
F20. Tailor clinical teaching to the student's level of competence					
F21. Create opportunities for the student to give me feedback on the clinical teaching strategies being used					

Adapted from Messick, C., & Mormer, E. (May 2012). *Bringing evidence to clinical teaching.* Invited presentation Communication Sciences & Disorders Department of the University of Utah, Salt Lake City, UT; Palomo, M. (2004). *Development and validation of a questionnaire measure of the supervisory relationship.* Unpublished doctoral clinical thesis, Oxford University, Oxford, England; and Palomo, M., Beinart, H., Cooper, J.J. (June 2010). Development and validation of the Supervisory Relationship Questionnaire (SRQ) in UK trainee clinical psychologists. *British Journal of Clinical Psychology, 45*(Pt. 2), 131-149.

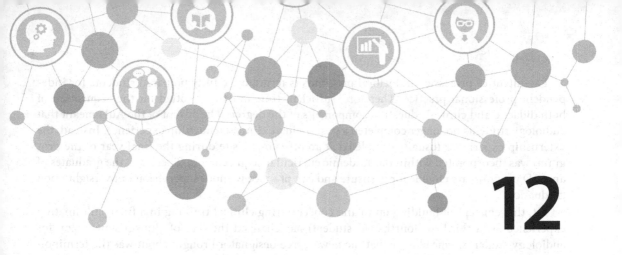

12

Supervision of Audiology Students

Donna Fisher Smiley, PhD, CCC-A, F-ASHA and
Cynthia McCormick Richburg, PhD, CCC-A

Brief History of Clinical Education and Supervision in Audiology

Changes in clinical education for students in audiology programs throughout the United States have come about over the past 25 years. The entry-level degree for the profession of audiology has moved from a master's degree to a professional doctorate, known as the Doctor of Audiology (AuD). Doctor of Audiology programs were meant to educate students beyond the master's-level degree by adding more courses, broadening course content, and by adding significantly to the clinical experiences obtained by students entering audiology programs.

One of the driving forces behind this move to a doctoral degree was created by the perception that more time and clinical experiences were needed to teach all of the knowledge and skills necessary for best practices. Additionally, the professional doctorate (also termed clinical doctorate) was meant to foster greater professional autonomy and increase credibility within the health care arena. Discussions began in the late 1980s and culminated in the mid 1990s with the Council of Higher Education granting authority to the American Speech-Language-Hearing Association (ASHA) to accredit professional doctoral programs in audiology. ASHA developed new standards based on results from a practice analysis study conducted by Greenberg and Smith (1987) and a skills validation study conducted by the Educational Testing Service (Tannenbaum & Rosenfeld, 1996). These standards have been updated several times over the years in an attempt to better prepare audiologists for today's technological and scientific advances.

McCrea, E. S., & Brasseur, J. A. *The Clinical Education and Supervisory Process in Speech–Language Pathology and Audiology* (pp 361-372).
© 2020 Taylor & Francis Group.

The intent of professional doctoral programs is to graduate fully prepared students for independent professional practice. Therefore, sufficient time must be allotted for the acquisition of both didactic and clinical education components of the degree. The advent of the AuD meant that audiology students no longer completed a postgraduate clinical fellowship experience. Instead, the externship experience (usually completed at an off-campus site during the final year of the program) was incorporated within the academic curricular requirements. Therefore, the graduates of an AuD program are eligible for licensure and can practice without supervision or oversight upon graduation.

Yet, this concept of building up to and concentrating clinical training in a final, culminating experience (as a third- or fourth-year student) has changed the face of clinical supervision for audiology students. One change that the new degree designator brought about was the terminology associated with clinical supervision, specifically the terms *preceptor* and *preceptorship*; that is, in addition to the traditional instructor in the classroom and supervisor in the university clinic, the new concept of preceptor was introduced. Likewise, in addition to the more traditional externship term, the use of the term preceptorship was introduced. Preceptor was first used in the 15th century, and it meant "tutor" or "instructor" (Pierce, 1991). Preceptorships have been used as a method of clinical teaching in several health-related professions. Preceptor, as a medical or health care term, refers to a skilled practitioner who supervises students in a clinical setting with the goal of obtaining practical experience with patients. More specifically, preceptorships emerged in health care to transition students from the educational phase to the professional phase of their lives. Preceptorships can be described within the realm of clinical education as one-on-one learning and teaching interchanges between a student and a professional who acts as a role model, mentor, and resource provider (Mantzorou, 2004). In the final year of an audiology student's academic program, the person in charge of transitioning that student from the educational phase to the professional phase is now called "preceptor." A student may have more than one preceptor, depending on the setting or job requirements in that externship placement. However, the term preceptor (adopted at the Consensus Conference on Issues and Concerns Related to the 4th-Year AuD Student; Mashie & Mendel, 2005) refers to the licensed audiologist providing clinical education to the extern. The preceptorship (or externship) is the designator used for long-term clinical training outside of the university. It is this preceptorship or externship that is informally referred to as the "fourth-year placement."

Similar to the former master's-level clinical experience in audiology, and typical still in speech-language pathology programs, AuD students obtain a semester-long clinical experience in university-based clinics, as well as off-site placements, prior to completing the externship with a preceptor. The American Academy of Audiology (AAA) has developed a list of roles and responsibilities (Table 12-1) that a preceptor should embody (AAA, 2014). In addition, professionals wishing to become preceptors adhering to AAA recommendations should be licensed audiologists with 3 years of experience (AAA, n.d). Currently, ASHA does not have a requirement for preceptor experience. However, AuD students applying for ASHA certification after January 1, 2020, will need to be supervised by preceptors who have a minimum of 9 months of experience post-certification with ASHA. Several university programs have also developed manuals or online sites with information for preceptors who take their students in externships (e.g., Ball State University in Indiana and Pacific University in Oregon; see the "Preceptor Manual," 2007 and "School of Audiology," n.d., respectively). Professionals engaging in preceptorship supervision should arm themselves with the descriptions and expectations used by the university in which the student is enrolled.

TABLE 12-1
THE AMERICAN ACADEMY OF AUDIOLOGY'S (2014) ROLES AND RESPONSIBILITIES OF THE PRECEPTOR

Clinical preceptors will have sufficient time, sufficient depth and breadth of experience, and the personal qualities necessary to:

- Promote and facilitate clinical skill development
- Serve as a role model for professionalism
- Provide timely and constructive feedback to the student and university, including formative and summative assessment
- Model and teach best practices in clinical audiology using an evidence-based approach
- Facilitate the personal and professional growth of the student
- Ensure that the ethical and legal practices of the profession are upheld
- Emphasize the need for lifelong learning by encouraging continuous professional education and pursuit of knowledge through research and professional literature
- Assure that the student holds the needs of patients and their families in highest regard
- Promote the development of administrative skill in the student, including effective record keeping, report writing, and knowledge of reimbursement issues
- Facilitate the student's ability to set clinical goals
- Encourage self-assessment on the part of the student
- Maintain a balance in the triadic system of patient, preceptor, and student
- Encourage the student's independent clinical practice
- Seek continuing education in clinical mentoring and the supervisory process

Adapted from American Academy of Audiology. (2014, June 5). *Roles and responsibilities of the externship site, preceptor, and universities.* Retrieved from http://www.audiology.org/education-research/education/externships/roles-and-responsibilities-externship-site-preceptor-and.

CLINICAL EDUCATION AND PRECEPTORSHIPS IN AUDIOLOGY TODAY

In addition to the differences between the master's-level clinical fellowship and the AuD externship, there are differences in the number of clinical contact hours and the type and amount of supervision required for speech-language pathology and AuD students who want to be certified. It is important for a potential preceptor in audiology to familiarize themselves with these differences, keeping in mind that the students' desires for a specific certification (ASHA, American Board of Audiology [ABA], or neither) need to be addressed. For a comparison of the differences in certification requirements, refer to Table 12-2.

Application of Anderson's Model to Audiology Preceptorships

As described in earlier chapters of this book, Anderson (1988) has a conceptual model describing the supervisory process in communication sciences and disorders. A continuum of

Table 12-2

Comparison of Certification Requirements for Students in Speech-Language Pathology Master's Programs and Students in Doctor of Audiology Programs

	SPEECH-LANGUAGE PATHOLOGY STUDENTS (CCC-SLP)	DOCTOR OF AUDIOLOGY STUDENTS (CCC-A)	DOCTOR OF AUDIOLOGY STUDENTS (BOARD CERTIFIED IN AUDIOLOGY)
NUMBER OF CONTACT HOURS	• Total of 400 hours of supervised clinical practicum 375 hours in direct patient contact, 25 hours of clinical observation • Up to 20% of direct contact hours may be obtained through clinical simulation	• As of January 1, 2020, there will be no minimum number of supervised clinical practicum hours required. University programs and applicants will have to ensure that clinical experiences meet CAA standards.	• 2,000 hours of "mentored professional practice" (AuD student externship or internship hours may be used)
SUPERVISION REQUIREMENTS	• Not less than 25% of the student's total contact with each patient • Must take place periodically throughout the practicum • Wording states, "Supervision must be sufficient to ensure the welfare of the patient… must be commensurate with the student's knowledge, skills, and experience."	• Specific percentage not mentioned • Wording states, "Supervision must be sufficient to ensure the welfare of the patient and the student in accordance with the ASHA Code of Ethics… must include direct observation, guidance, and feedback to permit the student to monitor, evaluate, and improve performance and to develop clinical competence • Amount of supervision must also be appropriate to the student's level of training, education, experience, and competence	• Specific percentage not mentioned • No descriptive wording found

continued

TABLE 12-2 (CONTINUED)

COMPARISON OF CERTIFICATION REQUIREMENTS FOR STUDENTS IN SPEECH-LANGUAGE PATHOLOGY MASTER'S PROGRAMS AND STUDENTS IN DOCTOR OF AUDIOLOGY PROGRAMS

	SPEECH-LANGUAGE PATHOLOGY STUDENTS (CCC-SLP)	DOCTOR OF AUDIOLOGY STUDENTS (CCC-A)	DOCTOR OF AUDIOLOGY STUDENTS (BOARD CERTIFIED IN AUDIOLOGY)
SUPERVISOR OR PRECEPTOR REQUIREMENTS	• Must have CCC-SLP • Must have at 9 months of full-time work experience • Must complete 2 hours of professional development/ continuing education in clinical instruction/supervision	• Must have CCC-A • Must have 9 months of experience post-certification • Must have 2 hours of professional development in the area of supervision	• Must be a state-licensed audiologist • Does not have to hold ABA or CCC-A
DEFINITION OF SUPERVISED CLINICAL EXPERIENCE OR CLINICAL PRACTICUM	"Assessment, diagnosis, evaluation, screening, treatment, family or client consultation, and counseling"	"Direct patient contact, consultation, record keeping, and administrative duties relevant to audiology service delivery"	• No definition found

Note: CCC-SLP indicates Certificate of Clinical Competence in Speech-Language Pathology obtained through the Council for Clinical Certification within ASHA; CCC-A indicates Certificate of Clinical Competence in Audiology obtained through the Council for Clinical Certification within ASHA; Board Certified in Audiology indicates certification obtained through the American Board of Audiology.

understanding, planning, observing, analyzing, and integrating information, coupled with the goal of moving students from being reliant on the supervisor to becoming independently capable of executing clinical practice, is useful as a guideline for the preceptors of today. In addition, Anderson described the supervisor's role as one that transitions over time from Direct-Active, to Collaborative, to Consultative.

Anderson's (1988) description of *understanding* within the supervisory process includes discussion of that process as it relates to respective roles, expectations, and objectives between the supervisor and supervisee (in the case of audiology, the preceptor and student). At the beginning of the preceptorship, the preceptor and student should sit down together to discuss the expectations that the specific setting mandates (whether in a hospital, private practice, or free-standing clinic). As is the case in most clinical education situations, it is important for the preceptor to lay out his or her expectations for the role of the audiology student and to explain to the student that the balance of their roles will shift from preceptor in the dominant role at 90% and the student at 10% to become the preceptor at 10% and student at 90%. Following this discussion, the preceptor should obtain information about the student's current clinical competencies and outline a means by which to move that student towards independence. For example, if the student has knowledge of hearing aid verification techniques yet has not performed those techniques with an actual patient, this information would assist the preceptor and student in their discussion for what skills need to be developed next.

Planning in the Anderson model (1988) refers to two sets of interaction for shared development of the clinical process; the interaction between the patient and student clinician, as well as the interaction between the supervisor (preceptor) and supervisee (student). Using the previous hearing aid verification example, the preceptor should help the student plan for the interaction with the patient by discussing the protocol of that setting. Then the preceptor and student should continue the planning by delineating the level of involvement that each will play in the clinical interaction. Planning these interactions should depend on the level of the student's knowledge and skills.

Anderson (1988) describes *observing* and *analyzing* within the supervisory process as gathering, documenting, and interpreting data by both the supervisor (preceptor) and supervisee (student). The data being recorded should be objective when possible and should include reflection of the student's own performance. The hearing aid verification example would allow the preceptor to observe and document the performance of the student, as well as allow the student to reflect on his or her own abilities. This process of evaluation can be used to strengthen the student's skill set.

The final stage of Anderson's (1988) model describes the *integrating* of all components at various points throughout the supervisory experience. Therefore, the experience of the hearing aid verification interaction would give the preceptor and student the opportunity to assess the student's current level of functioning for this particular skill and plan for further development to move the student towards independent practice. Table 12-3 describes this supervisory process for an audiology student at three different stages of a preceptorship. The goal for the student in the case example illustrated in Table 12-3 is to progress from dependence upon the preceptor to independent practice in obtaining a complete audiological evaluation on a pediatric patient.

ADDITIONAL CONSIDERATIONS FOR PRECEPTORSHIPS

It would be imprudent not to mention additional considerations that preceptors need to keep in mind as they agree to mentor students and future audiologists. The example of supervision for the hearing aid verification case does not describe much about the timing for providing feedback to audiology students. Yet, feedback gives the student the necessary information needed to reflect, improve, and move forward. It is not always easy to give a student feedback in the presence of the patient or patient's family members. Caution must be taken not to jeopardize the relationship between the patient and provider (in this case, the student). There are times in which the student

TABLE 12-3		

AUDIOLOGY EXAMPLE USING ANDERSON'S MODEL OF SUPERVISION (ANDERSON, 1988)

THE CLINICAL GOAL IS TO OBTAIN A FULL AUDIOMETRIC EVALUATION ON A 4-YEAR-OLD USING CASE HISTORY, OTOSCOPY, IMMITTANCE, PLAY AUDIOMETRY, SPEECH, AND COUNSELING TECHNIQUES

	BEGINNING OF PRECEPTORSHIP (DIRECTIVE-ACTIVE)	MIDDLE OF PRECEPTORSHIP (COLLABORATIVE)	END OF PRECEPTORSHIP (CONSULTATIVE)
UNDERSTANDING	Student has knowledge of play audiometry, but no skills or experience.	Student has gained skills and experience with children with typical hearing.	Student has gained skills and experience with children with varying degrees of hearing sensitivity.
STUDENT AND PATIENT PLANNING	Preceptor will complete the evaluation while the student observes.	Preceptor will assign the student to see patients with known hearing loss in this age group.	Student develops the plan for patient contact and executes testing.
PRECEPTOR AND STUDENT PLANNING	The preceptor will describe the clinic's protocols and discuss the techniques used during the evaluation.	Preceptor and student have a meeting to discuss strategies and techniques for using play audiometry with a patient this age. Conversation should encompass the presentation of information to the family (e.g., counseling).	Student is now responsible for evaluating the case and reviewing the outcomes of the evaluation with the preceptor. More of the discussion will occur post-appointment instead of pre-appointment.
OBSERVING	Student is observing and collecting information while the preceptor performs the evaluation.	During the evaluation, the preceptor notes the student's proficiency of diagnostic skills.	Preceptor uses less direct line-of-sight supervision; therefore, student is more responsible for reporting objective data about his or her performance.

continued

TABLE 12-3 (CONTINUED)

AUDIOLOGY EXAMPLE USING ANDERSON'S MODEL OF SUPERVISION (ANDERSON, 1988)

THE CLINICAL GOAL IS TO OBTAIN A FULL AUDIOMETRIC EVALUATION ON A 4-YEAR-OLD USING CASE HISTORY, OTOSCOPY, IMMITTANCE, PLAY AUDIOMETRY, SPEECH, AND COUNSELING TECHNIQUES

	BEGINNING OF PRECEPTORSHIP (DIRECTIVE-ACTIVE)	MIDDLE OF PRECEPTORSHIP (COLLABORATIVE)	END OF PRECEPTORSHIP (CONSULTATIVE)
ANALYZING	Preceptor works with the student to evaluate the test results, formulate a diagnosis, and develop a plan for how the student will obtain the skills needed for use with future patients.	Preceptor rates the student's proficiency (e.g., emerging, present, independent). Student analyzes his or her own proficiency.	Student demonstrates more depth (e.g., self-awareness of strengths and weaknesses) in the analysis of his or her clinical skills.
INTEGRATING	Preceptor and student develop a skill-set check sheet in which the student will show mastery of skills needed to evaluate patients of this age.	Preceptor and student formulate a plan to work with patients in this age group with unknown hearing status.	Student and preceptor have a discussion about how the student will apply the knowledge and skills he/she possesses for difficult and complex cases in the future.
FINAL OUTCOME	Student writes a reflective paper on the experience.	Student is able to complete appropriate tests in collaboration with the preceptor.	Student is capable of completing the testing and counseling independently on all children in this age group; preceptor provides consultation as needed.

Note: The reader must realize that there are many additional scenarios that can be added to the above table. The suggestions provided are by no means exhaustive.

will need immediate feedback in order to provide appropriate care for the patient. However, at other times, feedback can be withheld until patient care is completed and more summative information can be given.

Another consideration that must be addressed is the pre-planning phase of service delivery. The practice of audiology does not lend itself to as much pre-planning for a student prior to delivery of patient services as it does with other health-related professions (e.g., speech-language pathology). A student doing a preceptorship in an ear, nose, and throat clinic may have very little information about a patient prior to obtaining the case history during the initial contact with the patient. In other words, a patient may be in the clinic to see the physician who then determines that the audiologist needs to complete an audiological evaluation in order to assist with a diagnosis. Therefore, very little pre-planning can occur between the preceptor and the student for that patient.

When considering becoming a preceptor for an audiology student, one must contemplate how to balance the responsibility to the patient with the responsibility to the student. It is necessary to ask oneself which is more important: obtaining an accurate result or educating a future professional? This balancing act may change from case to case, but ultimately, the preceptor is the person who has to make the decision about how much patient care to release to the student.

Finally, most of what an audiologist does is diagnostic in nature. Depending on the practice setting, patients may be seen only once (e.g., ear, nose, and throat clinic, speech and hearing clinic) or seen once a year after being fit with hearing aids (e.g., school setting, private practice). In contrast, speech-language pathologists see patients more frequently due to the therapeutic nature of the profession. A preceptorship can be affected by the frequency with which a patient is seen. That is, an audiology student cannot track the development of his or her skills with the same patient over a period of time. For an audiology student, the set of patients seen on one day is very different from the set of patients seen on the next. This difference in the frequency of contact with an individual patient has an impact on the preceptorship in that the preceptor cannot evaluate the student on his or her skill set development across time with a specific case.

PRECEPTORSHIP CHALLENGES

Since the profession of audiology transitioned to the professional doctorate, audiology students must have many more hours of clinical experience than ever before. Academic programs now depend more and more on off-site clinical experiences. The necessity for preceptors to provide and document these experiences, as well as students' clinical competencies, has increased exponentially. With this increased dependence on preceptors, several challenges have to be recognized and addressed. The following topics are not meant to be presented in order of urgency or severity. Instead, the authors wish to bring about awareness and some understanding for persons interested in becoming a preceptor.

Paid Versus Unpaid Preceptorships

The first challenge that must be acknowledged concerns the idea of payment or reimbursement for a fourth-year extern. The idea to pay fourth-year externs may have arisen from the past paradigm used with clinical fellows, although the two models were not meant to be the same. Most people would not consider a payment or stipend to be problematic. Who would not want to be paid for completing billable services, especially after a long and expensive education program, when paying externs could help to offset the cost of that education? Yet, paying a student still enrolled in his or her educational process brings about several problems (including conflicts of interest) for the academic programs, as well as the preceptors involved in the clinical education component of those programs.

First, some sites have the resources to pay students while others do not. Therefore, an extern might try to obtain a preceptorship at a site that can pay although that site may not be the best fit for strengthening the student's knowledge and skills, or for helping the student pursue his or her own professional interests. The idea of paying a fourth-year student can also hurt the externship site because for those facilities that do not have an adequate funding source, the ability to recruit well-qualified students is diminished. The most alarming problem brought about by this concept of payment is the idea that some preceptorship sites use the student as "cheap labor," as opposed to really maintaining the experience as an educational one. Therefore, preceptors need to bear in mind their obligations to the code of ethics for their profession.

Reimbursement Considerations

Sometimes regulations imposed by third-party payers will affect how supervisory processes and preceptorships are handled. For example, Medicare Part B requires "line-of-sight supervision of students" to bill for services (Center for Medicare & Medicaid Services, 2019). This policy dictates that preceptors must be in the room and involved 100% of the time when a student is seeing a patient. The preceptor must not be engaged in any other task or distracted from the student-patient interaction (ASHA, n.d.-a). Therefore, a person interested in becoming a preceptor needs to become familiar with the regulations set forth by insurance companies and third-party payers in their specific practice.

Availability of Certified Preceptors (To C or Not To C)

For many years, academic programs in audiology have expressed concern over securing enough preceptors with appropriate credentials to supervise their students. In part, this problem has arisen as some audiologists have opted to become board certified in audiology with the ABA instead of maintaining or obtaining certification with ASHA. Additionally, other audiologists are opting not to become certified by any organization and are obtaining state licensure alone.

For audiology students who wish to apply for the ASHA Certificate of Clinical Competence in Audiology (ASHA CCC-A,) following graduation from their academic program, this means that they have needed to obtain 1,820 hours of clinical experience supervised by audiologists who also hold the CCC-A. Therefore, the availability of audiologists who hold their Cs impacts the availability of an appropriate preceptorship for a student who also wishes to obtain his or her Cs.

Many academic programs in audiology are utilizing creative teaching methods, such as simulated patients and cases, to address the increase in the number of hours that AuD students need in order to obtain ASHA certification. Simulations have been used in medical education for many years and range from the use of clinical skills labs, to standardized patients, to computer-based avatars and mannequins. The use of simulations does not necessarily reduce the need for well-trained, certified preceptors, but it does assist with reducing the number of hours needed for that preceptor and the site to generate for each student. This creativity ultimately helps students reach their required clinical hours with on-campus faculty and clinic supervisors, and it saves the preceptorship for exposing the students to actual (live) patients.

As alluded to earlier in this chapter, beginning on January 1, 2020, any person who applies for the CCC-A from ASHA will come across two changes that have been made to current certification standards. These changes appear to address the issue of finding preceptors with their CCC-A to supervise audiology students. First, a specified number of supervised clinical practicum hours will no longer be required; that is, the current mandatory number of 1,820 clinical hours will no longer be the "magical number" students are required to obtain. Applicants and their academic programs will only be obligated to "ensure that the student's experience meets CAA standards for duration, and for depth and breadth of knowledge" (ASHA, n.d.-b). It will be up to the individual university to determine what "ensures" that depth and breadth of knowledge. The second change that will take place in 2020 will be the provision that applicants who do not complete their entire supervised clinical experience under an ASHA-certified preceptor can make up the remainder of their experience post-graduation to meet ASHA certification standards. This means that a student can graduate with the depth and breadth of knowledge required by their academic program and then continue to obtain clinical experience supervised by another professional who has ASHA certification in order to become ASHA certified themselves. With this scenario, preceptors may be contacted by a colleague, not a student, to help that person obtain certification.

Training Programs for Preceptors

Professionals interested in becoming preceptors now have the option of obtaining training specific to the topic. This training, meant to prepare today's audiologists for the professional expectations of a preceptorship, can be obtained at state and national conferences or with online modules, similar to the traditional methods used for continuing education/professional development. Academic programs have discussed developing day-long seminars to offer to their supervisors and preceptors as a means for improving and strengthening the clinical education experience for both the student and the preceptor (E. Clark, personal communication, October 12, 2017).

The ABA has developed an "assessment-based, standards-driven certificate training program" for individuals who provide clinical education for students in their externship/fourth-year placement (ABA, n.d.). Based on results from a 2012 training-needs survey that ranked the development of preceptor training as a top priority, the ABA Board of Governors approved the development of the training program, which contains four, 2-hour long modules in an online format. At the conclusion of the training program, participants are awarded a certificate that designates the professional as a Certificate Holder-Audiology Preceptor (CH-AP). These certificates expire 5 years after the completion of the training. University programs looking for preceptors who hold this special certificate can go to the National Registry of Audiology Preceptors maintained by the ABA to search for licensed audiologists who hold the CH-AP certificate.

ASHA has also acknowledged the need for better-prepared preceptors and supervisors. The organization has developed a webinar entitled "Nine Building Blocks of Supervision." Professionals interested in obtaining more training on the topic of supervision can sign up for the 2 hours of continuing education. Topics covered in this webinar include assessing a students' competencies upon entrance to a clinical experience, establishing and modifying goals, and evaluating progress across the clinical experience.

Continuing Education Requirements for Preceptors

As a final consideration for professionals interested in becoming a preceptor, there are additional recommendations coming about in January 2020 regarding requirements for AuD students applying for ASHA certification; that is, for audiology students interested in obtaining their Cs, the preceptors who supervise them will not only need to have ASHA certification, but will also have to have had a minimum of 2 hours of professional development in the area of supervision post-certification. These new recommendations are part of a multiphase plan that includes requiring a minimum of 2 hours in supervision training for every 3-year cycle of certification maintenance with ASHA. For more information on these future plans, refer to the full report of the ASHA Ad Hoc Committee on Supervision Training (ASHA, 2016).

Some state licensure boards (in audiology and speech-language pathology) are beginning to require licensees to obtain specialized continuing education related to the topic of ethics. Predictions are being made that, over time, state licensure boards will also require specialized continuing education for the topic of supervision, if ASHA requires these as a part of their certification maintenance. Preceptors will need to stay current on forthcoming requirements.

PRECEPTORSHIP IN THE FUTURE

To conclude, changes made within the educational realm of the profession of audiology (e.g., the move from a master's-level degree to a clinical doctoral degree) have transformed the way we clinically educate our students. These transformations will continue to occur as more experience with the machinations of the professional doctorate are encountered and changes to the educational needs of students become more apparent.

Our profession relies on volunteerism from practitioners. Our profession also relies on the knowledge and skill base of those practitioners. Although time consuming, audiologists should consider the benefits of taking on students during their clinical education experiences. Those benefits are not only for the profession, but for the practitioner, as well. Preceptors are exposed to students who are learning the most up-to-date methods and ideas within the profession. Preceptors report that they often learn as much from the student as the student learns from them. With AuD degrees being offered at universities these days, it is important for practitioners to remember that a student attending a university's graduation ceremony on Saturday may well be a fully practicing audiologist at their clinical setting on Monday.

REFERENCES

American Academy of Audiology. (n.d.). *Clinical education guidelines for audiology externships*. Retrieved from https://www.audiology.org/publications-resources/document-library/clinical-education-guidelines-audiology-externships

American Academy of Audiology. (2014, June 5). *Roles and responsibilities of the externship site, preceptor, and universities*. Retrieved from http://www.audiology.org/education-research/education/externships/roles-and-responsibilities-externship-site-preceptor-and

American Board of Audiology. (n.d.). *Certificate programs: Certificate holder-audiology preceptor (CH-AP)*. Retrieved from www.boardofaudiology.org/certificate-programs.shtml

American Speech-Language-Hearing Association. (n.d.-a). *Medicare coverage of students: Audiology*. Retrieved from https://www.asha.org/practice/reimbursement/medicare/student_participation/

American Speech-Language-Hearing Association. (n.d.-b). *Certification standards to change in 2020*. Retrieved from https://www.asha.org/certification/certification-standards-change-in-2020/

Anderson, J. (1988). The supervisory process in speech-language pathology and audiology. Boston, MA: College-Hill.

American Speech-Language-Hearing Association. (2016, May). A plan for developing resources and training opportunities in clinical supervision [Report of the Ad Hoc Committee on Supervision Training]. Retrieved from http://www.asha.org/uploadedFiles/ASHA/About/governance/Resolutions_and_Motions/2016/Report-Ad-Hoc-Committee-on-Supervision-Training.pdf

Center for Medicare & Medicaid Services. (2019). *Medicare benefit policy manual: Chapter 15*. Retrieved from https://www.cms.gov/Regulations-and-Guidance/Guidance/Manuals/downloads/bp102c15.pdf

Greenberg, S., & Smith, I. (1987). *Evaluation of the requirements for the Certificates of Clinical Competence of the American Speech-Language-Hearing Association*. New York, NY: Professional Examination Service.

Mantzorou, M. (2004). Preceptorship in nursing education: Is it a viable alternative method for clinical teaching? *ICUs and Nursing Web Journal, 19*, 1-10.

Mashie, J., & Mendel, L. (2005). *The AuD externship experience: Summary document from the Consensus Conference on Issued and Concerns related to the 4th year AuD student*. Retrieved from http://www.capcsd.org/proceedings/2005/toc2005.html

Pierce, A. (1991) Preceptorial students' view of their clinical experience. *Journal of Nursing Education, 30*(6) 244-250.

Preceptor manual for off-campus clinical rotations and externships. (2007). Ball State University, Muncie, IN. Retrieved from http://cms.bsu.edu/-/media/www/departmentalcontent/spaa/docs/preceptormanual.pdf?la=en

School of audiology preceptor site. (n.d.). Pacific University Oregon, Forest grove, OR. Retrieved from https://sites.google.com/a/pacificu.edu/preceptor-guidance-2/

Tannenbaum, R., & Rosenfeld, M. (1996). *The practice of audiology: A study of the clinical activities and knowledge areas for the certified audiologist*. Princeton, NJ: Education Testing Service.

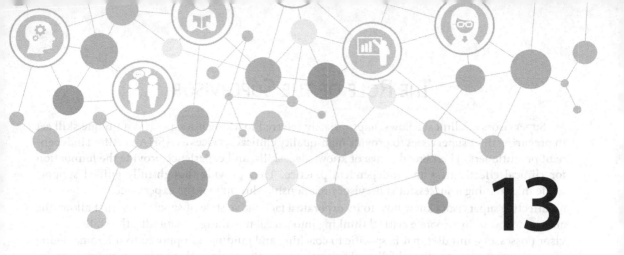

13

Clinical Education and Supervision of Clinical Fellows

Melanie W. Hudson, MA, CCC-SLP, F-ASHA

The clinical fellowship (CF) is a mentored experience leading to the Certificate of Clinical Competence in Speech-Language Pathology (CCC-SLP), a nationally recognized professional credential representing a level of excellence and professional credibility. Individuals who hold this credential have met the rigorous academic and professional standards established by the American Speech-Language-Hearing Association's (ASHA) Council for Clinical Certification in Audiology and Speech-Language Pathology (CFCC). These standards include a master's or doctoral degree from an accredited academic program, a passing score on the national examination, and the CF, supervised by an ASHA-certified professional (ASHA, n.d.-d)

The purpose of the CF is to integrate and apply theoretical knowledge from academic training, evaluate strengths and identify limitations, develop and refine clinical skills consistent with the scope of practice, and advance from constant supervision to independent practice (ASHA, n.d.-a). The successful completion of the CF signifies attainment of the essential knowledge, skills, and expertise required to provide high-quality clinical services as an independent practitioner.

What specific knowledge and skills must a supervisor possess to guide and support these new clinicians? What specialized skills should be acquired that support critical thinking and decision-making? What knowledge, insight, perspective, and wisdom can a supervisor share that will lead these new clinicians from constant supervision to self-supervision and independent practice? Supervisors of clinical fellows should seek the answers to these questions as they consider the roles and responsibilities that are part of this unique supervisory relationship.

McCrea, E. S., & Brasseur, J. A. *The Clinical Education and Supervisory Process in Speech-Language Pathology and Audiology* (pp 373-379).

THE ROLE OF THE SUPERVISOR

Supervisors of clinical fellows, appropriately referred to as mentors, possess a unique skill set in preparing their supervisees to provide high-quality clinical services as ASHA-certified independent practitioners. Their broad range of knowledge, skills, and experience provide the foundation for clinical effectiveness and independent practice. They provide thoughtfully guided support while maintaining a successful supervisory relationship throughout the experience.

Effective supervisors know how to incorporate a facilitative style of supervision that allows the clinical fellow to incorporate critical thinking into decision making. Essentially, the skilled supervisor possesses a mindset that is specific to coaching and guiding, as opposed to micromanaging the performance of the clinical fellow. They realize that their role in this unique supervisory relationship is not to "create a clone" of themselves as part of the process, and are skilled in promoting the use of reflective practice (Hudson, 2010). This often requires a shift in thinking for many experienced supervisors who may need to learn how to be less direct in their supervisory style. Effective supervisors fully comprehend the collaborative nature of this unique supervisory relationship and can establish clearly defined goals and outcomes for both themselves and their clinical fellow. This results in both parties "raising the bar" as goals are achieved while their insights and skills continue to grow. They are keenly aware of the importance of a trusting, confidential relationship based on mutual respect, and appreciate the role that communication plays in the relationship. They are skilled in active listening, asking purposeful questions, and responding appropriately to questions when asked. They are aware of the importance of communication style, both verbal and nonverbal, particularly when providing feedback.

Successful supervisors promote cultural competence awareness and sensitivity by using self-inventory tools and having open discussions (Anderson, 1992; Battle, 1993; Langdon & Cheng, 1992). They consider the learning styles and culturally based behaviors of their clinical fellows to improve interpersonal interactions. In addition, they provide opportunities to develop cultural competence and self-awareness for increased sensitivity and understanding of situations that may occur during the CF.

Supervisors are familiar with the ASHA (2016a) Code of Ethics and take their responsibility seriously in preparing the clinical fellow for a lifetime of ethical conduct. They model behaviors necessary for lifelong ethical practice and provide opportunities for discussion of ethical dilemmas. Supervisors recognize the extraordinary commitment of time and talent required to prepare these future professionals for successful careers as independent service providers. They are mindful of the fact they serve as role models, thereby providing clinical fellows with opportunities to observe and reflect on their own behaviors.

SKILL ACQUISITION AND THE SUPERVISORY PROCESS

The relationship between skill acquisition the supervisory process should be consistent with the various stages of professional growth and development. The Dreyfus Model of Skill Acquisition (Dreyfus & Dreyfus, 1986) ("Novice to Expert," 2005). describes a learning process consisting of five stages: novice, advanced beginner, competent, proficient, and expert. It is used to assess and support progress in skill development while providing a definition of acceptable performance levels for each developmental stage.

The *competent stage* of learning has been achieved upon completion of graduate coursework and clinical practicum in speech-language pathology. At this stage, the learner is typically able to plan with more independence, deliberately use analytical assessment to treat problems in context, view actions in terms of long-term goals, and incorporate conscious, deliberate planning to achieve those goals. This individual is also able to use standardized and routine procedures while recognizing their relevance to a given situation.

The development of critical thinking skills has played a major role in achieving the skills that define the *proficient stage* of learning. At this stage, the learner has achieved a holistic understanding and is able to view situations in terms of long-term goals. This improves decision making, as maxims are used for guidance and the individual is able to modify plans in terms of what should be expected. At this stage, individuals are able to perceive deviations from what is typical and, as a result, are equipped to make clinical judgments more easily. In addition, they can see what is most important in a situation and to take responsibility for their own decisions, the hallmark of an independent practitioner providing high-quality clinical services.

The Dreyfus model sets the stage for the CF to be viewed as the transition from the competent stage to the proficient stage of learning, the latter being attained by the end of the CF. The role of the supervisor, therefore, is to guide the clinical fellow in making this transition that leads to independent practice.

The effective supervisor facilitates this transition from the competent stage to the proficient stage by enabling an ongoing collaborative process. ASHA (2008) describes an effective supervisory relationship that is collaborative in nature, with shared responsibility for many of the activities throughout the supervisory process. These activities include the development of clearly defined goals, with an emphasis on the use of self-assessment tools as part of the feedback process leading to self-supervision.

Anderson's (1988) *continuum of supervision* allows for the eventual achievement of self-supervision while employing different strategies and styles during various stages of the supervisory process. The degree of involvement of both the supervisor and the supervisee shifts as they progress through each stage or point along the continuum. Anderson's *Self-Supervision Stage* is comparable to Dreyfus' *proficient·stage* of learning as supervisees have learned to self-analyze their clinical behavior while taking responsibility for their own decisions. At this stage, the supervisor no longer plays a dominant role in the supervisory process as the relationship between the supervisor and the supervisee becomes more of a peer interaction.

As clinical fellow supervisors guide these new professionals from the competent stage to the proficient stage of skill development, an effective supervisory model should be in place. Anderson's (1988) continuum illustrates that an effective supervisory model should have a framework for systematic development of the process of supervision. Lubinski and Hudson's (2013) CORE Model of Supervision and Mentoring incorporates the key components of such a framework including collaborative planning, observation and data collection, analysis of data, and evaluation and feedback. Although professional demands and responsibilities may vary from setting to setting, these key components are universal and not specific to any setting. Each of these components supports principles of critical thinking and reflective practice that lead to self-supervision and independence.

THE CLINICAL FELLOWSHIP: STEP-BY-STEP

Supervisors of clinical fellows should familiarize themselves with their roles and responsibilities (ASHA, n.d.-d) and the requirements for ASHA certification (ASHA, n.d.-c). These should also be discussed with the clinical fellow as part of the supervisory process, keeping in mind that the clinical fellow assumes ultimate responsibility for meeting the requirements for certification.

The CF requires 36 weeks of full time (35 hours per week) experience (or the equivalent part-time experience), totaling a minimum of 1,260 hours. Eighty percent of the time must be spent in direct clinical contact, including assessment, diagnosis, evaluation, screening, treatment, report writing, family and client consultation, and counseling related to the management of the disordered that fit within the ASHA Speech-Language Pathology Scope of Practice (ASHA, 2016c).

The supervisor must provide 6 hours of on-site observations of direct client contact per segment (with each segment being one third the length of the fellowship) and six indirect monitoring activities per segment, including review of written reports and other record keeping, observation of participation in team conferences and other similar professional activities, and consultation with colleagues or clients and their families. If alternative methods of observation and mentoring activities are to be used, prior approval must be obtained from the CFCC.

At the very beginning of the CF, the supervisor and the clinical fellow should discuss how the monitoring activities will be completed, including frequency and method of documentation of those activities. Supervisors should also use this time to discuss preferred modes of communication (e.g., email, text, phone) and workplace policies and procedures directly related to the success of the CF (e.g., dress codes, time and attendance policies, etc.). This is also an appropriate time to discuss any pet peeves that the supervisor deems necessary to share with the fellow, such as checking personal email during treatment sessions and the like.

It is also important to review the Clinical Fellowship Skills Inventory (CFSI) at the beginning of the CF (ASHA, n.d.-e). Both parties should be familiar with the descriptions provided for each of the 18 skill areas described on this assessment tool prior to the first segment Evaluation-Feedback session. The skill areas may also provide the basis for the establishment of goals to be addressed as part of the supervisory process during the CF.

Supervisors must balance helping their clinical fellow's plan both for their clients and for their own clinical and professional growth as part of a collaborative planning process that includes the establishment of performance goals. Fredrickson and Moore (2014) cite the importance of clarifying expectations and discussing discrepancies early on as an important strategy. Breakdowns in communication during this planning process may give rise to long-term difficulties in the supervisory relationship and delay or even prevent the successful completion of the CF.

McCrea and Brasseur (2003) describe the concept of "fourfold planning" for all participants, including the client, the clinician, the supervisee, and the supervisor, as the foundation of the ongoing supervisory process. The needs of each of these participants should be considered and addressed appropriately when establishing goals. Supervisors should provide guidance as the clinical fellow self-identifies measurable goals that serve as a guide for action and as a source of motivation. The clinical fellow is more likely to achieve targeted goals if the supervisor offers continued support and recognizes effort and success while promoting critical reflection along the way.

Direct observation of clinical work is a required monitoring activity of the CF and may include observations of any direct clinical contact activities. The purpose of an observation is to collect data on predetermined aspects of the fellow's work. Anderson (1988) described observation as the point at which supervision changes from being solely an art to more of a science, and stressed that it must be an active process if it is to be of value. She also stated that "observation without data is a waste of time" (p. 123).

A supervisor maintains objectivity through observation and relevant data collection. Data collection should correspond to established goals and skill areas that have been discussed as part of the collaborative process. Clinical fellows should also be provided with opportunities to take data and reflect on their own performance as part of the self-assessment process. Pultorak's (1993) Critical Reflection Checklist is an excellent tool designed for this purpose. The checklist consists of six questions that may be answered by the supervisee and discussed with the supervisor following the completion of a clinical or related activity.

Analysis of collected data affords an opportunity for supervisors to observe how their actions may influence behavior and performance. Cogan (1973) cited that one of the purposes of analyzing data is to determine a database for the rest of the supervision program. This provides the information needed by the supervisor to provide objective feedback as progress in goal achievement is discussed.

The results of data analysis may also yield information that informs the clinician whether certain clinical procedures are effective. This provides an opportunity to engage in reflective practice while promoting accountability. In addition, the results of analyzed data may yield information that provide an opportunity for supervisors to improve their interactions and become more effective in facilitating self-assessment, a crucial skill to be acquired by the clinical fellow.

The purpose of a performance evaluation is to provide the clinical fellow with feedback that is objective, data based, verifiable, and systematic. Evaluations should be a continual process in which the supervisee is encouraged to describe and measure his or her own progress and achievement as part of this process (ASHA, 2008). The use of self-assessment tools places the evaluation component of the supervisory process in the proper context to support a collaborative supervisory relationship. As such, the supervisor relies on the results of analysis of objective data as part of the evaluation process, and input based on critical reflection on the part of the clinical fellow. The effective supervisor has developed expertise in critical reflection and should provide regular opportunities for guided activities to facilitate this important skill (Hudson, 2010).

The ability to assess one's own performance is an important characteristic of successful independent practice, and supervisors play an important role in promoting this skill as part of the evaluation process. Dowling (2001) states that "supervisee self-evaluation fosters the development of clinical competence and a sense of professional self" (p. 87).

The CFSI supports self-assessment, with feedback and guidance from the supervisor at the end of each of the three segments of the CF (ASHA, n.d.-d). The 21 skill areas targeted for assessment include a performance rating from 1-3, with 3 being the highest. A score of 2 or higher on each of the skill areas in the final segment is required for successful completion of the CF. The clinical fellow should be encouraged to assign a rating to each skill area, assess his or her own level of performance, with applicable feedback and guided reflection from the supervisor. If feedback and critical reflection have been ongoing and part of a collaborative process, there should be no unanticipated outcomes when the supervisor and the clinical fellow complete the CFSI together. If specific skill areas are identified as needing improvement, the supervisor should support the clinical fellow in developing new goals or refining already-established goals and implementing strategies that target these skills.

Mandel (2015) discusses how being aware of the perceptions and expectations of supervisees allows supervisors to target areas of need in supporting professional growth. If the supervisor has any reason to believe that the clinical fellow will not meet the requirements for successful completion of the CF, it is the supervisor's responsibility to counsel the clinical fellow accordingly. It is important to maintain documentation of contacts and conferences during this time period while addressing the areas of concern to achieve positive outcomes. If, however, positive outcomes are not ultimately achieved, and the supervisor does not recommend approval of the CF, the supervisor must indicate such on the Clinical Fellowship Report and Rating Form (ASHA, n.d.-b). Within 30 days of this decision, the supervisor must submit a letter of explanation and a signed Clinical Fellowship Report and Rating Form to the CFCC, which will then be shared and discussed with the clinical fellow. At that time, the clinical fellow may complete an entirely new CF, a portion of the CF, or request an appeal by the CFCC.

SELF-ASSESSMENT AND PROFESSIONAL DEVELOPMENT FOR SUPERVISORS

Supervisors also need to consider their own self-assessment and professional development as an important component of the supervisory process. The ASHA (2016b) Ad Hoc Committee on Supervision Training (AHCST) developed a self-assessment tool for supervisors to rate their competencies for specific knowledge and skills in supervision. This tool is designed to assist supervisors in developing training goals to improve their abilities in supervision. There are specific sections for each of five constituent groups, including supervisors of clinical fellows. The competencies identified specifically for CF supervisors include establishing goals through a collaborative process, providing ongoing assessment, providing opportunities to achieve independence, incorporating reflective practice and critical thinking, navigating the workplace and becoming part of a team, maintaining professional boundaries, and developing advocacy skills. It would benefit the supervisory relationship for supervisors to discuss their own goals for improvement with the clinical fellow as part of the growth process for both parties.

In addition to identifying their own competencies in supervision, supervisors need to be familiar with current ASHA certification standards and state licensure requirements. Current ASHA certification standards require that CF mentors hold up-to-date ASHA certification throughout the fellowship and may not be related to the clinical fellow. In 2020, supervisors will also be required to have to have a minimum of 9 months of practice experience post-certification before supervising a clinical fellow (ASHA, 2018). In addition, CF supervisors will be required to have completed 2 hours post-certification of professional development in supervision.

Supervisors of clinical fellows need to ensure compliance with state specific requirements for supervision of provisionally licensed supervisees. For instance, state licensure requirements for amount of on-site supervision may differ from ASHA's requirements for certification, and supervisors and supervisees alike need to be aware of these differences for purposes of compliance.

As previously stated, supervisors need to be aware of their ethical obligations to clinical fellows (ASHA, 2017). Inappropriate supervision may lead to severe consequences for both the clinical fellow and the supervisor. The issue of *vicarious liability* describes the supervisor's responsibility concerning the behavior of the supervisee (Newman, 2001). Supervisors must always consider the welfare of the patient paramount, including confidentiality and privacy, and documentation in keeping with principles of ethical practice. They recognize the power they hold over the clinical fellow and maintain an appropriate balance of power throughout the CF. See Chapter 9 for a more in-depth discussion of ethics in clinical education and supervision.

There are many other areas in which supervisors may consider improving their knowledge and skills relevant to the professional growth and development of the clinical fellow, including adult learning styles, interprofessional practice, accountability, the use of technology, dealing with stress and burnout, time management and organization, policies and procedures in the workplace, conflict management, maintaining professional boundaries and appropriate relationships, and fostering professional identity and engagement. It is not enough to assume that a supervisor is able to provide expert coaching and guidance in each of these related areas simply due to length of experience as a practitioner.

The CF marks the beginning of a long-term career path for speech-language pathologists and plays a major role in establishing and maintaining professional standards. Supervisors of clinical fellows hold the keys as gatekeepers of our profession and bear the responsibility as role models for these new professionals. If they are prepared to meet the challenges and share the joys that this unique supervisory opportunity provides, they are investing in a commitment to lifelong learning and the future of our profession.

REFERENCES

American Speech-Language-Hearing Association. (n.d.-a). *Clinical fellowship.* Retrieved from http://www.asha.org/Certification/Clinical_Fellowship

American Speech-Language-Hearing Association. (n.d.-b). *Clinical fellowship report and rating form.* Retrieved from https://www.asha.org/uploadedFiles/SLP-CF-Report-Rating-Form.pdf

American Speech-Language-Hearing Association. (n.d.-c). *General information about ASHA certification.* Retrieved from https://www.asha.org/Certification/AboutCertificationGenInfo/

American Speech-Language-Hearing Association. (n.d.-d). *Information for mentoring clinical fellowship (cf) SLPs.* Retrieved from https://www.asha.org/certification/CFSupervisors/

American Speech-Language-Hearing Association. (n.d.-e). *Clinical fellowship skills inventory (CFSI)*. Retrieved from https://www.asha.org/uploadedFiles/2020-Clinical-Fellowship-Skills-Inventory.pdf

American Speech-Language-Hearing Association. (2008). *Knowledge and skills needed by speech-language pathologists providing clinical supervision* [Knowledge and skills]. Retrieved from www.asha.org/policy

American Speech-Language-Hearing Association. (2016a). *Code of ethics*. Retrieved from https://www.asha.org/code-of-ethics/

American Speech-Language-Hearing Association. (2016b, May). *A plan for developing resources and training opportunities in clinical supervision* [Final report of the ASHA Ad Hoc Committee on Supervision Training]. Retrieved from www.asha.org

American Speech-Language-Hearing Association. (2016c, May). *Scope of practice in speech-language pathology*. Available from https://www.asha.org/policy/SP2016-00343/

American Speech-Language-Hearing Association. (2017). *Issues in ethics: Responsibilities of individuals who mentor clinical fellows in speech-language pathology*. Retrieved from https://www.asha.org/Practice/ethics/Responsibilities-of-Individuals-Who-Mentor-Clinical-Fellows-in-Speech-Language-Pathology/

American Speech-Language-Hearing Association. (2018). *Certification standards to change in 2020*. Retrieved from https://www.asha.org/Certification/Certification-Standards-Change-in-2020/

Anderson, J. L. (1988). *The supervisory process in speech-language pathology and audiology*. Austin, TX: PRO-ED.

Anderson. N.B. (1992). Understanding cultural diversity. *American Journal of Speech-Language Pathology, 1*, 11-12.

Battle, D. (1993). *Communication disorders in multicultural populations*. Boston, MA: Butterworth-Heinemann.

Cogan. M. (1973). *Clinical supervision*. Boston, MA: Houghton Mifflin.

Dowling, S. (2001). *Supervision: Strategies for successful outcomes and productivity*. Boston, MA: Allyn & Bacon.

Fredrickson, T. &, Moore, S. (2014). Key factors of influence in clinical educator relationships. *Perspectives on Administration and Supervision, 24*, 12-20. Retrieved from http://sig11perspectives.pubs.asha.org/article.aspx?articleid=1918821&resultClick=3

Hudson, M. (2010). *Supervision to mentoring: Practical considerations*. *Perspectives on Administration and Supervision, 20*, 71-75. Retrieved from http://dx.doi.org/10.1044/aas20.2.71

Langdon, H. W., & Cheng, L. (1992). *Hispanic children and adults with communication disorders*. Gaithersburg, MD: Aspen.

Lubinski, R., & Hudson, M. (2013). *Professional issues in speech-language pathology and audiology*. Clifton Park, NY: Delmar Cengage Learning.

Mandel, S. (2015). Exploring the differences in expectations between supervisors and supervisees during the initial clinical experience. *Perspectives on Administration and Supervision, 25*, 4-30. Retrieved from http://sig11perspectives.pubs.asha.org/article.aspx?articleid=2381513&resultClick=3

McCrea, E., & Brasseur, J. (2003). *The supervisory process in speech-language pathology and audiology*. Boston, MA: Allyn & Bacon.

Newman, W. (2001). The ethical and legal aspects of clinical supervision. *California Speech-Language-Hearing Association Magazine, 30*(1), 10-11, 27.

Novice to Expert: the Dreyfus model of skill acquisition. (2005). Retrieved from https://frrl.files.wordpress.com/2012/03/dreyfusmodelofskillacquisition.pdf.

Pultorak, E. G. (1993). Facilitating reflective thought in novice teachers. *Journal of Teacher Education, 44*(4), 288-295.

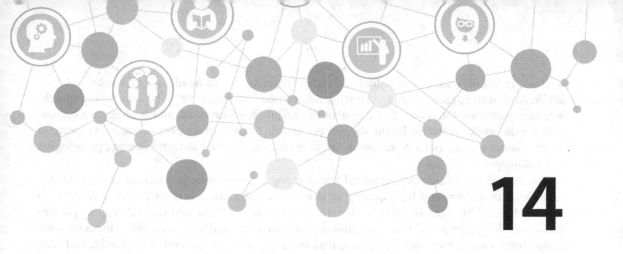

Supervision of Support Personnel

Heather L. Thompson, PhD, CCC-SLP

For many years, there has continued to be an increased need for professionals who provide services for the treatment of communication disorders (Teas, 1991). From 2016 to 2026, employment for speech-language pathologists is anticipated to grow by 18%, which is substantially faster than the national average for all occupations (7%; U.S. Bureau of Labor Statistics, 2018). Many variables may account for the shortage of speech-language pathologists and audiologists, including an aging population, a demand for multilingual service providers (Goldberg, Williams, & Paul-Brown, 2002), and a lack of speech-language pathologists entering doctoral programs with the potential to train future speech-language pathologists and audiologists (Myotte, Hutchins, Cannizzaro & Belin, 2011).

Other challenges impact the provision of speech-language pathology services. There is an increased need for speech-language pathology services in remote or rural locations (Paul-Brown & Goldberg, 2001). Individuals may depart the field following employment dissatisfaction associated with a high workload (Edgar & Rosa-Lugo, 2007). Other factors such as role ambiguity (Edgar & Rosa-Lugo, 2007; O'Brien, Mitchell, & Bryne, 2017), financial constraints (Edgar & Rosa-Lugo, 2007), or organizational changes (De Bortoli, Arthur-Kelly, Foreman, Balandin, & Mathisen, 2011) can contribute to concerns with service provision. Speech-language pathologists may be perceived as having insufficient time to work with clients or collaborate with other professionals as a consequence of departmental procedures (De Bortoli et al., 2011). These barriers to service have warranted a need for creative solutions and effective problem solving to ensure all individuals with communication disorders receive high-quality, timely, and appropriate care (Teas, 1991).

One way that speech-language pathologists can allow all individuals with communication concerns to receive appropriate services is by working with support personnel. Support personnel are individuals who perform prescribed tasks and duties under the supervision of licensed or

McCrea, E. S., & Brasseur, J. A. *The Clinical Education and Supervisory Process in Speech–Language Pathology and Audiology* (pp 381–400).
© 2020 Taylor & Francis Group.

certified speech-language pathologists and audiologists (American Academy of Audiology [AAA], 2018a; American Speech-Language-Hearing Association [ASHA], 1996). The supervising speech-language pathologist and audiologist assigns duties, provides direction, and is ultimately responsible for the work completed by the support personnel. The use of support personnel is meant to be an adjunct to, and not a replacement for, licensed and certified speech-language pathologists and audiologists.

The availability of support personnel allows many organizations to continue to provide efficient, high-frequency, and high-quality services while negotiating various financial constraints (ASHA, 1996). Through careful delegation of tasks and activities to well-trained support personnel, speech-language pathologists and audiologists have increased time available to focus on diagnostic, intervention, and caseload management tasks requiring a high level of knowledge and skill, thereby allowing professionals to spend time working at the "top of the license" (McNeilly, 2018; Wheat, 2018). By transferring some routine tasks to highly skilled assistants, client populations can be best served (Boyle, McCartney, O'Hare, and Forbes, 2009).

There continues to be an increase in the utilization of speech-language pathology support personnel in the United States as well as in other countries (O'Brien Byrne, Mitchell, & Ferguson, 2013). O'Brien et al. (2017) conducted semi-structured interviews with 20 speech-language pathologists working in local health districts in New South Wales, Australia, and found that 65% had exposure to or experience working with support personnel. While the literature evaluating the outcomes of services provided by support personnel is small, results are positive. For example, Boyle et al. (2009) examined the language outcomes of 161 children from 6 to 11 years old who received intervention from either a speech-language pathologist or a speech-language therapy assistant or who were assigned to a usual-therapy control group. Results of the study showed nonsignificant differences in Clinical Evaluation of Language Fundamentals-3^{UK} test scores for children in the two experimental groups at the end of the intervention period and at a 12-month follow up appointment. Results of Boyle et al.'s study demonstrate the effectiveness of intervention provided by support personnel. However, additional research is needed to determine if the intervention effects observed are consistent across populations or for different ages of clients.

Among professionals in the field, there are differing viewpoints regarding the use of support personnel (Bach, Kessler, and Heron, 2007; McCartney et al., 2005; O'Brien et al., 2017). Once speech-language pathologists begin to work with speech-language pathology assistants (SLPAs), however, they have reported to be pleased with the collaborative relationship (Millican, 2015; Peters-Johnson, 1998; Polovoy, 2011; Rowden-Racette, 2011). Given the rapid growth of the profession and the acknowledgment that changes to practice require a period of adjustment, speech-language pathologists and audiologists are encouraged to explore information about the utility of support personnel to determine if having the assistance through this professional designation may facilitate the care of patients in a given workplace.

This section provided information on the need for services in the communication sciences and disorders. In the next section, types of support personnel will be described. Following a description of support personnel positions, information regarding the history of support personnel in the field of communication sciences and disorders will be provided. Finally, roles and responsibilities of support personnel and their supervisors will be discussed.

DEFINITION OF SUPPORT PERSONNEL, SPEECH-LANGUAGE PATHOLOGY ASSISTANTS, AIDES, AND TECHNICIANS

Within the field, many different terms may be used to describe support personnel, including *audiology assistant, audiology technician, communication aide, communication (communicative) disorders assistant, communication health assistant, health care assistant, paraprofessional, paratherapist, paraeducator* or *para-speech educator, rehabilitation assistant, service extender, speech-language pathology assistant, speech aide, speech technician, therapy assistant,* or *therapist assistant* (Aguilar and Ostergren, 2016; Ostergren & Aguilar, 2015; Speech-Language and Audiology Canada, 2018). Internationally, multidisciplinary therapy assistants may be employed to address health care needs following concerns with high staff turnover in the health care field in general or following the need for services over a large geographical region (Lin & Goodale, 2005).

ASHA defines SLPAs as "support personnel who, following academic coursework, fieldwork, and on-the-job training, perform tasks prescribed, directed, and supervised by ASHA-certified speech-language pathologists" (ASHA, 2018a). A speech-language pathology aide (SA) is a position that generally requires less formal training than an SLPA. The position is defined by the State of California Speech-Language Pathology & Audiology & Hearing Aid Dispensers Board as an individual who "assists or facilitates while the speech-language pathologist is evaluating the speech and/or language of individuals or is treating individuals with a speech-language and/or language disorder...and is registered by the supervisor with the Board and the registration is approved by the Board" (Department of Consumer Affairs [DCA], 2014, ASHA, 2018b). The position of an SA generally requires a high school diploma or equivalent. However, some SAs may have completed college coursework or obtained a bachelor's degree without receiving formal clinical training. SAs can be used when employment of an SLPA is not feasible in a given work place (ASHA, 1996). Finally, a speech-language technician (ST) provides educationally-based services and requires less supervision than an SLPA or SA. However, STs are only recognized in a few states, and individuals must meet specific criteria (e.g., continuing education requirements) in order to remain employed (Arizona Speech-Language-Hearing Association [ArSHA], 2011).

The State of California Speech-Language Pathology & Audiology & Hearing Aid Dispensers Board defines an audiology aide or audiometrist as "a person who assists or facilitates while an audiologist is evaluating the hearing or vestibular function of individuals and/or is treating individuals with hearing or balance disorders...and is registered by the supervisor with the Board and the registration is approved by the Board" (DCA, 2014). Similar to the role of the speech-language pathologists, the AAA indicates that the role of the audiology aide is to support the audiologist by performing routine tasks and/or procedures to enable the audiologist to spend time performing activities which are more complex and require additional education to complete (AAA, 2018b). Finally, a teleaudiology clinical technician (TCT) is an individual who works in the Veteran's Administration health care system and provides patient/equipment support under the supervision of a licensed and certified audiologist (ASHA, 2018c).

BACKGROUND

Support personnel have worked in the field of speech-language pathology since the 1960 and 1970s (Scalero & Eskenazi, 1976). Over the years, changes have been made in how support personnel are regulated and supervised, with much variability among the states. In 1969, ASHA (1970) created its first set of guidelines to delineate the utilization of support personnel. Revisions to these guidelines took place in 1981 and 1988 (ASHA, 1996; Moore & Pearson, 2003, p. 8). In 1995, a position statement was developed that outlined activities such as training, credentialing, and use of support personnel (ASHA, 1996). The guidelines were revised again in 2000 (Moore and Pearson, 2003, p. 9). In 2002 to 2003, ASHA began a voluntary registration program for SLPAs (Appler, 2002), and, in 2004, the legislative council subsequently passed additional documentation that included a position statement, a technical report, guidelines, and curriculum content for support personnel. In 2011, the ASHA associate's program was initiated to allow all SLPAs and audiology assistants to be considered ASHA affiliates with the stipulation that the support personnel professional must pay dues and be qualified to practice in his or her state (ASHA, 2018d). The affiliate must also adhere to ASHA's principles of ethics and be employed and work under the supervision of an ASHA-certified speech-language pathologist with at least 2 years of experience following his or her clinical fellowship year and at least 10 hours of continuing education in the area of supervision.

In 2013, the SLPA Scope of Practice was finalized (ASHA, 2013a). This document provided information about ethical considerations and roles and responsibilities for clinical practice of SLPAs (ASHA, 2013a). In 2015, the associate's program migrated to an ongoing ASHA program and decisions were made to increase the standardization of SLPAs and audiology assistants through a proposed ASHA program for assistant certification. This proposed program will be launched by the end of 2020 and will involve the development of SLPA and audiology assistant standards for roles and scope of practice, establishment of a certification exam, and the development of guidelines for service reimbursement (ASHA, 2018e). In November 2017, ASHA's Board of Directors approved the assistant certification program for SLPA and audiology assistants.

The field of audiology has also experienced a significant transformation over the years, demonstrating increased usage of support personnel. In 1997, the AAA published a position statement and guidelines for the use of support personnel. This document delineated the qualifications of support personnel in audiology, the nature of the training, the roles and responsibilities of support staff, and the supervision required (AAA, 1997). ASHA's Scope of Practice in audiology was updated in 2004. Currently, audiologists provide program administration and supervision of support personnel (ASHA, 2004). Advances in technology (e.g., hearing implantation and the availability of personal listening devices), telehealth, hearing loss prevention, and educational audiology practice, have created a need for revisions to the scope of practice in audiology. In 2018, an ad hoc committee was formed; a new scope of practice document was developed. As part of the 2018 update, audiologists who provide assessment and intervention services for young children with hearing loss under the Early Hearing Detection and Intervention Act provide training and supervision to audiology support personnel.

EDUCATIONAL REQUIREMENTS AND FEDERAL REGULATIONS OF SUPPORT PERSONNEL

Support personnel have been regulated since the 1970s. Throughout the United States, the educational requirements vary (ASHA, 2018f). For example, for the position of an SLPA, 19 states require an associate's degree or equivalent and 24 states require a bachelor's degree with or without additional hours of training at the graduate school level (ASHA, 2017a). Information about requirements within each state is available on ASHA's website (www.asha.org; ASHA, 2017a).

In 2013, the ASHA board approved the Scope of Practice for SLPAs (ASHA, 2013a). This document provides guidelines and recommendations for the minimum qualifications for support personnel. In February 2016, ASHA developed model regulations for the professions that included state licensure for audiology assistants and SLPAs (ASHA, 2016a). In this document, it was delineated that SLPAs must complete academic coursework that includes the completion of an associate's degree from an SLPA program or a bachelor's degree in speech-language pathology or communication sciences and disorders, or the equivalent. In addition to the educational requirements, SLPAs must complete 100 hours of field work under the supervision of a speech-language pathologist, or the equivalent, and must demonstrate competency in skills required to work as an SLPA (ASHA, 2013a). Finally, the individual must agree to adhere to state laws to meet requirements for licensure and/or certification and subsequently obtain appropriate documentation for licensure and/or certification (ASHA, 1996; ASHA, 2016a).

SLPAs who are registered or licensed will often be required to obtain regular continuing education hours. The number of hours and the interval for obtaining them vary according to state (ASHA, 2017a; 2017b). Increasingly, there are resources available for SLPAs wishing to obtain continuing education advancement. A number of these resources are available electronically and are presented in Appendix 14-1.

There are essentially two tiers of support personnel who differ in the degree of training received, their knowledge, and the amount of supervision required when interacting with clients (ASHA, 1996; ASHA, 2018a). Generally speaking, SLPAs have more training, and as such, more responsibility than SAs. While SAs may have a high school diploma or equivalent or a college degree, training for SAs is generally provided by the supervising pathologist while on-the-job (ASHA, 1996; ASHA 2013a).

STs are only recognized in a few states and their employment responsibilities depend on the state in which the individual is employed. For example, in Arizona, STs must have a bachelor's degree in speech-language pathology, speech-hearing sciences, or communication sciences and disorders and have completed 50 hours of supervised observation and 150 hours of clinical experience under the supervision of a master's level speech-language pathologist (ArSHA, 2011). After that initial qualification, STs can only be employed in school settings and do not require supervision by speech-language pathologists. Every 6 years, STs must acquire at least 180 clock hours of graduate level coursework in the field of speech-language pathology or professional development in articulation, voice, fluency, language disorders, low incidence disabilities, professional issues and ethics, or service delivery models, to be permitted to renew certification with the Arizona Department of Education (ArSHA, 2011).

There is some variability in the scope of practice of support personnel outside of the United States. In Canada, SLPAs complete a diploma program and a fieldwork experience and are trained specifically to work with children in an educational setting. Communicative disorders assistants (CDAs) must have completed a postsecondary diploma or 4-year university degree with a focus in communication disorders, human anatomy and physiology, linguistics, social sciences, or human services, prior to completing a 1-year CDA program with multiple clinical fieldwork placements (CDAAC, 2018). CDAs can then work with individuals across the lifespan and can apply for membership with the Communicative Disorders Assistant Association of Canada (CDAAC, 2018). Currently, SLPAs are not eligible for membership with the CDAAC.

Audiology assistants (support personnel in audiology) must be at least 18 years old, have a high school diploma or equivalent (AAA, 2018a), demonstrate knowledge and skills to be able to carry out assigned tasks, and provide written notification of the name of the ASHA-certified audiologists under whom he or she works (ASHA, 2018g). Teleaudiology clinical assistants (TCTs) may be licensed vocational nurses or nurses who have earned a bachelor's degree (ASHA, 2018c). An audiology aide must complete a training program established by the supervising audiologist (ASHA, 2018b).

STATE REGULATION OF SPEECH-LANGUAGE PATHOLOGY ASSISTANTS

Regulations, policies, education, and training of support personnel vary widely among states (Aguilar & Ostergren, 2016; Ostergren & Aguilar, 2015). It is the responsibility of the supervisor (SOR) to obtain accurate information from the state association, board of education, or licensing board where the supervisee (SEE) is employed, and to be aware of the licensure, certification, and registration requirements of the support personnel with whom he or she works (Aguilar and Ostergren, 2016). Due to the significant variability across the United States, SLPAs are also encouraged to research the state regulations for employment to determine the necessary process for achieving licensure or certification, if available. ASHAs state advocacy team has provided information and resources for professionals interested in learning about state-specific regulations (ASHA, 2018f).

Many states require regulation with the state licensing board to practice in the role of support personnel. In 2017, ASHA provided a summary of school support personnel and reported that 8 states license support personnel (Arizona, Illinois, Kentucky, Louisiana, Maryland, Tennessee, Utah and Wisconsin), 8 states register support personnel (Alaska, Arkansas, California, Georgia [registration for speech-language pathology aides is not required if fees are not charged for service], Indiana, Kansas, Maine and North Carolina), and 8 states certify support personnel (Alabama, Florida, Georgia, Louisiana, Missouri, Nebraska, Oklahoma and Oregon; ASHA, 2017a). Outside of the school setting, 13 states license support personnel (Arizona, Colorado, Idaho, Illinois, Louisiana, Maryland, Massachusetts, New Mexico, Ohio, Oklahoma, South Carolina, South Dakota and Texas), 18 states register support personnel (Alabama, Alaska, Arkansas, California, Delaware [audiology aides only], Indiana, Kansas, Maine, Massachusetts, Mississippi, Missouri, Montana, Nebraska, North Carolina, Pennsylvania [SLPA or audiology assistant], Rhode Island, Tennessee and West Virginia), and 4 states certify support personnel (Florida, New Hampshire, North Carolina [audiometric technicians only], Oregon; ASHA, 2017b). There is also variability among states regarding the nature of the fieldwork experience. While some states require fieldwork that is part of an SLPA training program, other states allow on-the-job-training or do not specify the nature of the clinical training required.

ROLES AND RESPONSIBILITIES OF SPEECH-LANGUAGE PATHOLOGY ASSISTANTS, AIDES, AND TECHNICIANS

There are several roles and responsibilities one must adhere to when moving into a support personnel position. In this section, the roles and responsibilities for several support personnel positions will be described. After the roles and responsibilities of support personnel are discussed, the requirements for SORs of support personnel will be presented.

According to ASHA's SLPA Scope of Practice (ASHA, 2013a), SLPAs must:

- Present oneself as an SLPA to clients, families, and colleagues, in verbal and written form, and with a title on name badges
- Comply with the Health Insurance Portability and Accountability Act (HIPAA) and Family Educational Rights and Privacy Act (FERPA) regulations
- Only work in an employment setting where regular and systematic direct and indirect supervision are provided by an ASHA-certified or licensed speech-language pathologist
- Adhere to responsibilities for SLPAs as specified in ASHA's SLPA Scope of Practice and do not perform any tasks or activities that are the sole responsibility of the speech-language pathologist
- Only perform tasks delegated or assigned by the supervising speech-language pathologist
- Adhere to state licensure laws and rules applicable to support personnel within the field of speech-language pathology including those related to practice, licensure, and registration
- Exhibit ethical behavior within the scope of practice for an SLPA. Ethical behavior guidelines are described in ASHA's Code of Ethics document (ASHA, 2016b)
- Actively collaborate with the pathologist throughout the process of supervision
- Secure liability insurance, as needed
- Obtain hours to support continuing education and professional development

Following completion of the SLPA fieldwork and clinical hours, SLPAs can perform the following tasks and activities that are focused in three main areas including: 1) service delivery, 2) administrative support, and 3) prevention and advocacy (ASHA, 2013a, pp. 4-5). In the area of service delivery, SLPAs may:

- Assist the speech-language pathologist with speech, language, and hearing screenings without interpreting screening assessment data
- Assist the speech-language pathologist during assessment sessions without administering and/or interpreting assessments
- Document client performance by tallying data, preparing charts and/or records and reporting information to the supervising speech-language pathologist
- Assist the speech-language pathologist with bilingual translation during screening and assessment activities (without interpretation)
- Follow documented treatment plans developed by the speech-language pathologist without modifying them
- Provide guidance and treatment via telepractice to clients as deemed appropriate by the speech-language pathologist
- Program and provide instruction on the use of augmentative and alternative communication devices
- Demonstrate and share information with patients, families, and staff regarding feeding strategies as developed by and under the direction of the supervising speech-language pathologist

In the area of administrative support, SLPAs may:

- Assist with clerical duties such as scheduling and materials preparation
- Assist in maintaining equipment by performing checks and/or ordering supplies
- Assist with departmental operations such as scheduling and record keeping

In the area of prevention and advocacy, SLPAs may:

- Provide information regarding the prevention of communication disorders to at-risk individuals or groups, and promote the need for early identification and early intervention within the community
- Provide advocacy through education and training to promote and facilitate community members' full participation in communication
- Provide information to emergency personnel for individuals who have communication and/or swallowing disorders
- Advocate at the local, state, and national levels for public policies connected to funding for services and research
- Support the supervising speech-language pathologist in presentations and programs for research, education, public relations, and marketing
- Actively participate in professional organizations

Similarly, there are a number of tasks and activities that are outside the scope of practice for an SLPA. It is the responsibility of the SEE and the SOR to ensure that the SLPA does not engage in activities which are not permitted. According to ASHA (2013a), SLPAs *may not*:

- Present him or herself as a speech-language pathologist
- Conduct standardized or non-standardized diagnostic evaluations, formal or informal tests, or swallowing screenings
- Perform procedures requiring a high level of skill
- Tabulate or interpret results of feeding and swallowing evaluations performed by the speech-language pathologist
- Participate in formal meetings or interdisciplinary conferences without a speech-language pathologist
- Provide interpretive information to the student, client, patient, or family, or other individuals, regarding the status or service of the patient
- Write, develop, or modify a client's treatment plan

- Assist with students/clients without following the plan established by the supervising speech-language pathologist or provide services without appropriate supervision
- Sign any formal documentation
- Select clients for service, discharge clients, or make referrals for additional service
- Disclose clinical or confidential information via the oral or written modality to anyone other than the supervising speech-language pathologist unless mandated by law
- Develop or determine swallowing strategies
- Treat medically fragile patients independently
- Design or select augmentative and alternative communication systems

Individuals are encouraged to review information presented in the Speech-Language Pathology Assistant Scope of Practice (ASHA, 2013a).

Roles and Responsibilities of Speech Aides

When compared to SLPAs, SAs are significantly different in terms of the scope of practice and responsibility and the amount of supervision required. SAs can complete work that does not involve direct patient contact and may include activities such as setting up treatment rooms, preparing assessment or treatment materials, or ordering supplies (ASHA, 1996; Longhurst, 1997). SAs may not "independently diagnose, treat, or advise clients of disposition" (ASHA, 1994, p. 24).

Roles and Responsibilities of Audiology Assistants

The AAA (2018a) delineated guidelines for audiology support personnel and those employed for the purpose of conducting infant hearing screenings. Audiology support personnel must be at least 18 years old and have a high school diploma or the equivalent, in addition to the following characteristics:

- Have current immunizations and be free of communicable diseases
- Be able to work independently to complete procedures
- Demonstrate competency in performing specified tasks consistently
- Be willing to adhere to hospital policies, regulations, and procedures
- Communicate with staff reliably and maturely
- Exhibit the ability to meet the physical demands of the screening process
- Be able to remember a precise sequence of instructions for the screening protocol
- Be able to operate the equipment to be able to perform the screening (AAA, 2018a)

Guidelines for audiology support personnel delineated by AAA (2018a) are not intended to replace those regulations established by licensing or state-level regulatory bodies.

Suggested duties for audiology support personnel who perform newborn hearing screening include (AAA, 2018a):

- Reporting to the hospital nursery on time each week
- Selecting and preparing infants for screening based on program policies
- Operating the screening device according to procedures dictated by the manufacturer and training
- Recording data through records or logs, as required, and conveying results to supervising audiologist
- Maintaining client confidentiality
- Interacting appropriately with infants, parents, and caregivers

- Recognizing the occurrence of potential problems and reporting them to appropriate supervisory personnel
- Adhering to infection control procedures by ensuring that screening supplies are cleaned and materials are disposed of appropriately

ROLES AND RESPONSIBILITIES OF SUPERVISORS OF SUPPORT PERSONNEL

In 2012, the ASHA (2013b) Board of Directors appointed an ad hoc committee on supervision. The committee included speech-language pathologists and audiologists who had expertise in clinical education, as well as representatives from the Council of Academic Programs in Communication Sciences and Disorders (CAPCSD). The committee was developed to establish training requirements for individuals who provide supervision for five different types of (emerging) professionals including: 1) students completing on-campus internships in communication sciences and disorders programs, 2) supervisors of off-campus graduate student interns, 3) practitioners who supervise support personnel such as SLPAs, 4) clinicians who supervise clinical fellows, and 5) clinicians who supervise credentialed colleagues who are transitioning to a new area of clinical practice (ASHA, 2013b). The work of this committee also resulted in ASHA's (2013a) SLPA Scope of Practice.

Supervision of SLPAs can take place following adequate preparation by speech-language pathologists. Some states require a minimum number of hours of education for speech-language pathologists supervising support personnel. Currently, it is recommended by ASHA that supervising speech-language pathologists have current ASHA certification and/or a state license, at least 2 years of work experience following completion of the clinical fellow year, and have received at least 10 hours of education in the area of supervision (ASHA, 2013a). After the initial hours, continuing education requirements vary according by state. Continuing education can be obtained in a variety of ways, such as through supervision workshops, attendance at state or national conferences, participation in online webinars, and/or through self-study such as by reading articles or accessing ASHA's (2016c) resources. Information regarding continuing education opportunities for SORs is presented in Appendix 14-2.

Speech-language pathologists are highly trained professionals who possess a graduate degree in speech-language pathology or communication sciences and disorders. However, to provide supervision, SORs require knowledge and skills in a variety of areas that extend beyond training as a speech-language pathologist. ASHA's Ad Hoc Committee on Supervision (2013b) indicated that speech-language pathologists providing supervision require knowledge regarding how to supervise collaboratively and have an understanding of theories of adult learning and the roles and responsibilities for each member of the support personnel dyad (ASHA, 2013b). As the speech-language pathologist or audiologist is responsible for directing and supervising SEEs, the SOR must have knowledge of ASHA's (2016b) Code of Ethics and also be able to develop a plan for supervision that protects the welfare of clients, patients, and students, maintains a high quality of care, and adheres to rules regarding the documentation of supervision (ASHA, 2017c).

The Ad Hoc Committee on Supervision also indicates there a number of skills required for supervision. SORs must provide information to the SEE about the supervisory process. They must facilitate a trusting and supportive relationship with the SEE, allowing him or her to become aware of his or her personal strengths and needs, and over time, exhibit an ability to collaborate in decision making, as appropriate (ASHA, 2013b). The SOR must demonstrate clear expectations regarding requirements for the SOR–SEE relationship, exhibit excellent interpersonal communication skills, and be able and willing to address differences in communication style (ASHA, 2013b).

Other essential skills include a high level of cultural competence and the ability to make appropriate accommodations for SEEs with disabilities (ASHA, 2013b).

SORs must exhibit a number of behaviors when supervising support personnel (ASHA, 2013a). SORs are required to adhere to applicable licensure laws for the practice of speech-language pathology, ASHA's Code of Ethics, and retain legal and ethical responsibility for the clients served (ASHA, 2013a). Therefore, SORs must provide ample supervision of the SEE, and be able to access technology, as needed, to provide appropriate supervision (ASHA, 2013b). SORs must observe sessions conducted by the SEE, review paperwork and documentation, collect data, and assess the performance of the SEE by providing specific and objective feedback (ASHA, 2013b). The SOR should evaluate the SEE's performance while paying close attention to the presence of patterns of behavior that can be focused areas for improvement (ASHA, 2013b). The SOR can assist the SEE to continue to improve by giving feedback in a way that is motivating, by asking questions, by encouraging self-reflection, and adjusting the nature and style of the supervision to respond to SEEs needs (ASHA, 2013b). It is expected that the SOR will complete evaluations of the SEE to ensure that she or he has met competency for required skills. A number of resources are available to assess competencies for SLPAs employed in medical or educational settings, available through ASHA (e.g., ASHA, 2008).

SORs must develop goals for the SEE that allow him or her to develop high-level critical thinking skills and problem-solving abilities, while understanding the majority of clinical decision-making resides with the speech-language pathologist. SORs can create a plan for improvement through goal setting and delineating tasks and activities through which the SEE can improve in their skill set. Regular meetings can take place to allow both the SOR and SEE to reflect, and subsequently discuss clinical practice and collaboration to further develop the working relationship.

SORs must also identify continuing education opportunities that are appropriate for the SEEs given their area of work and job requirements (ASHA, 2013a). Of the states that require continuation education for support personnel in school settings, the number of hours can range from 8 to 30 every 2 years; most require that SLPAs complete 10 hours of continuing education per year (ASHA, 2017a). The SOR is encouraged to remain up to date on continuing education opportunities and subsequently recommend continuing education opportunities that would be appropriate for, and of benefit to, the SEE and the client populations served.

SORs are responsible for making all case management decisions, and developing, reviewing, and modifying treatment plans for clients served by the SLPA. Adjustments to treatment plans can be made during regular supervisory meetings with the SLPA. Speech-language pathologists and SLPAs are encouraged to develop a plan for how best to communicate changes to treatment plans to ensure comprehension of how a given plan should be executed.

To continually improve in supervision, SORs must also set personal goals for him or herself. This involves the SOR asking self-reflective questions about what he or she could do to improve in the area of supervision. The SOR is encouraged to obtain continuing education in the area of supervision of support personnel in order to maximize skill level.

The ASHA Ad Hoc Committee on the Scope of Practice in audiology is currently revising the audiology scope of practice document (ASHA, 2018h). Within this scope of practice, audiologists who supervise support personnel should: 1) have skills in service delivery and professional practice needed to supervise support personnel, 2) obtain advanced knowledge in the practice of supervision, and 3) establish collegial and supportive working relationships that provide guidance while promoting growth and increased independence (ASHA, 2018h). ASHA recommends that supervision for TCTs be provided through real time or recorded audio-video technology (ASHA, 2018c).

ETHICAL CONSIDERATIONS FOR SPEECH-LANGUAGE PATHOLOGY ASSISTANTS

In 1952, ASHA formulated the first version of the Code of Ethics in response to the desire to establish, in writing, expectations for clinical and research practices within the profession. The Code of Ethics also provides guidance on what behaviors are valued within the field for members and non-members of ASHA holding the Certificate of Competence or individuals applying for the Certificate of Competence. The most recent update to the Code of Ethics that took place in 2016 provides clear wording for Principles of Ethics in four domains, including (I) responsible conduct with those served through clinical practice or when involved in research, (II) responsibility for professional competence, (III) responsibility to the public, and (IV) responsibility to professional relationships (ASHA, 2016b). Supervisors of support personnel should ensure that they have knowledge of the current Code of Ethics and have shared the document with those supervised.

SLPAs working under the license of the speech-language pathologist and audiologist should also be knowledgeable of ASHA's Code of Ethics so they can be sure that they are practicing within the guidelines and are not exhibiting any behaviors that would violate the Code of Ethics and subsequently place the SORs license, certification, or credential, at risk. Supervising practitioners are responsible for ensuring that the support personnel supervised are performing duties and providing services in a way that adheres to the Code of Ethics. Additionally, it is important for the SOR to remember that work should only be delegated to support personnel if the quality of care and level of professionalism will not be compromised (ASHA, 2013a).

For those individuals providing bilingual interpreting or translating services, it is important for support personnel to be aware of skills and competencies needed to do so competently. Within the practice portal, ASHA has several documents with information in these areas, including *Bilingual Service Delivery* (ASHA, 2018i), *Collaborating With Interpreters* (ASHA, 2018j), and *Cultural Competence* (ASHA, 2018k). The California Speech-Language Hearing Association (CSHA; 2017) has also published a position paper. Individuals working with culturally or linguistically diverse populations should become knowledgeable of information contained in these resources.

SUPERVISION STANDARDS

SORs must provide adequate supervision for support personnel to ensure that services are of high quality. Supervision includes direct and indirect supervision. Direct supervision is defined by ASHA as the speech-language pathologist providing observation and guidance during assigned activities while they are on site and in view of support personnel (ASHA, 1996, 2013a). The frequency/intensity of the supervision is dependent on the needs of the SEE (Havens, 2013) and is inversely related to the amount of training and experience of the support personnel. Indirect supervision is defined as the speech-language pathologist providing observation through electronic means (ASHA, 2013a). For example, the SEE can be evaluated through the review of audio-recorded or video-recorded sessions, or interactive media technology (ASHA, 1996).

Requirements for Supervision of Speech-Language Pathology Assistants

Currently, ASHA recommends that during the first 90 days of employment, an SLPA must be supervised for 30% of the week, where 20% is direct supervision and 10% is indirect supervision. Further, the amount of direct supervision should be at least 20% of the SLPA actual client contact time. ASHA recommends that direct supervision be scheduled in advance and structured so that the SOR is able to see clients once every 2 weeks. Supervision time should be flexible so that the supervising speech-language pathologist can see all clients on the caseload and that direct supervision is provided to each client once every 60 calendar days (ASHA, 2018a). Direct supervision hours should be documented using a log form such as the one available through ASHA (2008). Each week, the data for each client should be reviewed by the supervising speech-language pathologist.

Following the initial 90-day period, the SLPA must be directly supervised for at least 1 hour per week, with as much indirect supervision as is necessary, based on the skill set of the SEE. The amount of supervision should be inversely proportional to the amount of training and/or experience, with judgment by the speech-language pathologist for situations in which additional supervision is required. For example, new or challenging cases may require additional supervision (Ostergren & Aguilar, 2015). Individuals who are medically fragile require 100% direct supervision (ASHA, 2013a). Essentially, the supervising speech-language pathologist must determine that the individual being supervised has met appropriate competencies and has acquired the skill set to be able to provide appropriate care.

Of the states that provide guidance, most indicate that two full-time SLPAs can be supervised by one speech-language pathologist. Occasionally, a state restricts practice to one SLPA per speech-language pathologist (e.g., Minnesota; ASHA, 2017b), while a couple of states allow up to four in the case of non-school settings (e.g., Oregon and Texas; ASHA, 2017b). Other states indicate that a total of three full-time support staff can be supervised, with a maximum of two SLPAs out of that number (e.g., California). Supervisors are encouraged to contact their state agencies to determine the rules and regulations for the number of support personnel permitted to be supervised at one time. In general, one speech-language pathologist supervises one SLPA, and while multiple speech-language pathologists can supervise one SLPA, it is recommended that one speech-language pathologist is identified as the primary SOR and that all SORs communicate with each other to provide ample supervision (ASHA, 1996).

Requirements for Supervision for Aides

Aides have less training than SLPAs, and as such, require more supervision when interacting with clients/patients. For example, when providing direct service, registered aides in California require 100% direct supervision, unless another plan for supervision has been approved by the Speech-Language Pathology & Audiology & Hearing Aid Dispensers Board (DCA, 2014). For duties that do not require direct client contact, the aide can be indirectly supervised. Supervisors of aides should to reach out to appropriate state organizations to ensure compliance with supervision standards for the region where the aide is practicing.

QUANTITY OF SUPERVISION

The primary role of the speech-language pathologist is to provide high-quality care for clients, patients, students, and their families. This role is equally as important when support personnel are providing intervention via a protocol designed by the supervising speech-language pathologist. When support personnel provide direct services to clients, the speech-language pathologist must ensure that the quantity and type of supervision provided is appropriate for each and every client interaction.

Hagler and McFarlane (1994) developed a strategy for determining which tasks performed by support personnel involving direct client contact require high levels of supervision and which tasks require less supervision. Variables in their strategy depend on the required task and take into consideration 1) the degree of client contact, 2) the complexity of the specific client within the contact, and 3) the degree of interpersonal interaction required by the client contact. Based on these variables, Hagler and McFarlane (1997) suggest four task levels that consider the amount

		TABLE 14-1	

GUIDELINES FOR ASSISTANT SUPERVISION BY TASK BY HAGLER AND McFARLANE (1994)

	NATURE OF TASK	AMOUNT OF SUPERVISION	TYPE OF SUPERVISION
A	• Extensive contact • Highly complex or technical or requires a high level of interpersonal interaction	20% to 80%	Direct only
B	• Extensive contact • Less complex and less technical and requires minimal interpersonal interaction	20% to 60%	Minimum of 5% direct or a combination of direct and indirect
C	• Without extensive contact • Highly complex and technical and requires high levels of interpersonal interaction	10% to 40%	Minimum of 5% direct or a combination of direct and indirect
D	• Without extensive contact • Minimally complex and minimally technical and requires minimal interpersonal interaction	0% to 20%	Indirect only or a combination of direct and indirect

Adapted from Hagler, P., & McFarlane, L. (1997). Collaborative service delivery by assistants and professionals (Rev.). Edmonton, Alberta, Canada: Albert Rehabilitation Coordinating Council.

and nature of the supervision required, referred to as Guidelines for Assistant Supervision by Task (Table 14-1). They state that tasks requiring extensive patient contact that are complex and technical require substantially more supervision than tasks without extensive patient contact or that are minimally complex or technical.

McCrea & Brasseur (2003) noted that the levels of supervision suggested by Hagler and McFarlane (1994) are not the same as those delineated by ASHA (1996) with regards to direct and indirect supervision percentages. They suggested that because of the range in the ratio of assigned assistants in various settings (1:1 to 1:4) and the flexibility implied by Hagler and McFarlane's task analysis to determine the quantity and type of supervision, it is important for SORs to provide education to those responsible for making personnel assignments about the need for balance in the assignment of support personnel to supervisors (McCrea & Brasseur, 2003). For example, an SOR who employs support personnel to aid with clerical work related to service delivery could likely supervise three SLPAs appropriately. However, an SOR who employs an SLPA to work directly with clients in complex and/or interpersonally challenging situations should probably not assume responsibility for three or four SLPAs because of the requirements of his or her employment position in addition to minimum supervision requirements for direct client contact for multiple support personnel. Each SOR will need to decide on the appropriate supervision parameters upon considering the caseload dynamics and the competency of the SLPA.

Ostergren and Aguilar (2015) administered a survey to 64 speech-language pathologists who supervised support personnel and asked participants about how they typically determine the level of supervision for SLPAs. Participants indicated they determined appropriate supervision based on the skill level of the SLPA (51.6%), the complexity of the population served (20.8%), the laws and regulations (10.9%), and the tasks assigned (5.4%). Based upon these survey responses, Ostergren and Aguilar concluded that decisions regarding supervision for SLPAs aligned with ASHA's recommendations for supervision.

PREPARING FOR SUPERVISION

A number of factors should be considered once a professional decides to work with support personnel. Due to the supervision required as part of this close working relationship, one of the first objectives is to ensure that the supervising speech-language pathologist is involved in the hiring and/or selection of the SLPA (McCrea & Brasseur, 2003). Employers are encouraged to understand the scope of practice for these positions. SORs can work with administrative staff to develop a position description so that individuals with the appropriate credentials are aware of the available jobs. The position should be posted in a way that clearly delineates the category of support personnel sought, the role and responsibilities of the position, and the anticipated salary, keeping in mind that SLPAs have greater knowledge and skill than other support positions and therefore should be compensated at a higher rate than support personnel with less knowledge and expertise. Example SLPA position descriptions are available through resources such as *Practical Tools and Forms for Supervising Speech-Language Pathology Assistants* (ASHA, 2008). To ensure that support personnel adhere to the Code of Ethics, employers should seek to hire SLPAs from ASHA accredited/ approved programs that offer SLPA training (McCrea & Brasseur, 2003). Once available, employers should endeavor to hire SLPAs who are registered through ASHA's assistant certification program (Paul-Brown & Goldberg, 2001). Because of the additional training required to become an SLPA, individuals who have an SLPA license or certificate should be hired as an SLPA rather than an SA. Finally, it is important to remember that just because the scope of practice for SLPA delineates roles and responsibilities that an SLPA can perform, it does not mean that it is appropriate for the SLPA to perform all tasks in all settings. Some settings may require more or less supervision, and it is important for the SOR to collaborate with workplace administrators to make decisions on the position roles and responsibilities in advance of the hire.

As many factors beyond qualifications can impact a working relationship, supervising speech-language pathologists should ensure, at minimum, that they review the applicant's materials and have had the opportunity to participate in the interview and/or meet with the candidate (McCrea & Brasseur, 2003). Interviewers may wish to ask questions that assess the candidate SLPA's knowledge of the scope of practice, critical thinking and problem-solving abilities, and how he or she may handle various situations that individuals are likely to encounter while working. To ensure fairness in the hiring process, individuals on the hiring committee are encouraged to ask all applicants the same set of questions so that responses can be compared across applicants. Finally, speech-language pathologists should be given the opportunity to provide feedback to the hiring committee regarding his or her preference prior to the selection of the candidate (McCrea & Brasseur, 2003).

Once the candidate is hired and he or she accepts an offer of employment, training on the duties and expectations should commence. SORs can refer to ASHA (2008) for information that could be included as part of a new SLPA orientation. SORs may wish to review aspects of the position including physical work environment, location of different required materials, office/clerical work or safety, and emergency procedures (ASHA, 2008). The SOR should also provide information on the caseload to be served, documentation used, and specific departmental policies (ASHA, 2008). Training provided for a SEE should be documented in writing (Coufal, Steckelberg, & Vasa, 1991). Finally, the SLPA should be provided with information regarding how and when his or her performance will be evaluated.

Once the individual has started working in the position, it is important for the SOR to reserve time that will be dedicated to performing supervisory activities and convey the need for protected time for supervision to the administrative staff. SORs will require time to plan sessions and observe, evaluate, and meet with the SEE (Goldberg et al., 2002).

DUTIES PERFORMED BY SPEECH-LANGUAGE PATHOLOGY ASSISTANTS

SORs are encouraged to read and review current research in supervision of SLPAs to ensure the support personnel's skill set is optimized within a given employment setting. Ostergren and Aguilar (2015) obtained survey data from speech-language pathologists who work with support personnel and determined that while SLPAs frequently provide intervention by following established treatment plans or protocols and regularly document client performance, many never provide bilingual or interpretive services for clients/families whose first language is not English. SLPAs also rarely (or never) engage in prevention or advocacy work for the profession or provide guidance or intervention via telepractice. As bilingual service provision and prevention and advocacy work are SLPA practice domains, these results support the need for SORs and SEEs to consider opportunities for these skill sets to be utilized.

RESOURCES AND CONTINUING EDUCATION FOR SUPERVISORS OF SUPPORT PERSONNEL

Although the use of support personnel has been described in the literature for almost 50 years and there is a great deal of research in the area of supervision (McCrea & Brasseur, 2003), there is relatively little information on the supervision of support personnel. While in graduate school, speech-language pathologists and audiologists spend a great deal of time learning to perform tasks within their scope of practice. Oftentimes, however, there a lack of formal training in supervision of support personnel. University programs are beginning to include didactic and clinical instruction on the topic of supervision.

One way to support graduate training in supervision of support personnel is to match graduate and undergraduate students who have completed coursework in communication sciences and disorders through a mentor program as part of an in-house university clinical practicum. Undergraduate students can act as "assistants," aiding with various aspects of graduate-student-provided intervention such as organization of the session or the collection of data during session activities (Goldberg et al., 2002). Opportunities for graduate student leadership early in students' careers can scaffold later supervision roles, leading to increased preparedness upon entry into the workforce.

Speech-language pathologists who have been practicing in the field for many years are encouraged to seek out continuing education opportunities on the topic of supervision to be aligned with ASHA's guidelines for continuing education in the area of supervision. SORs are referred to Chapter 2 for a review of the supervision literature from related disciplines, a description of supervisory approaches in the field, and information regarding Anderson's Continuum of Supervision. SORs are also referred to Chapter 3 for helpful information. Additionally, speech-language pathologists who are members of ASHA can obtain information through ASHA's Special Interest Group 11, Administration and Supervision. Through this special interest group, members can obtain information on issues related to supervision, ask questions of group members, and learn about short courses on continuing education opportunities. CAPCSD (2018) has online courses in supervision on the topics of effective student-clinical educator relationships and foundations of clinical education. Several courses are also available. For example, Alexandria Technical & Community College offers a 10-hour, 11 module, self-directed online course for speech-language pathologists supervising SLPAs (see www.alextech.edu/customizedtraining.) Several resources for continuing education are also presented in Appendix 14-2.

SUMMARY

Due to the shortage of professionals in the field and an increased need for service providers, creative solutions for service provision are required for the field of communication sciences and disorders. Support personnel, when knowledgeable of their scope of practice and dedicated to continually learning, can assist speech-language pathologists and audiologists to increase the frequency of services while maintaining a high level of care. This chapter provided a description of support personnel, and described roles and responsibilities and state and federal regulations for practice of support personnel and supervisors of support personnel. It is hoped that as a result of this chapter, speech-language pathologists and audiologists who already collaborate with, or are considering working with support personnel, will have increased knowledge and skill to be able to provide a collaborative and productive work environment that best supports the patient's need for improved communication.

REFERENCES

Aguilar, S. M., & Ostergren, J, A. (2016). Finding answers regarding the 2 r's of speech-language pathology assistants (SLPA) supervision: Regulations and recommendations. *Perspectives of the ASHA Special Interest Groups, SIG 11*(Part 2), 86-91.

American Academy of Audiology. (1997). *Position statement and guidelines of the consensus panel on support personnel in audiology*. Retrieved from https://www.audiology.org/publications-resources/document-library/position-statement-guidelines-consensus-panel-support

American Academy of Audiology. (2018a). *Considerations for the use of support personnel for newborn hearing screening, AAA Task Force of Early Identification of Hearing Loss*. Retrieved from https://www.audiology.org/publications-resources/document-library/considerations-use-support-personnel-newborn-hearing

American Academy of Audiology. (2018b). *Audiologist's assistant*. Retrieved from https://www.audiology.org/publications-resources/document-library/audiologists-assistant

American Speech and Hearing Association. (1970). Guidelines on the role, training, and supervision of the communication aide [Report of the Committee on Supportive Personnel]. *Asha, 12*, 78-80.

American Speech-Language-Hearing Association. (1994). ASHA policy regarding support personnel. *Asha, 36* Suppl. 13), 24.

American Speech-Language-Hearing Association. (1996). Guidelines for the training, credentialing, use and supervision of speech-language pathology assistants. *Asha, 38*(Suppl. 16), 21-34.

American Speech-Language-Hearing Association. (2004). *Scope of practice in audiology* [Ad Hoc Committee on Scope of Practice in Audiology]. Retrieved from https://www.asha.org/policy/SP2004-00192/.

American Speech-Language-Hearing Association. (2008). *Practical tools and forms for supervising speech-language pathology assistants*. Rockville, MD: American Speech-Language-Hearing Association.

American Speech-Language-Hearing Association. (2013a). *Speech-Language Pathology Assistant Scope of Practice*. Rockville, MD: American Speech-Language-Hearing Association.

American Speech-Language-Hearing Association. (2013b). *Knowledge, skills and training consideration for individuals serving as supervisors*. Rockville, MD: American Speech-Language-Hearing Association.

American Speech-Language-Hearing Association. (2016a, February). *Model regulations for state licensure of audiologists, speech-language pathologists, and audiology and speech-language pathology assistants*. Retrieved from https://www.asha.org/uploadedFiles/A-Plan-for-Developing-Resources-and-Training-Opportunities-in-Clinical-Supervision.pdf

American Speech-Language-Hearing Association. (2016b). *Code of ethics* [Ethic]. Retrieved from: www.asha.org/policy

American Speech-Language-Hearing Association. (2016c). *A plan for developing resources and training opportunities in clinical supervision* [Ad Hoc Committee on Supervision Training]. Retrieved from http://www.asha.org/upload-edFiles/ASHA/About/governance/Resolutions_and_Motions/2016/Report-Ad-Hoc-Committee-on-Supervision-Training.pdf

American Speech-Language-Hearing Association. (2017a). *Support personnel requirements in school settings.* Retrieved from https://www.asha.org/uploadedFiles/Support-Personnel-Requirements-School-Settings.pdf

American Speech-Language-Hearing Association. (2017b). *Support personnel excluding school settings.* Retrieved from http://www.asha.org/uploadedFiles/Support-Personnel-Excluding-School-Settings.pdf

American Speech-Language-Hearing Association. (2017c). *Issues in ethics: Speech-language pathology assistants.* Retrieved from https://www.asha.org/Practice/ethics/Speech-Language-Pathology-Assistants/

American Speech-Language-Hearing Association. (2018a). *Frequently asked questions: Speech-language pathology assistants (SLPAs).* Retrieved from https://www.asha.org/associates/SLPA-FAQs/#a2

American Speech-Language-Hearing Association. (2018b). *California support personnel requirements.* Retrieved from https://www.asha.org/advocacy/state/info/ca/california-support-personnel-requirements/

American Speech-Language-Hearing Association. (2018c). *Teleaudiology clinical technician.* Retrieved from https://www.asha.org/Practice-Portal/Professional-Issues/Audiology-Assistants/Teleaudiology-Clinical-Assistants/

American Speech-Language-Hearing Association. (2018d). *ASHA's associate affiliation category.* Retrieved from https://www.asha.org/Members/Associate-Affiliation/

American Speech-Language-Hearing Association. (2018e). *Assistants certification program.* Retrieved from https://www.asha.org/associates/assistants-certification-program/

American Speech-Language-Hearing Association. (2018f). *ASHA state-by-state.* Retrieved from https://www.asha.org/Advocacy/state/default/

American Speech-Language-Hearing Association. (2018g). *Audiology assistants.* Retrieved from https://www.asha.org/Practice-Portal/Professional-Issues/Audiology-Assistants/

American Speech-Language-Hearing Association. (2018h). *Scope of practice in audiology* [Scope of practice]. Retrieved from www.asha.org/policy.

American Speech-Language-Hearing Association. (2018i). *Bilingual service delivery.* Retrieved from https://www.asha.org/Practice-Portal/Professional-Issues/Bilingual-Service-Delivery/

American Speech-Language-Hearing Association (2018j). *Collaborating with interpreters.* Retrieved from https://www.asha.org/Practice-Portal/Professional-Issues/Collaborating-With-Interpreters/

American Speech-Language-Hearing Association. (2018k). *Cultural competence.* Retrieved from https://www.asha.org/Practice-Portal/Professional-Issues/Cultural-Competence/

Appler, K. (2002). Assistance on assistants: ASHA's registration program for speech-language pathology assistants. *SIG 11 Perspectives on Administration and Supervision, 12,* 12. doi:10.1044/aas12.3.12.

Arizona Speech-Language-Hearing Association. (2011). *Navigating the maze of speech therapy licensure in Arizona.* Retrieved from https://www.arsha.org/documents/AZ_SLP_Licensure_Maze.pdf

Bach, S., Kessler, I., & Heron, P. (2007). The consequences of assistant roles in the public services: Degradation or empowerment? *Human Relations, 60*(9), 1267-1292.

Boyle, J. M., McCartney, E., O'Hare, A., & Forbes, J. (2009). Direct versus indirect and individual versus group modes of language therapy for children with primary language impairment: Principal outcomes from a randomized controlled trial and economic evaluation. *International Journal of Language & Communication Disorders, 44*(6), 826-846.

California Speech-Language-Hearing Association. (2017, September). *Collaborating with interpreters and translators* [Position paper, CSHA Task Force on Collaborating with Interpreters]. 1-33. Retrieved at: https://www.csha.org/Member-Center/Position-Papers

Communicative Disorders Assistant Programs. (2018). *CDAAC position statement.* Retrieved from https://cdaac.ca/about/education/

Coufal, K. L., Steckelberg, A. L., & Vasa, S. F. (1991). Current trends in the training and utilization of paraprofessionals in speech and language programs: A report on an eleven-state survey. *Language, Speech, and Hearing Services in Schools, 22,* 51-59.

Council of Academic Programs in Communication Sciences and Disorders. (2018). *CAPCSD eLearning courses.* Retrieved from http://www.capcsd.org/clinical-education-courses/

De Bortoli, T., Arthur-Kelly, M., Foreman, P., Balandin, S., & Mathisen, B. (2011). Complex contextual influences on the communicative interactions of students with multiple and severe disabilities, *International Journal of Speech-Language Pathology, 13*(5), 422-435.

Department of Consumer Affairs. (2014). *Title 16 Division 13.4. Article 5. Speech-language pathology & audiology aides.* Retrieved from http://www.speechandhearing.ca.gov/forms_pubs/interested_parties.pdf

Edgar, D. L., and Rosa-Lugo, L. I. (2007). The critical shortage of speech-language pathologists in the public school setting: Features of the work environment that affect recruitment and retention, *Language, Speech, and Hearing Services in Schools, 38,* 31-46.

Goldberg, L. R., Williams, P. S., & Paul-Brown, D. (2002). Leading the change effort: I. real and perceived challenges in working with speech-language pathology assistants. *Communication Disorder Quarterly, 23*(4), 193-201.

Hagler, P., & McFarlane, L. (1994). *Supervision of support personnel in audiology and speech-language pathology* [Short course:].American Speech-Language-Hearing Association Convention, New Orleans, LA.

Hagler, P., & McFarlane, L. (1997). *Collaborative service delivery by assistants and professionals (Rev.).* Edmonton, Alberta, Canada: Albert Rehabilitation Coordinating Council.

Havens, L. (2013). Bottom line: Who can bill medicaid for services in schools? *The ASHA Leader, 18,* 24-25. doi:10.1044/leader.BML.18082013.25. Retrieved from https://leader.pubs.asha.org/article.aspx?articleid=1785879

Lin, I., & Goodale, B. (2005). Improving supervision of therapy assistants in Western Australia. *Rural and Remote Health,* 6(1), 479. Retrieved from https://www.rrh.org.au/journal/article/479

Longhurst, T. M. (1997) Idaho's three-tiered system for speech-language paratherapist training and utilization, *Journal of Children's Communication Development, 18*(1), 57-64.

McCartney, E., Boyle, J., Bannatyne, S., Jessiman, E., Campbell, C., Kelsey, C.,…O'Hare, A. on behalf of the trial collaboration. (2005). "Thinking for two": A case study of speech and language therapists working through assistants. *International Journal of Language & Communication Disorders, 40*(2), 221-235.

McCrea, E. S., & Brasseur, J. A. (2003). *The supervisory process in speech-language pathology and audiology.* Boston, MA: Allyn & Bacon.

McNeilly, L. (2018). Why we need to practice at the top of the license. *The ASHA Leader, 23,* 10-11. Retrieved from https://leader.pubs.asha.org/article.aspx?articleid=2671812

Millican, A. K. (2015, March 24) *An SLPA eases a school SLP's load. Leader Live.* Retrieved from https://blog.asha.org/2015/03/19/the-help-of-an-slpa/

Moore, S. M., & Pearson, L. (2003). *Competencies and strategies for speech-language pathology assistants.* Clifton Park, NY: Thomson Delmar Learning.

Myotte, T., Hutchins, T. L., Cannizzaro, M. S., & Belin, G. (2011). Understanding why speech-language pathologists rarely pursue a PhD in communication sciences and disorders, *Communication Disorders Quarterly, 33*(1), 42-54.

O'Brien, R., Byrne, N., Mitchell, R., Ferguson, A. (2013). Rural speech-language pathologists' perceptions of working with allied health assistants, *International Journal of Speech-Language Pathology, 15*(6), 613-622.

O'Brien, R., Mitchell, R., & Byrne, N. (2017). Paradoxical perceptions towards the introduction of assistants in speech-language pathology and potential impact on consumers. *Scandinavian Journal of Caring Sciences, 32*(1), 1-11. doi:10.1111/scs.12437

Ostergren, J., & Aguilar, S. (2015). Speech-language pathology assistant supervisor survey. *Contemporary Issues in Communication Sciences and Disorders, 42,* 226-245.

Paul-Brown, D., & Goldberg, L. R. (2001). Current policies and new directions for speech-language pathology assistants. *Language, Speech, and Hearing Services in Schools, 32,* 4-17.

Peters-Johnson, C. (1998). Action: School services. *Language, Speech, and Hearing Services in Schools, 29,* 120-126.

Polovoy, C. (2011). California SLP-SLPA team forge successful partnership. *The ASHA Leader, 16.* Retrieved from https://leader.pubs.asha.org/article.aspx?articleid=2279131

Rowden-Racette, K. (2011). Dynamic duo forges smooth relationship. *The ASHA Leader, 16*(8), S3. Retrieved from https://leader.pubs.asha.org/doi/10.1044/leader.SOA1.16082011.np Retrieved from https://leader.pubs.asha.org/article.aspx?articleid=2279130

Scalero, A. M., & Eskenazi, C. (1976). The use of supportive personnel in a public school speech and language program. *Language, Speech, and Hearing Services in Schools, 7,* 150-158.

Speech-Language and Audiology Canada. (2018). *Communication health assistant academic programs.* Retrieved from https://www.sac-oac.ca/students/supportive-personnel-academic-programs

Steele, C. M., Barton, D., Meissner Fishbein, B., Meltzer, A., Pennock, T., Soucie, M., & Wagner, S. (1996). *Journal of Speech-Language Pathology and Audiology, 20*(4), 256-261.

Teas, B. (1991). *A countrywide program for expanding speech-language services in the elementary schools* (Dissertation/theses). Nova University, Fort Lauderdale, FL.

U.S. Bureau of Labor Statistics. (2018). *Occupational outlook handbook.* Retrieved from https://www.bls.gov/ooh/healthcare/speech-language-pathologists.htm

Wheat, K. (2018). Supervising for success: Working with an assistant can help ease—not add to—your responsibilities, *The ASHA Leader, 23,* 36-38. Retrieved from https://leader.pubs.asha.org/article.aspx?articleid=2671839

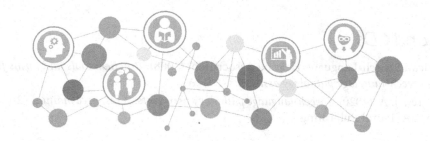

APPENDIX 14-1
RESOURCES FOR CONTINUING EDUCATION FOR SUPPORT PERSONNEL

Electronic Resources to Assist in Training

1. Master Clinician Network. Available at masterclinician.org
2. SimuCase. Available at www.Simucase.com
3. Speech Pathology. Available at www.speechpathology.com

Resources for Speech-Language Pathology Assistants

1. American Speech-Language-Hearing Association. (2013). *Practical tools and forms for supervising speech-language pathology assistants.* ASHA.
2. Kraemer, R., & Bryla, J. (2018). *Clinical workbook for speech-language pathology assistants.* San Diego, CA: Plural Publishing.
3. Ostergren, J. A. (2020). *Speech-language pathology assistants: A resource manual.* (2nd ed.). San Diego, CA: Plural Publishing.

APPENDIX 14-2
RESOURCES FOR CONTINUING EDUCATION FOR SUPERVISORS OF SUPPORT PERSONNEL

Electronic Resources

1. Alexandria Technical and Community College SLP/SLPA Supervisory 10-hour course. Retrieved from https://www.alextech.edu
2. Council of Academic Programs in Communication Sciences and Disorders (CAPCSD) Online Learning. Retrieved from http://elearning.capcsd.org
3. Supervision CEU Courses for speech-language pathologists. Retrieved from https://www.speechpathology.com/slp-ceus/supervision/

Books and CDs

1. American Speech-Language-Hearing Association. (2008). *Practical tools and forms for supervising speech-language pathology assistants.* ASHA.
2. Ostergren, J. A. (2020). *Speech-language pathology assistants: A resource manual.* (2nd ed.). San Diego, CA: Plural Publishing.

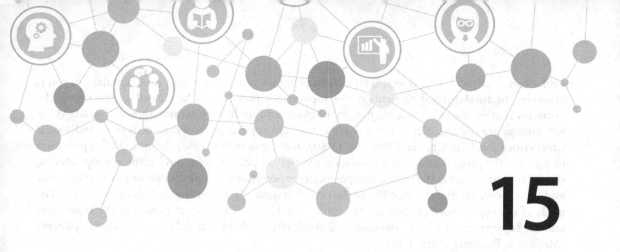

Supervision of Professionals in Transition

Mary L. Casper, MA, CCC-SLP, F-ASHA, FNAP

Speech-language pathologists and audiologists have many work settings from which to choose. Typical employment settings for audiologists include physician practices, private practices, university clinics, public school settings, hearing aid and cochlear implant manufacturers, military settings, and industrial sites. Similarly, speech-language pathologists have a variety of work settings to consider: K-12 public and private schools, early childhood development centers, adult and pediatric acute and post-acute health care settings, long-term care, skilled nursing facilities, inpatient rehabilitation facilities, physician practices, and private practices. The U.S. Department of Labor, Bureau of Labor Statistics (n.d.) indicated that, in 2016, most audiologists worked in health care facilities while about two out of five speech-language pathologists worked in schools.

A website, School SLP 101 (n.d.), states "one of the best things about being an SLP [speech-language pathologist] is the flexibility to work in a variety of environments. You can choose from clinic, SNF [skilled nursing facility], hospital, early intervention or school. If you're switching from a school-based SL job from another position, you'll be faced with IEPs [individualized education programs], Common Core, teacher collaboration, group therapy and scheduling in ways that you've never experienced." This website also includes a series of video modules in support of transition to a school-based speech-language pathology position.

Professionals who serve those with communication disorders may, over the course of their careers, find reason to leave their profession for a brief or extended period of time for reasons including parental leave, burnout, layoff, or relocation. They may also change practice settings because of a new area of clinical interest, potential of higher wages, or opportunity for promotion. Changes in practice setting or clinical population may take place immediately, seamlessly moving from one position to another, or occur over a period of time. Whenever and however they occur, changes of this nature have the potential to create challenges for the supervisory process.

McCrea, E. S., & Brasseur, J. A. *The Clinical Education and Supervisory Process in Speech-Language Pathology and Audiology* (pp 401–409). © 2020 Taylor & Francis Group.

Professional, clinical, and operational demands across practice settings and populations vary; however, the fundamental elements of the supervisory process can be viewed as remaining the same no matter where speech-language pathology and audiology services are delivered. What will change are the specifics of the process as they are applied to meet the needs of an individual supervisory dyad. McCrea and Brasseur (2003) used Anderson's (1988) definition of supervision to describe the process as one that consists of a variety of patterns of behavior, the appropriateness of which depends upon the needs, competencies, expectations and philosophies of the supervisor and the supervisee, and the specifics of the situation (task, client, setting and other variables). The goals of the supervisory process are the professional growth and development of the supervisee and the supervisor, which it is assumed, will result ultimately in optimal service to clients/patients (McCrea & Brasseur, 2003, p. 12).

CLINICIANS IN TRANSITION

To help examine some of the supervisory process considerations for those in professional transition, two examples of clinicians and their supervisors will be provided. They will be used to illustrate relevant concepts regarding professionals in transition throughout the remainder of this chapter.

Hope completed a master's degree in speech-language pathology and worked as a speech-language pathologist in a school setting for 4 years before taking time off to be a full-time mother to three young children. Over the next 5 years, Hope let her Certificate of Clinical Competence (CCC) lapse due to financial considerations within a young family. Her family moved to a new state when her youngest child was starting kindergarten and she investigated the necessary steps she would need to complete in order to resume her profession. First, she learned that she had only a short time frame to reinstate her CCC through continuing education within her maintenance interval and satisfy her lapsed fees, or she would be subject to new educational standards when seeking to reinstate her certificate. Hope considered options for new employment and determined that her best path would be pro re nata work in a skilled nursing facility. Since this was not her previous area of practice, she first sought continuing education courses in dysphagia, dementia, and reimbursement. Second, she discovered that the state license she carried with her previous position was specific to schools and did not translate to the license she needed to work in a health care setting. She contacted the state board in her new location to learn the necessary elements of and process for obtaining the license she would need to practice. By the time Hope sought employment, she had reinstated her CCC, obtained her license, and strengthened her knowledge base in the adult population she was going to serve.

Jessica is an audiologist who, like Hope, is transitioning from her previous employment in a school setting to practice in a major medical setting. Anita is the supervising audiologist in the new setting and responsible not only for the day-to-day management of the audiology services but all of the administrative, financial, and personnel management activities important to the success of the audiology practice. In successfully supervising Jessica, Anita will need to consider her own current professional responsibilities as well as develop a plan to accommodate Jessica's specific professional needs as she transitions from a school-based setting to the medical setting, (e.g., policy and procedures, electronic health record system). Anita will also need to thoughtfully consider continuing education opportunities to support Jessica in her new setting.

The American Speech-Language-Hearing Association (ASHA; 2013) Ad Hoc Committee on Supervision (AHCS) identified the knowledge and skills needed by supervisors to support the transition of professionals in new work settings:

> The supervisor will explore existing skills and knowledge, including transferable skills; identify the need for continuing education and training and develop a plan for achieving necessary skills/knowledge; assist in the development of workplace navigation skills;

including becoming part of the team and adhering to policies and procedures of the facility; promote self-reflection to learn new skills and hone existing skills; and provide ongoing collaborative assessment. (p. 12)

The ASHA Ad Hoc Committee on Supervision Training (AHCST) developed a detailed plan (2016a), including topics for supervision training, for the five unique supervision constituencies identified in the 2013 AHSC, one of which was professionals in transition (2016b). The broad categories of training targets identified by the AHCST include: supervisory process and clinical education; relationship development and communication skills, establishment and implementation of goals; analysis and evaluation; and clinical performance decisions. (Specific topics for supervision training relative to professionals in transition are elaborated on further in the full document; see ASHA, 2016b.)

SUPERVISORY PROCESS AND CLINICAL EDUCATION

The supervisor of the professional in transition should understand the supervisory process and the provision of clinical education especially as it is set out in the definition of supervision (Anderson, 1988; McCrea & Brasseur, 2003). The core knowledge and skills of particular relevance to the supervision of professionals in transition are identified by ASHA's (2008a) AHCS and include:

- Preparation for the supervisory experience
- Interpersonal communication and supervisor-supervisee relationship
- Development of supervisee's critical thinking and problem-solving skills
- Development of supervisee's competence in assessment
- Development of supervisee's clinical competence in intervention
- Supervisory conferences and meetings of teaching teams
- Evaluating the growth of the supervisee both as a clinician and as a professional
- Diversity
- Development and maintenance of clinical and supervisory documentation
- Ethical, regulatory, and legal requirements
- Principles of mentoring

ASHA's (2008b) AHCS released a technical report that discussed supervision across settings, which is applicable in many respects to the supervision of professionals in transition:

These supervisors also have an obligation to provide clinical teaching to supervisees at all levels of their career. Clinical education may be managed directly by the supervisor, facilitated as a collaborative activity by the supervisor, or delivered in peer training formats (e.g., through literature review and discussion or continuing education). Methods may vary according to the needs of the clinical population, developmental level of the supervisee, supervisor and supervisee teaching/learning styles and preferences, economics, and practice setting. The objective of professional growth and development for both supervisor and supervisee remains at the core of the supervisory process. (pp. 4-5)

Falender and Shafranske (2007), writing about supervisor training in psychology, described steps to achieve supervisory competence. These same strategies are consistent with the ASHA's (2008) AHCS knowledge and skills and can also inform the practice of supervisors of professionals in transition:

- The supervisor examines his own clinical and supervision expertise and competency.
- The supervisor delineates supervisory expectations, including standards, rules and general practice.

- The supervisor identifies setting specific competencies the trainee must attain for successful completion of the supervised experience.

- The supervisor collaborates with the trainee in developing a supervisory agreement or contract for informed consent, ensuring clear communication in establishing competencies and goals, tasks to achieve them, and logistics.

- The supervisor models and engages the trainee in self-assessment and the development of metacompetence (i.e., self-awarenesss of competencies) from the onset of supervision and throughout (p. 238).

Hudson (2010) described practical considerations for supervisors of clinical fellows, moving their practice from direct supervision to mentorship. The argument may be made that there are parallels between the supervision of clinical fellows and that of professionals in transition. Hudson describes mentorship as a strategic partnership in which "proper consideration is given to the influence held by the mentor" (p. 74). Insight to the supervisory process is essential for those supervisors of professionals in transition, as those supervisees are often farther along in their careers and may believe that supervision is unnecessary. A mentor-mentee relationship may be more desirable and achieved relatively quickly. Tailancich-Klinger and Cooperson (2017) compared practices and beliefs of novice vs. expert clinicians as supervisors. They suggested that the "ideal situation would be for a speech-language pathology student to be supervised by an expert clinician and supervisor because of an expert's amount of supervision and service delivery experience" (p. 8). As with clinical fellows, students are not the same as professionals who are in transition; however, observations about their supervision relative to the experience of the supervisor are informative.

To address the clinical education component for professionals in transition, the supervisor will need to review the supervisee's existing knowledge and skills. An audiologist who stopped working for a period of time may not have kept with advances in technology or current best evidence for practice. A speech-language pathologist moving from school-based practice to a medical setting (or vice versa) may or may not have taken continuing education courses to prepare for the transition or the speech-language pathologist may be anxious about the change in setting and be full of questions. It is important that the supervisor have the necessary knowledge, skills, and strategies to thoughtfully consider whether a training, mentoring, or coaching approach is needed to ensure that the transitioning professional meets performance expectations in the new setting. ASHA's (n.d.) Practice Portal can provide a wealth of resources on a variety of disorder areas as well as professional topics including documentation, service delivery, and evidence-based practice. For example, as Anita is supervising Jessica while she makes the transition from school-based practice to practice in a medical setting, Anita might decide to provide resources to her from the Practice Portal if she determines that Jessica needs more information regarding documentation of service (for examples, see www.asha.org/Practive-Portal/Professinal-Issues/Documentation-of-Audiology-Services/).

Some of a clinician's existing skills and knowledge may serve to enhance her/his performance in a new setting. In her undergraduate honors thesis, Fortson (2014) discussed perceived keys to success in private practice for speech-language pathologists. The survey identified a "variety of factors in both the decision to pursue a private practice and the preparation necessary to become a successful private practitioner. Education, clinical experience, conferences, and personal drive were all subjects of discussion" (p. 19). In addition, Fortson notes, "many felt that their experience in other areas of the field contributed the most to their success in private practice" (p. 15). This study suggested that transition in a clinician's career may actually position them to achieve success in a new setting and that the existing skills possessed by a clinician in transition may be sufficient to meet clients' needs. The supervisor of the professional in transition should not assume that skills are lacking simply because of a long period away from the profession or by practice in a new setting.

Employers and supervisors may need to conduct a gap analysis for the individual in transition, comparing the job description, performance appraisal, business objectives, and future organizational needs with the current capabilities of the individual. When gaps are identified, the supervisor can provide mentoring, coaching, education, and training to the individual to strengthen their skills. Education can be provided to teach theories and concepts, building on already established foundations of knowledge. Training is geared toward implementation of new equipment or improving skills or practical application of a particular treatment technique.

Supervisors will have insight to the needs of the clinical population in their setting and after conducting analysis of the clinician's capabilities as compared to the needs of the patients, the supervisor will need to develop a plan for continuing education and training. In a blog post, Tactus Therapy (n.d.-b) suggested ways to continue one's professional education, including participation in social media, following blogs, reading journals, joining groups, learning online or in person, and teaching. Hope was proactive in this regard. Before seeking employment in a new work setting and with a new population, she had completed a number of continuing education courses that she believed to be relevant, yet Hope's supervisor may find additional areas of need that need to be supported. Hope's supervisor may direct her to the ASHA Practice Portal regarding documentation in the health care setting (for examples, see www.asha.org/Practice-Portal/Professional-Issues/Documenation-in-Health-Care/).

The professional in transition may benefit from completion of continuing education courses in a live or online format. Training on specific skills or systems can also be conducted online or face-to-face. In a busy work setting, microlearning may be an effective training methodology in the plan for the transitioning supervisee. Microlearning is short, focused training with the intent of achieving a specific learning outcome. It may be formal, such as a handout, quick reference guide, or flipbook; or informal, such as a brief discussion or demonstration by the supervisor.

RELATIONSHIP DEVELOPMENT AND COMMUNICATION SKILLS

A supervisor of a clinician in transition needs to assist the clinician to assimilate with her or his colleagues in the department and participate effectively with the interprofessional team. In addition to an orientation that would be conducted for any new staff member, the supervisor should focus on differences in expectations from the clinician's previous position when it comes to aspects of process and performance expectations.

Professional issues may be of heightened importance for a clinician in transition. Employers of speech-language pathologists and audiologists may be reluctant to provide time for professionals to develop and enhance skills requisite to the new position. Employers have varying degrees of company, department, and role-specific orientation time available to new employees. Broadly speaking, the transitioning professional needs to be able to demonstrate clinical competence within the new setting and should use the orientation period to acquire exposure to setting policies, electronic health records, reimbursement, scheduling, and compliance considerations. To be most successful, the transitional supervisee needs to demonstrate adequate skills for planning and prioritizing, flexibility, and building professional and peer relationships, thus, setting the stage for supervisory relationship to flourish.

The supervisor may need to discuss aspects of workplace culture with the transitional supervisee. Attitudes about professional collaboration, professional communication and courtesy, methods of sharing new ideas and mechanisms for achieving systematic change should be topics of interest for the supervisee. For example, in a residential health care setting, the speech-language pathologist may need to access food and liquid in order to conduct a clinical assessment of swallowing. The request for the food and liquid might need to be made in advance or submitted on a certain form. The transitioning clinician's awareness of the demands on dietary staff during the hour before each meal is served will be of value in establishing cordial relationships rather than being perceived as interrupting a routine process during a critical time. If the supervisee has transitioned from a setting where this task or time is not as important, it will be important that the "ground rules" are made clear by the supervisor.

Self-reflection on the part of the supervisee should be supported by the supervisor. In a blog post, Tactus Therapy (n.d.-a) discussed the transition from a school-based setting to a medical setting, highlighting fears and concerns that might be experienced by a transitioning clinician. Professional considerations that might come into play include familiarity with the needs of the client population and current, evidence-based intervention methods. In developing her process of returning to the profession, Hope identified areas of need based on self-reflection and her awareness of some aspects of the clinical population she might serve in a skilled nursing facility. Jessica was encouraged by Anita to analyze her own areas of strength and need in the context of her new setting and to use them as a basis for their dialogue together.

Hudson (2010) described the importance of mentoring and supervision in fostering self-reflection and an examination of "one's own values, tastes, and preferences" (p. 72). Self-awareness on the part of the supervisor helps with establishing a strong relationship with the supervisee or mentee, fostering trust, learning, and setting the stage for the positive pursuit of any difficult conversations should they become necessary.

ESTABLISHMENT AND IMPLEMENTATION OF GOALS

The supervisor and transitioning professional should work together to establish performance goals to support not only the continued development of clinical skills of the supervisee in the new setting but the adjustment of the supervisee to the new organization. Goals may relate to the successful completion of the orientation period (typically 30 to 90 days) during which time the supervisee must complete educational modules regarding organizational systems and processes. Clinical skill goals may include obtaining advanced education on a particular clinical procedure. Supervisors should address opportunities for supervisees to achieve ongoing competence in clinical practice beyond the first 30 to 90 days of employment. Often, goals are an expected component of the performance appraisal but may also occur at more frequent intervals. For professionals in transition, setting goals may not be a linear activity where one goal is achieved and the next one established. The supervisor will need to adjust the approach to goal-setting based on the individual learning style and identified needs of the supervisee.

Upon hire, Jessica spent 2 days with Anita to review relevant policies and procedures, reimbursement and regulatory considerations, technology available for her use, and access to internal resources. During Jessica's first months of employment, Anita observed her completing various audiological procedures and reviewed her documentation for at least one patient per week. Anita subsequently made suggestions about aspects of wording within her notes and reports and about different assessment approaches for her to consider.

In order to meet the needs of a specific transitioning professional, a supervisor may find the need to establish goals to enhance their practice within the supervisory process. Chapter 4 details this process thoroughly; however, the use of scaffolded questions to support critical thinking and problem solving, the provision of feedback, or the use of data to support observation and analysis might all be areas of supervisor performance important to the success of the supervisory relationship and process.

ANALYSIS AND EVALUATION

The supervisory process and relationship should present an opportunity for regular feedback and exchange between the transitioning clinician and the supervisor. As Hope transitioned back into the workforce, even though she identified gaps in her skills and sought continuing education opportunities pertinent to her new desired work setting and clinical population, she needed to work closely with her supervisor to confirm that her performance was meeting expectations. Prior to her actual employment in a medical setting, Hope could not be certain of what her day-to-day work would consist of, so regular checkpoints and open dialogue are key factors to her success. Anita and Jessica, the audiology supervisor and supervisee, will be expected to deliver efficient and effective services despite Jessica's lack of experience in the medical setting. Their regular collaboration regarding Jessica's perception and performance are important to her success and achievement of a positive outcome.

Vinson (2009) suggests that feedback may be objective or evaluative. "Evaluative feedback is the most traditional manner of feedback and is frequently warranted in the early stages of a supervisee's employment. However, in providing evaluative feedback, the supervisor is in a position of judging the appropriateness of the clinician's behavior and performance" (p. 232). Evaluative feedback may also limit self-evaluation and collaboration because of the supervisee's perception of being judged. In contrast, objective feedback "should be the goal as the supervisee progresses" (p. 234). Through the performance appraisal process, supervisors and supervisees can validate agreement of perception about performance and set goals for ongoing competence and identification of additional needs.

CLINICAL AND PERFORMANCE DECISIONS

This area encompasses all of the previously discussed aspects of supervision in support of the transitioning supervisee as the supervisee moves toward proficiency following the move to a new work setting and reentrance into the workforce, most especially those focused on the use of feedback and reflective practice to modify and enhance performance. In addition, ethical decision making pertains to documentation; reimbursement; confidentiality; licensure and certification requirements; local, state and national standards and regulations; and preferred practice patterns (Hudson, 2010).

Documentation must be timely and accurate, reflecting the services delivered and meeting the payer requirements. Documentation should show evidence of clinical decision making and adherence to preferred practice patterns. The supervisor will likely take a role in documentation review as part of her or his job responsibilities and the supervisee should anticipate receiving constructive feedback regarding the content of the notes and reports.

When a clinician returns to the workforce or changes practice settings, documenting the necessary and correct professional qualifications is fundamentally important. Supervisors will be expected to verify the status of certification and licenses necessary to meet the requirements for practice in the state and setting. A publication from the Arizona Speech-Language-Hearing Association (2011) points out:

> Currently, the gold standard for speech and language practitioners in the public schools is a Master's degree in Speech-Language Pathology and the Certificate of Clinical Competence (CCC) awarded by the American Speech-Language-Hearing Association. However, each state has different titles for practitioners and different requirements as to what is required to work in the public schools. As a result, there is confusion regarding the titles of various practitioners and requirements set forth by the Arizona Department of Education (ADF) and the Arizona Department of Health Services (ADHS). These

agencies also differ in the practitioners' titles. For example, the Arizona Department of Education recognizes a Speech-Language Pathologist (SLP) and a Speech-Language Technician (SLT). The Arizona Department of Health issues regular, limited, and temporary licenses depending upon the level of education and credentials one has in speech-language pathology. (p. 2)

This example illustrates the understanding and attention to detail that must be observed when a clinician seeks to make the transition back to work or into a new work setting. Hope experienced this when going through the process of reinstating her CCC and obtaining a license to practice in health care in a new state. Her supervisor needed to be certain that her professional qualifications would allow her to provide services and be reimbursed for her service in a skilled nursing facility.

SUMMARY

The goal of the supervisory process specific to professionals transitioning to a new area of practice or reentering the workforce is to "facilitate the acquisition of knowledge and skills needed" for a successful transition (ASHA, 2013). The achievement of this goal occurs with supervisory insight to the particular needs of the clinician and to the supervisory process itself. Attention to job-specific requirements will allow for assessment of current clinical and professional capabilities and identification of training and educational needs. Structured orientation and on-the-job training may require longer than expected to complete when the professional has been out of the workforce for an extended period. In situations when the clinician previously worked in a different setting, it is imperative that no assumptions are made about adequate licensure and credentials to practice in the new setting. Supervisors must introduce supervisees to organizational culture and expectations of team members, sorting through previous work patterns and myths to align with the needs in the current position.

The example of Hope illustrates the value of self-reflection and reinforces the need for her supervisor to have the ability to collaboratively set goals, give realistic feedback, identify Hope's training needs and modify supervisory style when necessary. Because of Hope's diligence in the process of returning to work, she will likely have a quicker path to proficiency than someone who did not take the same approach. Anita and Jessica's supervisory relationship should provide the needed support for Jessica to acclimate to the medical setting and make the most of her previous experience as an audiologist. Jessica is likely to demonstrate some gaps in her skill set relative to the use of technology and will need to develop insight into the culture and practices in her new setting. Anita can serve as a mentor in their collaborative relationship as Jessica gains experience.

Ultimately, the supervisor of the professional in transition plays a key role in achieving the desired outcome for the transitioning clinician as well as for the individuals being served through the application of needs assessment, coaching, delivering feedback, providing open communication, and encouraging self-reflection.

REFERENCES

American Speech-Language-Hearing Association. (n.d.). *Practice portal: Documentation of audiology services.* Retrieved from: www.asha.org/Practice-Portal/Professional-Issues/Documentation-in-Health-Care/

American Speech-Language-Hearing Association. (2008a). *Knowledge and skills needed by Speech-language pathologists providing clinical supervision* [Final Report of the Ad Hoc Committee on Supervision]. Retrieved from https://www.asha.org/policy/KS2008-00294/

American Speech-Language-Hearing Association. (2008b). *Clinical supervision in speech-language pathology* [Technical report of the Ad Hoc Committee on Supervision]. Retrieved from https://www.asha.org/polilcy/TR2008-00296/

American Speech-Language-Hearing Association. (2013). *Knowledge, skills, and training considerations for individuals serving as supervisors* [Final report of the Ad Hoc Committee on Supervision]. Retrieved from http://www.asha.org/uploadedFiles/Supervisors-Knowledge- Skills-Report.pdf

American Speech-Language-Hearing Association. (2016a). *A plan for developing resources and training opportunities in clinical supervision.* [Final report of the Ad Hoc Committee on Supervision Training]. Retrieved from https://www.asha.org/uploadedFiles/A-Plan-for Developing-Resources-and-Training Opportunities in Clinical Supervision.pdf

American Speech-Language-Hearing Association. (2016b). *A plan for developing resources and training opportunities in clinical supervision.* [Final report of the Ad Hoc Committee on Supervision Training, Appendix A]. Retrieved from http://www.asha.org/uploaded Files/Topics-for-Supervision-Training.pdf

Anderson, J. (1988). *The supervisory process in speech-language pathology and audiology.* Boston, MA: College-Hill.

Arizona Speech-Language-Hearing Association. (2011). *Navigating the maze of speech therapy Licensure in Arizona.* Retrieved from https://www.arsha.org/documents/AZ_SLP_Licensure_Maze.pdf

Falender, C. A., & Shafranske, E. P. (2007). Competence in competency-based supervision practice: Construct and application. *Professional Psychology: Research and Practice, 38*(3), 232-240.

Fortson, M. K. (2014). *Private practice in speech-language pathology and audiology: Experience, Preparation and confidence levels of practicing professionals* (Unpublished undergraduate honors thesis). University of Arkansas, Fayetteville, AR. Retrieved from http://scholarworks.uark.edu/rhrcuht/28

Hudson, M. W. (2010). Supervision to mentoring: Practical considerations. *SIG 11 Perspectives on Administration and Supervision, 20,* 71-75.

McCrea, E. S., & Brasseur, J. A. (2003). *The supervisory process in speech-language pathology and audiology.* Boston, MA: Allyn and Bacon.

School SLP 101. (n.d.). *School SLP 101 enrollment is open.* Retrieved from https://www.thespeechroomnewspd.com/p/school-slp-101

Tactus Therapy. (n.d.-a). *Changing course–transitioning from school to medical speech therapy.* Retrieved from https://tactustherapy.com/transition-to-school-to-medical-slp/

Tactus Therapy. (n.d.-b). *7 Ways to continue your education–a guide for adult-focused SLPs.* Retrieved from https://tactustherapy.com/continuing-education-ceus-adult-slp/

Taliancich-Klinger, C. & Cooperson, S. (2017). Clinical supervision in a medical setting: A Preliminary study about the practices and beliefs of expert and novice clinician supervisors. *Perspectives of the ASHA Special Interest Groups, 2*(SIG 11), 7-16.

U.S. Department of Labor, Bureau of Labor Statistics. (n.d.). Retrieved from: https://www.bls.gov/ooh/healthcare/speech-language-pathologists.htm

Vinson, B.P. (2009). *Workplace skills and professional issues in speech-language pathology.* Englewood Cliffs, NJ: Prentice-Hall.

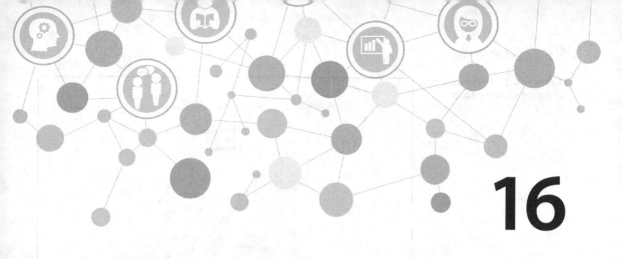

16

Research and the Clinical Education and Supervision Process

Sarah Ginsberg, EdD, CCC-SLP, F-ASHA and
Mark DeRuiter, MBA, PhD, CCC-A/SLP, F-ASHA

In the previous chapters of this book, you have read about various aspects to consider in becoming an effective supervisor and providing supervision to your speech-language pathology and audiology graduate students, clinical fellows, assistants, or other professionals. Much of what we already know about how to be effective supervisors is based on research that has gone before. In our fields, we have an expectation of practicing as clinicians using evidence-based practice (EBP). As is the official policy of the American Speech-Language-Hearing Association (ASHA), EBP means that we rely on input from three critical sources: we must take into consideration the needs of the clients that we work with; we must develop our own knowledge and skills that will allow us to judge the appropriateness of literature-based approaches; and we must rely on "high-quality" EBP literature that has been made available through public dissemination (ASHA, 2005). By relying on EBP in our clinical practice, we ensure that the clients that we work with are receiving the best standard of care which will deliver the best outcome feasible for the client and their circumstances. The Dolloghan (2007) model applied EBP to communication sciences and disorders in a way that is now familiar to many of us. In Dolloghan's E^3BP model, she outlined that our clinical expertise comes from relying on: 1) external evidence, 2) internal evidence, and 3) client preferences.

In the same vein that clinicians endeavor to provide clients with the highest quality of care through the use of EBP, supervisors must provide students with the highest quality education to achieve their best learning. How do we know what methods are effective in helping a student learn how to administer an informal assessment of a child's language or the best method for teaching them how to administer an audiological screening to an older adult? We must rely on evidence-based education (EBE; Ginsberg, Friberg, & Visconti, 2012; Williams & Brown, 2015). The original model of EBE was oriented toward classroom teaching and learning and consisted of 1) literature about teaching and learning (referred to as "scholarship of teaching and learning" [SoTL]; Boyer,

McCrea, E. S., & Brasseur, J. A. *The Clinical Education and Supervisory Process in Speech-Language Pathology and Audiology* (pp 411-426).
© 2020 Taylor & Francis Group.

Figure 16-1. Evidence-based education-clinical education.

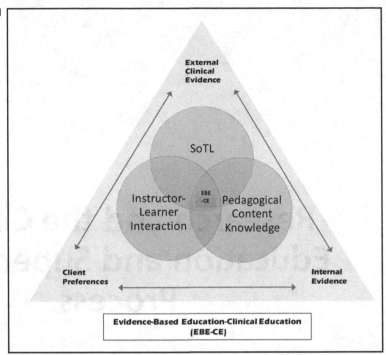

1990; Shulman, 2004); 2) pedagogical content knowledge (Shulman, 1998), which reflects the instructor's content knowledge and how to impart that to students; and 3) interactions between the teacher-learners.

In considering how supervisors adapt both EBP and EBE to their own purposes, we might alter the model to reflect the keen observations of teaching and learning that are made concurrently with observing student clinicians interact with clients while simultaneously moving the clients' development or recovery forward. The effective supervisor must balance the three components of EBP—internal evidence, external clinical evidence, and client preferences—to support the client's therapeutic progress, with the three components of EBE—SoTL, instructor-learner interactions, and pedagogical content knowledge—to support the student's learning progress. Thus, Figure 16-1 depicts a model of evidence-based education-clinical education (EBE-CE) might best reflect the complexity of what the supervisor brings to this process.

This new model best represents the significantly complex process which demands much of the skilled supervisor's attention and expertise to two constituents at the same time. For the purposes of research that will be focused on improving the teaching and learning process for audiology and speech-language pathology students, this model allows us to consider a variety of aspects of the clinical supervision and education process so we can identify characteristics that we would like to learn more about in our research. Research can be used to investigate a variety of interactions that can be observed in the EBE-CE model. The question then is, what does that research look like?

SCHOLARSHIP OF TEACHING AND LEARNING RESEARCH

In 1990, Boyer expanded the notion of the research that academics conducted from being focused solely on scientific discovery to include a variety of aspects of academic work, including what he referred to as the research category of the "scholarship of teaching" indicating that the process of structuring teaching and learning only becomes valued and important when it is understood by others (p. 23). Shulman (2004) took up this mantle and went on to suggest that in making the teaching and learning process understood by others, research must be systematic, disseminated in a public forum, and held up to the scrutiny of our peers as any other form of disciplinary research would be. In this manner, Boyer and Shulman facilitated the establishment of a body of literature that would allow us to make our teaching efforts as grounded in the literature as our clinical practices are.

CLINICAL RESEARCH COMPARED TO SCHOLARSHIP OF TEACHING AND LEARNING RESEARCH

At the heart of the research question, there is a great deal of similarity between clinical research and SoTL research in that both begin with a problem as observed by the professional. In the clinical arena, queries are often focused on which modality of treatment yields the best outcome for a set of patients. In the clinical supervision arena, questions are likely to be focused on questions such as which model for fostering growth of clinical skills is effective or the interaction between the processes of clinical and educational outcomes. For example, a research question focusing on a model for clinical education might ask what impact participation in an immersion language environment, such as an aphasia camp, might have on the graduate student's knowledge or abilities in the treatment of aphasia. In contrast, a research question that examines the intersection between clinical and educational outcomes might ask how students' clinical skill growth impacts the client's progress toward achieving language goals.

There are a variety of approaches that can be taken into consideration when examining both clinical and educational progress, which will be addressed below. The most important aspect for supervisors to consider is that having a problem that needs to be solved is a positive scenario rather than a negative one. Bass (1999) highlighted a paradox for many educators: Having a clinical problem that needs to be solved is a great opportunity to conduct disciplinary research, identify new knowledge, and share it with one's professional community, but having a teaching problem is often not viewed with the same opportunistic mindset. As educators, we might see a student's failure to learn or make progress in developing their clinical skills as a reflection on our own shortcomings. Surely if we were more effective as supervisors, we would be able to help this student learn how to treat this patient without so much difficulty, right? Bass suggests that we see the problems in our teaching and learning experiences as opportunities for systematic research and learning, in the same way as we view clinical problems. We have all had the experience, as supervisors, of becoming frustrated when a student appears unable to learn how to develop clinical writing skills despite our best efforts, for example. While it is tempting to struggle with this and only share the problem with trusted colleagues, Bass (1999) and Shulman (1998) both argue that by investigating the teaching and learning process, we not only improve our own students' outcomes when we share our new knowledge with our colleagues through public dissemination, we create a body of literature in which our colleagues can also improve their students' teaching and learning. This makes us more effective supervisors and supervisors across the disciplines.

While the identification of a problem is key to successful scholarship of discovery and scholarship of teaching, the research processes may look different in each area. Often in SoTL we attempt to adhere to research methodologies that are compatible if not consistent with our disciplines' broader research methodologies. However, the application of "gold standards" of research practice may not be feasible or even desirable in SoTL research. Consider, for example, the highly regarded, rigorous Level Ib, a well-designed, randomized controlled study (ASHA, n.d.). While clinical trials often seek to run studies, which are double blind or randomized to avoid bias in the interpretation of results and control for external variables, it is not often feasible to have controlled or randomized studies in clinical learning settings. This is due to the fact that flexibility is likely limited by site, number of students at each site, and the number of supervisors providing clinical education. In SoTL research, we must consider the best model for research design, which may be a Level III, well-designed, nonexperimental study that seeks to increase our understanding of the process by which our students develop clinical skills. Maxwell (2005) suggests that in identifying the best research design for our SoTL research, we identify the methodology that will yield the best quality of information to answer the research question. Conducting SoTL research is valuable but should never be designed or implemented in a way that might jeopardize the students' learning. In the following section, we will discuss some of the options for best practices in SoTL research for clinical education and supervision.

QUANTITATIVE METHODOLOGY

Quantitative statistical methodologies are effective for answering questions that are looking for numerical measures. Often quantitative methods appear to be heavily weighted when we consider clinical research and outcomes data. These "numbers" tell us which treatment is "best" and give us confidence in our approach to a patient population. In addition, clinical assessments and the evaluation of treatment outcomes are typically conducted using numerical data. Likewise, we could consider quantitative analyses as the best way to measure the effectiveness of student learning. This may lead the supervisor to believe that most everything they do is quantitative, and therefore, quantitative measures will be used in nearly every instance of SoTL. However, quantitative statistics can be abused under the best of circumstances, regardless of the question. Challenges within inferential statistics include: 1) which type of inferential statistics to use; 2) the importance of inferential statistics when compared with other kinds of statistical measures; and, fundamentally, 3) whether inferential statistics are appropriate in the first place.

Conducting work in SoTL adds to the challenge of quantitative analysis. There are multiple factors to consider here. Under the best of circumstances:

1. Inferential statistics are used when there are random group assignments (experimental and control groups).

2. Random sampling is required when we consider survey research that is generalizable to a population at large.

The aforementioned statements pose the challenge and the controversy. How do we meaningfully use quantitative statistical methods in SoTL? In most clinical education instances, we do not have the opportunity to randomly assign our participants to groups. This can be due to challenges such as a lack of a sufficient number of participants, the ethical obligation to provide students an educational experience that we believe will benefit them, or, an inability to randomly sample from a population at large.

Other challenges include the development of survey instruments to assess learning or experience that have not been subjected to the rigors of assessment for their validity or reliability. Surveys that utilize interval scaling are also not often validated. Therefore, we do not know whether our respondents' answers to numbers such as "1 = *not likely at all* to 5 = *very likely*" have meaningful steps within their intervals. We also may not have a clear understanding of whether our method for coding these responses is appropriate in the first place. This coding, in essence, straddles both data collection and analysis. This creates a challenge when using parametric statistics, where the assumption is that the data come from a population that follows the population distribution. These latter challenges can pose a clear barrier to some who wish to conduct quantitative research in SoTL.

Does this mean that all is lost? The answer is a clear no. However, most statistics textbooks will provide information regarding quantitative analyses in a very cut-and-dried manner. This presentation leads the reader to believe that quantitative measures are appropriate in nearly every instance. However, those conducting research within SoTL must consider the fundamental, best-circumstance statements above regarding inferential statistics. It is highly likely that neither assumption can be met. Does this mean quantitative methods should never be used? Some will argue yes, whereas others may argue that quantitative methods can be appropriate with the appropriate disclaimer. For example, Dudding and Pfeiffer (2018) conducted a quantitative analysis of clinical decision-making in graduate students enrolled in a graduate speech-language pathology program. These researchers performed quantitative analyses, displayed means, and conducted statistical analyses in the context of describing the limitations in their data (e.g., small sample size that was mostly female). The end result was a meaningful contribution to our knowledge base of student learning.

So, where do we take this from here? A conservative avenue is to begin by using descriptive statistics when discussing your work in SoTL. Often the means, standard deviations, and other appropriately displayed data can relay a message of significance to an audience, with the understanding that more work must be conducted in order to perform quantitative analyses.

QUALITATIVE METHODOLOGY

In contrast to quantitative research questions that attempt to seek numerical measures as indicators of outcomes, qualitative methodologies are most effective at answering research questions that seek to gain insights or understanding about how or why given methods work. Qualitative SoTL research often seeks to understand how a teaching or learning process influenced the students' thinking, the students' perspectives on a learning experience, or why students function as they do in an educational setting. Where quantitative research seeks to answer which method of teaching is best, qualitative research seeks to understand why and how the teaching method worked for the learners (Eisner, 1998; Ginsberg et al., 2012). It is not uncommon to explore students' satisfaction with or perceptions of learning with a particular pedagogical approach in an effort to understand how teaching strategies might influence both cognitive and affective learning (Bloom, 1956; Krathwohl, Bloom, & Masia, 1964).

In qualitative research there are several different approaches that can be taken (Bogden & Biklen, 2007; Creswell, 2014; Glesne, 1999). Qualitative research may reflect an ethnographic perspective, which attempts to describe processes or relationships, for groups of individuals, such as students. Phenomenological research seeks to understand the participants' perspectives regarding a phenomenon, such as clinical learning through one-on-one supervision. The grounded theory approach seeks to generate theories about processes or perspectives that can then potentially be applied to explain current and future related circumstances. While each of these qualitative approaches varies slightly, they all have commonalities.

Qualitative research is particularly applicable to investigations related to teaching and learning in classroom and clinical contexts. At the heart of qualitative research is seeking an understanding about the nature of relationships between the participants in an event or a setting.

Qualitative researchers do not typically seek to create an artificial context or control for variables in order to isolate a variable, as might be seen in quantitative research. Rather, the researchers typically examine interactions or learning in the context in which they actually happen, sometimes referred to as naturalistic settings (Creswell, 2003). Additionally, the value of keen observation, language, and reflection is emphasized as qualitative research views all the participants humanistically, as a source of insight and perspective that can be valuable for others. For qualitative SoTL research, the focus is on how teaching and learning happen for our students, rather than taking a measure of the effectiveness of teaching or learning.

Qualitative data collection can take a variety of forms. The individual or group interview is often a key method for collecting data in qualitative studies. In the interview, participants can be asked to describe their perceptions regarding their learning experience in their own words, which are the data. Responses can be explored in a relatively unstructured way such that, much like our patient interviews, we can allow the interviewee to lead the discussion in the direction of what they feel is critical. By listening carefully and analyzing systematically, the researcher can understand what the experience was like for the learner and how it impacted the learner's view of the process. Purves, Petersen, and Puurveen (2013) used semi-structured interviews with individuals diagnosed with aphasia who agreed to work with students in a learning and mentorship role, to identify how both the learning for the students and the quality of life for the mentors was transformed through participation in a mentoring program. Supervisors might find the use of interviews effective when trying to ascertain the perspective of a group of clients and or students who have experienced a unique model of treatment. For example, supervisors engaging with student clinicians working with a population in a residential context, such as inpatient rehabilitation clients, might interview the clinicians to identify how their views of the clients changed over time or how their view of themselves as clinicians was altered as a result of participation in a high intensity therapy program.

Another form of data collection that can be valuable for supervisors is a think-aloud (TA) process. In a TA, study participants are asked to verbalize steps as they work through how to solve a problem (Bernstein, 2010; Ericcson & Simon, 1993; Wineburg, 1991). This approach to studying how an individual solves a discipline specific problem can be particularly useful for those seeking to understand how a group, such as graduate student clinicians, solves a problem in comparison to another group, such as experienced clinicians. This approach was used by Ginsberg, Friberg, and Visconti (2016) to compare how graduate student clinicians with limited clinical experience and highly experienced clinicians approached diagnostic reasoning tasks. This was done to help gain a better understanding what reasoning skills might be purposefully taught to graduate students to make clinical teaching more effective. This method of investigating the thinking process can be applied to any level of clinician in virtually any context. To use in a more naturalistic setting, for example, the student could be shown a video recording of a client he is about to see and asked to identify how he would plan therapy goals based on the client's observed speech and language characteristics. V. E. Boyer (2013) combined the TA process with pre- and postclinical experience interviews to ascertain the impact of a clinical experience with English language learners on the students' self-efficacy and their knowledge acquisition. By asking a student to problem solve aloud, their thinking becomes identifiable to the supervisor. This gives the supervisor the opportunity to learn about the students' thought patterns in order to take a more informed approach to teaching a new way of thinking.

Written feedback can be focused and shaped to provide the qualitative SoTL researcher insights into the teaching and learning process as well. Written feedback can take a variety of forms, including journaling, written reflections shaped by the researcher's prompts, or open-ended surveys. Written feedback from students who have completed a specific learning or clinical experience can be beneficial for researchers as the data can be gathered anonymously, after a period of delay, and in a manner that allows the participant to take their time in contemplating their responses. Wallace (2017) employed the strategy of collecting delayed written feedback in her study of students' perceptions of an interprofessional education (IPE) workshop. Using a questionnaire that was distributed to participants one year after they participated in the study, the researcher was able to learn that the students experienced connections between their learning in the IPE workshop that took place prior to their clinical experience. Because of the phenomenological nature of the qualitative data, she was able to learn how the students' learning had specifically benefited from workshop participation. Hemmerich, Hoepner, & Samelson (2015) used preflection and reflection writing assignments to learn how undergraduates participating in an instructional internship program made gains in clinical and professional practices. Having students and clinicians engage in these types of written tasks can be beneficial for everyone. Asking students to respond to questionnaires or to write reflectively about a clinical learning experience not only helps supervisors to understand the students' perspective on that experience, it helps the supervisor understand how to improve it, as well as sharpens the students' focus on the value of clinical practice reflection, a habit of mind that can help them be more effective for many years beyond their education (Falk, 1995; Schon, 1983).

MIXED METHODS RESEARCH

Mixed methods are utilized when a researcher has the opportunity to blend both quantitative and qualitative analyses to make the strongest case possible. One way to conceptualize this is through the elements of a creative dinner dish. Perhaps each item on its own is satisfying by itself. However, cooking the ingredients together makes for the most satisfying experience because of the way the different foods might complement each other, much like a good soup or stew. When working with mixed methods the researcher may analyze the same data set with both qualitative and quantitative analyses, or, use complementary data sets and analyze them using both modes of analysis to create the strongest argument possible. A full explanation of mixed methods is beyond the scope of this chapter. However, they are often used in the SoTL works to examine both a correlational view of learner change and the meaning of the experience by understanding the learners' perspectives. One example includes an investigation of how a study abroad experience enhanced students' cultural competence (Krishnan, Masters, Holgate, Wang, & Calahan, 2017). In this study, the authors used a quantitative Likert-type scale to measure changes in intercultural sensitivity. Results from this measure were analyzed using traditional statistical analysis methods. Qualitative data was also collected in the form of students' reflective papers which were then analyzed using typical qualitative coding techniques to understand how the intercultural experiences impacted the students' views of the experience and how their learning was changed based on the model of education that they were exposed to. By combining both methods of research, the research identified both a measurable change in the students' learning and developed an understanding of the nature of the change.

SINGLE SUBJECT DESIGNS

Single subject designs, also often called functional analysis, time-series, within-subject, and single-case designs, offer a powerful, doable research method that will provide answers to functional questions. Single subject experimental designs allow clinical researchers to identify cause-effect relationships without large total number of cases (i.e., N), sophisticated statistical data analysis, big budgets and more time to their already demanding schedules. Yet, these studies allow us to identify what makes a difference using our everyday practice with just a bit more pre-planning, data collection, and analysis than we ordinarily do. Furthermore, unlike large group designs, these allow for examining intersubject and intrasubject variability. Individual variation in learning, level, and trend often provide more compelling evidence for clinicians and clinical educators than does statistical significance between or among groups.

Ingham and Riley (1998) noted that "single subject" is a misnomer, as researchers usually employ more than one participant. Because each participant serves as a replication within a single investigation, the researchers determine the exact number. Typically, three to six participants constitute the subject pool. All single subject designs include two fundamental time segments: baseline (A) and treatment (B). Baseline measures a behavior over time with no intervention, changing of conditions, or manipulation of the independent/treatment variable. A reasonably stable baseline is fundamental to be able to demonstrate experimental control but does not necessarily infer zero change, rather a small range of variability (e.g., 5%). After the baseline is established, treatment (B phase) is introduced and observed and measured. This manipulated variable (the independent variable), for example, might be a supervisor's use of convergent and broad questions in regular conferences, decreasing supervisor talk-time in scheduled meetings with the supervisee, or teaching the supervisee to use a specific clinical self-assessment tool. Direct measurements of the treatment behavior are taken over time. McReynolds and Thompson (1986) described the four typical kinds of dependent measures used in single-subject studies: frequency, rate of occurrence, duration of occurrence, and percentage.

Two basic types of single subject experiments employ reversal and multiple baseline designs.

A basic reversal design includes a baseline (A), treatment (B), and withdrawal of treatment (A) phase. In a SoTL example, a supervisor may work with a student and offer no input to a student as she or he is working with the patient. The supervisor can track student success with a client without input to determine a baseline phase. Here, the supervisor might track the number of utterances the patient produces during the session. This might occur over several sessions. Then, the supervisor might introduce an independent variable such as verbal reminders/cues to the student during the session. The supervisor can then track changes that occur during the sessions where the supervisor has provided the input. Do the number of utterances increase? If so, one could argue that the experimenter (i.e., the supervisor) was able to gain stimulus control over the patient utterances by giving the student verbal reminders to encourage the patient to speak.

In this case, the supervising clinician is measuring the number of utterances produced by the patient at baseline, with a verbal cue to the student clinician, and with no cue. This creates an A-B-A design.

Figure 16-2 gives an example of the design. It adds an element where the supervisor removes the cue, to make certain that the behavior is under stimulus control. Therefore, we are dealing with an A-B-A design, where A is a baseline or no treatment (no cues given to student) and B indicates our intervention (cues to student given). Again, because there is an additional A, we have a treatment withdrawal situation (no cues given to student), which helps demonstrate the experimental control, assuming that there are no other variables we are unaware of in this situation regarding the number of utterances produced by the patient.

Multiple baseline designs do not require a return to baseline in order to demonstrate experimental control. These designs replicate across behaviors, subjects or settings. By introducing treatments in a staggered manner, effects can be replicated and a functional relationship between intervention and outcomes demonstrated.

Gillam, Strike-Roussos, and Anderson (1990) used a multiple baseline across behaviors design with counterbalanced order of treatments to explore if supervisees altered their clinical behaviors as a direct consequence of joint data analyses. Dependent variables (outcomes) included clinician explanations, informative feedback and directive responses to off-task client utterances. In a multiple baseline across-subjects investigation, Strike (1988) taught supervisors to use broad questions and then examined the cognitive level of questions and supervisee and supervisees' level of thinking. A hypothetical multiple baseline across-settings investigation could focus on training certain interpersonal behaviors such as empathic understanding, genuineness, and or concreteness to clinical educators in a university clinic, a medical setting, and school setting, and measuring the impact of the degree and amount of these facilitative behaviors on supervisee self-exploration and reflection.

Other single-subject experimental designs (SSDs) include: changing criteria, multiple treatment, alternating treatments, and adapted alternating treatments. Interested readers are encouraged to explore resources provided at the end of this chapter. There are many different ways to consider SSD in your practice in SoTL. SSD is a broad area and this chapter only scratches the surface of the many different designs that you might implement this method into your research. Barlow, Nock, and Hersen's (2009) and Kazdin (2010) are two reasonable places to find more about SSD. They provide intricacies of SSD and prompts for applying it to SoTL practice. While there has been little published research in SoTL using SSD, they have been popular designs in research on treatment of articulation and phonological disorders, fluency disorders, and autism disorders

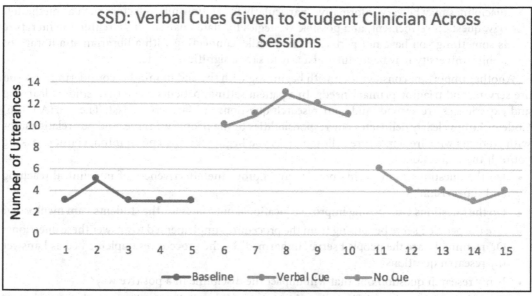

Figure 16-2. Hypothetical single subject design data representation. In this case, the supervising clinician is measuring the number of utterances produced by the patient at baseline, with a verbal cue to the student clinician, and with no cue. This creates an A-B-A design.

to mention just a few. Finding published SoTL examples of SSD in communication sciences and disorders is more challenging, however.

GETTING STARTED

Given that professionals providing clinical education and supervision in all contexts usually have more than their fair share of work to do as they balance clients' therapeutic needs and students' learning needs, why would they want to engage in research? The medical model, and indeed much of academia, would have us believe that the ability to contribute significant EBP or EBE is the purview of academics. However, the concept of "evidence to practice and practice to evidence" rejects the notion of academics and quantitative, gold-standard studies being the source of all knowledge (Isaac & Franceschi, 2008). Case studies and qualitative studies may shed more light on the actual supervisor's practice than any large scale, randomized, control group study can. Therefore, supervisors have an opportunity to bring a unique perspective to EBE-CE and contribute to the growing body of literature.

One intention of this chapter is to inspire you to consider conducting your own work relative to research in the science of supervision. In the sections below, we offer tips and suggestions for a successful start. Keep in mind—starting on a small scale may be the most rewarding for you as you begin this journey.

1. *Begin with the end in mind.* Unfortunately, this first suggestion can be the one that is most challenging. Often we have good ideas, and, if we are fortunate, we also have an enthused team or partners. However, it is important to determine the exact question you wish to answer, why the question is important, and what work might already exist relative to the question you are asking. At the time of this writing, the discipline of communication disorders has a relative paucity of research relative to EBE-CE in clinical environments. A field such as nursing or teaching may have many more offerings. It is important to gain clarity around your question and search broadly in the literature for any relevant work that may exist. Work from other

disciplines may be very informative, particularly in relationship to factors such as methodology, question refinement, and possible strategies for data analysis. If searching the literature is something you have not performed in a while, connecting with a librarian at a library or public university may be useful and a way to save a significant time.

Another important consideration with beginning with the end in mind is considering who you are serving and triaging primary needs. In a patient setting, patients come first, student learning and experiences are second, and your research questions are factored in last. The ASHA (2016) Code of Ethics clearly delineates our responsibilities to the people we serve, and our relationships with students who are our future colleagues. As you begin with the end in mind, consider asking yourself these questions:

- Do the questions I am posing potentially improve the effectiveness of my clinical teaching and supervision?
- Do the questions I am posing improve educational outcomes for the students I am mentoring?
- Are the people I serve benefiting from the procedures implemented to answer these questions? Or, minimally, are the people I serve "unharmed" by the procedures implemented as I answer my research questions?
- Is my research question one that will impact the discipline in a positive way?

2. *Consider your resources.* Clinical and supervisory research questions can be stimulating! Many clinicians relish the opportunity to think beyond the day-to-day routine and explore something new and exciting. This can mean talking with your colleagues about "grand plans" to answer questions that are exciting and new, with the assumption that the work will be devoured by your peers.

Realistically, our dreams can go far beyond our means. When conducting supervisory research, one must consider that resources may be at a premium. Do you have the time to make certain that the data collected are meaningful and collected with consistent methods? Is there a plan for statistical analysis, especially if you do not have the expertise yourself? Do you have the capacity to collect sufficient data for any statistical analysis you propose to conduct? Will you have the resources to disseminate the work? (Note: We will cover dissemination options in a subsequent section). Dissemination of resources could mean time for writing, designing a poster, traveling to a meeting, and more. Will you be developing your plan and collecting your data on your own time? Or, is your employer supportive of your plan and providing you time to move forward with the project?

Another important resource consideration can be financial funding for the work. Does the work require a specific set of funds to pay participants? Or, are the costs "time and energy"? Occasionally you may find that your work can be funded through grants. Grants may be obtained internally through your own organization, philanthropic organizations, or some professional associations. Typically, grants are competitive in nature. Researchers who are not awarded grants may be given the gift of feedback on the proposed work. This feedback can be used to write stronger proposals in the future. No matter the case, finances may be an important element of your work that should be considered as early in your process as possible.

3. *Consider "ownership" of the work early.* This consideration cannot be stressed enough! Groups will often engage in research and not completely understand the role of each of the "players" in moving the project forward. For example, imagine you are working with two graduate students and examining different modes for providing feedback to the students after their clinical encounters. You are conducting this work because the students noted you have different modes of feedback across your clinical instructors at your facility and the students thought it might be a great idea to study this topic. Are the graduate students the subjects? Are they the coauthors? If they are coauthors, does this confound your data collection and interpretation in some way? Additionally, if you plan to disseminate your work in a peer-reviewed paper, who are the authors? Are all of the players involved authors? If so, in which order? Or, are only a subset of the team on any final publication or presentation? Having these conversations early,

and consistently, can avoid uncomfortable conversations later. Stating the work, the owner-ship, and future authorship in a written document that is agreed upon by the team is best.

4. *Do you need institutional review board approval for your research?* This extremely important consideration is not one to take lightly. The rights of all parties in research must be protected and any potential harm must be minimized, if not eliminated (Protection of Human Subjects, 2009). Institutional Review Boards are established to guide researchers and confirm that risks are appropriately mitigated, subjects understand and consent to research, the institution itself has put into place any required procedural safeguards for the research, and the research is con-ducted ethically. If you find yourself working in a large organization, you may find a review board within your workplace. In other instances, you may need to reach out to your adminis-trators to determine next "best steps" before conducting your research. Finally, ASHA's (2016) Code of Ethics requires researchers to conduct their work ethically. Obtaining appropriate approvals for the work is part of the process.

5. *How will you disseminate your work?* Taking the time to conduct research can be rewarding and tiring! If you spend a great deal of time refining your question, determining ownership of the work, staying within your resources, obtaining the appropriate approvals, collecting the data, and analyzing the work, you should share it. How do you plan to do so? Is your plan to make people within your own organization aware of your results? If so, how? Do you plan to write a paper? Who will write it and where will it be submitted for publication? Do you plan to present the material to a local, state, or national audience? What will the venue be—a poster; a formal presentation?

Although this is a long list of questions, you will want to consider your options early on, and keep assessing them as your work moves along. Sometimes we find a negative result (i.e., what we thought might be a significant finding did not happen in the research you conducted). Is the work still worthy of dissemination to your peers? Continually considering your dissemination options, in the context of your results, is an important consideration for both yourself and anyone else on your team. See the following resource section.

Concluding Thoughts

Although this is a long list of questions and considerations, it is not meant to discourage you and your work. Instead, these questions are presented to get you thinking about the scope of both your questions and your resources. Starting a large project and watching it dwindle can be very discouraging. This can have a compounding effect if you have experienced disappointment in multiple projects. Often starting on a smaller scale, and testing your capacity, can be a fruitful path forward. These suggestions are provided to give you a framework before you move beyond the capabilities of yourself, your supervisees, your team, or your institution. Begin with the end in mind by developing a clear question/s that you can clearly articulate. Then, ask yourself about the points addressed in the "Getting Started" section.

Support

If after having read about the joys and challenges of conducting EBE-CE research you are still ready to move forward, you will want to consider what resources are available to support you in the process. The first step to consider if this is your first foray into research is probably to find a good research methods textbook. You might have one in your possession from your graduate program, or you might be in need of a more user-friendly guide. Many of us learned quantitative methods in graduate school, however qualitative methods historically have been less commonly taught in communication sciences and disorders programs. If you are looking for a quantitative text, it will depend upon your level of foundational knowledge. Consider Fox's (2009) *A Mathematical Primer for Social Statistics* if you are a beginner. However, there are many others that may suit your needs. If you are thinking that a qualitative study is more suited to your research question, you might consider Bogden and Biklen's (2006) *Qualitative Research for Education: An Introduction to Theories and Methods*. Both texts are reader friendly and will help you with both understanding and applying the research methods of your choosing. Additionally, consider picking up a copy of Creswell's (2014) *Research Design: Qualitative, Quantitative, and Mixed Methods Approaches*. This text is very oriented toward the development of written materials and has many excellent examples and checklists that are useful. Orlikoff, Schiavetti, and Metz (2015) *Evaluating Research in Communication Disorders* (seventh ed.) is a popular basic text for examining research from the consumers' perspective.

In addition to gathering a textbook or two, you might search the web for useful information about conducting research. Look for web pages that have been developed by universities and have ".edu" in their address. These web pages are often created by faculty who specialize in the research area, or by universities that have developed the publicly viewable pages to support those who are conducting research. Additionally, the Web Center for Social Research Methods hosts a web page, https://www.socialresearchmethods.net/kb/qual.php, that provides materials, from research background to design ideas, that are very useful.

Access to journals, both in our disciplines and in related disciplines can be very useful to the development of your research project. Consider journals that are specific to the topic of communication sciences and disorders, which may be publishing work related to your area of intended research and which might be good places for you to disseminate your work as well. If you have already searched to see what research has been done related to your question, as noted above, you have probably found these journals already. Reading how other researchers have designed and conducted their studies can be informative and help shape your thinking about what has been done and about how you might go forward with your own work. Outside of our discipline specific journals, consider journals that are related to our field, such as journals of medical education, nursing education, teacher education, physical therapy education, and teaching psychology. These journals often showcase research done by supervisors in related fields that will also give you excellent ideas. Finally, consider journals that are not discipline specific, but rather share the common interest in SoTL. In the United States and internationally, there are many high-quality journal publications that might be publishing clinical education research that can inform our own research. Familiarity with these journals can have the added bonus of providing you with more dissemination options beyond the scope of our own field for your future work.

If reading about research methods is not your preferred way to learn or you have done the reading and would like to talk to someone, consider reaching out to university faculty. This recommendation is not intended to promote a hierarchical structure that implies academics are necessary for completing the research, but rather to promote community building. Many academic faculty in communication sciences and disorders programs are interested in conducting EBE-CE research and will be interested in your ideas. If they are interested in your topic, ask if you can meet with them to discuss your research and questions you might have about design and implementation. You might find that in talking to them, you gain an advocate and supporter of you as a researcher, if not a person who might be willing to be actively involved in your project at no cost. Consider contacting faculty at your alma mater that you have had a good working relationship with or contacting faculty at a university in your local area. If they send their students to you for clinical experiences, they may be more than happy to repay your kindness with a professional research consultation.

Recommended Resources

We have listed below a variety of resources that might be useful to you if you are considering contributing to the body of EBE-CE literature. These resources are listed in the reference list, but they are organized by focus here for you. These lists are not intended to be exhaustive, but to give you support as you begin exploring if you are new to this work.

Scholarship of Teaching and Learning (SoTL) Resources

- Bass, R. (1998). The scholarship of teaching: What's the problem? *Inventio, 1*(1). Available from https://my.vanderbilt.edu/sotl/files/2013/08/Bass-Problem1.pdf
- Ginsberg, S. M., Friberg, J. C., & Visconti, C. F. (2012). *Scholarship of teaching and learning in speech-language pathology and audiology: Evidence based education.* San Diego, CA: Plural.
- Sackett, D., Straus, S. E., Richardson, W. S., Rosenberg, W., & Haynesl, R. B. (2000). *Evidence-based medicine: How to practice and teach EBM* (2nd ed.). Edinburgh, Scotland: Churchill Livingstone.
- Shulman, L. (2004). *Teaching as community property: Essays on higher education.* San Francisco, CA: Jossey-Bass.
- Shulman, L. (2000). From Minsk to Pinsk: Why a scholarship of teaching and learning? *Journal of Scholarship of Teaching and Learning, 1*(1), 48-53.
- Weimer, M. (2006). *Enhancing scholarly work on teaching & learning.* San Francisco, CA: Jossey-Bass.

Research Methods Resources

- Barlow, D., Nock, M. & Hersen, M. (2009). *Single case experimental designs: Strategies for studying behavior change* (3rd ed.). Pearson.
- Bogden, R., & Biklen, S. K. (2006). *Qualitative research for education: An introduction to theories and methods* (5th ed.). Boston, MA: Pearson.
- Byiers, B. J., Reichle, J., & Symons, F. J. (2012). Single-subject experimental design for evidence-based practice. *American Journal Speech Language Pathology, 21*(4), 397-414. doi:10.1044/1058- 0360(2012/11-0036)
- Connell, P. & Thompson, C. (1986). Flexibility of single-subject experimental design. Part III: Using flexibility to design or modify experiments. *Journal of Speech and Hearing Disorders, 51,* 214-215.
- Creswell, J. W. (2014). *Research design: Qualitative, quantitative, and mixed methods approaches* (4th ed.). Thousand Oaks, CA: Sage.
- Eisner, E. W. (1998). *The enlightened eye: Qualitative inquiry and the enhancement of educational practice.* Upper Saddle River, NJ: Prentice-Hall.
- Fox (2009). *A mathematical primer for social statistics.* Thousand Oaks, CA: Sage.
- Kearns, K. (1986). Flexibility of single-subject experimental design. Part II: Design selection and arrangement of experimental phases. *Journal of Speech and Hearing Disorders, 51,* 204-214.
- Maxwell, J. (2005). *Qualitative research design: An interactive approach* (3rd ed.). Thousand Oaks: Sage.
- McReynolds, L., & Thompson, C. (1986). Flexibility of single-subject experimental design. Part I: Review of the basics of single-subject designs. *Journal of Speech and Hearing Disorders, 51,* 194-203.
- Web Center for Social Research Methods (https://www.socialresearchmethods.net/kb/qual.php)

Dissemination Resources

- Presentations
  - American Speech-Language-Hearing Association Annual Convention (www.asha.org)
  - Council of Academic Programs in Communication Sciences and Disorders Annual Conference (http://www.capcsd.org)
  - Lilly Conference Series on College and University Teaching and Learning (http://lillyconferences.com/)
  - State speech-language-hearing association conferences
- Publications
  - *International Journal of Speech-Language Pathology* (http://www.tandfonline.com/loi/iasl20)
  - *Teaching and Learning in Communication Sciences & Disorders* (www.tlcsdjournal.com)
  - *The Clinical Supervisor* (http://www.tandfonline.com/loi/wcsu20)
  - *Journal of the Scholarship of Teaching and Learning* (https://josotl.indiana.edu)
  - *Journal of Applied Behavior Analysis* (https://onlinelibrary.wiley.com/journal/19383703)

SUMMARY

Conducting research based on your experience as a supervisor can be time consuming and hard work, but it can be extremely rewarding as well. You might have questions about the effectiveness of how you structure learning for students. SoTL research can be valuable for investigations about clinical education and student learning in specific clinical contexts, or with specific client-student interactions. As our professions expand the various models we use for students gaining clinical experiences, the opportunities to conduct SoTL investigations about the interactions between all of the aspects of the EBE-CE model also expand. SoTL research allows you to gather more evidence about the clinical education and supervision process. In addition to learning answers to questions that may have plagued you as an educator, such as "Why *do* students do that?" you will often have an immediate benefit in that the results will inform your practice and make you a more effective supervisor while improving student learning and patient treatment outcomes.

Further, dissemination of the results through publication or presentation at state and national venues will inform other practitioners of clinical education, both in communication sciences and disorders and possibly in related professions. Recall that Shulman indicated that without holding our EBE-CE research up to the scrutiny of peer-review through dissemination, we have not truly engaged in SoTL research as its adequacy and generalizability cannot be judged by our colleagues. Our SoTL work needs to not only be evaluated by our colleagues, but also shared with them so that they may benefit from our learning and avoid recreating the research wheel to answer the same questions. Finally, recall that the primary purposes of SoTL research across settings are to improve the effectiveness of the teaching we provide and improve the learning that our students experience. While engaging in SoTL represents hard work, the benefit for us, for our colleagues, and for our students is that we are all empowered with more knowledge than before we began our study

REFERENCES

American Speech-Language-Hearing Association. (n.d.) *Steps in the process of evidence-based practice. Step 3: Assessing the evidence*. Retrieved from https://www.asha.org/Research/EBP/Assessing-the-Evidence/

American Speech-Language-Hearing Association. (2005). *Evidence-based practice in communication disorders* [Position statement]. Retrieved from https://www.asha.org/policy/PS2005-00221/

American Speech-Language-Hearing Association. (2016). *Code of ethics*. Retrieved from www.asha.org/policy/

Barlow, D. H., Nock, M. K., &Hersen, M. (2009). *Single case experimental designs: Strategies for studying behavior change* (3rd ed.). Pearson.

Bass, R. (1999). The scholarship of teaching: What's the problem? *Inventio: Creative Thinking About Learning and Teaching, 1*(1), 1-10.

Bernstein, J. L. (2010). Using "think-alouds" to understand variations in political thinking. *Journal of Political Science Education, 6*(1), 49-69. doi:10.1080/15512160903467695

Bloom, B. S. (1956). *Taxonomy of educational objectives: The classification of goals: Handbook I: Cognitive domain*. New York, NY: Longmans, Green.

Bogden, R., & Biklen, S. K. (2007). *Qualitative research for education: An introduction to theories and methods* (5th ed.). Boston, MA: Pearson.

Boyer, E. L. (1990). *Scholarship reconsidered: Priorities of the professoriate*. San Francisco, CA: Jossey-Bass.

Boyer, V. E. (2013, October). Graduate students working with English language learners: Impact on self efficacy and knowledge acquisition. *SIG 10 Perspectives on Issues in Higher Education, 16*, 63-70. doi:10.1044/ihe16.2.63

Creswell, J. W., (2014). *Research design: Qualitative, quantitative, and mixed methods approaches* (4th ed.). Thousand Oaks, CA: Sage Publications.

Dollaghan, C. A. (2007). *Communication evidence-based practice in communication disorders*. Baltimore, MD: Paul H. Brookes.

Dudding, C., & Pfeiffer, D. (2018). Clinical decision-making in speech-language pathology graduate students: Quantitative findings. *Teaching and Learning in Communication Sciences and Disorders, 2*(1), 2. Retrieved from https://ir.library.illinoisstate.edu/tlcsd/vol2/iss1/2/

Eisner, E. (1998). *The Enlightened Eye*. Upper Saddle River, NJ: Prentice Hall.

Ericcson, K. A., & Simon, H A. (1993). *Protocol analysis: Verbal reports as data*. Cambridge, MA: MIT Press.

Falk, D. (1995). Preflection: A strategy for enhancing reflection [Evaluation/Reflection]. Paper 22. Retrieved from http://digitalcommons.unomaha.edu/slceeval/22

Fox, J. (2009). *A mathematical primer for social statistics*. Thousand Oaks, CA: Sage.

Gillam, R., Strike Roussos, C., & Anderson, J. (1990). Facilitating changes in supervisees' clinical behaviors: An experimental investigation of supervisory effectiveness. *Journal of Speech and Hearing Disorders, 55*, 729-739.

Ginsberg, S. M., Friberg, J., & Visconti, C. (2012). *Scholarship of teaching and learning in speech-language pathology and audiology: Evidence-based education*. San Diego, CA: Plural.

Ginsberg, S. M., Friberg, J. C., & Visconti, C. F. (2016 Spring). Diagnostic reasoning by experienced speech-language pathologists and student clinicians. *Contemporary Issues in Communication Science & Disorders, 43*(1), 87-97.

Glesne, C. (1999). *Becoming qualitative researchers: An introduction*. New York, NY: Longman.

Hemmerich, A. L., Hoepner, J. K., Samelson, V. M. (2015). Instructional internships: Improving the teaching and learning experience for students, interns, and faculty. *Journal of the Scholarship of Teaching and Learning, 15*(3), 104-132. doi:10.14434/josotl.v15i3.13090

Ingham, J. C., & Riley, G. (1998). Guidelines for documentation of treatment efficacy for young children who stutter. *Journal of Speech, Language, and Hearing Research, 41*, 753-770.

Isaac, C. A., & Franceschi, A. (2008). EBM: Evidence to practice & practice to evidence. *Journal of Evaluation of Clinical Practice, 14*(5), 656-659. doi:10.1111/j.1365-2753.2008.01043.x

Kazdin, A. (2010). *Single case research designs: Methods for clinical and applied settings*. Oxford, England: Oxford University Press.

Krathwohl, D.R., Bloom, B.S., & Masia, B.B. (1964). *Taxonomy of educational objectives: The classification of educational goals handbook II: Affective domain*. New York, NY: David McKay.

Krishnan, L. A., Masters, C., Holgate, H., Wang, C., and Calahan, C. A. (2017). Structured study abroad enhances intercultural competence. *Teaching and Learning in Communication Sciences & Disorders, 1*(1), 5. Retrieved from http://ir.library.illinoisstate.edu/tlcsd/vol1/iss1/5

Maxwell, J. (2005). *Qualitative research design: An interactive approach* (3rd ed.). Thousand Oaks, CA: Sage.

McReynolds, L. V., & Thompson, C. K. (1986). Flexibility of Single-Subject Experimental Designs. Part I: Review of the Basics of Single-Subject Designs. *Journal of Speech and Hearing Disorders, 51*(3), 194-203. doi: 10.1044/jshd.5103.194

Orlikoff, R., Schiavetti, N., & Metz, D. (2015). *Evaluating research in communication disorders* (7th ed.). Boston, MA: Pearson.

Protection of Human Subjects, 45 C.F.R. § 46. (2009)

Purves, B. A., Petersen, J., & Puurveen, G. (2013, May) An aphasia mentoring program: perspectives of speech-language pathology students and of mentors with aphasia. *American Journal of Speech-Language Pathology, 22*(2). S370-S379.

Schon, D. (1983). *The reflective practitioner: How professionals think in action.* New York, NY: Basic Books.

Shulman, L. S. (1998). Introduction. In P. Hutchings (Ed.), *The course portfolio: How faculty can examine their reaching to advance practice and improve student learning* (pp. 5-12). Sterling, VA: Stylus.

Shulman, L. S. (2004). *Teaching as community property: Essays on higher education.* San Diego, CA: Jossey-Bass.

Strike (Roussos), C. A. (1988). *Supervisors' implementation of trained information regarding broad questioning and discussion of supervision during their supervisory conferences in speech-language pathology* (Doctoral dissertation). Retrieved from ProQuest Dissertations and Theses Global. (Accession No. 8824185) http://proxyiub.uits.iu.edu/login?url=https://search.proquest.com/docview/303572273?accountid=11620

Wallace, S. E. (2017) Speech-language pathology students' perceptions of an IPE stroke workshop: A one-year follow up. *Teaching and Learning in Communication Sciences & Disorders, 1*(1), 4. Retrieved from http://ir.library.illinoisstate.edu/tlcsd/vol1/iss1/4

Williams, B. & Brown, T. (2015). *Evidence-based education: Promoting best practice in the teaching and learning of health professional students.* London, England: Radcliffe Publishing.

Wineberg, S. S. (1991) On the reading of historical texts: Notes on the breach between school and academy. *American Educational Research Journal, 28*(3), 495-519.

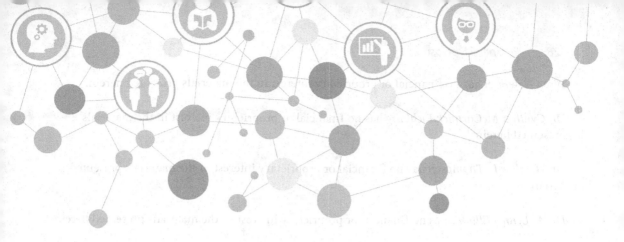

Financial Disclosures

Dr. Mindi Anderson has received grants from the National Science Foundation and UCF LIFE; has received a previous grant from UCF on intraprofessional simulation; was an invited speaker on content: Anderson, M. (2017, November); The Scholarship of Teaching and Learning (SoTL) in clinical education and supervisio; was an invited keynote at the Researcher-Academic Town Meeting, American Speech-Language-Hearing-Association Convention, Los Angeles, CA.

Dr. Judith A. Brasseur has no financial or proprietary interest in the materials presented herein.

Mary L. Casper is an employee of HCR ManorCare.

Dr. Mark DeRuiter is an employee of the University of Arizona.

Dr. Donna Fisher Smiley is an employee of Arkansas Children's Hospital.

Dr. Sarah Ginsberg has no financial or proprietary interest in the materials presented herein.

Melanie W. Hudson is an empolyye of EBS Healthcare.

Dr. Elizabeth S. McCrea has no financial or proprietary interest in the materials presented herein.

Dr. Cheryl Messick has no financial or proprietary interest in the materials presented herein.

Wren Newman has no financial or proprietary interest in the materials presented herein.

Dr. Cynthia McCormick Richburg has no financial or proprietary interest in the materials presented herein.

Dr. Heather L. Thompson has no financial or proprietary interest in the materials presented herein.

Dr. A. Lynn Williams has no financial or proprietary interest in the materials presented herein.

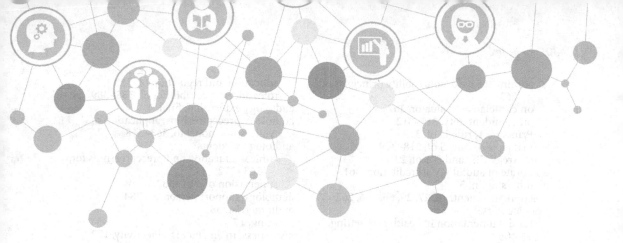

Index

Printed in the United States
by Baker & Taylor Publisher Services